SIR THOMAS BROWNE

A life

Sir Thomas Browne: A Life is the first full-scale biography of the extraordinary prose artist, physician, and polymath. With the help of recent archival discoveries, the biography recasts each phase of Browne's life (1605–82) and situates his incomparable writings within the diverse intellectual and social contexts in which he lived, including London, Winchester, Oxford, Montpellier, Padua, Leiden, Halifax, and Norwich. The book makes the case that, as his contemporaries fervently believed, Browne influenced the intellectual and religious direction of seventeenth-century England in singularly rich and dynamic ways.

Special attention is paid in the biography to Browne's medical vocation, but also to his place within the scientific revolution. New information is offered regarding his childhood in London, his European travels and medical studies, the setting in which he first wrote *Religio Medici*, his impact on readers during the English civil wars, and the contemporary view of his medical practice. Overall, the image of Browne that emerges is far bolder and more cosmopolitan, less complacent and provincial, than biographers have assumed ever since Samuel Johnson doubted Browne's claim that his life up to age thirty resembled a romantic fiction filled with miracles and fables.

Reid Barbour is Professor of English at the University of North Carolina, Chapel Hill.

Sir Thomas Browne

A life

REID BARBOUR

OXFORD
UNIVERSITY PRESS

OXFORD
UNIVERSITY PRESS

Great Clarendon Street, Oxford, OX2 6DP,
United Kingdom

Oxford University Press is a department of the University of Oxford.
It furthers the University's objective of excellence in research, scholarship,
and education by publishing worldwide. Oxford is a registered trade mark of
Oxford University Press in the UK and in certain other countries

First published 2013
First published in paperback 2016

Published in the United States of America by Oxford University Press
198 Madison Avenue, New York, NY 10016, United States of America

British Library Cataloguing in Publication Data
Data available

Library of Congress Cataloging in Publication Data
Data available

ISBN 978–0–19–967988–1 (Hbk.)
ISBN 978–0–19–877835–6 (Pbk.)

For Tillie and Ginger: Noble Quincunx, Brave Monster

Acknowledgements

In undertaking this biography of Sir Thomas Browne in 2003, I found myself embraced by the warmest and most collaborative family of scholars that I have ever encountered. The people in this family are as generous as they are inspiring in their own pursuits of scholarly excellence. I am especially mindful of Brooke Conti, Achsah Guibbory, Kevin Killeen, Mary Ann Lund, Antonia Moon, Kathryn Murphy, Brent Nelson, Graham Parry, Claire Preston, and William West. Katie has been an indispensable resource for and honest critic of this project. As for Claire, my debts are astonishingly steep and numerous, as are those for the future readers of Browne, since we have Professor Preston to thank for assembling the editorial team for the new Oxford edition of Browne and for designing, stocking, and captaining that massive vessel.

With each chapter I have received assistance in my attempts to keep up with Browne's vast learning and innumerable interests. I am especially indebted to Sarah Parker for help with the archives in Montpellier; Cynthia Klestinec with anatomy theaters and education in Italy; Victoria Moul with Browne's Latin poetry; Debora Shuger with Browne's religion; Mary Ann Lund with theology's relation to medicine; Antonia Moon with Browne's notebooks; Rebecca Bullard with Dorothy Browne; Rhodri Lewis with Browne's reception; Richard McCabe with Joseph Hall's library; James Rosenheim with the Townshend family of Norfolk; Brent Nelson with Browne's collection of curiosities and his dried plant book; Anne Dunan-Page with Adam Abrenethy; Jeremy Bangs with religious culture in seventeenth-century Leiden; Charles Webster with Henry Power; Paul Grendler as well as Edward Muir with the Jesuits; and Clive Davies with Christopher Wren's commentaries on Browne. I am very grateful indeed to Dan Albert for sharing with me some Montpellier medical manuscripts, at that time in his private collection; Steven Watkins Wolfe for his photographic skills; John Renton for help with Browne's overmantel; Allen Boyer for advice on writing biography; Rachel Lightfoot for information about Norwich School and Browne's sons; Suzanne Foster for advice on the records at Winchester College; Frank Grace for help with Samuel Duncon and the Quakers; Derek Keene for answering my questions about Cheapside and St Michael le Querne; Charles Noble, Keeper of the Devonshire Collection; and Tom Lockwood on the attribution of an ekphrastic poem.

Research on this book has taken me far and wide, from Iceland to Italy, from Quebec to California. Along the way, I have been especially assisted either in person or by way of email by Clive and Freda Wilkins-Jones (Norwich); Pat Sewell (Calderdale, West Yorkshire); Jenny Watts and Philip Gale (National Archives, Kew); Marilyn Ainsworth (Cheshire Record Office); Christopher Lyons (Osler Library, Montreal); Julian Reid, Michael Riordan, Tessa Shaw, Jennifer Thorp, Lucie Walker, Timothy Yu, and Simon Bailey (all in Oxford); Crystal Smith, Anne Myers, and Stephen Greenberg (all at the National Library of Medicine in

Bethesda, Maryland); Meg Sherry Rich (Princeton); Arlene Shaner (the New York Academy of Medicine); Franceso Piovan (Centro per la storia dell'Università di Padova); Guðrún Ása Grimsdóttir (Arne Magnusson Institute, Iceland); Matthew James Driscoll (Den Arnamagnæanske Samlung, Denmark); Susan Bourne and Tony Kitto (Towneley Hall, Lancashire); Richard McFarlane (Bankfield Museum, Halifax); Katrina Coopey (Cardiff Central Library); Krister Őstland (Uppsala University Library); John Sharp (archdiocesan archives, Birmingham); Mike Bevan (Royal Museums Greenwich); Phillipa Grimstone (Pepys Library, Magdalene College, Cambridge); and Jane Ruddell (Mercers' Hall). I would especially like to thank OUP editor Jacqueline Baker, the two anonymous readers for OUP (who helped me, among so many other things, to reduce a gargantuan manuscript down to size), and Brendan Mac Evilly for his copy-editing expertise. All remaining mistakes and misprisions are my responsibility.

Chapter 5 is reworked from "Atheists, Monsters, Plagues, and Jews: Tares in the Garden of Thomas Browne's Padua," in *Writing and Religion in England, 1558–1689*, eds. Roger D. Sell and Anthony W. Johnson (Farnham: Ashgate, 2009), 327–46. Copyright © 2009, and reused by permission of the Publishers. A version of chapter 6 appeared as "Discipline and Praxis: Thomas Browne in Leiden," in Kathryn Murphy and Richard Todd, eds., *'A man very well studyed': New Contexts for Thomas Browne* (Leiden: Brill, 2008). An early and truncated version of chapter 7 appeared as "Charity, Halifax, and Utopia: The Disadvantageous Setting of Thomas Browne's *Religio Medici*," in *Renaissance Papers 2007*, ed. Christopher Cobb and M. Thomas Hester (Rochester, NY: Camden House, 2008), 17–31. The Quaker section of chapter 9 appeared in a more extended form as "Thomas Browne, the Quakers, and a Letter from a Judicious Friend," in Anne Dunan-Page and Clotilde Prunier, eds., *Debating the Faith: Religion and Letter Writing in Great Britain, 1550–1800* (Dordrecht: Spinger, 2013), 37–48. I am grateful to the publishers for permission to use work that originally appeared in these volumes.

My doctoral students have offered a constant fund of support, advice, and material for this book. This is especially the case with Robert Erle Barham, Melissa Caldwell, Kathleen Curtin, Evan Gurney, Pablo Maurette, Sarah Parker, Adair Rispoli, William Russell, Nathan Stogdill, and Joseph Wallace. My undergraduates at the University of North Carolina have very kindly tolerated my reports from the archives but more than this, they have demonstrated quite brilliantly how Browne still moves readers today and that the future of Browne studies has never been brighter.

My work has been indebted from start to finish to Browne readers and scholars of the past, from the very earliest (Dean Christopher Wren in the seventeenth century) to Browne's first important editor, Simon Wilkin in the nineteenth. On so many occasions I have been thankful for the industry and dedication with which scholars in the twentieth century have sought the traces of Browne's life in their attempts to understand his incomparable writings, including crucial work by Charles Williams, Jeremiah Finch, Frank Huntley, C. A. Patrides, Norman Endicott, Trevor Hughes, Anthony Batty-Shaw, Geoffrey Keynes, and Jonathan Post. Standing like Janus in the field of Browne studies as I do, I want to assure future scholars that (of course) there is more to be found and understood. For instance, I did my very best to find Browne's letters to his Icelandic correspondent Þorður Jónsson, letters that I suspect were filled with rare insight into Browne's life, attitudes, and mind. It is entirely possible that these letters no longer exist, but until Clio descends and pronounces them irrevocably lost, I hope that Browne students will continue to look.

Jessica Wolfe has been my constant companion and guiding light over the decade in which this book was written, beginning one summer when we were happy transplants in California with our two dachshunds. As for those two Muses of my dedication: in both cases Browne anticipated the little wonders of the world.

A note on dates: I have modernized dates so that the new year begins on January 1 rather than on March 25.

Table of Contents

List of Illustrations

Introduction

"my life . . . a peece of Poetry"

In *Religio Medici*, thirty-year-old Thomas Browne claimed that his life so far had proved a wondrous affair, "a miracle" whose narration would strike the average person not as fact but "fable," not as "History" but "a peece of Poetry."[1] On the face of it, this testimonial seems overblown. Born into a London merchant's family in 1605, Browne had been educated at Winchester College and Oxford University before spending the early 1630s on the Continent in pursuit of his MD. While composing his *Religio Medici*, Browne was living in remote Halifax, West Yorkshire, in order inconspicuously to accrue vocational experience and to pass the time required before he could incorporate his Leiden medical degree at Oxford in 1637. He had no way of knowing that he would become the famous Dr Browne of the *Religio Medici* as well as of *Pseudodoxia Epidemica*. Unlike Milton, who in 1642 predicted his own future greatness as a national poet of epic, tragedy, and ode, Browne was declaring that his heretofore largely unproductive life was already extraordinary.

Nor did Browne know at age thirty that from the late 1630s until his death in 1682, he would confine the physical boundaries of his life to the city of Norwich and the county of Norfolk on the eastern shore of England. Yet increasingly over the course of these decades, Browne's contemporaries in England and on the Continent came to agree that his was a most extraordinary life, one simultaneously unique and vividly indicative of a European culture undergoing across-the-board transformation. Browne's life involved him in no courtly, clerical, or parliamentary office; yet his contemporaries near and far judged his authorship intensely deserving of praise, debate, emulation, and even infamy. This is the first biography of Browne to take seriously his own and his contemporaries' consensus that his was a remarkable life. To capture the poetry of Browne's life, this book will not only tell its story from start to finish but, far more substantially, recreate in detail the intellectual, social, and otherwise cultural and physical contexts in which Browne moved and on which he focused his exceptional learning and powers of perception.

[1] *Sir Thomas Browne: The Major Works*, ed. C. A. Patrides (New York: Penguin, 1977), 153; further citations of this edition will be made parenthetically.

Even factoring in the extraordinary events of early modern history from 1605 to 1635—the Gunpowder Plot in the year of his birth, for instance, or the pervasive religious and dynastic wars on the Continent—Browne's early life has never struck even his most sympathetic readers as anything other than commonplace. To be sure, his unusual claim for a miraculous youth might rank among the other bold paradoxes in *Religio*, for instance, the ones wishing that we could procreate like trees and that religion might prove even more mysterious than it is, or musing that all human beings are cannibals. Yet if Browne's claim to a fabulous life was meant to be strange, this did not mean that he expected or desired his readers to discount it. As a paradox, the claim might make good sense according to a wisdom that ran contrary to the expectations of the world. Looked at from the right perspective, a seemingly uneventful life might qualify as extraordinary.

In expressing awe over the miracle of his life, Browne quickly conceded that his regard for "the world" outside the self was low—earth was, he insisted, "not an Inne" for a traveler "but an Hospitall, and place, not to live, but to die in." What this disregard for the external world meant for the miracle of Browne's life was that its fabulousness depended in some measure on his regarding the "selfe . . . the Microcosme of mine owne frame." That is, whereas Browne might study the external world "but like my Globe, and turne it round sometimes for my recreation," it was the unlimited expansion within the capacity of the singular "minde" that converted history into poetry (Patrides, 153). Yet early in his life, then increasingly over its course, Browne was not one to embrace contempt for the world for very long. By conceiving of the self as a little world, Browne believed that the miracles of the inner life thrived on the intense and irreducibly various experience of the great world. So one's travels from London to Winchester and Ireland (1605–23), from Oxford (1623–31) to Montpellier, Padua, and Leiden (1631–34), one's intimate conversations in the barren, distant world of West Yorkshire (*c.*1634–37), one's observations of flora and fauna, one's loss of a parent or experiences with cadavers and patients, one's vast intellectual treasures found in books, discussions, and lectures—all these features of one's life would have a twofold value that might readily be missed. First, these contexts external to the self were for Browne far more vivid and stimulating than a slumbering or contemptuous traveler through life might notice, and second, the imaginative and intellectual alchemy that took place within the self could convert the world's already precious material into gold. Yet as Browne and his contemporaries recognized, not all that Brownean alchemy produced was golden; Browne himself struggled with—and some of his earliest readers denounced in his writings—those mental and spiritual monsters against which he assumed leadership in healing the epidemic of human error in the fallen world. More complexly, Browne's position as a lay theologian in *Religio Medici*, but also his physician's combination of gentle learning and manual labor illustrate how he tended to operate in some of the most troubling interstices of early modern culture.

This book operates on the conviction that the worlds in which Browne lived and learned were distinctively and accumulatively stimulating to his imagination and intellect, and that this was the case in dynamic and rich ways over the course of his entire life. In taking Browne at his word that his life was wonderful, I resist two assumptions that previous biographers have often made. The first is that while Browne's early life might indeed prove highly interesting, we lack the documents with which to reconstruct it. The second is that while Browne's later life is richly documented, it simply was not eventful enough to be interesting. Indeed, previous studies of Browne have operated on the assumption that when it comes to the events of Browne's existence on earth, the title of his biography might match that of Harold J. Cook's recent work on Joannes Groenevelt: *Trials of an Ordinary Doctor*.[2] Much as early twentieth-century anthropologists worried about the disappointing shape of Browne's skull, biographers have fretted about Browne's ordinary life, so much so in fact that at times they have refashioned it, for instance, insisting that Browne wrote *Religio Medici* in Oxford when it is patently clear that he did not.[3] As I hope to show, there are a sufficient number of vivid leads—some of them considerably surprising—that guide us in the reconstruction of Browne's early life in London, Winchester, Ireland, Oxford, Montpellier, Padua, Leiden, and Halifax. If one can rarely say that Browne did *x* on day *y*, one can nonetheless find out a great deal about the highly specific contexts with which he interacted—and this in ways that help to make fuller sense of what he cared about and wrote. What is more, newly discovered documents—such as the one identifying Browne's dissertation topic or others pertaining to his status as an orphan, his involvement in a witch trial, the success of his medical vocation, and what may have been an imprisonment by pirates—assist us in seeing anew those emphases that pervaded his life and thought. As for Browne's later life, not only is it richly documented with letters, notebooks, and works, but also, despite and sometimes even because of Browne's hunkering down in Norwich, it reveals a thinker and writer passionately and singularly engaged with the many dimensions of early modern life and culture, from politics, religion, and social dynamics to natural and historical studies. And as his later writings testify, Browne himself believed that every phase of life, old age as well as youth, had a distinctive part to play in our understanding of what it means to be human. All of Browne's environments help us to discern his life and mind more clearly and vividly, but this is not to suggest that the contextual "backdrop" justifies the biography; rather, it is the conviction of this book that never in history has there been another person quite like Sir Thomas Browne.

The dilemmas faced by biographers of Sir Thomas Browne were articulated early on by that brilliant practitioner of biography, Samuel Johnson. Attached to the second edition of *Christian Morals* in 1756, Johnson's life of Browne began with an account of biographical motives that gives us every reason not to expect too much:

> Though the writer of the following Essays seems to have had the fortune common among men of letters, of raising little curiosity after his private life, and has, therefore, few memorials preserved of his felicities or misfortunes; yet, because an edition of a

[2] Harold J. Cook, *Trials of an Ordinary Doctor: Joannes Groenevelt in Seventeenth-Century London* (Baltimore, MD: Johns Hopkins University Press, 1994).

[3] For the skull, see Miriam L. Tildesley, *Sir Thomas Browne: His Skull, Portraits, and Ancestry* (London, 1923); for Oxford, see the discussion of Frank Livingstone Huntley, *Sir Thomas Browne: A Biographical and Critical Study* (Ann Arbor: University of Michigan Press, 1962) in chapter 7 of this volume.

> posthumous work appears imperfect and neglected, without some account of the author, it was thought necessary to attempt the gratification of that curiosity which naturally inquires, by what peculiarities of nature or fortune eminent men have been distinguished, how uncommon attainments have been gained, and what influence learning has had on its possessors, or virtue on its teachers.[4]

In general, then, "men of letters" fail to inspire passionate interest in their daily existence or workaday concerns which, lacking the heroic dimension of great warriors or rulers, are essentially all that their lives comprise. Perhaps we simply do not want to know that great thinkers had petty problems or annoying foibles, but even if we did, Johnson avers, there will be little documentation for us to go on. Johnson's provision of a biography comes across here as a dull scholarly convention or marketing ploy for the curious.

When Johnson turns to the dearth of records regarding Browne's travels, however, the biographer's sense of loss is more acute, even if the desire to know more about those travels is treated as an instance of the vanity of human wishes (6). Johnson proceeds to explain why great minds such as Browne's tend to neglect reportage of their travels through the world, "either because it is more pleasing to gather ideas than to impart them, or because to minds naturally great, few things appear of so much importance as to deserve the notice of the publick" (6). Whatever else one might say about Browne's sense of his public, Johnson had Browne's predilections backwards—and not just because the biographer failed to grasp the physical, intellectual, and spiritual dangers of seventeenth-century travel: for Browne, all the world, the local as well as the foreign, was simply fascinating, and all of it, from ditches and insects to celestial bodies and divine providence, was worth sharing with others. Indeed Johnson missed the most obvious truth of the *Christian Morals*, not to mention the *Miscellany Tracts*, *The Garden of Cyrus*, *Hydriotaphia*, *Pseudodoxia Epidemica*, and *Religio Medici*: that for Browne, the smallest, seemingly slightest detail of God's world could offer the attentive observer with a paradise of delight, instruction, and inspiration. One of the pictures that hung in the adult Browne's household captured the humble cottage of Ovid's Baucis and Philemon, an elderly and profoundly loving married couple who showed the very gods themselves what it meant for the divine to take up residence in the humblest of places.[5]

For the earlier chapters of this book, the ones following Browne from London to Winchester and Ireland, then onward to Oxford, the Continent, and Halifax, I have taken Browne at his word that he experienced wondrousness in the places through which he had journeyed. I have also made the case that the mood, ethos, culture, and customs of these sites interacted with one another in Browne's imagination in complex and compelling ways, whether it was the intellectual daring of Padua, the specter of historical decay in Winchester, or the sobriety of social reform in Halifax. Following Browne's own anecdotal and intellectual leads, and with the

[4] See S. C. Roberts, ed., *Sir Thomas Browne's Christian Morals* (Cambridge: Cambridge University Press, 1927; reprinted New York: Kraus Reprint Co., 1969), 3.

[5] *The Works of Sir Thomas Browne*, ed. Geoffrey Keynes, 4 vols. (London: Faber & Faber, 1964), 3.281. Further citations of this edition will be parenthetical by volume and page number.

help of archival discoveries over the past few decades, I have tried to recreate as fully as possible these contexts. Yet oftentimes a detailed portrait of the contexts in which Browne lived and learned has been facilitated by stories, citations, preoccupations, and images that have been available to Browne's readers, often from the seventeenth century but at the very least since Simon Wilkin's great edition of the nineteenth century. As for Browne's Norwich years, despite the cache of personal letters and notebooks from the last decades of his life, treatments of Browne's life which have acknowledged the stimulus of Browne's travels have usually reneged on taking a close look at how the little world of Norfolk on the eastern coast of England supported the cabinet of curiosities that was Browne's brain as well as his house. In essence, biographers have simply refused to take Browne and his contemporaries at their word when they claimed that the little and local world could be more layered and larger in its historical and scientific importance than its physical dimensions or social boundaries might lead one to suppose.

For the most part Browne's biographers have regarded his life with that feeling of anticlimax that one of his earliest biographers, his friend John Whitefoot, described regarding one's first encounter with the man himself. "They that knew him no more than by the Briskness of his Writings," Whitefoot remarked in the *Posthumous Works* (1712), "found themselves deceived in their Expectation, when they came in his Company, noting the Gravity and Sobriety of his Aspect and Conversation; so free from Loquacity, or much Talkativeness, that he was something difficult to be engaged in any Discourse."[6] At times, Browne's laconic, careless way with the facts of his own life—was he born on October or November 19?—surely makes the earnest biographer wish for a certain loquacity. Yet Whitefoot proceeded to observe that when one got Browne talking, "it was always Singular, and never Trite or Vulgar." This is not entirely true: Browne's domestic letters can be movingly simple in their human concerns and anxieties. But the characterization has proved a model for this biography: what we find to be uninteresting in a superficial encounter with Browne's life proves to be fundamentally misleading. Whatever he undertook—parenting, medicine, encyclopedic study, or the observation of social, political, and natural phenomena, Browne lived out his days with uncommon intensity. As Whitefoot aptly observed of him, Browne was "Parsimonious in nothing but his Time, whereof he made as much improvement, with as little Loss as any Man in it; when he had any to spare from his drudging Practice, he was scarce patient of any Diversion from his Study; so impatient of Sloth and Idleness, that he would say, he could not do nothing" (*Posthumous Works*, xxxi). In his devoted care to his patients, in the record that he left of his medical practice and ongoing medical education, even this "drudging" centerpiece of his life proves fascinating, not least for what it teaches us about the history of disease and of natural studies more broadly in the second half of the seventeenth century. And in the last years of his life, his "Study" increasingly concerned itself with the world outside as well as inside books, though with Browne, what made education espe-

[6] See John Whitefoot, "Some Minutes for the Life of Sir Thomas Browne," in *Posthumous Works* (1712), xxxi.

cially complex was that the two worlds were always cross-fertilizing one another. For the years in which Browne dwelled in Halifax and Norwich, this biography attends more extensively to his social connections or networks together with his intellectual development, though in some striking cases—his stepfather Thomas Dutton, his Winchester school master Hugh Robinson, or his Oxford teachers Thomas Lushington and Robert Hues, for instance—the earlier chapters will also assess the impressions that social interactions and personalities made on his life.

The recent dialogue between literary scholars and historians about the nature of biography has been a fruitful one in clarifying and expanding the boundaries in which we might reconstruct the lives of the past. Blair Worden has pointed out the limits of the "life records" approach, according to which scholars start with "the documents that mention the name of an author, or fix him in time and place, or illustrate his social or professional relationships," then nervously work outward from there. Worden proposes that "if the relationship of writers to their times is to be more amply illuminated, an alternative method is needed. We need to reconstruct the wider life of politics or society or ideas: the life to which literature has belonged, and which it can illuminate, but which in main measure can be examined independently of it."[7] Whereas Worden has pursued this approach in a trinity of lives—those of John Milton, Andrew Marvell, and Marchamont Nedham—other scholars have taken a similar tack in the more traditional course of a single life. In giving us a rich new understanding of the Laudian Peter Heylyn, Anthony Milton has made the case that "we need to take more seriously and strive to understand the people in history who seem less than heroic or agreeable." Over the course of this book, I intend to make the further case that in contemporary terms, the same Browne whose life has seemed to his biographers so lacking in adventure nonetheless came to embody a certain type of heroism. Like Milton, I offer a life study that "is neither a straightforward biography, nor an intellectual study of [the subject's] works, but seeks to combine elements of both genres" as the best means of characterizing what makes Browne both distinctive among his contemporaries yet so central to their devices and desires.[8] As Wyman H. Herendeen remarks, while reconstructing as fully as possible the historical and material circumstances in which subjects lived, biographers should seek to demonstrate how their subjects proved "agents in" as well as "illustrations of the subtle but manifest changes in the intellectual history of the period."[9]

In unfolding Browne's circumstances, mental worlds, contexts, and writings, I have aimed to write what literary scholars and historians alike have referred to as a "cultural biography," in which texts are understood as events, their authors understood as active cultural agents within a series and network of social, political,

[7] Blair Worden, *Literature and Politics in Cromwellian England: John Milton, Andrew Marvell, Marchamont Nedham* (New York: Oxford University Press, 2007), vii.

[8] Anthony Milton, *Laudian and Royalist Polemic in Seventeenth-Century England: The Career and Writings of Peter Heylyn* (Manchester: Manchester University Press, 2007), ix, 5.

[9] Wyman H. Herendeen, *William Camden: A Life in Context* (Rochester, NY: The Boydell Press, 2007), xi. Cf. Cook: "one cannot fruitfully separate the world of ideas from the world of circumstance" (*Trials of an Ordinary Doctor*, xvii).

religious, and intellectual domains.[10] From start to finish, my efforts to describe Browne's complexities and peculiarities have benefited from recent scholarship on, among other matters, church history, the history of science, and the English civil war, since longstanding and rigid categories in each one of these fields have rarely worked well with Browne.[11] At long last, it has never helped very much to declare that Browne is Anglican, latitudinarian, Royalist, conservative, heterodox, a "true" scientist or no scientist at all, an Aristotelian or a Platonist. While there is a certain truth in each one of these labels, what that truth is—but also how all these labels *can* be true—in the case of Browne requires a dynamic, nuanced, and comprehensive reconstruction of the contexts of his life. Situated between the thick descriptions of micro-history, the rhetorical analyses of literary and intellectual history, and the chronological impetus of straightforward biography, the three parts of this study follow Browne from the workaday activities of parenting and earning a living through his far-reaching meditations on monsters, quincunxes, and the concentric circles of our lives.

The irreducibly complex responses to *Religio Medici*—both to Browne's English and to the Latin translation that quickly followed the first editions—clarify that this county physician instantly then persistently provoked his contemporaries into a stocktaking of their most deep-seated assumptions. Sometimes this shock to the reader's system brought Dr Browne a heroic celebrity; sometimes it brought him condemnation and scorn; at still other times it produced violently opposed reactions in individual readers who left extensive marginalia in their copies of the work and often tried somehow to stabilize or to correct it. Once Browne quickly added to his canon the Baconian invitation to his readers to join him in the reformation of learning (*Pseudodoxia Epidemica*), then published a decade or so later the stunningly learned yet also idiosyncratic, conflicted, and profoundly moving meditations of *Hydriotraphia* and the *Garden of Cyrus*: once these works were available leading into the 1660s, the man who spent the last decades of his life principally attending to the sick in the English county of Norfolk had intervened in—and altered—the discourses and tones of early modern culture in a way that his contemporaries considered a brand unto itself. More privately, in notebooks and letters, Browne matured in his engagement with the human and natural circumstances of life on earth right through his last days in the autumn of 1682. If Samuel Johnson could not understand Browne's claims for a poetic life, this was partly because Dr Johnson lacked information to be sure; but it was also because by the middle of the eighteenth century, assumptions about wonder, poetry, and biography had drastically, irreversibly changed.

The power and complexity of Browne's role in the shaping of seventeenth-century culture began with his bold embrace of a relatively new and controversial form of authority, the lay theologian. Browne was hardly alone among

[10] See, for instance, W. A. Sessions, *Henry Howard, The Poet Earl of Surrey: A Life* (New York: Oxford University Press, 1999), ix.

[11] For this state of affairs and its role in the resurgence of Browne studies, see Reid Barbour and Claire Preston, introduction to *Sir Thomas Browne: The World Proposed* (New York: Oxford University Press, 2008), 1–10; and Kathryn Murphy's introduction to *"A man very well studyed": New Contexts for Thomas Browne*, ed. Murphy and Richard Todd (Leiden: Brill, 2008), 3–12.

seventeenth-century writers in inventing this profile.[12] An anecdote, however, one recorded in the years after Browne's death but reaching back to the early days of his childhood, serves to illustrate how the modest and responsible physician of Norwich struck his contemporaries as extraordinary. Sometime over the course of his life, Thomas Browne or those family members closest to him came to associate a formative memory of his childhood with the youth of the controversial church father Origen. In a memorandum that she lent to Bishop White Kennett in 1712, Browne's favorite daughter Elizabeth reported that "His father used to open his breast when he was asleep, and kiss it in prayers over him, as 'tis said of Origen's father, that the Holy Ghost would take possession there."[13] One cannot be sure whether the parallel with Origen was Elizabeth's, her father's, or indeed her grandfather's, the giver of the remembered kisses. But Elizabeth was the person with whom in his last years Sir Thomas most intimately shared his love for books—by his own report, she read aloud to him an astonishingly ambitious set of volumes, especially history, travel, and sermons, but also "Many other Books, Treatises, discourses of severall kinds" (Keynes, 3.331–2). Although the classic account of Origen and his father Leonides appeared in Eusebius's *Ecclesiastical History*, it may be that the father and daughter shared the memory of—and made the connection regarding—Browne's father during their reading of Foxe's *Actes and Monuments* (included in the list of books that Elizabeth read to her father), in which the episode with Origen and his father was featured amongst the heroic deeds of the church father. As Martin Holmes points out, it was customary for a London citizen to bless his son "in his shop or counting house" at the commencement of a new school day.[14] But the blessing received by Thomas Browne was no ordinary valediction: it suggests a deeply felt celebration and confirmation of a child elected by God to experience his daily life with extraordinary spiritual and intellectual gifts in tow. The memory also suggests that Browne himself had been aware of those gifts from an early stage, then discovered an association of the paternal blessing with Origen that anticipated a controversial future in writing and exegesis that such gifts were apt to generate.

Given the premium that Origen placed on love as well as on the skeptical, speculative, allegorical spirit with which he explored the mysteries of his faith, the story of Browne's father kissing the breast of his soon-to-be orphaned son was either

[12] For this phenomenon see especially Amos Funkenstein, *Theology and the Scientific Imagination from the Middle Ages to the Seventeenth Century* (Princeton, NJ: Princeton University Press, 1986). For Browne's England, see Marc L. Schwarz, "Lay Anglicanism and the Crisis of the English Church in the Early Seventeenth Century," *Albion* 14 (1982), 1–19. More recently, there is Guy G. Stroumsa, *A New Science: The Discovery of Religion in the Age of Reason* (Cambridge, MA: Harvard University Press, 2010).

[13] The source of this anecdote is circuitous: one C. D. divulged it to the *European Magazine*, vol. xl, p. 89 on the basis of "a copy of the works of Sir Thomas Browne, printed in 1686, which formerly belonged to Dr. White Kennet, Bishop of Peterborough," in which might be found a memorandum in Kennett's hand to the effect that "In the time of my waiting in Windsor, in the latter part of November 1712, Mrs. Littleton, a daughter of Sir Thomas Brown, of Norwich, lent me a short account and character of her father, written by John Whitefoot," to which Elizabeth Lyttleton added her own appendix regarding her father's life. See Simon Wilkin, ed., *Sir Thomas Browne's Works* (London: William Pickering, 1836), 1.cx.

[14] Martin Holmes, *Elizabethan London* (London: Cassell, 1969), 26.

prescient on the part of a parent, a development in Browne's own self-identification, a posthumous but apt invention, or somehow all three at once. As with one contemporary's comparison between Browne and the Venetian Paolo Sarpi, who boldly assailed the prerogatives of the Catholic church,[15] Browne's supposedly uneventful life scarcely concealed from those that knew or read him just how exciting, transformative, and even disquieting his life had been. With the father's kiss, a Saturnine disposition,[16] and an education at Winchester College, Browne would seem destined for a life in the clergy. The fact that he achieved enormous fame in lay divinity, in "secular" learning, and in the vocation of medicine only just begins to explain what made his life a heroic venture.

[15] See chapter 6 in this volume.

[16] Marsilio Ficino, for instance, passed along the warning to avoid Saturnine physicians (*Three Books on Life*, ed. and trans. Carol V. Kaske and John R. Clark (Binghamton, NY: Center for Medieval and Early Renaissance Studies, 1989), book 3, chapter 10). I owe this reference to Jo Nixon.

PART I

SEEDS

1

London, 1605–1616

Not just Browne's Origen-like precocity but even his affection for his parents would prove a complex matter in *Religio Medici*. Like Origen, Browne lost his father at an early age, and as records from the Court of Orphans show, he would find that orphanage had considerable perils, even if the financial catastrophe was not so bad as some of Browne's earliest biographers opined. Having thanked his parents for his "mercifull disposition, and humane inclination," he also purveyed a discontentment with filial obligations, insisting that his religious faith is not owed exclusively "to those principles my Parents instilled into my unwary understanding," and more brashly declaring that true friendship trumps blood relations in the apportioning of his love (Patrides, 133, 61, 142–3). Over the course of his life, Browne would come to see childhood as a highly distinctive stage in human development as well as an intriguing subspecies of medical learning; and in the vivid memories that he recorded of his own early days, Browne left us evocative clues to the ways in which his London upbringing shaped him. When set together with the known facts about his childhood, these memories lead us into the layered and dynamic city into which Browne was born the son of a Mercer (Thomas Sr.) and his wife Anne Garraway.

1. BIRTH IN THE CITY

In *Religio Medici* Browne meditated on the astrological import of his birth in 1605. "At my Nativity," Browne explains, "my ascendant was the watery signe of *Scorpius*; I was borne in the Planetary houre of *Saturne*, and I think I have a peece of that Leaden Planet in me."[1] On this occasion, Browne stresses that at least in dreams, when he is freed from and transcendent over his normal self, he resists the influence of the planets and stars. For even if he is "no way facetious, nor disposed for the mirth and galliardize of company," his dreams are often comical. Yet Browne might also attribute certain modifications of his saturnine melancholy to his ascendant Scorpio. An "ascendant" was "the zodiacal sign on the eastern point or ascendant 'house' of the natal horoscope"; according to some astrologers, the ascendant was

[1] Text from Vittoria Sanna, ed., *Religio Medici: Edizione Critica con Introduzione e Note*, 2 vols. (Caligari: Annali delle Facoltà di Lettere-Filosofia e Magistero dell'Università di Cagliari, 1958), 165; the error in MSS, 1642, and even 1643 of speaking of Scorpio as "earthie" or "earthly" when it was famously associated with water was corrected in the errata of 1643.

more powerful than the planetary hour, which involved "daily periods of time between sunrise and sunset and between sunset and sunrise, each 'hour' being under the rulership of one of the seven planets (in the so-called 'Chaldean order'; i.e., the sun, Venus, Mercury, the moon, Saturn, Jupiter, Mars)."[2] Indeed, at other points in the *Religio*, Browne imagines his natural proclivities as opposites, with an inclination toward passionate worship running at cross-purposes with the austerity and rigidity of his "common conversation" and "behavior."

The most significant point about Browne's nativity was that, astrologically, it was singularly unfortunate—no wonder, then, that Browne "looked upon each day of his life as a special gift of Providence that stayed his natural destiny."[3] Melancholy was famously a mixed blessing, in keeping with Browne's associations with an Origen who was at once spiritually and intellectually gifted yet also on a collision course with heresy. A saturnine nativity may have prompted Browne's obsession with circularity, for it was associated with the "serpent biting its own tail" as well as with "time, the year, the universe, and the completion of the alchemical process" (Huntley, 3). But it also reinforced his sense of being bashful, reclusive, and singular; a scholarly embodiment of the embarrassing *pudor rusticus* against which he would later warn his sons (Keynes, 4.4, 5, 14). By contrast, Scorpio might help Browne account for his amiability—"For my conversation, it is like the Sunne's with all men, and with a friendly aspect to good and bad" (Patrides, 151)—and for his love of cheerful company in mitigation of an asocial and a self-involved melancholy. But Scorpio offered its own dreadful prospects. On the one hand, it was better that Saturn be aligned with watery Scorpio than with an earthly Taurus, Virgo, or Capricorn, for the latter "would add its dulling effect to the earthly qualities of Saturn."[4] On the other, though, with threats of "malignancy, horror, and death," Scorpio also accrued a vicious and debased association with the genitals, fundament, and bladder, and withal fornication. It might bring good fortune and hardiness, but it also might help to account for Browne's excessive ceremonialism, for, according to astrological lore, a man of Scorpio would gladly serve images.[5]

London merchants (such as Browne's father) customarily made a big affair of the casting of their children's nativities, for such a ceremony counted among those rites of passage that included baptism, apprenticeship, and marriage.[6] The date of his birth was either October or November 19, that is, either weeks just before or just after the Gunpowder Plot and the first publication of Bacon's *Advancement of Learning* (both November 5, 1605).[7] For the child whose father kissed him on the breast

[2] Johnstone Parr, "Sir Thomas Browne's Birthday," *English Language Notes* 11 (1973), 44–6.

[3] Huntley, *Sir Thomas Browne*, 3.

[4] Don Cameron Allen, *The Star-Crossed Renaissance: The Quarrel about Astrology and Its Influence in England* (Durham, NC: Duke University Press, 1941), 174. For Browne as a "moderate astrologer," see 104, 145.

[5] Alexander Barclay, *Shepheards Kalender* (1656 edition), chapter 52.

[6] Richard Grassby, *The Business Community of Seventeenth-Century England* (Cambridge: Cambridge University Press, 1995), 325.

[7] The evidence for November comes from Browne himself in a 1672 letter to John Aubrey (see Keynes, 4.374), but Browne could be careless about biographical details. For October we have the anonymous life in *Posthumous Works* (a1r) but also the testimony of his daughter Elizabeth Lyttleton

then departed this world of travail, there was much ahead to do in deciphering the interworkings of divine will, the beauties and properties of nature, the workaday business of money and trade, the Pauline concerns with salvation and grace, and the specter of premature death. From an early age, Browne was attentive to learning how the diverse constituents of his London would come together, mature, and metamorphose.

Browne's mother was born Anne Garraway, the daughter of Paul Garraway (or Garroway), whose onetime residence in Lewes, Sussex, is known to us thanks only to her son's own memory of it. Writing to his son Edward in the last winter of his life, Browne confirmed his son's decision "not to hazard your self at that time by such a journey to Lewys, whereof a part is very bad waye. I remember when I was very yong & I thinck butt in coates, my mother carryed mee to my Grandfather Garrawayes howse in Lewys. I retaine only in my mind the idea of some roomes of the howse and of the church" (Keynes, 4.203). As Finch has pointed out, "This must have been before [Browne] was six years old, for his grandfather Garraway remarried in 1611 and removed from Sussex to Bedfordshire";[8] indeed "coats" refers to the petticoats worn by small children. Born in Acton, Middlesex, in February 1553, Paul Garraway died in Tingriffe, Bedfordshire, though he was buried at St Martin's in the Fields, London, on January 24, 1620.[9] He married Browne's grandmother at the parish church of St Peter-le-Poor in London.[10] So far as records show, Anne Garraway had two brothers Philip and John: the first, a bachelor, apparently died overseas sometime after writing his will in 1624 or 1625, while the second lived until the early 1660s. Anne also had a sister, Mary, who wedded John Brockett, Esquire, of Hertfordshire sometime prior to January 1625, when she and Browne's mother were included together in the will of their half-brother Edward Britridge. For grandfather Paul's additional marriage to Alice Britridge meant that Browne's mother Anne also had half-brothers, Edward and Francis Britridge, the latter a Merchant Tailor who would play a role in the execution of Thomas Browne Sr.'s estate in 1613–14.

There is no record of how Browne's parents met, and none of what they looked like.[11] Thomas Sr.'s will suggests an affection for and trust in his wife, the posthumous disputes over his legacy notwithstanding. Of Browne's sisters, we know

(C. D., *European Magazine*, 90), though this might reflect a desire to make his life perfectly circular. His monument in St Peter Mancroft claims that he died in the seventy-seventh year "of his Age." For the calculation that his birthday was a Saturday, see *Religio Medici*, ed. William Murison (Cambridge: Cambridge University Press, 1922), 252. An argument for Wednesday is made in Parr, "Sir Thomas Browne's Birthday," 44–6.

[8] Jeremiah S. Finch, *Sir Thomas Browne: A Doctor's Life of Science and Faith* (New York: Henry Schuman, 1950), 27.

[9] For the Garraways see Charles Williams, "The Pedigree of Sir Thomas Browne," *Norfolk Archaeology* 15 (1904), 109–13.

[10] See notes on Browne's genealogical chart in Miriam L. Tildesley's *Sir Thomas Browne: His Skull, Portraits, and Ancestry.* Reprinted from *Biometrika* 15 for subscribers only, 1923, 69.

[11] Browne's daughter Elizabeth mentioned her father's "picture…at the Duke of Devonshire's house in Picadilly in his mother's lap" together with Browne's father and siblings (see C. D.'s letter to *European Magazine* 40 (August, 1801), 89). But the closest extant candidate for this picture, the so-called Dobson group, has been ruled out: see Tildesley, 28–30.

something of their marital fortunes: Anne was married to a Grocer named John Palmer in St Martin Pomeroy on Ironmonger Lane;[12] in either 1632 or 1633, having accompanied her mother to Ireland, Jane married Thomas Price, a London native but at the time of the marriage a resident of Drumlaham in County Cavan, and eventually the archbishop of Cashel; Mary wedded Nevill Craddock of Clifford's Inn on September 30, 1630 in St Michael, Paternoster Royal, in London;[13] and Ellen, having never married, remained with her mother in Ireland at least until 1642. Of these sisters, so far as we know, Mary played a role in Browne's later life, joining him in Norwich after the death of her husband in 1651 (Morris, 13). Browne's letters show an ongoing concern for the welfare of Thomas and Jane Price, as late as 1682 requesting that Edward remember him to the archbishop of Cashel (Hughes, 25). Indeed, Browne's letters to his own children later in life purveyed a concern that they treat one another with love and consideration, even if the *Religio* sometimes evinces a strident disregard for the nuclear family.[14]

For England in general and London in particular, the season of Browne's birth bore witness to a major turning point in history. He was born in 1605 in the West Cheapside neighborhood between the cathedral dedicated to Paul at the western boundary and a onetime shrine to Thomas à Becket at the eastern—the latter with special connections to the company of Browne's father, the Mercers. A neighborhood framed between two powerful but potentially conflicting civic and religious symbols; the early years of his life coincident with a national trauma—the Powder Plot—on the order of the conquest of the Spanish Armada in 1588; his birth attended by the launching of Bacon's revolution in knowledge; and the celestial regions casting down some of their gravest emanations: as he looked back on his youth, Browne had sufficient reason for believing that his times had been portentous.

Yet Browne remembered his early years in softer, simpler terms too. For a boy who would grow up to value peace, it is noteworthy that Browne's England was ruled by a king, James I, with a strong commitment to religious harmony. Browne's own memories of childhood are at times pastoral and provincial: a protected life of local plant-gathering, a visit to his grandfather, and curiosities such as ostriches or, more macabre, the "body wh. had been buried some hundreds of yeares in St Pauls" (Keynes, 3.340). Browne's earliest memories also resonate with the commercial context in which his father and Uncle Edward (a Grocer) operated. Writing to his son Edward in 1681, Browne recalled with striking specificity the "Two complaints I have heard of the East India company ever since I was a youth, that it was a very hard matter to gett their money out who putt any in, & that the considerable profitt went unto the officers"; Browne recalled not just how his uncle would "always" express regrets about his investment with this company but even

[12] J. Trevor Hughes, "The Childhood of Sir Thomas Browne: Evidence from the Court of Orphans," *London Journal* 23 (1998), 25.

[13] G. C. R. Morris, "Cradock, Amherst and Howell: A Link between the Selbys of Ightham and Sir Thomas Browne of Norwich," *Archaeologia Cantiana* 102 (1985), 11–18.

[14] See Keynes, 4.180 for instance.

the sum of the initial investment, £800 (Keynes, 4.189). London would also prove a city in which to experience loss: for his father would leave him orphaned at the end of 1613, and subject to the vicissitudes of care meted out by guardians who could not always be entirely trusted. The erasure of his father from his life is not something that Browne discusses in his extant writings; but as his adult correspondence shows quite clearly, he made sure that he was a loving and nurturing presence in the lives of his children, even when they were far away from home.

2. THE RELIGION OF A CHILD

The parish in which Browne was born, St Michael le Querne (or at the Corn), locates his childhood home close to the northern gate leading to St Paul's Cathedral. One document from his Winchester days mentions St Foster's as his parish, in other words, St Vedast's, the parish to which St Michael le Querne would later be joined.[15] It is possible that this anomaly is a mistake for Foster's Lane but also that young Browne identified his parish by a guardian—say, his uncle—as well as the home in which he was raised. But whether Browne's childhood belonged to one parish or two, it was rooted in the western part of Cheapside, officially in the ward of Faringdon. Like St Paul's and the Mercers' Chapel, Browne's parish church had evocative associations for a future antiquarian, since John Leland had died in the parish and was buried there. (See Figure 1.1.)

Browne's antiquarian sympathies were not fully awakened until the Civil War in the 1640s. Yet as a lifelong lover of sermons, he had occasion in his adulthood to remember not just the cathedral of St Paul's but Paul's Cross in particular. Describing the "green yard" in which sermons were preached at Norwich Cathedral, he remarked that, with the social and clerical elite provided for with galleries, "the rest either stood, or sat in the green, upon long forms provided for them, paying a penny, or halfpenny apiece, as they did at St. Paul's cross in London" (Keynes, 3.141). An observation in his notebooks appears to depend on personal recollection: "At the 2 howers sermons at St. Pauls crosse the preacher to refresh him & continue his voice was used to stoope downe in the pulpit & drinck" (Keynes, 3.268).

Browne's fascination with the sermon as a special case of religious rhetoric and epistemology began at the Cross; this is not surprising since, as Walsham remarks, "On children and adolescents prophetic rhetoric" at the Cross "could have an electrifying and intoxicating effect."[16] For Browne, performances at the Cross offered complex lessons in the experience of worship, for instance, driving home the irony that even the most iconophobic "Puritan" might rely on intense theatricality in the pulpit, no small lesson for a child who would grow up to write so extensively and brilliantly on religion's basis in imagination, reason, and the senses, but also on its

[15] See Tildesley, *Sir Thomas Browne*, 76.

[16] Alexandra Walsham, *Providence in Early Modern England* (Oxford: Oxford University Press, 1999), 324.

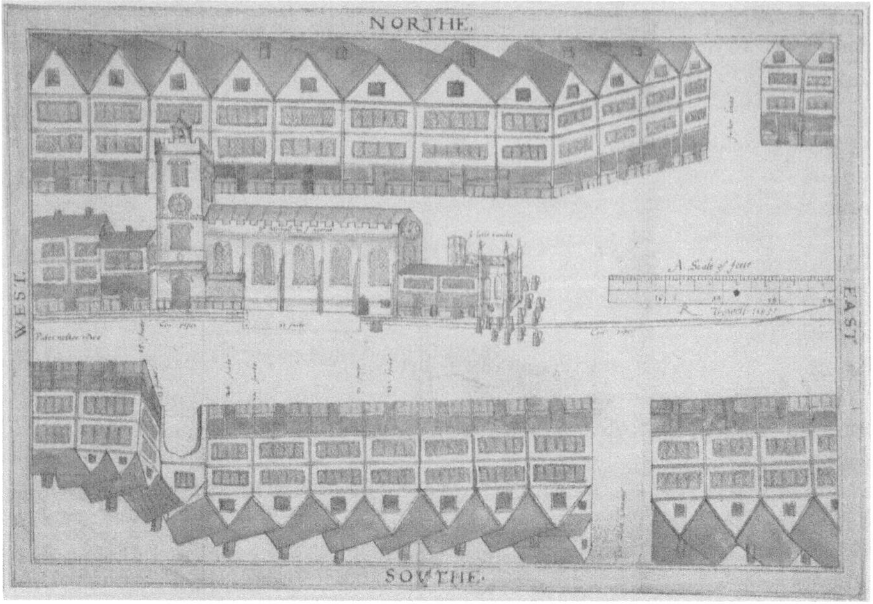

Figure 1.1 St Michael le Querne, in West Cheapside, from Ralph Treswell, pen and ink and watercolor on paper (1585): © The Trustees of the British Museum.

capacity for error. With regard to the natural world to which Browne would devote so much of his attention, Cross preachers explained the definitions and characteristics of providence; the scale of creation; the world as a mirror of the divine plan or as an operation executed by God's finger; the sympathy amongst creatures; the types of Christian mysteries such as the resurrection in creatures; metaphors of the relation between the creator (the potter) and the creation (the pot); hieroglyphs of eternity such as the "Egyptian serpent bended about into himselfe";[17] the various lives through which human beings pass; and the status of miniature creatures in God's plan—all issues to which Browne would turn as early as *Religio Medici*. If young Thomas Browne would have found doctrinal topics in the Cross sermons—on the relation of faith to works, for example—he also would have whetted his lifelong appetite for questions of interpretive method. In varying degrees, Cross preachers engaged the history of biblical scholarship and exegesis, whether in pursuit of the etymology of "angel" (about which Browne would later debate a Jesuit divine), in juxtaposition of the available biblical texts in a variety of languages, or in assessment of the various modes—literal and allegorical—of interpretation.

Especially significant for Browne's development was the fact that over the first years of his life, strong anti-papal prejudice poured from the orators at the Cross, their rhetoric intensified by the Gunpowder Plot. The consequent discovery of the

[17] William Hull, *Repentance not to be repented of* (1612), 3v.

conspiracy in the days just before its event was habitually credited to both the wisdom of James and the all-seeing providence of God. The latter assessment prompted comparisons to 1588, the former to James's protection from plots (such as Gowrie's) throughout his life: Browne himself would make such connections in the *Religio*'s praise for providential intervention in cases of "manifest disproportion between the powers and forces of two several agents" (Patrides, 82). Yet in the same passage, he typically resisted full-scale polemic; rather than single out England for special dispensation, he proceeded to argue that while the hand of God had directly intervened with miraculous disproportion in the Powder Plot, including its strange "miscarriage of the letter" in the year of Browne's birth, this event could not be wholly divorced from a tendency in nature toward circularity or revolution that would eventually reward all nations equally.

Given the fact that the rectors in Browne's own parish church were John Bowle and George Downame, we can be certain that Browne heard attacks on the papal Antichrist in St Michael le Querne as well: the former was happy to condemn the Pope as "the vicar of hell" while the latter was well known for his *Treatise Concerning Antichrist* published two years before Browne's birth. Antipopery pervades the sizable body of divinity that Downame published. But Bowle and Downame also modeled for Browne a complex or hybrid approach to English Protestantism that would prove formative for the author of *Religio Medici*.[18] Both Bowle and Downame had bishoprics in their future, but Downame in particular was noted, and controversial, in Browne's childhood for his defense of the apostolic basis and divine right of episcopacy, especially in two sermons preached at the consecration of James Montagu in 1608. By the time that he came to St Michael le Querne in 1613–14, Downame was under attack by critics of episcopacy such as the famous Puritan divine Paul Baynes.[19]

Yet despite his own penchant for polemic against the Antichrist and his generation of controversy regarding bishops, Downame embodied for a precocious young English Protestant such as Browne an appealing combination of serious theological learning, assiduous preaching, practical divinity, and a fervent promotion of peace and unity among Christian brethren. In his sermons he made judicious use of Hebrew and Greek, of the church fathers, and of standard Protestant authorities such as Luther and Calvin. Downame's views of salvation were moderate, for example as they are epitomized in a sermon published in 1607 in which Abraham's readiness to sacrifice his son at God's command serves to reconcile Paul's emphasis on salvation by grace with James's insistence (as Downame interprets it) that while faith in God's grace is our only means of salvation, it produces and is accompanied

[18] Information about the preachers and practices from Browne's parish church is derived from the churchwarden's account book, LMA P69/MIC4/B/005/MS02895/002. For overviews of the careers of Bowle and Downame, see the *ODNB* articles by C. S. Knighton and Kenneth Gibson respectively.

[19] In addition to Downame's *Two Sermons, The One Commending the Ministerie in Generall: The Other Defending the Office of Bishops in Particular* (1608), see Anthony Milton, *Catholic and Reformed: The Roman and Protestant Churches in English Protestant Thought, 1600–1640* (Cambridge: Cambridge University Press, 1995), 480–1.

by good works.[20] For Downame, Abraham was heroic for automatically obeying and believing in the legitimacy of a divine command that on the face of it might strike the Old Testament patriarch as contradictory. But Downame's Abraham also models those deliberate processes by which the patriarch worked out his convictions—processes that show an independence of mind not far removed from Downame's account of how he himself arrived at the divine right of episcopacy—a powerful message for the author of *Religio Medici*.

While Downame aimed to steer English Protestants between the extremes of the papists and the "carnal Gospeller" (that is, those radical Protestants who assumed that salvation relieved them of responsibility for good works),[21] he was also formative for Browne in focusing on practical divinity, not least with regard to the commercial practices with which Browne's family was confronted on a daily basis. While an essential lesson of Downame's *Lectures on the XV. Psalme* (1604) was that usury is evil, it took the preacher over two hundred pages to work out the complexities of and objections to that conclusion, not least because of a recent penchant to defend usurious lending. As will be seen with the case of Browne's orphaned estate, debt played a crucial role in his childhood prospects for a happy life.[22] Indeed, Downame's discussion of usury took up the cause of orphans in addition to its lingering examination of one of the chief concerns of *Religio Medici*, the criteria of charity. Perhaps most importantly of all, Downame took seriously not just his own vocation to preach and teach but also the future of that vocation, worrying that the bad mixture of the pains to be taken in becoming a godly minister with the paltry benefits of doing so was diverting bright young men to law and medicine.[23] For Browne, whose *Religio Medici* and *Christian Morals* alike oscillated between practical divinity and the learning of an arts education, an exposure to Downame at an early age—to a preacher who avidly promoted the logic of Peter Ramus and dedicated himself to nurturing and edifying his flock—was seminal.

The church warden's accounts from St Michael le Querne reveal more about the everyday life of Browne's parish church than just the identity of the rectors: it records the yearly expenses for holly and ivy at Christmas; for the mending of the physique of the church, especially in 1610–11 and 1614–15; for the scavengers who kept the north and south sides of the church clean; for the recipients of charitable donations, including poor scholars; for the washing of church linen; for the breakfast at the annual perambulation of the parish; for fetching the hook out of Foster's Lane when there was a fire in Lillypott Lane; and for the services required in the answering of visitation articles. The account books also recorded the receipts, of course, including the three shillings and four pence received for the tolling of the bell upon the death of Browne's father in 1613, a payment that does not include the breaking of the ground for his burial.

[20] George Downame, *Abrahams Tryall: A Sermon Preached at the Spittle, in Easter weeke, Anno Domini, 1602* (1607).

[21] Downame, *Abrahams Tryall*, A3r.

[22] See George Downame's *Lectures on the XV. Psalme: Read in the Cathedrall Church of S. Paule in London* (1604), 148–362.

[23] See Downame, *Two Sermons*, 87–8.

For Browne's religious education, the churchyard and precinct of Paul's involved more than the performance of sermons, penances, or book-burnings. For one thing, it was the heart of the London book trade. As such, the significance of the book trade for the propagation of reformed religion made the churchyard doubly evocative as a precinct of Protestantism. For another, the churchyard shared its eastern border with St Paul's school, a premiere grammar school for humanist learning and one of the most significant charges of the Mercers. More complexly, the cathedral itself comprised an oft-satirized mixture of profane business with sacred worship. Debts were frequently paid at its font; the destitute visited Duke Humphrey's tomb in search of a dinner invitation; and business deals were often negotiated in the nave. The threat that Mammon always posed to Christian worship in the business district of Cheapside emanated out from its obvious menace at Paul's to include the nearby medieval church of St Michael le Querne whose very name (*ad bladum*, in the corn market) smacked of commerce and whose proximity to shops and "verie indecent" buildings drew protestations in the 1630s.[24] This threat, however, also gave way to strenuous attempts on the part of the Cross preachers to mediate between the debts owed to Christ and those owed to commerce. In becoming a Christian and learned physician with potentially competing obligations and a vexed social status, Browne often reflected in his adult letters an anxiety about the value of money that was regularly vetted in the Cross sermons of his childhood. The complex calculus of values that Browne's family confronted on a daily basis was not simply spiritual in its reach; rather, the family's social position (for instance, its relationship to the gentry), its obligations to civic duty and charity, and its moral credentials: all these critical factors in the Browne family's identity were intensified by the ways in which "consumerism of the turn of the century focused anxieties along all the major faultlines within metropolitan society."[25] Later in life, as a moralist, physician, collector, and father in increasingly cosmopolitan Norwich, Browne weighed the rival claims of commerce, charity, prestige, and curiosity with a persistence and nuance that were indebted to a childhood in Cheapside among silks.

3. THE MERCERS ON CHEAPSIDE

As an avid book collector, Browne would always maintain a strong connection to the area around Paul's churchyard. But Browne's father had much closer ties to a building eastward down Cheapside, the Hall that the Mercers had constructed on the site of a complex associated with the martyr Thomas à Becket. The polemic of early Jacobean England might juxtapose the two buildings, Paul's and Thomas's, as a clear division between true religion and false; between a theology of grace and an

[24] Howard Colvin, "Inigo Jones and the Church of St Michael le Querne," *The London Journal* 12 (1986), 36–9.

[25] Ian Archer, "Material Londoners?" in Orlin, ed., *Material London*, 179–87, with quotations at 179–80, 186, and 187.

idolatry of works; between Tudor and Stuart London and papal Rome; between the sacred and the profane. In embracing "St *Pauls* Sanctuary" in *Religio*, Browne stressed the incomprehensibility of the divine, on whose grace we must rely (Patrides, 72). But, to reverse the polemic, Becket could be considered a courageous hero of his faith, one whose singular charity might chasten what Browne would dub the insolence of the zealous hypocrite.[26] For Browne, whose *Religio Medici* would promote and embody a reconciliation between faith and charity in a polemical culture that tended to divide them, this iconography was potent stuff.

Thus Browne did not have to travel abroad to experience the deeply rooted conflicts of contemporary religious culture. He was also privy to a certain level of international ecumenicalism close to home, insofar as the non-parochial status of the Mercers' Chapel but also the company's involvement in foreign trade led to a distinctive feature of the worship conducted there, namely, the permission to alien Protestant congregations, especially Italian, to have their services on site. With the ready supply of Italian teachers in this community, it is possible that Browne's knowledge of that language was initiated when he was a child.[27] By contrast, just next to the Mercers' Hall, the long and brutal London history of religious intolerance was evoked by the name of Old Jewry, where Jews had lived and worshiped in the city before their expulsion in the Middle Ages. Having received further impetus from his travels abroad in France, Italy, and the Netherlands, Browne recalibrated Christian and Jewish relations in writings from *Religio* and *Pseudodoxia* through *Hydriotaphia*.

To reach Paul's churchyard, Browne would have entered through the northern gate—Paul's or Cheap Gate—just across Cheapside and Paternoster Row from his parish church. To reach Mercers' Hall, the boy would have walked a short distance down Cheapside past Ironmonger Lane to one of the most striking buildings on the left hand side of one of London's most impressive streets. Streets running off to the north took a pedestrian in a few short steps to the wall and to the expansive fields beyond where young Browne might go simpling; to the south, tumultuous, close-packed streets led to the river which paralleled Cheapside.[28] In 1680, Browne recalled even the city traffic of his youth with a nostalgia suggestive of a bygone humility and simplicity, remarking to his son Edward that "I thinck you are in the right when you say that physitians coaches in London are more for state then for buisinesse, there being so many wayes whereby they may bee assisted and at lesser charge & care in London.... When I was a youth many great persons travelled with 3 horses, butt now there is a new face of things" (Keynes, 4.166).

In the city, shops of the kind that many Mercers maintained fronted the street but were connected to "larger establishments known as selds containing many

[26] For the charitable Becket, see Nathanael Carpenter, *Achitophel, or, the picture of a wicked politician*, 1629.

[27] For this possibility, see Gordon Campbell and Thomas N. Corns, *John Milton: Life, Work, and Thought* (Oxford: Oxford University Press, 2008), 49–50. For the Italian community see Stefano Villani, "The Italian Protestant Church of London in the 17th Century," in Barbara Schaff, ed., *Exiles, Emigrés and Intermediaries: Anglo-Italian Cultural Transactions* (New York: Rodopi, 2010), 217–36.

[28] John Stow, *A Survey of London by John Stow*, ed. Charles Lethbridge Kingsford, 2 vols. (Oxford: Clarendon Press, 1908), 1.76.

chests and trading stations from which goods were sold. Many of the shops probably performed a dual function in retail outlets and as places where goods were manufactured or processed."[29] Although some Mercers were principally involved in international commerce, others lived with their families above or behind their shops and warehouses. The very wealthiest might have a mansion but many would rent rather than own their own dwellings.[30] In 1617, Fynes Morison described the average citizen's house as "very narrow in the front towards the street, but... built five or six roofs high, commonly of timber and clay with plaster, and... very neat and commodious within."[31] During Browne's childhood, Cheapside was wealthy, dense in population, and in demand. The very street names and history of the area evoked trade, commerce, and crafts, including the spicers, shoemakers, ironmongers, goldsmiths, drapers, founders, wiredrawers, as well as mercers; in short, the physical and imaginative space of Browne's childhood was vividly material, commercial, and creatural.

Stow emphasized the street landmarks in his account of the Cheapside area: the little conduit by Paul's gate (on the spot of an ancient stone cross long since removed when St Michael le Querne was expanded), the Great Conduit (with water piped in from Paddington) directly across from Mercers' Hall, the Great Cross in memory of Queen Eleanor, and the Standard where, in olden times, corporal punishments were effected. Whereas each landmark accrued civic and religious significance, for instance when the conduits and standard, along with the houses and churches, were festooned with garlands at Christmas (Stow, 1.97), they also could become the vehicle of religious conflict. The Great Cross was a key site for the clash between iconoclasts and those supportive of monuments into the seventeenth century, with the erection of a timber cross covered with gild and lead, but the Virgin losing her crown and child, and being stabbed in the breast (1.267).

At the water sources especially, but really all throughout Cheapside, urban life was vibrant, densely packed, and indecorous (with rich and poor, high and low living side by side) but also pervasively stable, regulated, and habitual. Yet Cheapside was also the heart and soul of city pageantry and, therefore, of the urban myth-making that reflected and constituted London's moral, social, and spiritual identity. Browne's affection for civic pageantry in *Religio Medici* reflects his Cheapside childhood in the center of those allegorical processions that composed the

[29] Derek Keene and Vanessa Harding, *Historical Gazetteer of London before the Great Fire, Part I, Cheapside* (London: Institute for Historical Research, University of London, 1987), liv.

[30] For the basic features of the London merchant's home, see John Schofield, ed., *The London Surveys of Ralph Treswell* (London Topographical Society, Publication 135, 1987), 15–31. Extant accounts of properties rented by the various livery companies from the period are spotty, not least because while remaining account books record some rentals, often the books of the renter wardens are missing. LMA P/69/MIC4/D/008/MS00805 has deeds and leases from the Querne parish but the only Thomas Browne appearing in the records lived in the late eighteenth century. Records of the Merchant Tailors in the Guildhall Library record an assessment of a Thomas Browne in Watlinge Street but it is impossible to know whether this was Browne's father.

[31] Quoted in Lawrence Manley, ed., *London in the Age of Shakespeare: An Anthology* (University Park, PA: Pennsylvania State University Press, 1986), 43–4.

Lord Mayor's shows. As Anthony Munday clarifies in his comments on the 1609 pageant, children were commonly participants in the pageantry, not just spectators of it, sometimes to the dissatisfaction of the producers—yet the "weake voyces of so many Children" were "vrgently require[d]" in "such showes."[32] Children not only sang; they rode on chariots and ostriches amid a panoply of allegorical devices. For a young Browne, who would grow up to write one of Europe's major histories of symbolism in *Pseudodoxia Epidemica*, these pageants provided a vivid introduction. As a grandfather, he encouraged and delighted in his grandson Tomey's excitement about civic shows and pageantry.

As the son of a Mercer, Browne grew up under the presumption of civic status and surrounded by the resplendent fabrics that mere worms could produce. Even though there was an increase in the variety of shops to be found along Cheapside, the fame and impressiveness of its expansive way depended on the sheen of the artificial—on the silks of the Mercer for instance. Browne's father was embedded in the most sumptuous and impressive of civic institutions. The elaborate feasts held by the Company included major dignitaries among their guests (including ambassadors and court officials) and fervently cultivated the principle of decorum from the position of the tables to the proportions of red deer, quail, or capon that one received over the many, minutely regulated, courses of the dinner.[33] As Company records show, the freedom of the citizen was not always free, since the investment of the Mercers in the plantation of Ireland entailed that Browne Sr. invest money—two pounds, ten shillings—in that business.[34] There is evidence that Browne's father had some ambition in his Company. When Browne's father stood twice—albeit unsuccessfully—for office as either a Renter or Fourth Warden in 1612–13, this suggested, first, his willingness to risk expense in the affairs of the Company; it also meant that he ranked among the half-dozen leading liverymen of the Company in those years, with his competitors including leading citizens of London such as Lionel Cranfield.[35] But office in the Company could also be lucrative, and Browne Sr. may have wanted to enhance an estate that was saddled with the burdens of having extended credit to others as well as his own personal debt. Concerns about money, debt, and ambition never left Browne; in the letters that he wrote to his son Edward in particular, he persistently offered advice (and at times regret) about the handling of a physician's financial and social-cum-vocational standing. Indeed, Browne continued to worry about those commercial pressures that had occupied his father and that, he tells his sons, must concern all fathers: anxiety about one's capital intake and expenditures; assessment of the virtues and vices associated with trade practices; justification of an affection for expensive

[32] Anthony Munday, *Camp-bell, or the Ironmongers faire field* (1609), B2v. The children's singing is said to be better in Anthony Munday's *Himatia Poleos* (1614), 9, led as it is by the Master who directs the St Paul's boys' choir.

[33] Harding and Keene describe the courses in detail in *Historical Gazetteer*.

[34] Acts of Court 1595–1629, Mercers' Hall, London, f. 115.

[35] Acts of Court, Mercers' Hall, August 21, 1612 and September 3, 1613. Apprenticeship was not the only way to gain the liberty of London, but it was by far the predominant way over and above inheritance and "redemption."

rarities and curiosities with an appeal to the labors of vocation and scholarship; and uncertainty over the social status that results from the strange combination of luxury and labor.

As a Mercer who ran for office in the Company, Browne's father confronted tensions between godliness, commercial self-interest, and public duty. On the one hand, the early Jacobean promotion of a domestic silk trade offered a largely unprecedented support for the ethos of the Mercer, even if the financial effects of the project were stunted or uncertain.[36] On the other, the essential moral and spiritual dilemma for the Mercer was that he profited from the expanded sale of luxury items in a world in which preachers were apt to condemn luxury and in which sumptuary laws and rigid notions of natural and social hierarchy were dedicated to confining the consumption of luxuries to an elite few. In Browne's childhood, a mulberry-silkworm promotion was underway, with a series of publications and with the enlistment of foreign advisors. It is no wonder that over the course of his life, the silkworm's artistry and mystery would continue to figure prominently in the imagination of Browne's "sensible artist."

Silk came to Browne's childhood home on ships from afar, especially from Italy; its many varieties were evocative for an intellectually curious child; its complex moral lessons were provocative for an intensely spiritual one. Nothing demonstrates this combination more vividly than the simple fact that on October 8, 1613, a ship known as the *Greyhound* imported for Browne's father a bale of organzine, a type of silk known for its particular composition—"a strong silk yarn, made of single threads twisted together, folded into two, and twisted again in the opposite direction"—but also for its status as "Superfine...the best sort." It was a shipment that the Mercer would not live to sell, a potent emblem of the thin line between luxury and mortality in the youth of Thomas Browne.[37] Perhaps organzine's combination of strength and delicacy offered him an early lesson in how to reconcile the heavenly and earthly obligations between which for the rest of his life he persisted in mediating.

Browne's father had arrived in London from provincial Cheshire to transmute the landed past of his family into a mercantile future. Perhaps the most practical lesson that Browne learned from his commercial upbringing was the challenge of mediating the unstable social status accruing with one's vocation. In early Stuart London, much about a Mercer's status and profile was complex. In his daily business, a Mercer's success whether in retail or wholesale trade required that he have excellent relations with his customers and associates at home and abroad—Browne himself would develop an appealing bedside manner, an unfailing civility in professional correspondence, and an international reputation—but also that he understand and manipulate the intricacies and uncertainties of credit in those relations. Indeed apprenticeship in the

[36] Linda Levy Peck, *Consuming Splendor: Society and Culture in Seventeenth-Century England* (Cambridge: Cambridge University Press, 2005), 1. For the importance of silk in Jacobean England, see also Robert Brenner, *Merchants and Revolution: Commercial Change, Political Conflict, and London's Overseas Traders, 1550–1653* (Princeton, NJ: Princeton University Press, 1993), 25–30.

[37] National Archive, E 190/17/4 (3r), an impost log for ships. The definition of organzine's composition is the *OED*'s. For the variety of silk, see John Wheeler, *A Treatise of Commerce* (1601), 23; for the elite status of organzine, see *Philosophical Transactions of the Royal Society* (1699), 184.

Mercer's trade had a reputation for ranking amongst the most arduous. Even if a good education was only a desideratum rather than a necessity, he was obviously required to master the complex and changing material realities of textiles both commonplace and luxurious. Especially early in his apprenticeship he might be expected to hawk products from outside the store front. But the "incessant bawl" of such hawking was not always confined to the lowly apprentice: in addition to the "newer and less strenuous" advertisements to be situated in "an attractive display of goods on the shop-board," merchants habitually depended on their wives to strike up conversations with passers-by so that "the wit and beauty of these Cheapside wives became something of a legend."[38] Some Mercers, however, would have focused on international trade, not on the keeping of a shop.

As a Mercer, then, Browne's father was implicated in the ambivalent social status of seventeenth-century businessmen in general, a problem that Browne himself would encounter in his medical profession. Sir Baptist Hicks offended the city officials "when he kept shop after he had been knighted"; conversely, when he sought a good marriage, "he thought it advisable to emphasize that a mercer did not necessarily see a yard of silk" (Grassby, 119). As Grassby observes, however, "Sooner or later, a merchant had to feel a piece of cloth or put his hand in a barrel of fish" (120). For Browne, whose theological imagination struck contemporaries as sublime but whose natural historian's comfort with the lowliest creatures of the physical world was also famous, this need to touch as well as to think was a crucial ingredient of a Cheapside childhood. In the cases of medicine and business alike, social recognition required what William Birken has called a "struggle for respectability": thus young Thomas Browne, "who matriculated as a gentleman, was actually the son of a London mercer, but his father's death, and his mother's remarriage to a knight, made a gentleman out of the mercer's son at the time of his entrance."[39] When Browne's daughter Elizabeth Lyttleton remarked of her grandfather that he was "a tradesman, a mercer; but a gentleman of good family in Cheshire,"[40] the sequence of three characterizations ascended in status, with the third and final ascent taking an apologetic turn away from London trade to her grandfather's Cheshire, arms-bearing heritage.[41]

[38] For hawking and the Cheapside wives, see Dorothy Davis, *Fairs, Shops, and Supermarkets: A History of English Shopping* (Toronto: University of Toronto Press, 1966), 102, 109.

[39] William Birken, "The Social Problem of the English Physician in the Early Seventeenth Century," *Medical History* 31 (1987), 201–16; quotations on 204, 208; cf. Grassby, 124.

[40] Quoted in Wilkin, volume 1, xviii.

[41] For the significance of Cheshire in early modern England, see Robert W. Barrett, Jr., *Against All England: Regional Identity and Cheshire Writing, 1195–1656* (Notre Dame, IN: University of Notre Dame Press, 2009). See Charles Williams, "The Pedigree of Sir Thomas Browne," 109–13. For further information, see Trevor Hughes, "The Browne Family at Upton by Chester," *Cheshire History* 39 (1999–2000), 2–6. Their blazon consisted of "argent, two bends sable, in sinister chief and dexter base a pellet," the crest with a lion, sejant argent (Wilkin, I, pedigree 2; and Williams). As Hughes explains (2), Thomas Sr.'s maternal grandmother derived from "a celebrated Cheshire family, being the daughter of Henry Birkenhead of Huxley and Hackford, in that county, with Henry serving as Clerk of the Green Cloth in the mid sixteenth century." Browne never had the opportunity to meet his paternal grandparents, for they died before his birth: the grandfather in 1578, the grandmother in 1602. In the pedigree that he drew up for a visitation in 1664, he even mistook his grandfather's name as Richard Browne, the name of his great-grandfather. Browne's only record of a visit to Chester is a poem focused on the storm that he had just experienced in the Irish Sea, and says nothing about his responses to the city, two miles north of which lay Upton.

Despite the fact Browne's father straightforwardly apprenticed himself to Master Richard Barnes, paid three shillings and four pence for his freedom in 1594, then attained the livery in October 1604,[42] the Mercer bestowed on young Thomas a complex social identity with which he would be dealing for the entirety of his adult life, in his capacity as an educated, prosperous, and eventually knighted physician. In addition to the unclear or flexible social status of business and medicine, father and son also could appeal to a family tree that on the higher side ascended to Anne Keightley, the Countess of Devonshire, and via Thomas Sr.'s paternal grandmother to Norman knights, but on the lower extended to more modest roots among the fee-farmers in Cheshire.[43]

Although the Mercers were widely and deeply involved in the administration of grammar schools including their very own, Browne says nothing about any formal education that he may have received prior to Winchester and Oxford. Browne's education might have derived from any one or a combination of several sources. The initial education of London merchants' children was commonly undertaken at home. In the first decade of his life, Browne's own parents might instruct him in English orthography, reading, and writing, much as he himself guided his children in these matters. By his own account, they instructed him in the fundamentals of his faith to be found in available primers and catechisms as well as Psalters and the Bible itself; in the *Religio*, Browne credits them with instilling the "principles" of his faith into his "unwary understanding" (Patrides, 61). A family member (including his uncles) might also be called in to commence his work in Latin grammar. The most obvious choices for Browne's early education—whether as a "petty student" in English reading, writing, arithmetic, and religion, or as a Latin grammarian—would have been one or both of the two local schools overseen by the Mercers: one in Mercer's Hall itself, the other St Paul's.

The Mercers' School enrolled students—officially twenty-five at any one time—so that they might "receive a classical education, together with English, writing, arithmetic, merchants' accounts, and the useful appendages of geography and history."[44] The school was well established in St Thomas's Hospital prior to its occupation by the Mercers in the sixteenth century; Stow spoke of this "free Grammar schoole, as of old time had been accustomed" (1.269–70).[45] The Acts of Court for the Mercers' Company clarify that from 1606 onward, the expansion of the student body at the school was balanced by a renewed dedication to servicing children of the Company.[46] There is also the possibility that

[42] Recorded in List of Members of the Mercers' Company from 1347 (London, 1915, typescript, Mercers' Hall), 52.

[43] Williams, "The Pedigree of Sir Thomas Browne," 1. See also Tildesley. Cf. William Fergusson Irvine, ed., *A Collection of Lancashire and Cheshire Wills . . . 1301–1762*, The Record Society 30 (1896), for "The Will of Thomas Browne, of Hoole, dated 1572."

[44] William Herbert, *The History of the Twelve Great Livery Companies of London* (London, 1836–37), 275.

[45] See W. E. F. Ward, *A History of Mercers' School* (London: Old Mercers' Club, 1971).

[46] See Acts of Court 1595–1629, Mercers' Hall, 78r-v. For the first two decades of the seventeenth century, the schoolmaster at Mercers' Chapel was Richard Levesay, who appears to have suited the Company until, in 1612, he was "charged with 'sundry misdemeanours in oversuiting himself in

Browne attended St Paul's School.[47] Records from the Mercers' Company show that there may well have been connections between St Paul's School and Winchester College, if, that is, the Christopher Johnson working as an Under Usher until his retirement in 1614 was in fact the son of Christopher Johnson, Head Master of Winchester from 1560 to 1571.[48] There was also ongoing interchange between the two Mercer schools in Cheapside: William Muffit or Moffet is an example of a Mercer's son who studied at Mercers' Chapel School and St Paul's. In 1617–18, boys from Paul's staged a play at Mercers' Hall, a fact also suggestive of the interplay between the two locations.[49] But it is worth stressing that if Browne attended either or both of these schools, he made no mention of the fact at least in the extant record. It is almost as though formal education began for him when at ten years old he set out for Winchester in 1616, along with two other boys from his area: David Darnelly, eleven years old, of St Mary Woolchurch in London, and James Gosson, of St Leonard, Foster Lane.[50]

speeches to Sir Thomas Bennett, and in charging Thomas Dalby senior with slanderous and untrue speeches before Sir Thomas Bennett and the wardens'" (Ward, 14). According to Company records from the month, September, 1613, during which Browne's father stood for Third Warden for a second time in a row, Levesay was admonished to keep his class sizes down to sixty pupils, as well as to keep on an Usher only at his own discretion and cost. Despite this conflict with powerful officials in the company, Levesay continued to teach in the school, receiving a raise of ten pounds in 1616 "in commemoration of his old age and the charge he shall be constrained to be at in maintaining an usher" (Ward, 15). See Mercer Company Archive, Acts of Court, 1595–1619, September 3, 1613, 129v.

47 Since our knowledge of who attended St Paul's in the early seventeenth century depends on sources other than official school records, we have no certain means of knowing whether Browne studied there or not. If he did study there, it is likely that he had already received some petty and Latin grammar training; in order to be admitted, boys were expected to have some basic preparation in Latin and English which they received at petty school or from home tutors. For more, see Donald Lemen Clark, *John Milton at St Paul's School: A Study of Ancient Rhetoric in English Renaissance Education* (New York: Columbia University Press, 1948), 44.

48 Sir Michael McDonnell, *The Registers of St Paul's School, 1509–1748* (London: privately printed, 1977), xxiii for the meaning of "son of Mercer"; 96 for Christopher Johnson the younger, who was plagued by debt. It is worth noting that there were several Robinsons in the Mercers' Company with Browne's father, one of whom may have been a kinsman of Browne's headmaster Hugh Robinson at Winchester.

49 For Muffit, see McDonnell; for the play, see Clark, *John Milton at St Paul's School*, 50.

50 On September 30, 1620, Browne was required to swear his allegiance to the Winchester College statutes; listed as a member of the parish of St Foster's in London, he took this oath in the presence of John Harmar of London, a name with three strong connections to Winchester (Tildesley, editorial appendix). A man by that name had been headmaster then Warden of Winchester until his death in 1613. Obviously more important for our purposes is his nephew, a Winchester graduate considered "an excellent Grecian" and philologist if only a "tolerable Latin poet" by Wood. Having entered Magdalen College in 1611, "aged seventeen years or more," and entered holy orders in 1617, he went on to a noteworthy career in the field of education, not just as a schoolmaster but also as a pedagogue in print, starting with his *Praxis Grammatica* in 1622. He taught petty as well as grammar pupils, first at the school adjoining Magdalen then at St Alban's in Hertfordshire. Although he was an Oxford student until 1617, the year of his MA, Wood suggests that he was already teaching at the Magdalen School, and it is possible that Harmar earned extra money in those years as a private teacher, that he afforded the Cheapside boys of 1616 their connection to Winchester, and that this accounts for Browne's use of a John Harmar's notary services in 1620. According to Wood, Harmar was "happy in rendering Greek into Latin, or Latin into English, or English into Greek or Latin, whether in prose or verse; which we now call transversing and transposing" (Anthony Wood, *Athenae Oxonienses*, ed. Philip Bliss, 4 vols. (Hildesheim: Georg Olms, 1969), III.918). In addition to textbooks, epistles, poems, orations, and "De Lue Venerea, Libellus," he published over his long career a *Lexicon*

In addition to the obvious choices of Mercers' and Paul's, Browne might have received petty and grammar training from a licensed schoolmaster—including "parsons, curates and lay graduates"—who either worked at a more obscure school (for instance, the one at St Mary le Bow) or privately taught a handful of children at home or at the parish church.[51] But when Browne remembers the education that he received in London, its varieties are of the rather informal kind. The opportunities for informal education within the city were countless for a curious child who liked books and experience alike. From those Paul's booksellers who always afforded Browne with one of his key intellectual lifelines, a scholarly child of seven would have found available in 1612 two lovely books that Browne later singled out as amongst his favorites. In 1681, he wrote to Edward about "a prettie booke writt 1612 by Michael Drayton, a learned poet, in smooth verse called *Polyolbion*, & Mr. Selden writt a learned commentary upon it, though without his name" (Keynes, 4.194–5). This comment captures one of the earliest modes of access that Browne would have to the turning point at which the study of history found itself in his lifetime: between a fictional approach to the past that prized (and fashioned) monuments of moral, spiritual, and political value; and the antiquarian commitment to the accurate, evidence-bound reconstruction of the past as it was. Browne seems to have sensed that Drayton and Selden—both "learned"—wished a reconciliation between approaches that would prove elusive for them both. Then, in the last year of his life, Browne reminded his son of a particular edition of Plutarch's *Lives*: "Sr Thomas North translated his out of the French wch is that wch commonly passeth and dedicated it to Queen Elizabeth, which was that you & your brother Thomas used to read at my howse, and printed 1612, of a fayre & legible print" (4.211). As he worked with Edward on a new translation of Plutarch, Browne once again testified to a longing that the criteria of moral (if factually irresponsible) instruction and of rigorous accuracy might cohere. Also worth noting is the fact that in 1606, John Dee donated copies of his books, including the *Monas Hieroglyphica*, to the Mercers' Company, a testimony to the fact that by patrimony Dee was "a brother of this Companie." By way of his son Arthur, Dr Dee (as he was called) would continue to play a potent role in Browne's intellect and imagination as Browne helped his contemporaries to negotiate a natural philosophy at its own crossroads.[52]

Etymologicon Græco-Latinum, junctim cum Scapula, a 1652 version of which Browne owned. One of the several titles to which he laid claim over the course of his life was that of a BMed. There was yet a third John Harmar with Winchester connections, this one a companion of Browne's headmaster Hugh Robinson when the two matriculated a year apart at their grammar school in the 1590s. This Harmar, from Hackney and dubbed a gentleman of London in his matriculation at New College, Oxford, in 1603, was a Fellow of his College from 1605–10. It is possible that he is the notary of 1620 and, again, that he afforded the Cheapside boys with their entrée into Winchester.

[51] See Keene and Harding for St Mary le Bow; and John Lawson and Harold Silver, *A Social History of Education in England* (London: Methuen, 1973), 120, for a variety of private teachers. See also Arthur F. Leach, *Milton as Schoolboy and Schoolmaster* (1908, reprinted Folcroft, PA: Folcroft Library Editions, 1976), 1–8.

[52] Acts of Court 1595–1629, Mercers' Hall, 69r.

Browne's memories of London suggest experiential education as well. Writing to Edward in 1680, he recalled that he "knewe one Browne, an empericall practiser in London, who made a powder of Bezoar, musk & Amber & gave it to bee snuffed up into the nostrils in the toothach" (Keynes, 4.173). In his earliest recorded mention of Cheapside, in the *Religio*, Browne remembered his childhood access to herbs and "simples." In a passage intended to underscore his humility respective to his learning, Browne points out that "I know most of the Plants of my Country and of those about mee; yet me thinkes I do not know so many as when I did but know an hundred, and had scarcely ever Simpled further than Cheap-side" (Patrides, 147). In Browne's youth, literary herbalists such as Thomas Johnson tended to disparage the women who sold medicinal simples in Cheapside, complaining, for instance, that a certain plant has been "dayly by the ignorant women in Cheape-side sold to people more ignorant than themselves... Caveat Emptor. The danger that may ensue." Another scolded that "Cheapside is as full of these lying and forswearing Huswives as the Shambles and Gracechurch Street are of the shameless crew of Poulters wives."[53] But such learned snobbery was certainly not shared by the host of folks who found that they could afford herbs from these "unauthorised practitioners" far better than they could from the licensed shops. For his part, Stow noted simply that a woman had been selling "seedes, rootes and herbes" in a shop at the end of Soper Lane (1.268). A sixteenth-century parliamentary Act had made it legal for these female herbalists to ply their trade, and they were made the more affordable by the fact that "they often accepted payment in kind, such as food or service." According to one count, late Elizabethan London contained some two hundred and fifty of these women. In his recollection, Browne does not say whether he has in mind these women or, more respectably and expensively, the area "to the left of the Great Conduit" known as Bucklersbury "where the apothecaries and grocers sold herbs and spices, making a welcome change from the normal London stinks." With his uncle Edward gaining his freedom from the Grocers, Browne would have particular reason to know this gathering of about a hundred shops in which shoppers were greeted by delightful aromas and by curiosities such as stuffed alligators and strange animal skins. Like so many other companies, the Grocers had their own garden, theirs of course specializing in herbs.[54]

By noting that as a child he had "scarcely ever Simpled further than Cheapside," Browne implies what for Londoners was an obvious factor of everyday life: a day of simpling was always just an easy stroll away outside the walls of the city in virtually any direction but especially into the northern fields such as Moorfields, Finsbury, Bunhill, Spital, and Mallow. These expansive fields were particularly close to Browne's childhood home, just the other side of either Bishopsgate, Moorgate, or Aldersgate. In a more westerly direction, fields surrounded Gray's and Lincoln's Inns of Court as well as Covent Garden and Drury Lane. St Martin's was

[53] Johnson and Sir Hugh Plat quoted in Charles Raven, *English Naturalists from Neckam to Ray: A Study of the Making of the Modern World* (Cambridge: Cambridge University Press, 1947), 281.

[54] Liza Picard, *Elizabeth's London: Everyday Life in Elizabethan London* (New York: St Martin's Griffin, 2003), 107, 27, 74.

a field, not in one. Despite suburban growth to the east and south, countryside was readily accessible in those directions too, not least the delightful stroll along the south bank between Paris Garden and Lambeth. For the adult Browne, however, for whom youth and health were always shadowed by gruesome disease and decay, it was seminal that a stroll into the countryside might be interrupted by more macabre experiences, by the heads of traitors posted on Moorgate or the specter of madness at Bedlam hospital.

Although we do not know when Browne first encountered John Stow's description of London, the antiquarian's version of the scene of Browne's childhood continued to resonate with him in old age.[55] For Stow, degradation was everywhere apparent in his survey of London: in the loss of gardens, commons, and fields; in the preference of artillery over archery and fencing. Such antiquarianism may have lent itself to Browne's softened pastoral, sacralized, and provincial vision of city life. As for May Day, the setting for Browne's *Garden of Cyrus*, published in tandem with his antiquarian *Hydriotaphia*, Stow's Londoners "would walk into the sweete meddowes and green woods, there to rejoice their spirits, with the beauty and savour of sweet flowers, and with the harmony of birds, praysing God in their kind."[56] What matters for the childhood of Browne was that such a London was still available if also imperiled by intensive growth: for if Jacobean Londoners lived in the still readily accessible meadows and the still tightly knit communities of the city itself, they also fretted the death knell of this pastoral as their city became increasingly crowded and commercialized. In his old-age attempt to preserve Norwich Cathedral from historical erasure, Browne would remember Stow's ghastly image of supposed progress, the removal of bones from "the charnell howse of St. Paul, kept under a chappell in the north side of St. Pauls church yard" (Keynes, 3.140). Browne found this passage in Stow's survey of "Faringdon Ward within," even in Browne's last years the most moving account of the old neighborhood of his youth.

4. ORPHAN

In the *Religio*, the 30-year-old Browne's complex attitude toward the nuclear family of his childhood—at once reverential and dismissive—reminds us that what happened to Browne's household with the death of his father was the most perplexing event of his early youth. Between the Common Serjeant's book for the Court of Orphans and the repertories of the Court of Alderman, the major events in the adjudication of the father's estate are clear.[57] Having signed his will on September

[55] See for instance Keynes, 3.140, on "the charnell howse of St. Paul."

[56] Quoted in Holmes, *Elizabethan London* (London: Cassell, 1969), 48.

[57] Common Serjeant's book 1586–1614 (LMA CLA/002/01/1); Repertories 31, 36, 138, 40, Court of Aldermen (LMA). On fortunes of the estate of Thomas Senior, see further Hughes, "The Childhood of Sir Thomas Browne"; and N. J. Endicott, "Sir Thomas Browne as 'Orphan,' with Some Account of His Stepfather, Sir Thomas Dutton," *University of Toronto Quarterly* 30 (1960–61), 180–210.

29, 1613, Thomas Sr. must have died quickly for the will was probated on December 4. In a straightforward manner, his will followed London regulations in apportioning the estate into three equal parts: one for his wife; another for his four living children (Thomas, Anne, Jane, and Mary) as well as for "such child or children as Anne my now wife is great withal" (a girl, Ellen, was posthumous); and the final or "dead-man's" third for "such legacies and otherwise to dispose thereof as hereafter, in this my last will and testament, I have set down, nominated, and appointed the same." These latter bequeathals were relatively minor: twenty pounds to Bridget Smithwicke, daughter of Anne Smithwicke, "to be paid unto her at her full age of one and twenty years, or day of marriage"; twenty pounds to his brother William; and "the rest and residue" to his wife and children "equally amongst them to be divided."[58] Then the Mercer appointed his wife and his brother Edward to serve as his executors. Called a "brewer" in Thomas Sr.'s will, Uncle Edward was more importantly a Grocer (apprenticed 1587, freedom 1594, and livery 1604). Since he would bear primary responsibility for Browne's legacy and education in the years after Thomas Sr.'s death, it is significant that until 1618, the Grocers oversaw the apothecary trade, a state of affairs that would have given Browne an opportunity to "see what Apothecaries do," as he would later urge Henry Power (Keynes, 4.255).[59] Thrice married, he died on January 4, 1624, and was buried at St Werburgh's in Chester.

With the will having been probated to Anne alone on December 4, 1613, she was accompanied by her half-brother Francis Britridge when on December 9 she obliged herself in front of Cornelius Fish, the London Chamberlain, to produce the required inventory of the estate. The trouble for the orphans began when the widow was slow in producing the requisite inventory of the estate, which was supposed to include not just the assets but also debts owed by and to the estate (with an estimation of the likelihood, desperate or not, of collecting the debts owed) and including various recent expenses such as the funeral and the so-called widow's chamber owed to his wife.[60] When on March 10, 1614 the inventory was recorded in the Common Serjeant's Book, the estate was valued at £5 667½d; its debts at over £11 209.04.1; and the debts ("doubtful and desperate") owed to the estate at £11 514.11.9. Instructions were issued that there would be nothing for the widow or her orphans until payments had been rendered.[61]

[58] For the will see Charles Williams, "The Will of Thomas Browne, Mercer," *Proceedings of the Norfolk and Norwich Archeological Society* 16 (1906), 132–6.

[59] Browne's uncle Richard, who apparently matriculated at Brasenose College, Oxford, in 1579 and spent some time in the study of law at Clement's Inn in 1583, joined his brother Thomas in apprenticing with the Mercers. On Richard, see Joseph Foster, *Alumni Oxonienses* (Oxford: Parker and Co., 1891). Another brother, Henry, died at Oxford in 1680. In addition to other brothers (William, Ferdinando, Hugh, and Francis), about whom little to nothing is known, Browne's father had two sisters, Jane, who married Richard Hartley of Chester and died in 1627, and Anne, married first to John Smethwick, then to John Dutton.

[60] This included the widow's clothing, the bed and hangings of the couple's bedroom, the linen chest, and the widow's jewelry; cf. Charles Carlton, *The Court of Orphans* (Leicester: Leicester University Press, 1974), 45.

[61] LMA CLA/002/01/1, 417v. The inventory itself is no longer extant.

Soon thereafter, the problems and suspicions concerning the handling of the estate by Browne's mother and her new husband Sir Thomas Dutton became so evident that the London Court of Alderman took over the case. When, prior to July 1614, Anne Browne married Sir Thomas Dutton, the situation began to grow contentious between Edward Browne and the now Lady Anne Dutton, so much so that on July 14, with Mayor Thomas Middleton presiding, the Court of Aldermen took the advice of a subcommittee on the Browne case, with assistance from the servants and friends of the testator, and required a reexamination of the estate so that the orphans might not suffer from its mishandling.[62] In addition to the remarried widow and her husband, the people of "neerest blood and aliance" to the orphans were Uncle Edward, Francis Britridge, and Browne's grandfather Paul Garraway. The upshot of this investigation was that the initial assessment of an estate emptied by debt was not to be trusted; that the "Controversie" arisen between Dutton and Edward Browne needed to be resolved, by intervention of the mayor if necessary; and that, even if the figures pertaining to the estate had not been grossly distorted, the widow's care of the estate was still impeachable. Thus on July 14, with Lord Mayor Thomas Middleton presiding, Anne Dutton was said to have misappropriated—indeed, "wasted & consumed"—some £1 500 of "the debtes owing." According to the Aldermen, "it is likely and very much to be feared that unlesse somme speedy Course be taken for setling therof that very great losse will fall to the five orphans." And they deemed Sir Thomas Dutton a flight risk; even if he is "a very worthy gent," he was also a soldier who "may live beyond the seas, or in the Countrey, and so out of the iurisdiccion and power of this Court."[63] Anne and Thomas Dutton were not to meddle with the estate under any circumstance, not least since they had been paid off and protected from the deceased husband's creditors.[64] With Edward Browne taking over sole supervision of the estate by September, the controversy over the legacy was essentially over, and further records involving the five orphans express their satisfaction as each child reached majority. Browne acknowledged himself satisfied on November 19, 1629—this on the brink of his journeys abroad for a medical education in Montpellier, Padua, and Leiden.[65]

In the *Christian Morals* Browne would insist that childhood forms a separate stage in one's life and that the child is not necessarily the father of the man. In particular, bad beginnings can end happily in adulthood (Patrides, 440–1). "Confound not the distinctions of thy Life which Nature hath divided," he adds later,

[62] LMA Repertory 31, July 14, 1614, 372b–375.

[63] LMA Repertory 31, 373r.

[64] Even with a sum settled on the "medling" couple, they were back in court on August 4 in pursuit of more, claiming "that wares had been sold for £38 10s less than the sum at which they were valued, and giving further details of Anne's living expenses, including her lying in expenses, as Ellen had now been born" (Hughes, "The Childhood of Sir Thomas Browne," 24). Sir Thomas and Lady Anne Dutton would go on to have children of their own. As Endicott reports, they celebrated the christening of two daughters in the Isleworth parish church and mourned the death of one, this in 1622–23. Their two boys Thomas and William were still living as of 1634 (195). But in the early years of their marriage, there is no clear record of where the newlyweds were living.

[65] LMA Repertory 44, 20b–21.

"that is, Youth, Adolescence, Manhood, and old Age...Do as a Child but when thou art a Child, and ride not on a Reed at twenty" (453). There comes a time to put away childish things; Browne reflects on this assessment in the *Religio* as well, when he emphasizes one's capacity for maturation not just in spirituality but also in literary study, noting the importance of rereading Lucan so that one will be "able not onely, as we doe at Schoole, to construe, but understand" (114). From this vantage childhood involves a strictly limited if distinctive stage of preparation that we are expected to transcend as we embrace mature wisdom and divine purpose.

But the *Religio* is also pleased with, and haunted by, continuities between childhood and adulthood. The pleasure consists of Browne's tendency to think of advanced spiritual meditation as itself a godly form of innocent recreation. The dark side of continuity between childhood and maturity derives from Browne's commonplace notion that as we age, the sins of our fallen natures only get worse unless we simply lose the capacity to experience them. And Browne's own medical interests in childhood diseases, especially in morgellons and smallpox, make it clear how well he understood that childhood was no cakewalk. Included in the adult Browne's library was a 1613 copy of Petrarch's *De remediis utriusque Fortunae* which, while it may have been purchased long after the death of his father in that very year, nonetheless strikingly coincides with the date of Browne's new identity as an orphan facing an uncertain future and needing to cultivate self-control as he confronted the vicissitudes of fortune. Between such Stoic discipline and a fertile, imaginative interaction with highly diverse contexts, Browne's extraordinary contribution to early modern culture took shape. As Steve Rappaport has noted, however, his London had a way of assuring its citizens that they were already living in "worlds within worlds."[66]

[66] See Rappaport, *Worlds Within Worlds: Structures of Life in Sixteenth-Century London* (Cambridge: Cambridge University Press, 1989).

2

Winchester and Ireland, 1616–1623

Having convinced the examiners that he was sufficiently literate in English as well as corrigible in Latin, ten-year-old Thomas Browne was admitted for grammar study at Winchester College from the parish of St Michael le Querne on August 20, 1616, after which he in all likelihood began his studies with the post-Michaelmas term in late October.[1] On September 30, 1620, according to rubric 5 of the College statutes, he swore before John Harmar of London that he would obey all the statutes, with the register noting that Browne was from St Foster's parish in London. On August 10, 1622, positioned eleventh on the roll, he stood unsuccessfully for election to New College, Oxford, once more as a parishioner from St Michael. A year later, in keeping with Winchester rules, he left his "Grammar Learning"[2] at the age of eighteen, matriculating at Broadgates Hall, Oxford on December 5, 1623. In the extant records of his later life, Browne recalled his years at Winchester on just a handful of occasions. But the education that he received there played a lasting role in the development of his habits of reading, writing, and thinking—this, whether or not he considered a Winchester schoolboy's slang one of the "patois" (Patrides, 147) that he had mastered.[3]

Although Browne had come to Winchester in August 1616 as a commoner, he very quickly received a scholarship and lived at the college as a scholar until he left "of his own free will" for Oxford in 1623. In all likelihood, Browne had the recommendation of a powerful London merchant or of a Winchester alumnus such as John Harmar. Election for new students at Winchester and New College, Oxford, took place simultaneously and involved a "series of ceremonies and festivities."[4] According to the statutes, the New College members of the election committee were to visit Winchester between July 7 and October 1. In 1617, for instance, they arrived in mid-August. On arrival the visitors were met by an oration at the middle gate from a senior, a custom dating from 1615 when a benefactor provided funding for a Gunpowder Plot sermon as well as three orations. Election to Winchester owed more to nomination (and to having the £20 entrance fee) than to talent

[1] The year 1623 is missing in the election records in the Winchester College Muniments (WCM) but see WCM 21609 for Browne's unsuccessful bid for New College election in 1622. His admission is recorded in the Register of Scholars, WCM 21490A; his oath can be found in WCM 21851. All are transcribed in Tildesley, *Sir Thomas Browne*, 76.

[2] The phrase comes from Browne's anonymous biographer in *Posthumous Works*, ii.

[3] See Charles Stevens, *Winchester Notions: The English Dialect of Winchester College* (New Brunswick, NJ: The Athlone Press, 1998).

[4] A. K. Cook, *About Winchester College, To Which is Prefixed "De Collegio Wintoniensi" by Robert Mathew* (London: Macmillan, 1917), 390.

per se, though election to New College—as Browne would discover—depended at least in some measure on how many openings the Oxford college had.[5] In being elected for admission to Winchester, scholars without a connection to the founder faced an uncompetitive exam and were expected to be scholars in need of support for their education, "of good character and well conditioned, of gentlemanly habits, able for school, ... completely learned in reading, plain song and old Donatus."[6] In addition, "they were to be between eight and twelve years old, but might be admitted up to sixteen years old if they were sufficiently advanced to be able to be perfect in grammar by eighteen," at which age all but the founder's kin were obliged to leave.[7]

As early as *Religio Medici*, Browne was critical of the impoverished mentality that the wrong kind of grammar education was prone to produce. But the tendencies of his composition in prose and verse, together with highly specific memories of people and phenomena that he experienced while a Winchester student, corroborates the judgment offered by Samuel Sprott and Jonathan Post—that Browne's education between 1616 and 1623 proved an essential constituent of who he became.[8] And the considerable body of writing published by his master Hugh Robinson shows that at Winchester, Browne was introduced to a learned, dramatic, and inquisitive study of scripture within the context of world history that laid the foundation for the combination of deep piety, scholarship, and criticism on display throughout his published and unpublished works.

A few memories in his letters indicate that schoolboy outings at Winchester stimulated Browne's attention to natural phenomena. In a 1663 letter to John Evelyn, he still recalled "the very great yewe tree in Sutton church yard by Winchester" (Keynes, 4.281).[9] In early 1665, he explained to his son Thomas that the comet which he had seen in 1618 "began in Libra & moved northward, ending about the tayle of ursa major" (Keynes, 4.19). In 1680 he wrote his son Edward that "I never sawe a large & very long tayle of a comet since 1618, when I was at schoole" (Keynes, 4.175). A month later he elaborated on parallax as the means by which "Astronomers find out the comets distance from the earth, and in that of 1618 they found it to bee as farre above the moone as the moone is above the earth, & so find out its place or sphere it is in" (4.178). In yet another letter to Edward, Browne recalled what for him was an especially striking animal specimen, the

[5] See chapter 3.

[6] *The Victoria History of the Counties of England: Hampshire and the Isle of Wight* (Westminster: A. Constable, 1900–12), 1.269.

[7] Thomas Frederick Kirby, *Winchester Scholars* (London: Henry Frowde, 1888), 270.

[8] Samuel Ernest Sprott, *Tom Browne's Schooldays: A Study of the Education of Sir Thomas Browne at Winchester College* (Columbia, doctoral dissertation, 1954); Jonathan Post, "Browne's Life: A 'Cabinet of Rarities,'" *English Language Notes* 19 (1982), 313–35.

[9] As one observer has noted, "in the diocese of Winchester [yews] were so common that they were sometimes called the 'Hampshire weed'" (Cyril Ebor, archbishop of York, introduction to Vaughan Cornish, *The Churchyard Yew and Immortality* (London: Frederick Muller, 1946), 11). In his catalogue of yews, Cornish lists one at All Saints in Long Sutton, to be distinguished from Bishops Sutton. Long Sutton is farther to the northeast toward London from Winchester (about fifteen miles) than Bishops Sutton (about half that to the northeast of Winchester). For the Long Sutton yew, cf. John Lowe, *The Yew-Trees of Great Britain and Ireland* (London: Macmillan, 1897), 83; 191–2.

ostrich: "I sawe one in the latter end of K. James his dayes at Greenwich when I was a schooleboy" (4.156).

But Browne's memories of Winchester can also evoke more problematic and all-too-human associations. Writing to Edward, he noted the troubling political legacy of a fellow Wyckamite: "I knewe one Mr. Christopher Love, sonne unto Dr Love, warden of Winchester Colledge, who was an active man agaynst the King in the late warres and gott a great estate, butt I thinck hee was fayne to fly upon the Kings restauration" (Keynes, 4.156).[10] If the civil war had sprouted a Wyckamite supporter of regicide, it was more pertinent for Browne's development that in the first quarter of the century, Winchester had been more notorious for the conspiratorial, equivocating Jesuit Henry Garnet. As he looked to his future in 1623, Browne had reason to worry about what his Winchester background might mean for his vocational identity, especially since the most obvious course for him to take from his grammar education was a career in divinity.

Browne's clearest and most pervasive debts to Winchester College, however, were his classicism and the beginnings of his historicism, a training that informed his critical method, style, reading habits, and cross-disciplinary frames of reference. Above all, given Robinson's extensive historical writings, as well as the obvious decay of Winchester in its population, commerce, authority, and physical edifices, it is likely that between 1616 and 1623, Browne was inspired for the first time to consider two potentially competing approaches to the past, one skeptical and critical, the other commemorative and reverential. What is more, the storied past of the town itself, but also its current state of disrepair, ensured that Browne's Winchester days were as formative of his historical imagination as the college's curriculum was of his Latin. Winchester grammar was an educational tradition that Browne wished to thrive after his death: late in his life, not only did Browne contribute to the fund-raising drive for a new school at the college, but he exhorted his son Edward to "forgett not phrases scholæ wintoniensis," a reference to one of the handbooks published by Browne's own headmaster Hugh Robinson (Keynes, 4.197).

1. APPROACHES TO ANTIQUITY

According to its boosters, Winchester gave visitors a taste of the salubrious climate that Browne would come to enjoy some fifteen years later in Montpellier. In the 1630s, two-time mayor John Trussell celebrated the natural healthiness of his town and its environs. No doubt with the proximity of Winchester to a healthy sea air in mind, Trussell heralded a virtually golden-age, quasi-Mediterranean natural health and purity for a city in which "neither physitian, apothecarye or surgeon did ever growe rytch by their practise in this place."[11] Yet Trussell's panegyric scarcely informed a traveler to Winchester in the first decades of the seventeenth century

[10] During Browne's tenure in Winchester, the warden was Nicholas Love.

[11] Quoted in Tom Atkinson, *Elizabethan Winchester* (London: Faber and Faber, 1963), 218.

about a pronounced discontinuity with the city's famous past. Unlike Browne's London, which was growing and flourishing at an astonishing—some worried a detrimental—rate, his Winchester was suffering from decline in population, prosperity, and significance. Its renowned college was suffering too—its overseers and inspectors were on guard against the erosion of ancient customs and of the faculty's concern for and duty to the welfare of the student body.

By the early seventeenth century, Winchester could still pack a punch to a visitor whose historical imagination was alert to the vestiges and emblems of the recent and distant past. The past was monumentalized everywhere in Winchester. Most importantly for Browne, the college retained pervasive architectural and sculptural vestiges of its Catholic origins. Within the city walls, Winchester Cathedral boasted its fair share of monuments, including one for the college founder William of Wykeham.[12] Visitors to the cathedral learned that in one chest could be found the bones of Saxon kings, but also the Viking remains of the good Danish Canute.

Winchester's significance as an ancient center for the legendary sanctity of royal power was visibly preserved throughout its walled site on the Itchen River.[13] In addition to its career as the Roman Venta Belgarum, it was the chief city of the learned Saxon King Alfred, the place from which "he planned a kingdom that could defend itself" but also one with a rich and pious culture.[14] Here too was one of the capitals of early Norman England, though by the reign of Stephen (1135–54) its status as such was already slipping. Even in the sixteenth century, when Winchester's days as a royal capital were over, Tudor monarchs could call upon its legendary past for political effect: a painted ceiling from Winchester College, rediscovered in 1885, serves as testimony to this fact insofar as its probable purpose was "to celebrate the wedding of Mary Tudor and Philip of Spain in Winchester in 1554."[15] Visitors experienced the evidence and the legends of this exceptional history in such a variety of ways: for instance, the weather vane of the cathedral featuring St George and the dragon served as "a reminder that the bishops of Winchester were the prelates of the Order of the Garter."[16] Although the seat of the Order of the Garter was Windsor—further evidence that Winchester was no longer of any great value to the monarchy—the little George in heroic combat over the cathedral proffered in miniature a reminder of the sacred historical legacies of the town. But visitors also experienced the sacred monarchical traditions of Winchester in singular, impressive monuments such as could be found in the royal tombs of the cathedral but also over at the castle to the west, where a table on display was reputed to have been the round table of King Arthur.

[12] Rev. John Milner, *The History Civil and Ecclesiastical & Survey of the Antiquities of Winchester*, 2 vols., 2nd ed., corrected and enlarged (Winchester, 1809), 2.26.

[13] Milner, *Antiquities of Winchester*, 2.34, 37, 48, 182–3.

[14] Barry Shurlock, *The Winchester Story* (Horndean, Hampshire: Milestone, 1986), 12.

[15] See Elizabeth Lewis, "A Sixteenth-Century Painted Ceiling from Winchester College," *Proceedings of the Hampshire Field Club Archaeological Society* 51 (1995), 137–65.

[16] Graham Parry, *The Arts of the Anglican Counter-Reformation: Glory, Laud and Honour* (Woodbridge, Suffolk: Boydell Press, 2006), 54. See also, Martin Biddle, "The Bishop of Winchester and the Foundation of the Order of the Garter," in Martin Biddle et al., eds., *King Arthur's Round Table: An Archaeological Investigation* (Woodbridge, Suffolk: Boydell Press, 2000), 513–18.

The town's medieval heritage interlacing with its college curriculum, Winchester offered early seventeenth-century pupils a complex exercise in historical interpretation and valuation. Given the older Browne's profound engagement with rival methods of responding to the past, an extended habitation in one of the chief—and most imperiled—sites of English history was especially formative as the young scholar accrued the discursive means by which to analyze ancient evidence. The wooden antiquities of Arthur's table and of the yew tree (recalled in the letter to Evelyn) embodied two potential reconciliations to be gained from the Winchester experience and education to which young Browne came. Most simply, human and natural history offers an unbreakable bond between melancholy and hope: ritual ceremonies and natural hieroglyphs prove invaluable in our mediation between the tragic and comic. More complexly, our dealings with the created world—its human artifacts and natural phenomena—should never be reduced to one restrictive method or monolithic set of assumptions. Long before he wrote Evelyn of the yew in Sutton churchyard, Browne's adult attempt to synthesize competing approaches to natural and historical evidence had begun under the tutelage of Hugh Robinson at Winchester College, and among the sights and shadows of a once-glorious royal capital.

The palpable decline of Winchester was perfectly suited for the inauguration of Browne's engagement with monuments of the past and with their moral and spiritual significance. Yet even if the vestiges of the town's monumental past were in far greater peril and decay than the mostly flourishing classicism of the college, one event in the years 1616–1623 injected ecclesiastical life into the bishopric: in 1618, Lancelot Andrewes was translated to the see of Winchester. And while, as bishop, Andrewes spent little time in the town itself, oversight of student welfare in a time of heightened concern at the college devolved on him, and his rejuvenation of a liturgically rich style of worship served as a crucial model for all those younger members of the Church of England, including Browne, who sought to justify and to reinvent the beauty of holiness in the 1620s and 30s. For a bishop keen to maximize diocesan conformity, Andrewes faced the geographical challenge that Winchester "was very exposed to foreign influences," including "Protestant refugees from the Continent"—the Channel Islands were included in the diocese—as well as Roman Catholics.[17] But Andrewes's visitation articles for 1619 evince far more than simply his eagerness to minimize Puritanism and popery in the 362 parishes of the see, for every effort is made to ensure and to heighten the reverential decency of the church and the worship that takes place therein.[18] As for the parishioners, Andrewes's 1619 Articles also seek to guarantee their obedience to the king's sovereignty; their submission to the prelacy of the Church of England; their careful observance of the sabbath; and their decency of worship in matters such as the removal of all head covering during the service (*Works of Andrewes*, 11.116–19).

In Browne's years in Winchester, then, there was lively evidence that ceremonial worship was undergoing a revival, as well as impressive reminders such as the famed

[17] Paul A. Welsby, *Lancelot Andrewes, 1555–1626* (London: SPCK, 1958), 113.

[18] Lancelot Andrewes, *Works of Lancelot Andrewes*, 11 vols. (Oxford: John Henry Parker, 1854; reprinted in New York: AMS, 1967), 11.113.

Round Table that Winchester was the treasury of sacred institutional bond between royal authority and Christian piety. But in Winchester, there was also—more pervasively and obviously—an ambience of decay.[19] In August 1623, at the end of Browne's period of residence in Winchester, John Taylor the Water Poet toured the city and declared it dead: "An ancient city, like a body without a soule."[20] Looking back at this sorrowful period, Alderman Trussell himself lamented in the 1640s that his "truly ancient" and once glorious city "now hangs down its head and at this day presents herself *tanquam Carthaginis cadaver*, a body without a soul" (quoted in Rosen, 146). For Trussell, Winchester offered a study in the life span of all great cities, for "all and every city are subject to one and the same fate, that is to be visible in infancy, flourish in maturity, and decline and droop in decrepit age." Similarly, in *Religio*, Browne would apply such cycles to countries for which, according to providence, "there is a revolution and vicissitude of their greatnesse" (Patrides, 82). As Keene says, "the decay visible in the streets would have stood in obvious and bitter contrast to the wealth of the earlier medieval city, of which there were still impressive monuments," not least of course the cathedral and the college (*Winchester Studies 2*, 94). Inside and outside the city walls, Winchester's cadaverous nature was made all the more pronounced by the wreckage of sacred buildings wrought by the Reformation.[21]

Winchester's decay had a direct pertinence to the young Thomas Browne: the college itself was also beginning to experience decline in the form of faculty neglect, for the students were facing not just unwillingness on the part of their teachers to preserve some of the old customs but even a diminution of their daily food rations, a development apt to dismay all the pupils, not least a young orphan from London.[22] From the years of Browne's education at Winchester, the extant records of inspections tell the story of a struggling institution placed under injunctions aimed at the reform of some serious lapses.[23] Headed by Robert Pinke of New College, Oxford, the inspection teams discovered abuses ranging from the impoverished spiritual life of the community to the underfeeding of the boys. According to the 1617 report, the inspectors decried what Leach has called an "absolute disintegration of collegiate life" amongst the fellows: "The Fellows were to attend chapel, an observance, the visitors said, almost entirely neglected; also to dine in hall, where the High Table was only to consist of the Warden and four or five seniors, the rest, as in Rubric 14, to dine at a side-table." But some of the trouble was attributed to a recent expansion of the presence of commoners who were good for college finances but corrosive of college identity. More critically, however, the injunctions protested that the scholars' food was "not to be diminished, nor their joints... carried away by

[19] Adrienne Rosen, "Winchester in Transition, 1580–1700," in Peter Clark, ed., *Country Towns in Pre-Industrial England* (New York: St Martin's Press, 1981), pp. 143–95.

[20] Quoted in Derek Keene, *Winchester Studies 2: Survey of Medieval Winchester*, vol. 2, i, Part I (Oxford: Clarendon Press, 1985), 105.

[21] Milner, *Antiquities of Winchester*, 2.237.

[22] See WCM 266 and WCM 268 in the Winchester College archives (reports of annual scrutinies from 1617 and 1620–1).

[23] WCM 266 (1617); 267 (1619); 268 (1620–21); and 269 (1623).

any one before they are served."[24] Clearly many of the problems were resulting from the recent tendency of fellows to marry; the inspectors insisted that "the Fellows were to sleep in College," even if they were married: Bishop Andrewes was especially angry over the neglect of this office.[25]

According to the inspection of 1620, however, the scholars still needed protection. Thus, "in 1620 it was ordered that meat was to be given the boys 'of due weight, that they may not be driven to get their food elsewhere' "—that is, with their own funds (Leach, 330; Cook, 127). Again, in 1621, whilst the college clergy were required to attend to their offices with greater frequency and solicitude, and the college staff to dine in hall, the boys were still found to be physically undernourished.[26] The deprivation of the scholars proved a persistent concern (Leach, 330), so that the years of Browne's residence in Winchester bore witness to the erosion of community in the most visible and visceral fashion, from the offices of prayer to the solidarity and sustenance of meals, a change potentially disastrous for an institution in which "the corporate life was everything, the private nothing."[27]

2. COLLEGE AND CURRICULUM

Located just south of the city walls, Winchester College was experiencing a decay of its own in Browne's time there, but it persisted as one of the town's impressive medieval legacies. (See Figure 2.1.) Properly speaking, the College of St Mary nigh Winton belonged not to the City of Winchester but to the Soke, that is, to the jurisdiction of the bishop; its original focus was on the production of secular clergy in the wake of the Black Death.[28] With the coming of the Reformation, this collegiate identity was officially deceased but unofficially a pervasive element in the school's personality. By the time that Browne reached Winchester, the college was still thriving as a grammar school where one might receive a first-class education; but it was also suffering in two respects. From within, its staff was neglecting the customs of communal living that formed the very core of the college identity and experience. From without, Winchester College was suffering from its reputation as the seminary of obscure clerics in insignificant positions. It is true that Winchester produced its fair share of bishops (Thomas Bilson, for instance) and that future statesman Henry Wotton was sent to Winchester as a commoner (a paying student) for the "strict discipline and order"—"the method of living by rule"—that it might afford him. Yet the choice of Winchester College over, say, Eton, Westminster, Merchant Taylors', or Paul's often reflected a penchant for serious scholarship

24 Arthur F. Leach, *A History of Winchester College* (London: Duckworth & Co., 1899), 329–30.

25 See A. K. Cook, *About Winchester College*, 75.

26 WCM 268 (1621), points 4, 6, and 7.

27 J. D.'E. Firth, *Winchester College* (London: Winchester Publications, 1949), 20.

28 See Atkinson, 19–20; and Arthur F. Leach, *A History of Winchester College*, 103. See also *Victoria History*, 1.264, 266. Cf. Winfred A. Harwood, "The Household of Winchester College in the Later Middle Ages, 1400–1560," *Proceedings of the Hampshire Field Club Archaeological Society* 59 (2004), 163–79.

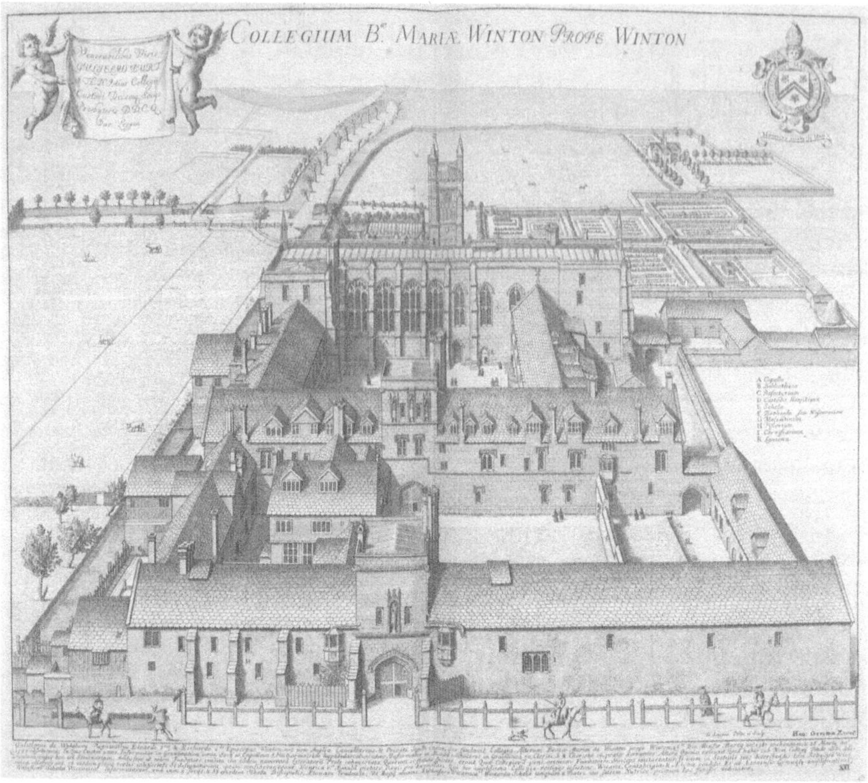

Figure 2.1 Winchester College, from David Loggan, *Oxonia Illustrata* (1675). Reproduced with the permission of the Anne and Jerome Fisher Fine Arts Library, University of Pennsylvania Libraries.

leading to a frequently minor clerical office.[29] Ironically, the tendency of the most eminent graduates of Winchester to botch their election to New College—Wotton as well as Browne suffered this fate—might be seen as "escaping the prevalent paralysis."[30] A further liability for the advancement of Winchester graduates was that, even if it produced Puritans and regicides by the middle of the century, the college shared with New College, Oxford, a tendency to be "surprisingly resistant to the Protestant Reformation."[31] The juvenile asceticism in the *Religio*'s declamation

[29] Izaac Walton on Wotton, quoted in Leach, *History of Winchester College*, 323. See G. E. Aylmer's "Seventeenth-Century Wykehamists," in Roger Custance, ed., *Winchester College: Sixth-Centenary Essays* (Oxford: Oxford University Press, 1982); quotation at 286. Also cf. Thomas Frederick Kirby, *Winchester Scholars*, 165–72.

[30] W[inchester] C[ollege] A[rchaeological] S[ociety], *Winchester, Its History, Buildings and People* (1913), 181–2.

[31] Patrick McGrath, "Winchester College and the Old Religion in the Sixteenth Century," in Custance, ed., *Winchester College: Sixth-Centenary Essays*, 229–80; see 229–30 and 278.

against human sexuality—but also Browne's sympathy for Catholic rites—surely owed something to the fact that the founder had devised rubrics ensuring that "a strong monastic strain runs through the code."[32]

From what Browne says about his youthful studies in *Religio*, we can infer that his self-identity as a severely chaste, theologically brilliant new Origen was already developing at Winchester. Bible readings were key features of chambers and hall alike, while the posted rules of behavior demanded that the boys show (as well as feel) reverence during services. But Browne's Winchester faced the challenge not just of nourishing earnest and learned piety; in the second decade of the seventeenth century, the college was also supposed to produce conforming and obedient subjects. As a counterbalance to whatever infamy Henry Garnet had brought to the school, the college received funding in 1614 for an annual Gunpowder Plot sermon, and Andrewes himself was famous, among other things, for the skill and equanimity with which he preached on this annual occasion. Of more daily significance to the scholars was the fact that Alexander Nowell's catechism was an essential ingredient of their education. Between Nowell's words and Andrewes's sometimes passionate oversight of the corporate solidarity of the college, Browne's Winchester aimed at instilling in its charges an understanding of and devotion to a Church of England rid of Jesuitical equivocation and Puritanical insubordination alike.[33]

Winchester schoolboys of Browne's generation were also required to master a theologically grounded political catechism complementary to their Nowell in a dialogue known as *Deus et Rex*.[34] In 1615, King James issued a proclamation "tending to the Vniuersall publishing and teaching, of a certaine Religious Treatise, compiled by Authority, and Intituled by the Name of GOD, And the KING," the treatise itself being published in both 1615 and 1616. In 1620, Winchester pupil John Hutton recorded his purchase of the book, together with his other school texts.[35] The thrust of the catechism was instruction in the legitimacy of and basis for the Oath of Allegiance; its relevance to Winchester among other grammar schools was underscored by the king's concern that the dialogue between Theodidactus (godly teacher) and his pupil, Philalethes (truth-lover) prepare the young to resist the "divers secret practises, and deuices" of Jesuits and other Catholics, including the tendency to take the oath "onely in dissimulation," the trickery made infamous by Winchester graduate Henry Garnet. Thus Browne's insistence on his obedience as a "sworne subject" in *Religio* (Patrides, 64) was instituted in—and partly motivated by—his training at Winchester.

An understanding of Browne's Winchester experiences is greatly assisted by two documents. For the nitty-gritty concerns of Browne's daily life at Winchester, there

[32] W. C. A. S., *Winchester, Its History, Buildings and People*, 153, 157, 163.

[33] It is impossible to say how much Browne would have known about Nowell's rocky career in the church. At Winchester, it was the catechism that mattered most.

[34] For the author of this dialogue, see M. A. Screech, ed. and intro., *Richard Mocket, Doctrina et Politia Ecclesiae Anglicanae: An Anglican Summa Facsimile, with Variants, of the Texts of 1617* (Leiden: Brill, 1995); and the *ODNB* article by Bertha Porter, revised by Glenn Burgess.

[35] James I, *A Proclamation for the confirmation of all Authorized Orders*... (1615); for Hutton's purchase see below in this volume, p. 44.

is the account of expenses kept from 1623 by John Hutton for each of the four annual terms—Michaelmas, then Christmas, Lady Day in March, and Midsummer.[36] In addition to living expenses (clothing, bedding, a shilling to have his urine examined), Hutton records his payment for books, including *Deus et Rex*, Ovid's *Metamorphoses*, a "sett of Ovids," Cicero's *De officiis* and *Tusculan Disputations*, a Greek grammar by Camden, a Lucan, Terence, a psalter, grammar, a Greek New Testament, and Nowell's catechism, plus ink and paper.

A second, crucial, document for information about Browne's Winchester takes the form of a poem written around 1647 by a student, Robert Mathew, whose aim was lovingly to capture the normal routine and curriculum of the school.[37] For the daily pattern of college life, Mathew notes the number of chambers (six for the scholars, one for the choristers), the wake-up call at 5:00 a.m., the hurried dressing, followed by the singing of a Latin psalm in chambers,[38] after which the scholars clean their chambers and their persons—all before a second bell at 5:30, when they retreat to chapel for prayer to each person of the Trinity for direction, illumination, and inspiration. At 6:00 the scholars are summoned to school until 9:00 and their breakfast in hall. Unless it was a Tuesday or Thursday—a "remedies" day—the rest of the schedule for a school day unfolded as follows: 9:30–11:00 books in chambers; 11–12:00 school; 12:00 dinner with readings by Bible clerk; 1–3:30 p.m. school; 3:30 bevers; 4:00–5:00 school; 5:00 prayers; 6:00 tea in the hall; 6:30–7:45 study in chambers; 7:45 supper; 8:00 chapel; 8:15 bedtime.[39]

At the south end of the poorly lit school were the elevated seats for the prefects while "On the northern wall is a map of the world," a feature for which ten shillings had been paid in 1614–15; this map was especially useful for the study of Robinson's synopsis of ancient history, published together with his rhetoric as the Winchester textbook (Cook, 7). On the eastern wall scholars read the so-called "table of Quintilian's Laws," which in fact had nothing to do with Quintilian but rather consisted of the college rules of behavior, for instance, the requirement that the scholars converse in Latin and that they demonstrate due respect to college authorities by removing their hats and bending their knees (Cook, 238–41). The Latin mottos on the western side of school reduced the scholar's choices in life to three: learn, leave, or be whipped. Those who learn are promised a bishopric in the form of a mitre and staff; those who leave are offered the far lesser career in law or the military.

[36] See *The Correspondence of Dr. Matthew Hutton, Archbishop of York*, ed. Sir Timothy Hutton and Matthew Hutton (Publications of the Surtees Society, 1843), 237–44. These accounts are excerpted in *William of Wykeham and His Colleges*, by Mackenzie E. C. Walcott (London: David Nutt, 1852), 166–9.

[37] Leach and Kirby wrongly attributed the poem to Christopher Johnson, a mid-sixteenth-century student and headmaster. The breakthrough for dating the poem to "not earlier and not much (if at all) later than the summer or early autumn of 1647" came with the discovery of another manuscript at Magdalen College, Oxford, which includes the name Robert Mathew at the end. A reference to the conduit also helps date the poem. See Cook, *About Winchester College*, 7.

[38] Cook (160) makes the case for this site for the Psalms, adding that they were compiled by Hugh Robinson.

[39] Based on *Victoria History*, 333–5, which derives its account from Mathew's poem.

At last Mathew turns to the curriculum for the various forms, which with slight modification (Cook, 283) is also Browne's. In tabular form, the main readings for the boys are as follows[40]:

Form	Monday	Wednesday	Friday	Saturday
Sixth	Martial's epigrams; Robinson's rhetoric	Martial; *Aeneid;* or Cicero	Homer; Terence	Nowell's Greek catechism; Musaeus; Hesiod; Virgil
Fifth	Martial; Cicero's *Tusculan Disputations*	Same as sixth	Theoginis; Horace's odes, satires or epistles	Same as sixth
Fourth	Cicero's *De officiis*; Ovid's *Fasti*	Same as Monday	Ovid's *Metamorphoses*	Nowell's Latin catechism; Ovid's *Tristia*
Second fourth	Ovid's *Tristia*; or Erasmus's *Colloquies*	Same as Monday	Same as fourth form	Ovid's *Fasti*

Martial's epigrams were especially prized at Winchester; as Robert Krueger has noted, "the most important epigrammatists of the 1590s were scholars together at Winchester," while Browne's own adult recourse to Martial and the epigram suggests that this legacy continued into his generation.[41] Whereas Mathew's curriculum centers on poetry, earlier evidence for the curriculum at Winchester offered by documents from 1530 purveys a more widely ranging course of reading. Although the page covering the sixth and seventh forms is missing, these records testify to the study of certain authors and texts missing or left vague in Mathew's account. It is clarified, for instance, that the fifth form reads Cicero's letters; that the fourth covers Cicero's paradoxes; and that the lower forms study Aesop and Lucian in Latin, and Cato's moral distiches. Records of the purchases made by Winchester scholar John Hutton in 1621 allow us to add another Latin writer of considerable interest to Browne: Lucan. With the 1618 Farnaby edition of this Stoic poet, the Winchester pupils would have had ready access to his great poem on civil war and the demise of republicanism.[42] Given the potential for this poem to incite the young to rebellion, it is noteworthy that according to Mathew, Nowell's catechisms were recited by heart.

Browne's library's holdings[43] from this period in his life offer possibilities of texts that the young scholar might have encountered, on his own or with Robinson.

[40] Based on Leach but modified.

[41] Robert Krueger, ed., *The Poems of Sir John Davies* (Oxford: Clarendon Press, 1975), xxvi. For Browne and the epigram, see for example Keynes, 2.275.

[42] See Matthew Hutton, *The Correspondence of Dr. Matthew Hutton*, 166–9.

[43] Jeremiah S. Finch, *A Catalogue of the Libraries of Sir Thomas Browne and Dr Edward Browne, His Son* (Leiden: E. J. Brill, 1986).

Some entries are likely candidates for Winchester purchases: the two-volume Greek/Latin edition of Plutarch from 1620; the 1621 Plautus, a 1618 orations of Themistius, and a 1619 gathering of Greek tragedians; a 1618 Statius; and a 1619 *Rhetoric* of Aristotle. There are also some highly intriguing entries that suggest Browne's precocious scholarship as encouraged by Robinson: a 1612 Athenaeus; Meursius's study of Greek festivals and cults (1619); the same scholar's translation of Plato's *Timaeus* (1617); a 1617 Tertullian (he of the "certum est quia impossibile est" advocated in the *Religio*); a 1619 theological lexicon from Altenstaig; a perilous *Amphitheatrum* by G. C. Vanini, executed for his heresies in 1620; a 1619 handbook to chronology beginning with the creation (from J. Behm); Spondanus's epitome of the annals of Baronius (1623); and a Greek/Latin edition of the skeptical philosopher Sextus Empiricus (1621). Given his testimonial to those expansive, prodigious "greener studies" in the *Religio*, this list of books offers a glimpse of the fields in which Browne, with Robinson's guidance, sowed the sophisticated, skeptical, and profoundly reverential scholarly habits that remained with him for the whole of his life.

Some of the texts on the grammar curriculum were relatively safe for youthful consumption: obvious examples include Cicero's clarion call to duty in *De officiis*, as well as his defense of divine providence and cosmic order against the Epicureans in the *Tusculan Disputations*. Given the Ovidian works chosen for the boys—the antiquarian *Fasti*, plaintive *Tristia*, and habitually allegorized *Metamorphoses*—that potentially corrupting poet offered little of danger. As the seventeenth-century expurgated editions of Martial make clear, the epigrammatist required some culling for the removal of obscene content; though neither the 1601 edition owned by Browne[44] nor the 1623 Farnaby edition removed the ruder poems, a schoolmaster would have little trouble offering relatively chaste material from the hundreds of little poems. Lucian was rather more problematic. In the *Religio*, Browne himself testified that Lucian embodied an unusually extreme penchant for "atheism" that amounted to "the Rhetorick of Satan" (Patrides, 87).

Of Sundays, Mathew says only that the scholars take notes on the sermon and copy them out into their notebooks. Tuesdays and Thursdays were recreational days provided that the students were permitted by the Headmaster to take to the nearby meadows and onward to St Catherine's Hill, or, if it were winter, to the fire in the hall where "they might amuse themselves with songs and other honourable solaces; they might soberly (*seriosius*) recite or listen to poetry, the chronicles of kingdoms, the wonders of this world, and such other things as befit the clerical state" (Cook, 379). On the Tuesdays and Thursdays when for some reason recreation was not permitted, the scholars studied their books in chambers. By contrast to the refreshment of remedies, Mathew jokes, Fridays are considered "bloody" by virtue of the fact that "all the sins of the past week are visited with a bloody punishment."[45]

44 *M. Valerii Martialis Epigrammatum Libri XIV* (Paris, 1601).

45 Quoted in Sprott, *Tom Browne's Schooldays*, 31.

With assistance from grammars and rhetorics written by schoolmasters such as John Stanbridge, William Lily, Camden, and Robinson himself, grammar education taught the scholars the rules of declension and conjugation (the "accidence"), of prosody and epistolary rhetoric. Beyond "parsing" the forms of words and the rote learning of "vocables" (memorization for the purposes of building vocabulary), boys learned to "construe" Latin syntax. To demonstrate their understanding of the rules, students were required not only to recite them from memory but also to employ them in translating Latin into English, and English into Latin (i.e. "vulgars").[46] Winchester was especially keen to teach syntax;[47] such continuing emphasis on larger grammatical and rhetorical units of meaning helped ensure that their education yielded the boys more than rules of accidence and syntax per se, an approach that helps to explain Browne's lifelong tendency to keep notebooks for revising the cadences of his prose. Ideally, grammar, rhetoric, and virtue matured together: for instance, Cato's distiches functioned as an entrée into the parts of speech or accidence, the construal of syntax, the accumulation of vocabulary, and the instillation of morals. In short, Latin grammar was not just a field of knowledge, a method of writing and reading, or a mine for copious phrasing; it was a stimulus to active thought and exploration, reinforcing old verities yet also yielding new ideas according to which the best ancients would prompt students to transform, even to move beyond antiquity. Thus Browne would have less trouble than one might expect in accommodating his Winchester training to the announcement in 1620 of Bacon's Great Instauration, with its appeal to experience, natural history, and a sweeping reform of education.

In composing poems, themes, and epistles, the scholars were generating variations of phrase always disciplined by decorum according to subject, audience, and speaker. According to a leading pedagogue, they were also mastering a copiousness of commonplace material including "short histories" such as Plutarch's, fables, adages, "Hieroglyphicks," "Emblems and Symbols," "Ancient Laws and Customs," "Witty Sentences" from compilations, florilegia, or enchiridions of moral philosophy, "Rhetorical exornations," "Topical places," and "Descriptions of things natural and artificial."[48] As this list suggests, in addition to reading the ancients themselves, the boys had access to any number of handbooks and dictionaries listing epithets, poetic flourishes, and oratorical phrases. The themes composed by the pupils were executed according to the norms of ancient rhetoric, with key guidance to be found in the *Progymnasmata* of Aphthonius, whose famous introduction to over a dozen exercises shaped Browne's ability to examine a subject from the vantage of competing perspectives. Headmaster Robinson clearly envisioned his charges as future orators whose wit would be cultivated by the exercise, imitation, and art that he bestowed on them by way of the rules and

[46] Arthur F. Leach, *Educational Charters and Documents 598 to 1909* (republished New York: AMS, 1971), 448–9.

[47] T. W. Baldwin, *William Shakspere's Small Latine & Lesse Greeke* (Urbana: University of Illinois Press, 1944), 1.136.

[48] Charles Hoole, quoted in Sprott, *Tom Browne's Schooldays*, 115.

examples of classical oratory.[49] As we learn from Mathew, not only did Winchester students learn the various types of themes and cases, the divisions of an oration into parts, and the "precepts for oratory and eloquence," but they frequently practiced their skills insofar as they "were accustomed to mount the rostrum in the schoolroom and declaim."[50] From his early days as a public orator at Oxford to those letters in which he helped Edward with the enunciation as well as the content of an important speech, Browne thought of rhetoric as an oral performance as well as a written composition. Even in the synopses of history and in the *Annalium* that he published posthumously, Robinson paid special attention to the historical role of speeches.[51]

The inclusion of "hieroglyphics" in the commonplace list widely used by schoolmasters in the sixteenth and seventeenth centuries has a special significance for a study of Browne, whose earliest major publication announces the author's fascination with this concept. In general terms, the relationship between the commonplace and hieroglyphic is complex. As Kathy Eden remarks, hieroglyphs belong together with proverbs as the "common property" of a rhetorical community—the lists of pedagogues clearly reflect this juncture.[52] The commonality of the language potentially afforded by hieroglyphs is heightened by explanatory textbooks such as the one by Valeriano, by the means of which codes are not so much deciphered as translated into terms that a community can master and share. This shared heritage was meant to fashion these students as future leaders and ideal subjects according to the "dominant cultural code."[53]

In two ways, however, this model of analysis is not sufficient. For one thing, the classical legacies of Greece and Rome, even the texts included in the standard reading list, could prove morally, spiritually, and politically subversive or corrosive. For another, enigmatic hieroglyphs offered a more elusive and perfectionist conception of language, one transcending the "common" altogether. Hieroglyphs, while potentially a language for the childishly illiterate if found in nature, amounted to a mysterious ur-language insofar as they encode a cosmos of realist symbols—that is, of symbols perfectly and essentially engaged with the reality of God's creation—that were obscured in the first instance with the fall of Adam and Eve, and in the second with the dispersion of languages at Babel. In a curriculum whose schoolmaster was harping on biblical history, hieroglyphs might prove more, or even other, than commonplace rhetorical language. While commonplaces might allow rhetoric to prosper in a specific community by accommodating the imperfection of its users, hieroglyphs beckoned the young scholar to dream of a mystical possibility: that scholarship might lead the way back to the unfallen language of paradise.

[49] Sprott, *Tom Browne's Schooldays*, 120.

[50] Sprott, *Tom Browne's Schooldays*, 121.

[51] Sprott, *Tom Browne's Schooldays*, 125; see p. 53 below for *Annalium*.

[52] Kathy Eden, *Friends Hold All Things in Common: Tradition, Intellectual Property, and the Adages of Erasmus* (New Haven, CT: Yale University Press, 2001), 153.

[53] Mary Thomas Crane, *Framing Authority: Sayings, Self, and Society in Sixteenth-Century England* (Princeton, NJ: Princeton University Press, 1993), 4.

No set of questions interested Browne more than this one posing the relationship between hieroglyphs and commonplaces. Sometimes he saw hieroglyphs as accentuating the value of the common—for instance, with the manuscript of Nature in *Religio Medici*. In *Pseudodoxia Epidemica*, Browne ventured to demystify the hieroglyphic. In the case of those aphorisms featured in his Hippocratic medical training, the commonplace could assume the enigma of the hieroglyph, while, in *Christian Morals*, Browne offered what he considered the guidance of universal moral principles. In the *Garden of Cyrus*, nature and art coincided in their inscriptions of hieroglyphs at once esoteric and ubiquitous. Winchester College was by no means the end of Browne's education in these semiotic concerns, but it afforded his young mind a stimulating beginning.

Shaped as his prose artistry and composition habits were by Winchester, Browne's most striking departure from Winchester rhetoric was his decision to write his major works in English, the circumstances for which emerged over the course of Browne's further maturation as a student of natural philosophy and an arbiter of English Protestantism in the decades after Bacon's Great Instauration. Yet regarding both moral vision and critical analysis, Browne's meditations on the world would continually reveal their seminal debts to his headmaster Hugh Robinson.

3. HEADMASTER ROBINSON

Since headmasters were prone to put their own stamp on grammar learning, we are fortunate in possessing firsthand information about the pedagogy of Browne's Hugh Robinson.[54] Unlike most Ramists, Robinson did not reduce rhetoric to the task of "speaking stylishly"; far from it, he held rhetoric to be far more integral to the art of persuasion and pervasive in all the stages of a grammar education. From an early age, Browne was taught that rhetoric was intellectual, moral, and spiritual in its full and dynamic dimensions, not just lifelessly cosmetic. One lived rhetoric rather than simply observed it behind glass from afar. Nor was rhetoric only business and duty; closely related to, yet still distinctive from, the seriousness of rhetorical purpose was an idea of linguistic play, whether it took the form of paradox stretching from Cicero through Erasmus; the form of copious inventiveness of such importance to the Erasmian tradition; or the recreational sense that literature afforded us a remedy from our sober vocations.

[54] The *ODNB* article is by Rosemary O'Day, who notes that Robinson's future offices in the church tend to reflect moderation. Born around 1584, with Nicholas Robinson, the bishop of Bangor, as his father, Hugh Robinson was himself a scholar at Winchester from 1596 to 1603, then at New College, Oxford, where he matriculated in December 1603, received his BA in 1607 and his MA in 1611. His poems appeared in three Oxford collections dated 1605, 1612, and 1613. Serving as Winchester's headmaster from 1613 to 1627, Robinson published a textbook for his pupils in 1616, with an outline of their training in grammar, rhetoric, and history. Then, receiving his DD in 1627, he took up office in the church full time. In the 1650s his Winchester phrasebook was published for the first time; the 1658 edition, edited by his son Nicholas, lets us know that Hugh Robinson has died. But his afterlife continued in the impressive form of Thomas Pierce's 1677 edition of the *Annalium mundi universalium*, a project that massively expanded the historiographical interests already on display in his 1616 textbook.

A student picking up Robinson's 1616 textbook would hold four instruments for making the most of his days in school. First were certain prayers in English, including a "morning prayer for a child in private" that celebrates the "most gracious and mercifull Father, which hast ordained that the mouthes of children should praise thee," and bestowed upon each child his soul, body, and breath. The prayers beseech that God will continue to "sanctifie my childhood... that from my youth vp I may grow in thy true feare, and learne to know thee, through my Lord and Saviour Iesus Christ."[55] As a model for Christian morals, Robinson's prayers accompany the child through his day, publicly before and after meals as well as privately during the evening. In keeping with the liturgical aims of public prayer, the mealtime utterances include thanks for the founder and the benefactors of the college, and prayers for the rulers of the holy commonwealth. The private vesper, a preparation for sleep, anticipates Browne's composition of a "dormative" in *Religio Medici*.

The grammar that follows these prayers offers the students directions for how to read:

> Reade distinctly to a Period, or at the beginning further, observing carefully: 1. All the points: 2. Proper names beginning with great letters: 3. Words included in a Parenthesis () which are to be construed by themselues: 4. The argument, matter, and drift of the place. 5. All the Circumstances, Quis, cui, causa, locus, quo tempore, Prima, sequela... Who speaketh in that place, what he speaketh, to whom, upon what occasion, or to what end, where, at what time, what went before in the next sentences; what followeth next after: 6. The principall verbe with the Nominatiue case, according to the rule in the Grammer.

Escorting his pupils through the parts of speech, Robinson reminds his charges that of course no one sentence is bound to comprise them all and also that a number of items will complicate the construal of syntax (12). Having earlier taken an overall view of the sense, students are not thereafter prohibited from attempts at deeper understanding; they are required rather to parse and construe as carefully as they can before venturing into a more probing authorial and contextual interpretation of the passage.

After these rules of parsing and construal, Robinson turns to the two kinds of themes or exercises, the *gnome* and the *chreia*, which amount to the difference between moral persuasion and bare representation or conceptualization, as one might also learn in Aphthonius. Essentially teaching the young composer to write simple fables and narratives (mythic or historical), these exercises encourage not so much elaborate eloquence as the virtues of "clarity, brevity, probability, and propriety of diction in the expression of their knowledge."[56] Given the sententious maxims of Browne's *Christian Morals*, but also the *Religio*'s delight in what it calls "the Apophthegme[s] of a wise man,"[57] it is especially significant that moral sentences

[55] Hugh Robinson, *I. Preces. II. Grammaticalia Quaedam. III. Rhetorica Brevis* (Oxford, 1616), 1–2.

[56] Sprott, *Tom Browne's Schooldays*, 117.

[57] See Patrides, 152; Harvard owns a copy of Erasmus's *Apophthegmatum* opus inscribed by one Thomas Browne and with this apophthegm written in by one of the book's readers.

were essential to such exercises. Above all else, Browne learned at Winchester that carefully wrought rhetoric was the means by which true wisdom exerted its influence on the world.

Robinson's textbook follows its analysis of the two introductory types of themes with guidelines for excising stylistic impurities such as language that is old-fashioned, too poetic, harsh, obscene, rare, or appropriated from another language, though there are occasions on which one might legitimately mix Greek with Latin, especially in pursuit of arts such as medicine. A further section helps the scholar to differentiate between words that seem alike, such as "cruore" and "sanguine." These types of linguistic discriminations were crucial to Browne's habits of carefully crafting and revising his prose. So too was Robinson's expectation that more advanced students pay increased attention to the rhythms of prose; the basis of periodicity, with its claims on a full, apt, and perfectly coordinated articulation of syntactic parts; and the classical gradations of style, including low, middle, and grand, with special attention to what he calls the "subtle" style. When Robinson warns that rhetoric faces many duties or demands and therefore cultivates a number of distinctive styles, he explains that acuity or subtlety pertains to the orator's judgment, which has a special role to play in the evaluation of evidence in proof and confutation.

Whereas Browne appears to have easily digested the milk of his alma mater's phrasebook, far more challenging were Robinson's approaches to and assumptions about biblical exegesis and history. Robinson was the first authority in Browne's life to accentuate questions about the role of skepticism in the Christian life. How critical, zealous, accommodating, moderate, or doubting could or should a Christian be? Was Christian truth always plain or was it sometimes dark? Could and should unorthodox positions be dismissed out of hand? That Robinson raised these questions in the "green studies" of Browne is clarified by the headmaster's historical writings, first in the textbook, then more elaborately in his *Annalium Mundi*. But it should be remembered that in and after 1618, as Europe plunged into the Thirty Years' War, as Protestants convened in Dort to address a major rift in itself, as an extraordinary comet blazed its way across the skies, and as King James embarked on a highly controversial strategy for delivering peace in Western Christendom: in these Winchester years for Browne, questions took hold in England about the relative merits of Christian moderation and zeal, about how to read biblical history, and about the marks of the true English Protestant. Robinson bestowed on his pupils a way to speak respectably about—or around—these difficult matters. But his historiography gave Browne a habit of questioning evidence that took him perilously beyond decorum.

In the synopsis of history in his textbook, Robinson begins with the traditional tripartite division of the earth into Europe, Asia, and Africa, then quickly adds that now there are the new worlds of the West Indies, Mexico, Peru, America, as well as "terra Australis incognita," and he invokes the name of Magellan. After chapters on geography, covering the various lines, circles, and zones used to measure and apportion the earth, as well as longitude and latitude, Europe, Africa, and Asia, Robinson begins a historical survey which interweaves an account of Noah, Nimrod and Babel, and the children of Noah with a consideration of the Scythians (said to have been established by Magog), of the Assyrians (including Zoroaster), and the Amazons who murdered male children and exercised with arms, horses, and hunting.

Robinson's narrative includes assessments of human motives—Nimrod oversees the building of Babel in search of a lasting monument—as well as strong insertions of divine providence, with God punishing such arrogance with the confusion of languages. Already there are obvious cross-references to Browne's later work—in the *Religio* he takes up the question of motivation with Babel when he states "That our Fathers, after the Flood, erected the Tower of Babell, to preserve themselves against a second Deluge, is generally opinionated and beleeved," then reminds the reader "yet is there another intention of theirs expressed in Scripture" and criticizes the common opinion's failure to account for the geography of the place itself (Patrides, 90). But Robinson's history also touches on minor details—the nature of bitumen—that reappear in one form or another in Browne's work, sometimes dangerously: indeed the devil himself is at work when Browne, "having seene some experiments of *Bitumen*," is tempted to doubt Old Testament miracles, even "to thinke the combustion of *Sodom* might be naturall, and that there was an Asphaltick and Bituminous nature in that Lake before the fire of Gomorrha" (Patrides, 85). The study of history can yield a deeper faith in providence but it can also produce sinister doubts about whether history should be understood providentially.

Early on the survey is interrupted by a chapter on the origin of superstition and idolatry in which Robinson editorializes about the nature of religious belief, on the one hand attributing the spread of idols to the desire of the politically prudent to restrain people with fear, and on the other insisting that the true God is one and unchanging. Eventually Robinson begins to interrupt his Old Testament focus for two other reasons: one is to interject the histories of other peoples, the Greeks and Italians, and the other to offer another narrative of origins—the origin of the liberal arts. Although Robinson is clearly willing to offer moral and spiritual commentary on history, he is far more interested in the juxtaposition of histories: on how the Babylonian captivity occurs whilst Solon is ruling justly in Athens, for instance. Indeed the text never returns to the ancient Jews, ending instead with tables listing the ancient types of money and with elegiac genealogies of ancient heroes. Whatever the moral and spiritual lessons to be gained from history, it is noteworthy that Robinson's textbook emphasizes the value of cross-cultural study and, at least toward the Roman end, gravitates toward the institutional and evidentiary concerns of antiquarianism.

Robinson's historiographical interests and methods encouraged bright young scholars such as Browne to consider the relationship between fables or fictions and rigorous history. In the *Annalium* especially, Robinson adds rhetorical artistry to his history when he invents speeches for characters such as Delilah. But this fictionalizing and the headmaster's pulsing questions about the Genesis narrative were regularly counterbalanced by a reverence for its Christian significance with help from Tertullian, one of Browne's favorite authorities in *Religio Medici*. Moreover, Robinson tended to retract himself from endless controversies bordering on vanity, such as the one about the location of Adam's grave.

Sometimes Robinson's questions, if not his answers, coincide with Browne's own interests: the question of the season in which the world was created, for instance, the way in which Absalom died, the reason for a decline in longevity (cf. Patrides, 114), or inquiries surrounding the doves that were sent from the ark and either never came back or returned to the ark with an olive leaf. "I can read the history of the Pigeon that was sent out of the Ark, and returned no more," Browne insists, "yet not question how shee found her mate that was left behind" (Patrides, 88). But Robinson is prepared to unpack the type of questions at which Browne only hints, so that the headmaster's scholarly commitments help account for the precocity, daring, and profundity with which the young Origen clearly entered into religious scholarship both theological and historical. In the *Religio*, Browne testifies that in the past he has ventured into the territory of juxtaposing scriptural with "humane history" and that, thanks to what he considers a silly instance of the results in Justin, has since left it behind as an illegitimate "curiosity." In other words, the method runs afoul by virtue of its implication that the Bible's authenticity must be tested and can be found wanting. In what appears to be the *Religio*'s willingness to dismiss non-scriptural histories as essentially untrustworthy, however, Browne continues to interject assessments of biblical history that sound incredulous. Robinson's posthumous *Annalium Mundi* clarifies how the headmaster contributed to Browne's complex response to the Bible and to ecclesiastical history, at once scholarly curious, literarily rich, and deeply pious. In one instance, the tome shows how the mature Browne returned the favor.[58]

One of the most pervasive and appealing tendencies of Robinson's annals is their inclusion of set rhetorical pieces comprising speeches and colloquies. These invented pieces play two pedagogical roles. The first is that they obviously render the chief players in biblical history more dramatic, immediate, and morally or spiritually compelling. In some cases, when God orates or converses, Robinson implicitly encourages his audience to believe that divine providence, for all its mysteries and circuitous means, offers a dispensation to which they have access. Only very rarely does Robinson remind his readers that God spoke to his chosen patriarchs in a spiritual, not a human language, as he does in the divine dialogue with Abraham (*Annalium mundi*, 167). At the moral level, this dramatically high-pitched, if also comforting, access is clinched by Robinson's lessons involving the punishment of evil and the rewarding of patient goodness even in this world. If Sodom is a simple example of evil punished, Joseph's resistance to Portiphar's wife offers an elaborate, highly wrought, instance of goodness rewarded after much adversity. Robinson's lingering over the temptation of Joseph, the exemplum of a young boy in extremis, is redolent of the Winchester origins of the annals. In such

[58] It is impossible to say when Robinson's words reached the final form in which they exist in the 1677 *Annalium*. Although the title page of the 1677 edition advertises Pierce's editorial interventions—he has cleaned up the text, filled lacunae, and worked hard to bring the text into print—the rhetorical features of the text (including its set speeches and colloquies) remain consistent throughout. Moreover, very few works on the surprisingly short list of sources postdate the years of Robinson's headmastership, and none is published after his death.

cases, when human characters speak, Robinson invites his audience to consider the psychological, moral, and spiritual circumstances in which famous biblical events unfolded. One experiences the effect of Joseph's inferiority as a slave in Egypt, his divinely inspired resourcefulness as an interpreter of dreams, as well as the moral resolve to which his agonized soliloquies finally carry him (221–2). We encounter the panic or anxiety that both the Egyptians and the Israelites must have experienced in the drama of the exodus; or the moral perplexity of an Old Testament hero whose inner monologue leads to clear resolution. The message of his history is always that the patiently good and godly should have hope and will prevail, even, or especially, if they are young and male.

The second role played by the speeches and colloquies is more vexed. As rhetorical set pieces indebted to classical historians such as Livy, they epitomize in style what for Browne was Robinson's most intriguing and controversial historical method: an insistence on interweaving biblical history with the non-biblical histories of the world. This is not necessarily the same thing as assessing biblical history according to the non-biblical history—curiosity about which Browne claims comically to have jettisoned in the *Religio*. Nonetheless, the underlying assumption of the *Annalium mundi* is that the chronologies of the various histories will and must cohere—the running tally in the margin of the date *anno mundi* is a constant reminder of this fact—whether or not their competing explanations of events such as the exodus agree.

Throughout his interlaced narratives, Robinson pursues two key goals. On the one hand, Robinson cultivates scholarly standards: in his use of ancient, medieval, and early modern sources from Strabo and Philo to Juan Vives and Lorenzo Valla, he is prepared to guide his readers when a source, whether Josephus or Sir Walter Ralegh, is misleading. On the other, Robinson is ready with pithy religious and moral lessons: idolatry depends on the notion that nothing can exist unless it can be seen; and the history of theology divides into the good—entailing the desire to do good—and the bad, with its basis in a fear of punishment (107). Both these lessons are written large in the *Religio*, with its celebration of sightless, extraordinary belief (Patrides, 70), and its strong distaste for fear as a motivator to piety (126).

Having begun a discussion of hieroglyphics in his account of the rise of idolatry (106), Robinson singles them out for attention in his history of writing. Differentiating sacred from profane writing, he notes that the sacred kind employed not words but images of animals or human body parts in the manner of Chinese characters. Then, having enlisted the church father Clement's tripartite division of writing into imitative, tropical, and enigmatic varieties, he separates hieroglyphs from all three. While hieroglyphs might share qualities with each one of these writing forms, the symbols of the hieroglyphic remain more secretive and difficult, more arduous to produce and less useful for popular instruction. Having introduced his pupils to the basic rules for identifying hieroglyphs, Robinson directs them to study Pierio Valeriano and Horapollo (109) for further guidance on the nature and history of this elusive form of representation.

As the annals expand into a full-scale narrative of the six-day creation, Robinson increasingly allows room for curiosity and controversy. The view of Thomas

Cajetan—that an angel and not the Holy Spirit was responsible for producing air and fire—must be refuted. The question of what embodied light at its initial creation leads to the concession that Moses tells us nothing about *how* things were done: knowing *that* they were done should satisfy pious readers and true Christians, Robinson remarks. The angels generate a panoply of questions, not least because the Bible is not always clear. There are questions about how many orders of angels God made, but also about the exact sin that led to their fall. There are questions about when in the six days the angels were created, a point on which Browne opines that he "cannot with those in that great Father securely interpret the worke of the first day, *Fiat lux*, to the creation of Angels, though (I confesse) there is not any creature that hath so neare a glympse of their nature, as light in the Sunne and Elements" (Patrides, 102–3). As for the good angels, their status as the executors of God's mandates in the world has prompted their very name, since "angel" means nuncio or messenger. On this etymological matter, Robinson makes a modest point that Browne has carried further into controversy according to the *Religio*. The headmaster states simply that, according to some biblical scholars, "many so-called angels" are "properly speaking, servants or officers" of the human variety, then he notes that famous ancient fathers and theologians have supported the existence of guardian angels chosen as protectors and representatives of important persons from birth to death. As an example, he includes Acts 12:7, 15. By contrast, in the *Religio*, Browne reports his use of the etymological lesson as a paradoxical reading of the Acts passage in a dispute with a Franciscan; as for guardian angels, Browne is inclined to believe in them even if they are "not manifestly defin'd in Scripture" (101) and the Roman church has taken liberties with Acts.

Robinson introduces and reviews such points of controversy and curiosity, but his gravitational pull is toward a clear didactic lesson. His strong tendency to dismiss or at least to get beyond "niceties"—what Browne calls "Quere's and objections," "captious" readings, "fantastick Quere's," "Atoms in Divinity... not worthy our vacant houres, much lesse our serious studies" (Patrides, 67–9)—is clearly on display in the *Religio*. Browne shows his schoolmaster's determination to resolve biblical complexity or obscurity into untroubled lessons in divine providence or maxims of moral virtue. But the schoolmaster's seed has grown into a fascination with and commitment to biblical scholarship that requires more sophisticated management, often a delicate balancing act between profound reverence and serious criticism, and at times a plunge into the postulates of faith against which the believer would be able to offer textual proof ("'Tis a postulate to me, that *Methusalem* was the longest liv'd of all the children of Adam, and no man will bee able to prove it; when from the processe of the Text I can manifest it may be otherwise" (Patrides, 90); the story of Samson is both singularly "fabulous" and, given divine providence, "an easie possibility" (87)). On several occasions, for instance, regarding the legal implications of Lazarus's resurrection, Browne articulates the very question for curiosity's sake that he expresses no believer's need to pose (88).

Robinson and his pupil are on the same page in the explanation of the Tower of Babel. As Robinson relates it, Josephus has claimed that the tower was built for the purpose of protection against a second flood, an opinion adopted by many others.

Like Browne in the *Religio* (Patrides, 90), Robinson deems this opinion unworthy of belief, for God relieved the world of this fear; the place itself gave no hope of such an escape (for it was the lowest part of a deep valley); and it was ridiculous to imagine that very many people could squeeze into the confines of a tower (Robinson, 86). It is obvious to both headmaster and pupil that the builders of Babel sought fame and glory; indeed, attentive readers of the annals can discover a similar lesson in the discussion of the pyramids and in the erasure from historical record of those men who founded and built them (*Annalium mundi*, 200; cf. Patrides, 310).

Nonetheless, especially on questions regarding the relative merits of natural and theological explanations of events, Browne in the 1630s is far more apt to express anxiety than his schoolmaster. So it is that in regard to the extraordinary fecundity of the Israelites in Egypt, Robinson notes Aristotle's argument that Egyptian women are prone to bear three or four children from any one pregnancy; but he dismisses this explanation with a caution that it is far better to attribute Jewish fertility to God's power rather than to the natural propensities of Egypt (253). On the presence of manna and bitumen in the Bible, Robinson purveys none of his pupil's eventual queries about the nature of the miraculous. Regarding the episode in which Moses consumed the golden calf with "an actuall fire," Browne but not his schoolmaster confesses a desire to know how he did it, "for that mysticall mettle of gold, whose solary and celestial nature I admire, exposed unto the violence of fire, grows onley hot and liquefies, but consumeth not" (Patrides, 124). Whatever the calf's evil, its gold should have resisted Moses's flame.

As a testimonial to his now famous pupil, Robinson enlists Browne himself as a source on the subject of portraits depicting "Jephthah sacrificing his daughter" (Robbins, ed., *Pseudodoxia Epidemica*, 1.404–6). Embracing the criticism of "our Browne, a very learned man" (*Annalium*, 519), Robinson approves of the careful, rational way that his pupil has with sources, languages, and arguments. What matters about Robinson's scholarship for Browne is not simply the learned comment but also the dramatic excitement for biblical study, the ideal balance of reverence and criticism, and the penchant to support axiomatic moral and spiritual conviction with a scholarship both comprehensive and curious. These tendencies and qualities permeate everything that Browne ever wrote, anxiously in the *Religio*, authoritatively in the *Pseudodoxia*, plaintively in *Hydriotaphia*, playfully in the *Garden of Cyrus*, and familiarly in the *Miscellany Tracts* (for instance, on plants in scripture), letters, and notebooks.

Throughout his adult life, Browne returned to his rhetorical training in composing Latin letters of praise and blame in which, albeit in prose, he purveyed considerable debt to Horace, Martial, and the Roman poets. For instance, from Norwich he addressed his "Amico Clarissimo, de enecante garrulo suo"—translated by Keynes as "to an illustrious friend on his wearisome chatterer"—to an unknown recipient who would appreciate Browne's adaptation of Horace's ninth satire on a garrulous parasite. In one respect at least, Browne's epistolary set pieces chafe at the limitations of grammar decorum and the guidelines set by Winchester handbooks and phrases: his defense of inventive barbarism and macaronics, an apologetic that derives from his interest in those writers both prior and posterior to the golden age of Latin antiquity encountered in grammar school as well as in satire understood as a miscellaneous hodgepodge with a penchant for Stoic paradox and stylistic obscurity. In his reading notes from Athenaeus, Browne declares that the older of the Latin writers were apt to be freer in their use of Greek, "in composing and forming words" without concern for their barbarity, provided that the inventions were "most apt to the sense."[59] As Browne praises Plautus as an example of a fertile writer willing to offer putatively barbaric concoctions such as "plagipatidas" and "ferritribaces," his own satire on the garrulous bore illustrates this hybridizing inventiveness as well, with "glossogastor," "famigerator," and "opisthographis." Browne's response to Athenaeus explains that the best writers have the courage to shape and expand the language that they use, without anxiety over the claims of commonplace or shared rhetoric in the stultifying comfort of which "the herd dares nothing new save by roundabout ways, and coldly paraphrases in fear of foreign forms." Browne is sufficiently guided by his education in classical propriety to warn composers away from useless archaism or innovation. Nonetheless, he formulates a version of the apology that his readers would have encountered in ancient and contemporary writers dedicated to the exploration and representation of truth over and above the utility of commonplace persuasion—that language must be reshaped to keep pace with the reality that human beings are coming to know (Keynes, 3.171).

What we know from the records of seventeenth-century Winchester suggests the following conclusions. For the most part Browne learned the moral and rhetorical proprieties widely offered in a grammar education for the purposes of training the ecclesiastical and civil officers and professionals of contemporary England. Nonetheless, at least in Browne's way of thinking, various texts outside high classicism in the grammar school curriculum, the invitation to hieroglyphics, and above all Robinson's own critical methodology in the examination of history: these factors of Browne's education between 1616 and 1623 make it likely that he learned to examine the insufficiency of propriety and commonplace in the course of internalizing the wit, power, and utility of the commonplace. For his "extravagant and irregular" brain, commonplace was both the defense against damnable monstrosity—"the Rhetoricke wherewith I perswade another cannot perswade my selfe" (Patrides, 66, 129)—and the manacle enchaining that "singular" wit who might honestly "play and expatiate with security and farre without the circle of an heresie" (69). At its best, the Winchester way provided that singular wit with guidelines by which intellectual paradox, inversion, and expatiation might be anchored to piety, obedience, civility, and cogency. At Oxford and on the Continent, where Browne came into closer, less controlled contact with natural philosophy, heresy, and even atheism, the Winchester way played a complex role: it went a long way toward helping Browne restrain extravagant thought within a politically obedient, morally constant, and religiously conformist framework; but it also provided the seeds of extravagance itself from Browne's "greener studies."

[59] Keynes's translation, 3.170–1. "*Antiquiores enim in componendis fingendisque vocabulis libere Græcissant, quibus voces sensui accommodatissimas proferre non erat barbare et cum Evandro loqui.*"

4. THE CLOISTER AND THE WORLD

In Browne's time, Winchester College was still designed as a self-sufficient economic and social unit, even if this meant that the porter might double as a barber. The cloistered nature of life at Winchester was reinforced by the fact that for holidays, boys often remained in college, especially at Christmas.[60] By the seventeenth century, this autonomy clearly persisted in the college and would resurface in the *Religio* as Browne's recasting of affective obligations away from the nuclear family toward friendship and the affiliations of learning and spirituality. Whatever the changes wrought by the Reformation, Winchester was still predominantly a seminary for future clerics. The pupils were mindful of charity as well as doctrine: for the years 1616–25, charitable contributions chosen by the scholars included donations to a "shipwrecked Pole" and two shipwrecked Scotsmen; the redemption of captives from the Turks; the rector of Bosham for the refurbishing of his church; "a poor Oxford scholar from Poole, whose father had been plundered by pirates"; "sundry destitute Irish"; "a soldier on his way back to Bohemia"; and Eleanor, the bishop of Cork's daughter (*Victoria History*, 310–11). Browne's own financial concerns persisted: on March 28, 1622, the Court of Orphans decided that Browne's uncle and protector, Edward Browne, required an action against him for his handling of the estate, a decision that probably resulted "in recognizances entered on April 30, 1622, by Edward Browne, grocer, Richard Browne, mercer (Edward's brother), Richard Archedale, draper (Edward's brother-in-law), Christopher Rotheram, mercer (Edward's son-in-law), for £300 and £200 owing to Thomas, Anne, Jane, Mary, and Ellen, children and orphans of Thomas Browne deceased."[61] In 1624, Uncle Edward's attempt to extract money from the estate may reflect the fact that his nephew had matriculated at Oxford in December 1623 without a scholarship.[62]

Arguably, Browne's career in medicine was something of a fluke, a result of a boy with sensitivity toward yew trees and comets failing to gain entrance into New College, and ending up at Pembroke with an appealing medical humanist called Thomas Clayton. But the theological and clerical obligations of the young Origen continued to make themselves felt in Browne's ethos: *Religio Medici* testifies to Browne's ongoing desire to reconcile the orientations of theology and natural philosophy.

The 1618 comet so clearly remembered many years later by Browne was widely interpreted on its appearance as an omen of the serious challenges, changes, and conflicts that England was facing as Browne confronted the uncertainties of his own future. For some commentators, the national drama doubled as a domestic one, insofar as the question at hand was often whether King James was a good

60 *Victoria History*, 278.

61 LMA, London Court of Aldermen, Repertory 36, ff. 101r-v and 122b; and Norman J. Endicott, "Sir Thomas Browne as 'Orphan.'"

62 LMA, London Court of Aldermen, Repertory 38, 181r; cf. Endicott, "Sir Thomas Browne as 'Orphan,'" 187.

father, not just of his subjects but also of his children, Princess Elizabeth, her husband Frederick, and the heir apparent Prince Charles. The translation of Lancelot Andrewes to the bishopric of Winchester signaled what Peter McCullough has called "a major shift in Andrewes's career" as well as "in James's reign," for "the death of several leading Calvinist bishops with strong court connections had opened the way for James to appoint men like Andrewes, Laud, and Buckeridge to more prominent posts where their liberal theology and views on European politics could be of advantage in his attempts to secure the marriage of Prince Charles to the Spanish Infanta."[63] Liberal theology, the rehabilitation of liturgy and ceremony, and an irenic rapprochement with Catholic Europe: all these eventual Brownean sentiments came to the forefront—and into a maelstrom of controversy—as Browne himself was fully settling into his studies in Andrewes's jurisdiction. The comet of 1618 struck many as portentous of the beginning of the Thirty Years' War, the start of the Synod at Dort, but also the lingering excitement and bemusement over the recent claims of the mysterious Rosicrucian brotherhood for a transformation of the world. In 1618, events seemed equally favorable for a new ecumenical unity on the one hand and an apocalyptic war to end all wars on the other, a choice between which began sorely to divide English Protestants over the future of their church and the peacemaking intentions of King James. During the last half of Browne's Winchester years, the news often reflected anxiety and even gloom over the English role in the problems facing Christendom in the Netherlands, Spain, Germany, Bohemia, France, as well as Ireland and Virginia. For the boys at Winchester College, much of this anxiety was brought home by those widespread charges that James was a negligent father. As Browne was growing and maturing, his England was beginning to slip into a highly polemical and inwardly contentious political and religious culture.

In the official papers covering all this strife, the provincial town of Winchester and its college were rarely mentioned. But no matter how shielded Browne may have been from the national anxieties over royal authority, the neglect of the Winchester scholars by their superiors served as an obvious microcosm of James's supposed neglect of and recklessness with his own children. The link was made explicitly when, on one occasion in August 1618, the world of the court came to Winchester College in the person of Prince Charles, whose visit was celebrated with a collection of Latin and Greek verses.[64] Since the poems are anonymous, it is impossible to know which, if any, was written by young Browne. Not even his later disregard in the *Miscellany Tracts* for "all affectation in Poetry" (Keynes, 3.67) precludes the possibility that he was assigned or responsible for the one shape poem (a sword), any of the several anagrams (which the adult Browne continued

[63] Peter McCullough, ed., *Lancelot Andrewes: Selected Sermons & Lectures* (Oxford: Oxford University Press, 2005), xxix.

[64] Bodleian MS Tanner 466; I am grateful to Kathryn Murphy for calling my attention to this manuscript. Among the verses whose vocabulary comes closest to Browne's own in his published poem for William Camden, one poem stands out by virtue of the fact that its genre, the Horatian ode, is identified in its title (54v–55r). But the Winchester ode's incorporation of several Horatian poems is so conventional as to resist any confident attribution to Browne.

to enjoy), chronograms (poems including the Roman numeration of 1618), or the one set of "latticed verses" in which numbered rows of words match each other both across and down the page (53r). Nor does any of the poems come especially close to Browne's 1623 verses for Camden in language, metaphor, or allusion. Several poems find ways to celebrate the Prince's heroic qualities, some elevating him over the famous Habsburg emperor Charles V, others dividing his virtues between the martial prowess of the prince's uncle, Christian IV of Denmark, and the holiness of his father James I. With these verses on the characteristics of Charles's heroism, the Winchester youth edged their words toward the realm of adult accomplishment—and controversy. Of all the poems in the collection, however, the most revealing of life at Winchester is also the one most concerned with the domestic troubles of that life, not with a fantasy of British imperial heroism. In a pastoral dialogue between Tityrus and Melibaeus, the shepherds debate the question of whether their welfare is wholly subverted by negligent or hostile guardians or recuperated by a glorious patron. In a barely veiled allusion to contemporary abuses at the college, Melibaeus complains that the shepherds are wretched in exile from their fathers' homes, while Tityrus responds that Apollo himself has afforded them their current leisure and security for study. In fact, he insists, the abuse and alienation lamented by Melibaeus would prove the impossible, that Apollo has allowed a violation of the sacred laws of nature. But Melibaeus has a lesser view of Apollo's reach: as just as Phoebus may be, he cannot see all things in the obscure shadows below him (46r-v). As much as the Winchester poets of 1618 might meditate on the heroic role of Charles in the international theater, this poem clarifies that for these boys, the visceral need for sustenance mattered far more than the Defenestration of Prague.

Oxford would bring Thomas Browne much closer to the discursive center of political and religious controversy as well as to a hub for the advancement of learning. Browne himself would enter into public discourse early in his Oxford years. For the young man who throughout his adulthood would have considerable interest in prognostication, 1623, like the year of the comet in 1618, was momentous. Among the papers of the Hutton family, whose John was attending Winchester with Browne, one finds a prophecy bearing the date of July 29, 1623 and concluding that "This shalbe a ffatall yeare to suche as be of quallitie and authoritie; one shalbe poissoned, deathe followinge another as his shaddowe. A prophet will arise, and be authure of some newe relligion never harde of before: great allteracions in religion, lawes, empires, and kingdoms: studyinges of negromancie" (*Correspondence of Dr Matthew Hutton*, 299). Here was summer stuff designed to intrigue a saturnine and orphaned schoolboy on his way from a depopulated town to a university community keenly attuned and responsive to the signs of "great allteracions"—in the death of old Elizabethan heroes, the dalliance of the Prince with the Spanish Infanta, a growing disgust at the favorite Buckingham, the fall of Bacon under charges of corruption, the outbreak of contentiousness in the church at home, and the strife of international Protestantism in France, the Netherlands, and Germany.

Seemingly far less auspicious was Browne's own transition to Oxford, for having failed to gain election to New College, he settled for Broadgates and no scholarship.[65] The sting of an adolescent having to make his own way in the world is still felt in Browne's observation in his notebooks that "I attained my purpose and came to reach this port by a bare wind, much labour, great paynes and litle assistance" (Keynes, 3.273). Browne's failure to earn a scholarship at New College would later become the stuff of rude anagrammatic jokes: "There was in my time two proctors of the same yeare in Oxford John Smith a man not well beloved and William Oldis a purblind dimme sighted, on whom these Anagrams were made: William Oldis silly dimme owl John Smith shyt on him" (Keynes, 3.274). In bidding farewell to this and other anagrams—"Valete Anagrammata. Nil mihi vobiscum"—Browne was also putting away child's play and old resentments. Thanks to his own rhetorical prowess, as well as his coincidence at Broadgates Hall with a leader in the advancement of natural and medical knowledge, Thomas Clayton, Browne defied augury in Oxford, found a vocation for his life, and interacted with adventurous men of letters such as Robert Hues who opened his horizons of expectations further than the commonplace rhetorical training at the center of the Winchester curriculum could have managed.

By landing at Broadgates rather than New College, moreover, Browne operated in rhetorical and poetic communities which necessarily expanded and multiplied. Browne's gravitational pull at Oxford shifted in the direction of Christ Church and Broadgates, with their politically complex group of wits whose miscellanies often reflect training at Westminster School, and with cultural heroes such as Richard Corbett and Thomas Lushington.[66] As Broadgates was reborn with the name of Pembroke College, the young Winchester graduate chosen to speak on that occasion was reborn as a public orator perhaps to be reckoned with. Nonetheless, no matter how cloistered Winchester College may have been, Browne's experience there enlarged his sense of community, history, and the natural world in which ostriches and comets could be variously—and contentiously—interpreted.

5. IRELAND

For the year 1623, the church warden for the London parish church of St Michael le Querne recorded that the parishioners had approved a payment for the ransom of six pence for a William Newman and "Thomas Browne, captyves by sea."[67] Four factors suggest that the ransomed Browne was the future author of *Religio Medici*. First, this parish church was the very one with which Browne continued to align himself, in December of that year identifying himself as its parishioner when he matriculated at Broadgates Hall, Oxford; and the parish would have a vested interest in the welfare of one of its own. Second, the most active pirate in the summer of 1623 was John Nutt, whose marauding affected virtually every vessel in passage

[65] Contrast the success of student John Potenger in *Private Memoirs of John Potenger*, ed. C. W. Bingham (London: Hamilton Adams, 1841), 28.

[66] For the miscellanies produced by these two Oxford traditions, see Mary Hobbs, *Early Seventeenth-Century Verse Miscellany Manuscripts* (Brookfield, VT: Scholar Press, 1992), 87–90.

[67] LMA P69/MIC4/B/005/MS02895/002, expenses for 1623.

between Dartmouth and Ireland; and Browne's most memorable trip prior to his continental voyage was to Ireland.[68] Third, while it has often been assumed that Browne took his Irish voyage after his graduation from Oxford, he clearly remembered that he had returned from Ireland by way of Chester at Michaelmas, a detail that would have stuck with him as a student facing the first term of his inaugural year at Oxford. Fourth, the stated purpose of the journey to Ireland, to survey the lands and properties in the care of his stepfather Sir Thomas Dutton, makes more sense in 1623, when Dutton is commencing his offices as Scoutmaster in Ulster and is explicitly concerned with just such a survey.[69]

Born in Isleworth, Middlesex, in 1575, the "worthy" Thomas Dutton, as Browne's daughter Elizabeth would call him, possibly knew Anne Garraway's family from their mutual association with Middlesex. Knighted by the new King James in 1603, he may have been admitted to Gray's Inn in 1605, but, as Hughes notes, he "turned to the Army, serving in the Low Countries, and in Ireland, where, in 1619, he was granted 2,000 acres in the Longford Plantation" (Hughes, "Childhood," 26). In some measure his royal favor would persist, not least when in 1610, King James bestowed on Dutton a lifelong office, Scoutmaster-General for Ireland, a position whose salary and perquisites were substantial. Dutton would develop a hostility toward the Catholics in Ireland, one that may well have initiated Browne's own rethinking of anti-papal polemic.[70] Browne, we will see, left very clear evidence that he objected to the most notorious event in the life of the braggart soldier who was his stepfather, namely, the fact that in 1610 he had killed Sir Hatton Cheke in a duel, from which Dutton received serious wounds whose scars must have been visible for the rest of his life.[71] More vexatious to Dutton himself were the persistence and size of his debts, a problem about which he often complained to his royal masters and employers.

The anonymous "Life of Sir Thomas Browne" included in the *Posthumous Works* states that Browne "took the Opportunity of seeing Ireland, by accompanying his Father-in-law in a Visitation of the Forts and Castles of that Kingdom," after which he departed for the Continent (Anon., "The Life of Sir Thomas Browne," ii). Browne's daughter Elizabeth confirmed that her father's stepfather "shewed him all Ireland in some visitation of the forts and castles."[72] As Endicott notes, "From 1620

[68] The State Papers make it clear that Nutt took not just the booty of many vessels in June 1623 but also a considerable number of "captyves." The episode proved embarrassing to the Jacobean government when a pardon sent to Nutt reached him only belatedly, and only after he had gone on a piratical rampage.

[69] A main reason for the assumption of a later date for the Irish trip is that the anonymous version of "Life of Sir Thomas Browne" included in the *Posthumous Works* states that after taking his Arts degrees, undertaking "the Physick Line," and practicing "that Faculty for some Time in *Oxfordshire*," Browne "took the Opportunity of seeing Ireland, by accompanying his Father-in-law in a Visitation of the Forts and Castles of that Kingdom" (ii).

[70] *Calendar of the State Papers Relating to Ireland... 1625–1632*, ed. Robert Pentland Mahaffy (London: Stationery Office, 1900), 498–9, 500–1, 528. But these views from the later 1620s probably reflect Caroline policy on the "Graces."

[71] See Arthur Wilson, *History of Great Britain, Being the Life and Reign of King James the First* (1653), 50. Thomas Wentworth, Earl of Strafford, mocked Dutton's pouting, threatening face with reference to the duel: *The Earl of Straffordе's Letters and Dispatches* (London, 1739), 1.144.

[72] C. D., *European Magazine*, 89.

we can follow [Dutton's] manœuvres to get control of a whole chain of inland forts stretching from Cloghowter in Cavan, near 1,000 acres of his own grant at Rathcline, to Toome in Londonderry, and Lifford in Donegal" (Endicott, "Sir Thomas Browne as 'Orphan,'" 197). But the manuscript evidence vividly demonstrates that a crucial moment in Dutton's assumption of his duties and of this property occurred from April 1623 through the summer. In 1622 he had "built a house of lyme & stone, 42 foot long, and 21 foot broad, 2 stories high slated...In which house the said Cap.t Dutton, his Wife, and Familie dwell."[73] On May 20, 1623, Dutton petitioned the Privy Council that he was now ready to claim the Irish properties granted him by James some three years past.[74] In July there was top-level discussion of the conditions of his contract, but also the recommendation that "if S:r Tho: Dutton will passe his lands, accordinge to his Ma:ts instruccons he may therein vse his owne libertie."[75] By September a survey of forts and castles was produced, with an account of how much money would be required to repair and strengthen them.

In the *Pseudodoxia* but also in letters to daughter Elizabeth and to Sir William Dugdale, Browne recalled sights or experiences from his Irish expedition, and he left two versions of a poem memorializing the stormy journey homeward across the Irish Sea. What is striking about these recorded memories is that they never directly touch on the human tragedy of colonization, though *Religio Medici*'s disinclination for polemic and persecution surely reflects that experience. Browne's recorded memories of Ireland concern themselves not with human activities, offices, and conflicts, but with natural phenomena of concern both to a curious natural historian and a meditative natural theologian. Especially given the poem in which Browne assails the practice of dueling, it would appear that his Irish trip with an infamously quarrelsome veteran of military action in the Low Countries had a capillary effect on Browne's defenses of peace in verse and prose alike, but also on his mature conviction that the study of nature had a way of uniting (and civilizing) the naturalists. If indeed Browne had commenced that trip from Winchester in the captivity of John Nutt, then savage violence could have even more profoundly disturbed the vacation between grammar school and university. Add to this the tempest at sea that Browne confronted on his voyage homeward to England, and this moment of transition in his life was sufficiently cataclysmic as to provoke the soon-to-be Oxford student to reconsider the clerical course of life to which Winchester scholars were so commonly directed.

The fortresses in question were numerous.[76] Indeed, as contemporary records attest, Dutton's holdings were even more extensive than the category "inland"

[73] BL Additional MS. 1756, f. 116v.

[74] SP 63/237, f. 54, May 20, 1623.

[75] SP 63/237, f. 94r-v.

[76] For a list of the properties, see Endicott, "Sir Thomas Browne as 'Orphan,'" 209. For a contemporary critique of the award as not in the royal interest, see George O'Brien, ed., *Advertisements for Ireland*, an extra volume of the Royal Society of Antiquaries of Ireland (Dublin: The Royal Society of Antiquaries of Ireland, 1923), 17. See also George Hill, *An Historical Account of the Plantation in Ulster at the Commencement of the Seventeenth Century, 1608–1620*, intro. John G. Barry (Shannon, Ireland: Irish University Press), 501–2.

comprises, since "the forts of Donnagall and Liffer be not inland but the one stands upon the sea and the other upon the river of Loughfoile."[77] From Dublin, Browne's journey to see these structures would have taken him (for example) northward for 90 or 100 miles through Armagh (with its two castles named) to Toome toward the top of the island in Antrim, then across the northernmost part of the province of Ulster to the fortresses in Donegal before descending to Enniskillen on Lough Erne, to the castles or forts in Monaghan and Cavan, then south still farther to the properties in the province of Connaght. Dutton's stone house in Rathcline was the southernmost point in the circuit. The forts or castles that they visited would not have been comfortable places in which to stay. One of the more dominant designs was the so-called tower-house, which was usually a cramped, thatched square keep.[78] Indeed, seventeenth-century visitors voiced their complaints about these tower-houses, though an English visitor, Luke Gernon, conceded that the hosts of the tower-houses could be amply hospitable.[79] By contrast to the sturdy tower-houses, forts such as Charlemont tended to feature more free-standing buildings of far greater transience.[80]

Much as he recalled the sight of a comet and an ostrich from his Winchester days, Browne tended to remember the fauna and flora of the Ulster colony. In the *Pseudodoxia*, the question arises whether Ireland is in fact devoid of venomous creatures and, if so, whether this benefit can be attributed to the sacred power of St Patrick. It was a question of concern to colonists from the Elizabethan and early Stuart periods, for instance, to Barnabe Rich, who in *A New Description of Ireland* (1610) marshaled evidence to the contrary of Catholic claims that the dearth of poisonous animals was a gift from God, as surely as their presence was a punishment for sin.[81]

Regarding spiders, Browne looks to Ireland with the curiosity of a natural historian which might offer a gentle antidote to the strife and violence all around him on a tour among castles and forts in Ulster. In a letter to Sir William Dugdale from November 1659, Browne's memory of the natural resources of Ireland is more personal and more evocative of the human capacity for feckless destruction. Dugdale has inquired about evidence taken from a number of eastern counties in England that fenland was "at first firme land, the sea having no recourse into it"; the "ocular testimony" includes certain fallen fir trees, "not cut of wth any Axe or such like thing, but burnt, the coale appearing upon the ends where they were so burnt asunder" (Keynes, 4.317). Admitting that the reason why trees "should have burnt bottomes, seemes very obscure," he offers the first of two explanations "from the

[77] Quoted by Endicott, "Sir Thomas Browne as 'Orphan,'" 196.

[78] Edward MacLysaght, *Irish Life in the Seventeenth Century* (Dublin: Irish Academic Press, 1979), 94; cf. L. M. Cullen, *The Emergence of Modern Ireland: 1600–1900* (New York: Holmes & Meier, 1981), 26–8.

[79] See Brian De Breffny, *Castles of Ireland* (London: Thames and Hudson, 1977), 18–19. For dimensions, see *Nicholas Pynnar's 1618–19 Survey of Ulster*, in W. Harris, ed., *Hibernica: Or, some Antient Pieces relating to Ireland* (1770).

[80] G. A. Hayes-McCoy, ed., *Ulster and Other Irish Maps c.1600* (Dublin: Stationery Office, 1964), 7.

[81] Barnabe Rich, *A New Description of Ireland* (London: 1610), 43–6.

custome of Barbarous nations abounding in wood & making little account thereof; who ordinarily cutt not downe their trees for fuell, but upon occasion make a fire about the bottome, & fire the tree about the lower part, wherin having served their turnes, they depart." Among such reckless consumers of woodland might be included "our uncivilized predecessors" in England, as well as natives of the New World whose "burnt trees" have been spotted by voyagers seeking "the North-west passage," and finally the Irish: "The like I have often observed in Ireland, where passing through large woods I have observed many hundred trees, burnt at the bottome, the trunke yet standing in many" (4.321). The burning of Irish natural resources comes, Browne avers, not from the more obvious source of fiery destruction in the "scorched-earth policy" carried out by the English military, but from the native Irish disregard for the value of that extensive woodland through which Browne had ample opportunity to travel on his tour of the north.[82]

If Browne never fully credits the Gaelic Irish with the capacity for civility, piety, and the advancement of learning, he seems unready to dismiss them as benighted savages. In a 1682 letter to Edward, for instance, his account of a book entitled *A Prospect of the State of Ireland, from the yeare of the world 1756 to the yeare of Christ 1652* borders on dismissal when Browne points out that its author is "a Romanist" whose sources are "2 preists" and whose decision to reprint the first part of the work without offering its completion in a second part leaves the reader with a text lacking in a certain believability. But Browne's way of putting his critiques is oblique and even hopeful. Without explaining just why, Browne concludes that "few will take any pleasure to read it who have not been in Ireland and is acquainted with the old histories of that country" (4.228).

Browne's most extended meditation on nature during his Irish travels comes in the form of a poem, left in two versions, about his experience of the stormy seas between Dublin and Chester. Writing to Elizabeth in September 1681, Browne seeks to console his daughter, now in Guernsey, when she has seen "such an uncomfortable sight, as to behold a ship cast away, so neer you" (Keynes, 4.200). Aside from Elizabeth's brother, the naval officer Thomas, who experienced heavy winds and seasickness in his career, father Browne remembers that "I came once from Dublin to Chester at Michaelmas and was so tossed, that nothing but milk and Possets would goe down with me 2 or 3 days after; yr self is not impatient, you will have noe Cause to be sad, give noe way unto Malencholy, wch is purely sadnes without a reasonable cause." The chain of associations between melancholy, a sense of helplessness in the face of natural disasters and diseases, and the need for a strong faith in divine dispensations, is also found in a poem that Browne wrote on his transition from Ireland back to England, a trip that is transitional in other ways as well. The stormy journey is also depicted as something of a dark night of the soul for the believer in divine providence, though its couplets and conceits retain an awkward self-regard for their own wit, artifice, and learning. The poem appears in

[82] For Irish woodland and the scorched-earth policy, see R. A. Butlin, "Land and People, c. 1600," in T. M. Moody et al., eds., *A New History of Ireland, III: Early Modern Ireland, 1534–1691* (Oxford: Clarendon Press, 1976), 142–7.

a fragmentary state together with a few other sets of verses in a manuscript addressed to an unknown inquirer. Its incomplete state Browne chalks up to the failure of his memory: "The rest I have utterly forgott." A fuller, supposedly complete text, was copied into Elizabeth's commonplace book.

Both versions question the winds about why they are so angry and each offers a variety of reasons for the anger: 1) the waves themselves have an aspiring arrogance, a desire to topple the natural order according to which the element of fire transcends that of water (both versions); 2) the stormy sea picks on each traveler "as though each man a Jonas were," though no implication is drawn from this everyman-a-resistant-prophet motif (both versions); 3) some pagan Fury or "malicious hagge" has magically unleashed the winds (full version); and 4) God is angry (both versions). The two versions differ, however, on how they express an angry biblical God. In the fragment, Browne addresses God directly with what might be a challenge to, or an expression of wonder at, the disproportionate effort made with the storm: "what paynes thou takst great god to kill | those who are nothing, at thy will" (Keynes, 3.234). Why *is* God causing so much trouble to punish men whom he might simply will into suffering? In the full version, the rhyme is altered so that God works "to drowne | Those who are nothing at thy frowne."

The biggest difference between the two versions is that in the longer one owned by Elizabeth, Browne concludes with a hopeful prayer: "In vayne we do the Pilot coart: | the bottome of the sea's our Port. | no Anckers in the sea wee cast; | Our Ancker is in heaven fast. | our only hopes on him wee Laye | to whom both Seas and winds obeye." According to the copy kept by Elizabeth, Browne wrote these words "at the Crowe Inne in Chester at his Coming from Ireland." Although he had survived the infamously stormy seas between the islands now long at war, he chose to depict the storm as in progress, and the passengers as resolving, in the crisis, to rely on God rather than on any heroic navigator.[83] The transitional, agonizing experience of the storm was what Browne wanted to capture, no doubt in part because he continued to experience it for days at the Inn in which he could keep nothing down but "milk and Possets." Rendered thus childlike in the homeland of his paternal ancestors and of Dutton as well, Browne sought to express his reliance on God through all the stormy transitions from birth to death but he also resorted to another resource, the "wit" of a Winchester education. If each man is a Jonas from whom God exacts a difficult office, then Browne will supplement his reliance on a sometimes strange, disproportionate God with a "Poetick knack" productive of laughter. The poem makes a case, not for the easy harmonization of the serious and the playful, but for the human need for the comfort of art and wit in the overwhelming nausea that the passages of life can concoct. In speaking of this experience as being "shipwrackt" in *Religio Medici* (Patrides, 133), Browne stressed the significance of this stormy voyage on the verge of his Oxford years as essential to his development of faith in a God who would protect him from danger,

[83] For the stormy travels of passengers between Dublin and Chester, see MacLysaght, *Irish Life*, 264–5. Dutton's letters in the State Papers are filled with complaints about the bad weather and contrary winds.

direct his vocation, and help him to make peace with a violent, contentious world. Throughout his later works, however, Browne evinced a specific knowledge of nautical and ship-rigging practices that emphasized beyond the level of mere convention how crucial it was for him to wrest control over the potentially wild or erroneous unfolding of his own days on earth.[84]

In a poem that he wrote on the evils of dueling, Browne laments how human beings so senselessly create their own storms. Addressing the storm on the Irish Sea, Browne wonders "what furie... hath now let Loose the Aeolian bag?" Addressing the duelist, he wonders "what furie ist to take deaths part | & rather then by nature, dye by Art" (Keynes, 3.236). Indeed, compared to the artificial violence of the duel, nature's afflictions are gentle: "Diseases are the armes whereby | wee naturally do fall & dye." Unlike the wild Furies and witches of "Upon a Tempest at Sea," the Fates that control the threads of life operate with a "gentle hand." Only the artful human agent, the one who thinks in codified, ritualistic terms of honor and protocol, brings "heedlesse villany" and cruelty into the world. If in the poem on the storm young Browne seems helpless to change the course of nature, in the poem on dueling he seems equally helpless to evade the cruelty of art: willing to let others live so long as "Jared or Methusala," he nonetheless concludes with a prayer to an unnamed authority: "o let mee never know the cruell | & heedlesse villany of duell, | or if I must that fate sustayne | Let mee bee Abel & not Cain." In both poems, Browne imagines that a higher power might have a plan for him in analogy with a biblical hero. In facing the weirdness of providence at sea, when human art is wholly abandoned by the navigator, he imagines a kind of ironic but living vocation as an unwilling prophet. In the face of what artful violence can yield, however, his only model is a pious victim. It is important, of course, that Browne imagines the dueling as a family matter; whether or not this is a poem "about" Dutton, it is unquestionably a poem about the ways in which a putatively cultured, civilized code of behavior creates furious destruction and anarchy in the family of humankind to be sure, but in much smaller family units too.

Jacobean debates over the religious, moral, political, and social implications of dueling reached a new intensity and complexity in the decade just prior to Browne's Oxford years, when he was a Winchester College schoolboy moving toward manhood.[85] The malicious "furie" unleashed on the Irish sea is matched by that generated from human art, and young Browne's best hope is that providence has a plan for both. Yet the poem of duels is obviously not a rejection of human art: the very decision to write about duels in verse suggests Browne's alignment with those Winchester-manuscript wits that chose artistic pen over bloody sword in expressing their values.

Ironically, the savagery of Dutton's duel would be difficult for youthful Browne to differentiate from the violence of outlaws such as the pirate Nutt. Although in no extant record do we find Browne narrating his encounter with pirates, he would

[84] I owe my appreciation of Browne's specific knowledge of nautical matters to Claire Preston.

[85] See Markku Peltonen, *The Duel in Early Modern England: Civility, Politeness, and Honour* (New York: Cambridge University Press, 2003), 12–14, 80–145.

always remain fascinated with violence at sea, not least of course because his son Thomas would join the navy. In a letter to his son Browne described "a print of Domenic Ottoman" who, as "one of Hibraim the grand seignors sonnes...was taken at sea by a shippe of Malta 1652 at 18 yeares of age" (Keynes, 4.18). In 1623, Browne himself turned eighteen years old. Perhaps he had more cause than we have previously known to suspect that the story of his life—its "escapes of danger" (Patrides, 81)—might sound fabulous to the casual listener.

3

Oxford, 1623–1631

On August 14, 1622, the visiting examiners William Oldys and Thomas Booth determined that Thomas Browne ranked eleventh among the twenty-three seeking a scholarship at New College, Oxford.[1] Over a year later, on December 5, 1623, Browne matriculated at Broadgates Hall, Oxford.[2] At eighteen years old, he was obliged by statute to leave Winchester College. If Anthony Wood is right about Browne's entering Broadgates as a commoner,[3] Browne was required, at least at first, to pay his own way, without scholarship. Since the election roll for 1623 is missing in the Winchester archives, it is unknown whether he stood for election once again that year and, if so, how he fared.

Browne's failure to reach New College could be attributed in part to the priorities that the founder had established, not just regarding his own kin but also in erecting a hierarchy of counties from which scholars might be chosen.[4] But the process was also infamously corrupt. On July 31, 1621, Bishop Lancelot Andrewes had directed a complaint to both Winchester and New Colleges about a long-standing record of graft and bribery surrounding the elections.[5] The matriculation of commoners was far more customary in the halls than in the colleges, though the trend in Oxford was definitely in the direction of relaxed rules from the colleges too.[6] As a commoner paying his own way and expected to behave like a gentleman, Browne would to some extent have been grouped with those young men from influential families whose privileges included permission to wear non-academic dress, an invasion of the fashionable world into the scholarly one which was unwelcome to university officials.[7] He would also have been permitted to make use of the servitors.[8]

[1] Winchester College Muniments 21611.

[2] Oxford University Archives (OUA) SP/2, 266v.

[3] Anthony Wood, *Athenae Oxonienses, Fasti*, ed. Philip Bliss, 4 vols. (1813–1820; reprinted Hildesheim: Georg Olms, 1969), 4.56.

[4] See Hastings Rashdall and Robert S. Rait, *New College* (London: F. E. Robinson, 1901), 43.

[5] Winchester College MS 23236. For details, see Penry Williams, "From the Reformation to the Era of Reform 1530–1850," in John Buxton and Penry Williams, eds., *New College, Oxford, 1379–1979* (Oxford: New College, 1979), 44–71, at 52.

[6] For the various criteria, see Stephen Porter, "University and Society," in Nicholas Tyacke, ed., *The History of the University of Oxford: Volume IV, Seventeenth-Century Oxford* (Oxford: Clarendon Press, 1997), 37.

[7] See Mark H. Curtis, *Oxford and Cambridge in Transition, 1558–1642: An Essay on Changing Relations between the English Universities and English Society* (Oxford: Clarendon Press, 1958), 36–41.

[8] Porter, in Tyacke, ed., *History of the University of Oxford*, 37.

Even if the Warden of New College, Robert Pinke, was not in fact wholly resistant to new, scientific learning,[9] his college as a whole ranked among those at Oxford with the greatest disaffection for change and growth (Williams, 44).[10] Browne's failure to secure a scholarship at New College helped pave the way for his turn to medicine; his failure to receive support upon matriculation at Broadgates served as an obvious reminder that for this orphan from the middling sort, strenuous effort was going to be required. And instantly Browne made that effort, not just in contributing a poem to a commemorative volume for William Camden but, more extraordinarily, in being chosen as the one undergraduate speaker at the gala inauguration of Pembroke College when, in 1624, it was reborn from the old Broadgates Hall.

Arguably, Browne's failure to reach New College changed the course of his life both professionally and intellectually, for Pembroke College was the center of medical and anatomical studies at Oxford. It employed brilliant philosophical and theological minds such as the Platonizing, anti-Calvinist Thomas Jackson and the controversial Thomas Lushington. Broadgates-cum-Pembroke was positioned across the street from Christ Church, where Lushington's associate Richard Corbett headed a complex cadre of wits whose poetic miscellanies leavened the political and religious controversies of the decade. Indeed the patron of Browne's college, William Herbert, third Earl of Pembroke, played a central, contentious role in these conflicts.

Unlike the town of Winchester, which was suffering from the effects of decay, the town of Oxford underwent an extended period of growth from the sixteenth through much of the seventeenth century.[11] Throughout the 1620s, the head of Broadgates and Pembroke, Thomas Clayton, was assiduous in recruiting funds for new construction and effective in overseeing its completion. Browne's own speech to the distinguished audience gathered for the transformation of Broadgates into Pembroke emphasized both rebirth from the ashes—appropriately, since the Principal-turned-Master Thomas Clayton was escorting the university into the modern age of anatomical and botanical studies—and also continuity with the past. Indeed Clayton's degrees and onetime professorship in music meant that he was expert in the writings of Boethius; and Clayton's approach to medicine, far from being simply modern, was grounded in the writings of the ancients. At Pembroke, the humanist discipline of history tightly connected past to present and future: the antiquarian Camden, together with Clayton's friend Degory Wheare, epitomized the reinvention of historical discourse as a more authentic enterprise than it had been at the outset of the Renaissance. Indeed in 1672, Browne wrote John Aubrey that "old Dr Clayton" had pointed out the great historian William Camden's affiliation with

[9] See Mordechai Feingold, *The Mathematicians' Apprenticeship: Science, Universities and Society in England, 1560–1640* (Cambridge: Cambridge University Press, 1984), 55.

[10] For a further seventeenth-century assessment see Thomas Baskerville's "Account of Oxford," ed. Humphrey Baskerville, *Collectanea*, 4th series (Oxford: Oxford Historical Society, 1905), 191.

[11] A. Crossley, "Early Modern Oxford," in Alan Crossley, ed., *The Victoria History of the County of Oxford. Volume IV: The City of Oxford* (Oxford: Oxford University Press, 1979), 74, 85, 97, 94.

Broadgates (Keynes, 4.374). It was in the 1620s, then, that Browne's Janus-like position—looking with equal attentiveness backward at history, and forward at the advancement of learning—was inaugurated.

1. THE DEATH OF CAMDEN

The year 1623 was momentous for the course (and discourse) of English history in the seventeenth century, and the students at Oxford University were fully aware of it and complexly involved in its tensions, subtleties, and volatilities. Nothing shows this state of affairs more clearly than the three collections of poems put together by the university that year: one regarding Prince Charles's safe arrival in Spain, another regarding his return to England, and a third (to which Browne contributed) on the death of Camden. But the heightened contentiousness of the time during which Browne arrived at Oxford was brought into the light even more powerfully by the trouble in which his tutor Lushington found himself over a sermon during Eastertide 1624. By making offensive remarks about the sitting Parliament, Lushington joined another Broadgates preacher William Knights in demonstrating the altered political climate of the early 1620s, though the trouble with Knights derived from a very different political attack—on the divine right of kings. During 1623–24, too, religious controversy was unleashed in Oxford as well as London over the emergence of the so-called Arminians, whose supposed positions on free will, reconciliation with the Roman church, the premium on ceremony, and the exalted status of the clergy were widely held responsible for betraying the great Elizabethan legacy of true, heroic religion and for pulling the Church of England back toward popery.[12] Over the course of the 1620s Arminian critiques of Calvinism would make deep inroads into Oxford, with Thomas Lushington and Thomas Jackson, both involved in instruction at Pembroke, as prominent thinkers in this endeavor but with powerful men such as William Laud presiding over its success.

At the center of the turbulence in 1623 was the Spanish Match, Prince Charles's reckless, romantic, and incognito journey to Madrid in pursuit of the Infanta's hand in marriage.[13] It was a year of what Thomas Cogswell has called a "self-induced crisis mentality, which perceived political liberty and the Reformation in grave danger."[14] The journey itself prompted anxieties over Charles's physical and spiritual welfare, but it also alarmed the many critics of the Jacobean tendency to let peace and diplomacy resolve the crisis over the war raging between the Catholic imperial Habsburgs and the forces supportive of James's own daughter Elizabeth and her German husband, Frederick. On both sides of the summer of 1624, and almost exactly coterminous with Browne's years in Oxford, 1623–29, stretched a

[12] Nicholas Tyacke, *Anti-Calvinists: The Rise of English Arminianism, c.1590–1640* (Oxford: Clarendon Press, 1987), 84–5.

[13] See Glyn Redworth, *The Prince and the Infanta: The Cultural Politics of the Spanish Match* (New Haven, CT: Yale University Press, 2003), 51–2.

[14] Thomas Cogswell, *The Blessed Revolution: English Politics and the Coming of War, 1621–24* (New York: Cambridge University Press, 1989), 68.

period of heightened melancholy, outrage, and polemic in which collegiate culture at Pembroke and Christ Church was inwardly divided and unsettled by the domestic and international news for which the inhabitants of the famous university town increasingly hungered. When the Earl of Pembroke in 1624, then Parliament itself in 1625, came calling on Oxford, the volatile political and religious culture of the 1620s was intensely, palpably present in the town. What all this meant for Browne was an education in the assets and liabilities of aggressive speech that supported the English heroic spirit with one hand while damaging the peace of the commonwealth with the other. At stake in this tense, volatile culture was the very identity of orthodoxy itself. By the end of the decade, Christ Church poets Zouch Townley and Richard Corbett would demonstrate quite forcefully how one Oxford college, right across the road from Browne's own, could be deeply divided in a politics whose simultaneous clarity and subtlety were captured by the metaphor of a game at chess. Among the manuscripts that he owned was a copy of Thomas Middleton's *Game at Chess*, the single most explosive literary document of the years just after the demise of the Spanish Match. Browne's complex reconstruction of English piety in *Religio Medici* matured on the Continent, but his sense of the need for such an endeavor was awakened at Oxford. Moreover, it was at Oxford that Browne's lifelong interest in the world at large, its news, politics, religions, wars, and practices was forged.

In 1623 the members of Oxford University compiled two collections of poetry responsive to the events of the Spanish Match. A far more complicated response to the events of 1623 than either the anxious *Votiva* or the exuberant *Carolus Redux* marked Thomas Browne's first entry into print: *Camdeni Insignia* (1624). Camden's path to Broadgates, like Browne's own, resulted from a failure to receive a fellowship elsewhere (at Magdalen College), the first in a long series of frustrations coming out of Camden's "complex, often troubled" relationship to Oxford University.[15] When in 1622 Camden established a history lectureship in his own name and chose Degory Wheare as its inaugural holder, he was expressing his enduring commitment to a university which had neglected him and whose ways and means were, in Camden's mature understanding, infested with partisanship and conflict. Camden was a historian whose publications were internationally renowned and whose critical antiquarian method—with its attention to material evidence (coins, inscriptions, fragments of pottery, topography) and to manuscripts—was helping to revolutionize the discipline as well as secure England's place in the humanist republic of letters. His foundation of a history professorship was as much an attempt to modernize Oxford as was the Tomlins lectureship in anatomy. Schoolboys such as Browne's Winchester contemporaries encountered Camden in another capacity, as the author of their Greek textbook. Yet more than this Camden was a hero of British national and regional identity, a holdover from the heroic days of Elizabethan England, and an international star in the pantheon of sophisticated historians. Indeed, the volume of elegies was rendered all the more politically complicated by virtue of

[15] See Wyman H. Herendeen's article on William Camden in *ODNB*, from which the following account of Camden's life is taken.

its contributors' tendency to deploy the memory of heroic Camden in the political and religious conflicts of 1623–24. In this high-powered context, the young Thomas Browne confronted the challenge of conceiving his own version of active, relevant scholarship that resisted the often partisan agendas of his contemporaries.

Last in a series of four Broadgates students—after Anthony Hungerford, Nathaniel White, and Francis Chaloner—comes a twenty-line poem by "Th. Browne Generos. Lateport," Thomas Browne, a gentleman of Broadgates Hall.[16] Its prosody indebted to Horatian iambics in the first ten epodes, the poem offers its largely conventional terms of praise with assistance from Senecan tragedy:

> Quid in remotis sacra Parnassi jugis
> Vatum sedetis numina:
> Sonora doctas plectra dum mulcent deas
> Molli sopore languidas?
> Quin intumentes horror obducit genas,
> Et ora squalor nubilus,
> Planctúsq[ue] vester vincit Heliadum dolor,
> Orbísq[ue] luctus numinis.
> Viduum coronâ flete Musarum caput,
> Lugete defunctum senem,
> Cujus labores ultimi Seres canunt,
> Flavíq[ue] Gangis incolæ:
> Et quisquis alius orbe consepto jacet,
> Quà Phœbus illustrat diem.
> Quòd si quod istis numen in chordis, deos
> Mulcete plectris inferos,
> Illi resurgat clara Mausoli pyra,
> Struatur alta Pyramis.
> Vivat sepultus, dura quid pateris mori,
> Quo tota vivis, Anglia?[17]

Two noteworthy points emerge from the poem, the first being the poet's clarion call to scholarly labor over indolence. Thus Browne exhorts English poets to come out of their distant gathering place and to give public voice to national sorrow. As matters stand now, he laments, any poet who grieves for the loss of Camden sits silently without exerting a duly sanctified influence on learning (*doctas... deas*) or on the goddesses whose soft sleep is reinforced, not interrupted by,

[16] *Camdeni Insignia* (1624), C3v, spelling slightly modernized; for another version, see Keynes 3.146.

[17] "Why do you laze around on the distant slopes of Parnassus, you sacred influences of the poets, whilst sonorous lyres soothe the learned Muses, languid in soft slumber? Why doesn't dread overspread your rounded cheeks, and cloudy mourning your faces? And why doesn't your grief surpass the laments of the Heliades, and the sorrow of the mournful god? Weep the head widowed of the Muses' crown, bewail the deceased old man whose labors the distant Seres sing, and the inhabitants near the yellow Ganges; and anyone else who lies in the walled-in world, wherever Phoebus illuminates the day. And yet if there be any divine power in your strings, soothe the gods below with your lyres, so that the famous pyre of Mausolus might arise again, and the lofty pyramid be built once more. Although he is entombed, let Camden live; why do you allow him to perish, obdurate England, by whom as a whole you live?"

the contemporary soundings of the poets. Sitting is clearly opposed to the laboring of Camden himself, but it is also haplessly complicit with the contemporary role of poetry which is said to soothe the Muses as they lie "languid in soft sleep." These lyrics might sound impressive but their narcotic effect is to induce or to sustain a state of indolence in the world of learning. Their sorrow should rival that of the Heliades, the sisters of Phaeton whose tears converted into amber, but their remote silence reneges on what ought to be their sacred influence in the wake of Camden's death and in continuation of his legacy. Strikingly, this is a loss in the family, for Phaeton's father Helios also mourns, and Camden's loss of his learned crown is figured as a widowing.

In exhorting the Oxford Muses to respond actively and appropriately to Camden's death, Browne's poem makes its second noteworthy claim, that Camden's legacy (in itself and as it is transmitted by others) can influence the world at large as well as England and Oxford closer to home. With important links to the burgeoning field of critical chronology, the study of geography was enjoying a vibrant period in 1620s Oxford, with Carpenter's "very important General Geography" of 1625 joining a spate of other work by Henry Briggs, John Bainbridge, John Gregory, Peter Heylyn, and Robert Hues, in lively interaction with scholars such as James Ussher who lived and worked elsewhere.[18] In Browne's praise for Camden, however, what matters is Oxford's effect on, not simply its study of, the peoples and places of the globe. In lines 11–14, Browne claims that Camden's historical labors are heralded by the faraway Seres (in other words, peoples beyond Scythia and India, the Chinese and their neighbors), by "the inhabitants near the yellow Ganges," and indeed by people around the globe. Other allusions bring the Near East (Mausolus had his tomb in Halicarnassas) and Egypt (the pyramids) into the framework. The world may be hemmed in (*concepto*) but Camden's influence is pervasive. In these lines Browne is gathering material from Seneca's tragedy *Hercules Oetaues*, in which Deïanira explains how "*triumphos ultimi Seres canunt | et quisquis alius orbe concepto jacet*" [Hercules's "triumphs the far off Seres sing, and whoe'er besides dwells in the whole known world"].[19] Camden's scholarly labors are thus mythologized and imperialized so that, in the years just after Bacon has advertised the excitement of *Plus ultra* on the frontispiece of his *Novum Organum* (1620), the great historian's movement through the intellectual pillars of Hercules now depends on the ceaseless, various labors of the young generation. Yet as Camden's discipline (history) and Browne's ancient models remind us, movements forward, backward, and around the world are intricately bound together in scholarly methods and aims.

[18] See E. G. R. Taylor, *Late Tudor and Early Stuart Geography, 1583–1650* (London: Methuen, 1934), 136–8. The networking of Oxford and Cambridge mathematicians and scientists with the wider world of learning is documented in Feingold, *Mathematicians' Apprenticeship*. For Gregory, see *Gregorii Posthuma: or, Certain learned tracts* (1650).

[19] *The Tragedies of Seneca*, ed. and trans. Frank Justus Miller, 2 vols. (Cambridge, MA: Harvard University Press, 1961), ll. 414–15, in 2.216–17. I am indebted to Victoria Moul for help with this point and the rest of the poem.

In exhorting the Oxford poets to give active voice to their grief, Browne shifts from female to male deities, from Muses to lower gods, as the recipients of the poems. Perhaps these gods are the leaders of the university, of the nation (facing in 1624 a critical juncture in its political, religious, moral, and cultural formation), or even of the republic of letters. Whoever they might be, Browne hopes for poetic influence, for "*numen*" or "*numina*" that is neither body nor soul but the vital spirit of wit. In the final lines, Browne converts a conventional argument for the monumental fame of Camden into an admonition and exhortation. As the circumnavigation of learning makes its way from the Far East around to Africa, Browne's poem seeks to ensure that Camden's fame is trumpeted around the world, his values kept alive in public policy and pedagogy, and his books preserved always in print.

At the end of the poem, Browne returns home to England with his strongest admonition, roundly chastising England for its obduracy or cruelty: Camden's beneficent influence on the English people—he has given them life itself—has not yet been rewarded by their celebration of his name, and the poem ends with Browne's shaming of this neglect by "*dura*...*Anglia*," who seem willing to let Camden's legacy perish with his body. What the poem values is neither softness nor obduracy but numinous influence, an energy that at once soothes the aggrieved and awakens the slothful. But it also values the ability of such influence to unify: while cruel or soft England might be broken or wounded, Browne suggests that an England filled with the influence of Camden and his followers will thrive as a whole ("*tota*"). Seeking harmony in an already contentious university town, Browne expresses his desire for Oxonians to be known around the world and to exert an enlivening, enlightening effect on their own country. In the context of the collection, however, the poems give Browne's chastisement of the English a sharper point. Strikingly, the poems rarely mention King James at all and, when they do, they measure him according to the Elizabethan heritage of which Camden is an integral part. Although Browne's poem is neither strident nor polemical, it adapts the conventions of eulogy so as to resonate with the overall tenor of the collection, that Camden's death symbolizes a turning point—and perhaps a source of unity—for English scholarship and manners. Indeed, often in the Oxford of the 1620s, students and professors on both sides of contemporary conflicts appear in the same poetic miscellanies.[20]

It is unknown how or why Browne came to contribute to the collection for Camden in the early weeks of his studies in Oxford. Perhaps it was simply the thing to do, in continuation of the mastery of witty, allusive verses that Winchester boys learned to write. But there can be no question that Browne impressed Clayton and the other inhabitants of Broadgates in the first year of his residence there, for when, later in 1624, a major public ceremony was held to christen the foundation of Pembroke College, Browne was the one undergraduate asked to speak, and it was his speech that opened the proceedings.

[20] See for instance Malone MS 19, which has Winchester and New College associations.

2. THE BIRTH OF PEMBROKE COLLEGE

Beginning with William Knights, Broadgates men in the early 1620s proved themselves to have an aptitude for producing controversy when they spoke in high profile forums.[21] In Browne's very first year at Broadgates, in April 1624, his tutor Thomas Lushington became the Hall's next cause célèbre with a sermon that was more frequently copied down and culturally significant than Knights's defense of a resistance to tyrants. Its political transgressions ran in a direction entirely contrary to those of Knights's (directly insulting Parliament rather than the monarch), though, with Prince Charles and Buckingham as eager as the godly sort of anti-Catholics for outright conflict with Spain, a slight on Parliament in April 1624 might just as well as double as an attack on the royal family.[22] But Lushington's problem was not reducible to politics, for the authorities were displeased by his rhetorical impersonations of biblical characters, especially "lower" ones, a performance greeted with delighted applause by the auditors at the university church of St Mary's. At stake in the sermon, then, was not just what, politically, one could say, but also how, in terms of the vexed notion of Christian decorum, one might make a religious argument.

For Browne, the relationship between peace, conformity, and volatile polemic would gain a prominent place in *Religio Medici*. Even more germane for Browne's education was the fact Lushington's sermons investigated the epistemology of religion—an interest that the preacher shared with Thomas Jackson—as well as the logical and rhetorical discourses that human beings put to use in the process of attempting to understand, to represent, and to worship the divine. Lushington's playful and exploratory approach to skepticism serves as his most palpable contribution to Browne's intellectual development. Above all, the Lushington episode was a powerful yet complex lesson in how experimental thought and playful rhetoric would always have to navigate between the extremes of toadyism and transgression.[23] Indeed he appeals to the liberty of philosophizing in a mediation between peaceful community and bold individual speculation that anticipates one of *Religio Medici*'s most vital concerns. Defending solitary conjecture in modification of the sermon's overall emphasis on corporate submission, Lushington urges that his university audience remember the value of the truth-seeking intellect:

> Let us not be thought over-weening for casting now and then a conjecture diverse from the common current. We are free Denisons of Christendom, and may challenge the liberty of our thoughts as well as out-landish men. Let their learning not out-look us, for where the Scripture leaves us, all learning lies lame, and her two truths are Criticismes and Conjectures. (1658, 79)

[21] For the Knights episode, see Bodleian MS Wood D. 18, f. 45r–46r; and Douglas Macleane, *A History of Pembroke College Oxford* (Oxford: Oxford Historical Society, 1897), 144–5.

[22] Huntley has worked most extensively with Lushington, in his biography of Browne but also in articles. For the biography, see especially 43–5; see also "Sir Thomas Browne and his Oxford Tutor: or, Academic Guilt by Associaton," *The History of Ideas News Letter* 2, no. 3 (1956), 50–3; and "Dr. Thomas Lushington (1590–1661), Sir Thomas Browne's Oxford Tutor," *Modern Philology* 81 (1983), 14–23.

[23] Cf. Corpus Christi College 288, 247r, with the 1658 edition, *The Resurrection Rescued from the Souldiers Calumnies*, 70–3.

Lushington's defense of the intellect, of its efforts by way of criticism and conjecture to boost our understanding when scripture abandons it, shows that Browne's tutor introduced his charge to the powerful, if discomforting, efforts of the singular mind on behalf of truth. Lushington also prods the officials in his audience with the element of shame, essentially making the case that Oxford had better not let foreign universities surpass them in what a fellow of Exeter College, Nathanael Carpenter, in a 1621 publication had termed "*philosophia libera*."[24] Browne would encounter other versions of the liberty of philosophizing on the Continent, but his first glimpse of its attractions and perils came by way of his Oxford tutor.

When in late summer 1624 Browne was invited to take part in the inauguration of Pembroke College, then, his stress on a phoenix-like rejuvenation of a Hall whose very name suggested the way to perdition was more significant than the young scholar's admirable lightness of touch and good humor might let on. In keeping with the role of collegiate society in general, the Pembroke statutes of 1624 emphasized that the College was to operate as "a well-ordered Family in the due subordination and mutual helpfulness of its different parts."[25] In Browne's case, the notion of a surrogate family was further complicated by the fact that his tutor was an infamous wit with a record of trouble with the authorities—a far cry, to be sure, from Browne's respectable biological father. One of the most curious and wholly unsubstantiated legends about Browne surely bears this stigma out, namely, that Oxford had expelled him for his debauched behavior and opposition to all religion.[26]

On August 5, 1624, the day on which the Gowrie plot was commemorated, the letters patent and Charter of Mortmain were read in hall, and the masters, fellows, and scholars of the new college were officially admitted before a distinguished company including Vice Chancellor John Prideaux, Lord Dormer and his brother William, Sir Francis Godolphin, Sir John Smith, Dr. Daniel Featly, and the mayor, recorder, and principal burgesses of the donor's hometown, Abingdon. The public speakers announcing and celebrating the transition from hall to college were eager to emphasize continuity—that a good body of learning was being made better and larger. Thus Clayton would slide from principal to master, taking a vigorous role in raising the numbers of entering students from just three to twenty-nine in his very first year as master.

It was to this theme of continuity within rebirth that young Browne applied his wit in the opening speech.[27] Identified as an undergraduate commoner of the college, Browne playfully projects on his auditors an excited anticipation of his verdict regarding the change from Broadgates to Pembroke. With the first sentence suspended

[24] Nathanael Carpenter, *Philosophia libera, triplici exercitationum decade proposita* (1621).

[25] For the statutes, see Macleane, *History of Pembroke College*, 185–9. For family, see James McConica, "The Collegiate Society," *History of the University of Oxford: Volume III, The Collegiate University* (Oxford: Clarendon Press, 1986), 666.

[26] Douglas Macleane, *Pembroke College* (a shorter and revised version of the other text, 108), reprinted by Routledge/Thoemmes Press, 1998, from an 1898–1903 edition; the legend is attributed to "Clement, keeper of the French King's Library (ob. *c.*1705)."

[27] The text of the speech, printed in Keynes, 3.148–49, is offered "with minor corrections" from its seventeenth-century appearance as *Natalitia Collegii Pembrochiani Oxonii* (1624) in Henry Savage, *Balliofergus, or a Commentary upon the Foundation, Founders and Affaires, of Balliol Colledge* (Oxford, 1668), 92.

while he reminds his fellow students that they are on the verge of, not quite through, their transformation, Browne jokes that some gloomy, mistaken auditors will treat the occasion as a funeral of tragic proportions. Turning to thank the honorific founder of the College, he explains that their house is not a dying elder but a lost and orphaned child whose foundation is really an adoption or even an authoring by a kindly surrogate father, the Earl of Pembroke. His tutelage will ennoble the hall's brick (punning on the Latin term for Broadgates and for brick, "*de Lateportensi*" and "*de lateritia*") into marble.

Pursuing a little further his playful chastisement of those captious auditors who might show ingratitude toward their patron, Browne turns to make his most rhetorically delicate gesture—toward a continuity with the past that nonetheless does not minimize the value of the gift. On the one hand, the change is nominal and slight at that. On the other, Broadgates has always been an ironic name suggestive of the road to perdition, but Pembroke by contrast is a splendid ("*magnificum*") name, and in any case the orphaned child will lose nothing and indeed has nothing of such considerable private value that a change for the common good does not trump. In making this more complicated, if still lighthearted, point about rights and privileges, Browne imagines that the private should and will readily submit not just to the common good ("*de communi boni*") but to Pembroke's public power ("*fasces*").

Browne's climactic conceit for praising the transformation of hall into college is his image of the phoenix rising "*ex Aulæ antiquæ ruderibus*," "from the rubble of the ancient hall." As the mythological bird whose rebirth can suggest circularity and continuity, Pembroke retains a kind of identity with Broadgates' past, the two together possessing uniqueness and durability. But the Pembroke phoenix as Browne depicts it is reborn not in flames or from its own ashes but from Broadgates' lifeless shambles. The transformation offers the students a new vitality, nobility, and aspiration onward and upward that in Browne's speech leave a ruined antiquity behind, one ironically lacking a serious or redemptive name. His word for the condition of rising, "*excitatam*," suggests an awakening or a dislodging from a state of lethargy, even a raising of a spirit from the dead. It can carry the sense, too, of being obligated to act, or of being flushed like a hunted bird from the brush. But as with the erected ears and eager expectation that Browne projects on his audience, so too with his rising phoenix: the young scholars of Broadgates are encouraged to see this ceremony as a rite of passage in which they, with the university, are roused, inspired, and provoked into a brilliant maturity. And they are activated into this brave future within the protected environs of a college with a patron who, as Browne puts it, should be allowed to enter their hearts as well as their hall. Just as in *Camdeni Insignia* Browne urges poets to rouse themselves to substitute labor for lethargy, so too (though more prominently) on the birth of Pembroke: Browne elevates the fervid, ennobling activity of learning over the value of protecting the shards of the past.[28] In both cases for young Browne, the study of the past itself has been and must be vibrantly transformed.

[28] Browne studies the legend of the phoenix over the course of a chapter in *Pseudodoxia Epidemica*, ed. Robbins, 1.202–8, making sure to clarify the arguments against its natural existence while continuing to detail its moral and rhetorical value.

As the leader of the new college, Thomas Clayton devoted enormous energy to making Pembroke a haven for and symbol of a rich pedagogical synthesis. In this amalgam could be found a revised version of the seven medieval liberal arts, together with the humanist recovery of classical texts and a shift of emphasis to moral philosophy, history, poetry, and natural philosophy. In tandem with these ingredients were Clayton's instigation and active pursuit of what can fairly be called a modernizing reinvention of Oxford's medical instruction. Finally, with the likes of Lushington and Thomas Jackson, Clayton opened Pembroke's doors to theological and philosophical thinking with a proneness to move beyond the commonplace. The contrast of such active reinvention with the degeneration of college community at Browne's Winchester is a stark one indeed; Oxford opened for Browne the possibility that his scholarly fate might achieve some type of heroic greatness that might transform even the wide world.

3. LEARNING AT PEMBROKE

Although we do not know how closely Browne worked with or came to know Principal then Master Thomas Clayton between 1623 and 1631 when the graduate departed for Montpellier, it is fair to say that Clayton's presiding influence and professional focus changed the course of Browne's life. As Wood noted, Browne "took the degrees in arts," then "as a member of [Pembroke] coll[ege] entred on the physic line, and practised that faculty for some time in these parts" before setting out for Montpellier, Padua, and Leiden.[29] There can be no question that Clayton guided Browne not just to medicine but toward particular habits of thought within the medical vocation.

For one thing, Clayton was well known for harmonizing medicine and divinity. According to Robert Burton of Christ Church, Clayton spoke persuasively in 1621 of a reconciliation between physical and spiritual medicine, arguing that an analogy obtains between the two medicines (even if the means and the object differ significantly) and that human nature is governed by interactions between the body and the soul, so that a divine may have an effect on the body, a physician influence the health of the soul.[30] Clearly the future author of *Religio Medici* found in Clayton an influential model. Clayton's renown for his piety as a physician found its witnesses both before and after the *Anatomy of Melancholy* first appeared in 1621. In 1612, John Day dedicated his "concio ad clerum" to Clayton, thanking this doctor of medicine for being the most attentive auditor of the sermon, and for excelling in his understanding that health of both body and soul requires our sedulous cultivation.[31] Even a potentially hostile witness, Henry Savage, eulogized Clayton in his profiles of Balliol men as, among other things, "a good Divine"

[29] Wood, *Fasti*, IV.56.

[30] Robert Burton, *The Anatomy of Melancholy*, ed. Floyd Dell and Paul Jordan-Smith (New York: Tudor, 1927), 29.

[31] John Day, *Concio ad Clerum, Preached at St Mary's Oxford, 1612* (Oxford: 1612), dedication.

whose "skill" in religion "he did so seasonably exercise towards his Patients, that it rendred him worthy of double honour."[32]

It was precisely this intimacy between religious and medical aims that defined the mission of the Tomlins lectureship in anatomy. According to the statutes of the lectureship, dated November, 1624, the foundation was premised on the conviction that "the knowledge and true understanding of mans body and the parts and faculties of the same doth much conduce to the honor and glory of God our mightie and wonderfull creator." What is more, anatomy "is also of great vse to the Professors of Diuinitie, Philosophy and all other good Literature" as well as "more particularly necessary for the faculties and Arte of Phisicke and Chirurgery, the perfection whereof doth much avayle to the safety health and comfort of the whole Com[m]on wealth in the conservation of theire persons."[33] Not only did Tomlins choose the Regius Professor of Medicine to undertake the first of the anatomy lectureships, but it seems probable that Clayton pursued the foundation in the first place.[34]

Even more than the recently instituted Savilian lectureships in geometry and astronomy (founded 1621), which for all their interest in cutting-edge work might be seen as an extension of the seven liberal arts of medieval fame, a lectureship in anatomy was medicine's version of the Camden lectureship in history, the Sedleian lectureship in natural philosophy (the first being Edward Lapworth), or the White lectureship in moral philosophy, that is, an extension of humanism's efforts to update, refocus, and transform the university curriculum. What is more, Bainbridge and Lapworth were themselves medical men with MDs, so that practically, intellectually, as well as socially, medicine intersected with the other areas of curricular revision and contributed integrally to one of the most exciting moments in the history of the university. The very fact that Clayton, a professor of medicine and not a divine, was in the position of a college head, indicates quite clearly that at the time of Browne's arrival in Oxford, medicine was undergoing an unprecedented promotion and infusion of energy.

To ensure that the anatomy lectures took place on a regular basis, the Tomlins statutes offered guidelines for their preparation, execution, and compensation. Immediately after the Lenten Assizes, the lecturer was to procure the sound body of an executed prisoner or some other body if no prisoner was available. The body was then to be dissected by an adept chirurgeon—Clayton chose Bernard Wright for this role—while the lecturer himself demonstrated "the Scituation, Nature, vse and office of the partes of the body" in four lectures over the next two days, each morning from between eight and nine, each afternoon at two, and in all four cases to last a duration of two hours. In conventional fashion, the lectures would proceed from the "natural" faculties—liver, spleen, stomach, guts, and their neighbors (two lectures on these)—to the "vital" parts on the following morning (heart, lungs, thorax),

[32] *Balliofergus*, 117; cf. MS Rawlinson D.810, f. 44r.

[33] Oxford University Archives NEP supra/register N, f. 194.

[34] Robert G. Frank, "Medicine," in Nicholas Tyacke, ed., *The History of the University of Oxford: Volume IV* (Oxford: Clarendon Press, 1997), 541.

followed in the afternoon of the second day by the "animal" parts and faculties, principally the brain. In addition, the anatomy lecturer was instructed to explain the skeleton in three lectures, but these were to take place every Michaelmas term at the usual hour of the medical lecture. For the sake of integrating anatomy into the medical curriculum, the Tomlins statutes also encouraged the lecturer to introduce and expatiate on anatomical points over the course of the entire year.[35]

With the first lecture taking place on March 12, 1625, Clayton appears to have been typically proactive and strenuous in his duties, synthesizing the humanist physician's double-bound duty to books and direct experience. If on the one hand Clayton was largely a traditional Galenic physician who premised all medical knowledge on a theory of physiology, on the other he was relatively "comfortable" working with the cadaver, as well as renowned for his clinical skill, and he was "mildly congenial" to changes in the field such as Harvey's discovery of the circulation, published in 1628 and defended by one of Clayton's students in 1633.[36] In overseeing the publication of Caspar Bartholin's *Anatomicæ institutiones* in 1633, Clayton showed himself vigilant in improving the instruction of anatomy, but also in reconciling textual and experiential learning. Under Clayton, this synthesis of book and body was still weighted in the favor of the former, with Galen and Hippocrates always serving as the lenses through which the body would be viewed.[37] But Clayton's leadership in establishing anatomy and botany in Oxford, as well as his eagerness to have students such as Browne study on the Continent, all testifies to a mentor whose traditionalism was at once energetic and flexible.

Equally important, Clayton's association with other Oxford intellectuals modeled for Browne a conception of the integrity or "round" of learning that Browne would pursue for the bulk of his adult life in *Pseudodoxia Epidemica*. In a letter dated August 6, 1621, Henry Briggs expressed this sentiment to Samuel Ward at Cambridge University when he noted that the new lectureships, including Sedley's in natural philosophy and White's in moral philosophy, were of a piece with the foundation of the physic garden in improving the curriculum at Oxford.[38] In his poem in a 1622 commemorative volume for Sir Henry Savile, Clayton expressed his focus on and enthusiasm for the future of the university by addressing the two inaugural recipients of the Savilian lectureships in geometry and astronomy, Henry Briggs and John Bainbridge.[39] The Master of Pembroke was also close to Degory Wheare and indeed was partly responsible for bringing Wheare to Camden's attention when it was time to elect the first of the Camden lecturers in history.[40] In

[35] OUA/NEP supra/register N, 195v–197v.

[36] Robert G. Frank, Jr., *Harvey and the Oxford Physiologists: A Study of Scientific Ideas* (Berkeley: University of California Press, 1980), 26.

[37] Frank, "Medicine," 521.

[38] Tanner MS 73/1, f. 68.

[39] *Vltima linea Savilii* (1622), F2r–F2v.

[40] My account of Wheare is indebted to J. H. M. Salmon's article in *ODNB* and to his "Precept, Example, and Truth: Degory Wheare and the Ars Historica," in Donald R. Kelley and David Harris Sacks, eds., *The Historical Imagination in Early Modern Britain: History, Rhetoric, and Fiction, 1500–1800* (Cambridge: Cambridge University Press, 1997), pp. 11–36. For Clayton's part in Wheare's election, see Salmon "Precept," 20.

letters to Clayton, Wheare tends to single out his friend's "*humanitas*."[41] By this term, Wheare means to praise more than just Clayton's kindness or consideration; the new Camden lecturer envisions his supporter Clayton as a leader in the republic of letters, one who understands which disciplines matter most, how they are implicated in one another, and the need to clarify and advance the method of studying them for the benefit of the commonwealth.

In keeping with both his medical learning and his antiquarian interests, Clayton did not neglect medieval history and culture. In *Balliofergus*, Savage praised Clayton for his ability to understand Avicenna "without an Interpreter" (*Balliofergus*, 117). Both Pembroke College and the Bodleian were recipients of medieval manuscripts donated by Clayton, with a special focus on illuminated medical texts.[42] Doubtless Clayton's strongest link to medieval learning, however, was his background in music, another point of significance to the author of *Religio Medici*.[43] If his musical interests were theoretical, then Clayton was a specialist in the influential treatise of Boethius, the *Institutio Musica*,[44] an expertise that would challenge any neat bifurcation in Browne's education between Clayton's medical focus on the transitory world and Lushington's abstraction into logic and Neoplatonic emanations. By coming under the influential sphere of a musical physician, Browne studied in a world in which it made perfect sense for a medical man to include among his beliefs the notion that "there is a musicke where-ever there is a harmony, order or proportion," and that the widest range of musical performances—from church to tavern, as it were—could teach "an Hieroglyphicall and shadowed lesson of the whole world, and Creatures of God, such a melody to the eare as the whole world well understood, would afford the understanding."[45]

The best glimpse of Clayton's leadership in an Oxford republic of letters is his consultation with George Hakewill, in which he joins forces with Bainbridge, Lapworth, and Briggs in representing Oxford and England as seminaries of progressive knowledge. In the testimonials to the argument against the decay of learning found in Hakewill's *An Apologie or Declaration of the Power and Providence of God in the Government of the World* (first edition, 1627), Clayton takes the more modest and

[41] MS Selden supra 81, 64v and 65v.

[42] The Bodleian collection includes MS Auct F.5.31 with texts including Dioscorides, Galen, Aristotle's medical advice to Alexander, French medical advice, and illustrations of herbs; MS. Bodl. 591, with more medieval medical material; and MS e. Mus. 19, including work by Rhazes, Avicenna, and several texts on chirurgery. This third manuscript was given to Clayton by Dr Anyan of Corpus Christi on April 17, 1627; it includes an opening set of images from the life of Christ, as well as images of surgical instruments and of various chirurgeons treating their patients. Its margins show a sprinkling of early modern notations. For Pembroke's collection of Clayton's medieval manuscripts, see *Sixth Report to the Historical MSS Commission*, appendix, 549–50. Clayton's interest in Rhazes and Avicenna through the 1620s may have sparked Browne's interest in treatments of smallpox.

[43] See C. F. Abdy Williams, *A Short Historical Account of the Degrees in Music at Oxford and Cambridge* (New York: Novello, Ewer and Co., 1893), 17–21. John Ward, *The Lives of the Professors of Gresham College*, facsimile of the 1740 edition (New York: Johnson Reprint Corporation, 1967); for Clayton, 208–11.

[44] Henry Chadwick, *Boethius: The Consolations of Music, Logic, Theology, and Philosophy* (Oxford: Clarendon Press, 1981), 85–101. See also P. M. Gouk's essay on music at Oxford in Tyacke, ed., *History of the University of Oxford: Volume IV*, 622–3.

[45] Patrides, *Religio Medici*,149–50.

central of two rival strands in the massive volume; for if at times Hakewill suggests that in learning as in religion, the moderns have advanced over the ancients, his main argument is that nature and its artistic manifestations remain the same through the course of time (C1r-C1v). As Robin Robbins has shown, the cautious progressivism of Hakewill's argument was deeply influential on Browne, whose *Pseudodoxia Epidemica* reworks both its more conservative and progressive strains of thought.[46]

Browne's own tutor, Thomas Lushington, purveyed a brilliant ability to illuminate traditions of logic, moral philosophy, metaphysics, and theology in a brave new light. In the 1620s, Lushington was sufficiently affable to win the favor of Richard Corbett, the festive, anti-Puritanical, pro-Buckingham poet and cleric who would take Lushington with him to Norfolk in the 1630s and whose drinking parties with Lushington became the stuff of legend. But even in the 1620s, no one would ever have accused him of innocuousness. In a text published in 1655, a former student is emphatic, if not entirely reliable, on the point that Lushington was a serpent in the Oxford garden for those youth attempting to find true religion:

> For my one particular, I think I have as great cause as any, to admire the goodnesse of the Lord herein; that when I came from the University a foe and not friend to his truth and people, having been trained up under Dr Lushington, an Atheisticall, Arminian, Popish Tutor, and now a Socinian and a Mortalist: yet then the Lord of his own free grace brought me amongst you, and set me at the feet of Learned, Pious, Orthodox Divines, who instructed me in the way of the Lord, and where the foundation of that little I have was laid.[47]

Even factoring in a degree of revisionist history here, it seems safe to say that the Lushington of the 1620s was leaning away from rigid predestinarian theology as well as toward a style of worship with an unabashed affection for ceremony. It is significant for the author of *Religio Medici*, however, that the master, Clayton, was not a strict and partisan Arminian; he was, for instance, also very good friends with strong Calvinists such as Thomas Anyan of Corpus Christi. No doubt what attracted Clayton to Lushington—and to Thomas Jackson for that matter—was that they brought a powerful exploratory intellect to questions of discourse, metaphysics, and theology, and that their tendencies (if loosely Arminian) were not so easily reducible to a label and certainly not identical with one another. As early as *Religio Medici*, Browne was interweaving the same tendencies toward probing skepticism, Platonism, and doctrinal flexibility that Lushington and Jackson had modeled, but he never wholly abandoned the Calvinist doctrine that he had imbibed as a boy in London.

Because logic was the cornerstone of the Oxford curriculum, Lushington's publication of *Logica analytica* is not surprising; though published in 1650, the work in all likelihood reflects Lushington's work as a tutor in the 1620s. It joins a number of other logic textbooks—by Robert Sanderson and Richard Crackanthorpe, for

[46] Robbins, ed., *Pseudodoxia Epidemica*, 1.xxiii–xxiv.

[47] Thomas Hall, *The Beauty of Holiness* (London, 1655), A4r–A4v.

instance—as guides to "the principles, rules, and use of right reason" according to the subtitle of Lushington's book. It is revealing, however, that Browne characterized the work as a treatise on "Logick after a new method" (Keynes, 4.376), and that his own views of logic in *Religio Medici* were critical and provisional. For, like so many other logicians of the period, Lushington believed that logic could retain its vital role in the university curriculum only if it was rigorously and carefully reformed. By the 1620s, the pressure for reform had accumulated from a variety of sources: early, from the humanist critique of scholasticism, then from Ramism, skepticism, and, most recently, Baconian induction. Logic needed to prove its utility in the commonwealth, its support for the rhetorical dispensation of civic, moral, and spiritual wisdom, and its greater flexibility in the face of the skeptical demolition of apodictic and "necessary" demonstration. For Lushington, the reformation of logic involved not so much innovation but the recovery, purgation, and clarification of a genuine Aristotelian logic. But in the process of this "recovery," Lushington evinced epistemological anxieties that recur in his theological and philosophical works and that capture the ways in which he attempted to help his students grasp the limits, aspirations, and problems of human discourse.

Lushington recovers and adapts Aristotelian logic in the service of a Neoplatonic mediation between the one and the many. In the 1630s, not only would Browne's *Religio Medici* raise the question of whether syllogisms can capture spiritual mysteries, but it would also frequently (yet variously) assert that the visible world of the many reflected the invisible reality of the divine. It is noteworthy, then, that Lushington's logic is preoccupied with establishing the progress between these very realms. And like his tutor, Browne is fascinated by the ways in which geometry collaborates with (or substitutes for) logic in guiding human beings between the divine and the creatural. For Browne, however, Lushington's skepticism about his own logical model—that is, his examination of the various degrees of certainty or doubt with which one might approve a statement—was of seminal importance, to be replayed in virtually everything Browne ever wrote.

In a letter to John Aubrey written in March 1673, Browne recalled that Lushington had left in manuscript a work "upon the Theologie of Proclus," though he was not sure whether anyone owned copies of this among the other works of his tutor (Keynes, 4.375). In all likelihood, the work in question was in fact a translation of the 211 propositions in Proclus's *Elementa Theologica*, a text extant as British Library Sloane MS 1838, and reported in a seventeenth-century catalogue of manuscripts as belonging to Edward Browne.[48] The "excerpts" from the *Elements*, taken from the 1583 edition of Francesco Patrizi, offer in eighteen folios Proclus's distillation of Neoplatonic theology into propositions but without Proclus's explications. Beginning with the basic distinction between the one and the many, Proclus steps the student through the grades of causation, the levels of reality, and the higher beings of the gods, the intelligences and forms, before returning to a focus on the

[48] See Edward Bernard, *Catalogus Librorum MSS. Angliae & Hiberniae* (Oxford, 1697), 2.111, and Simon Wilkin, ed., *Sir Thomas Browne's Works*. 4 vols. (London: William Pickering, 1836), 4.468.

soul as the "intermediate between the indivisible principles and those which are divided in association with bodies."[49]

In the "goodly new" schools quadrangle at Oxford, as Leonard Hutton praised it in 1625, logic found its place amongst astronomy, rhetoric, music, natural philosophy, medicine, civil law, moral philosophy, history, grammar, geometry-math, metaphysics, Hebrew and Greek, and divinity.[50] As Browne's tutor, Lushington had the responsibility of introducing his charge to the whole round of the university curriculum. In the simplest terms, this instruction was meant to reinforce the integrity of the curriculum (each of the disciplines relating to all the others), as well as the practicality of the instruction either for preparing the student to enter public service or in providing him a foundation for moving onward to a career in one of the professions, civil law, divinity, or medicine. Lushington's instructions in logic and natural philosophy would be essential in preparing the way for Browne to study medicine. In addition to his work on logic and metaphysics, Lushington was also said by Browne to have written a treatise on moral philosophy—on the passions as understood by Aristotle and Aquinas (Keynes, 4.375). Such a work would be seen as an integral part of the Oxford curriculum, as a reconciliation of classical and medieval legacies, and as a major responsibility of the tutor who served as a surrogate parent in managing the manners and morals of his charges.

Our most extensive access to Lushington's intellectual preoccupations in the 1620s comes from the sermons that were copied into manuscripts by Oxford auditors with whom he was a favorite. At every turn, these sermons anticipate Browne's abiding concerns in *Religio Medici*. From the outset of his sermon on John 20:15, "woman why weepest thou," Lushington calls attention to his own religious experience: "My Deuotions are but dull unlesse my love doth quicken them, and my loue is apt to misleade mee unlesse my faith direct her Course."[51] Faith substitutes for logic here in supplying rule and order at the foundation of experience, but love or charity provides the spirit and the life of devotion. Soon this sermon on a simple scene of human error offers Lushington an opportunity to explore the complex epistemology of faith. Lushington's reflexive examination of the means of human worship anticipates Browne's own personal interaction with rites and ceremonies in *Religio Medici*. In the case of Lushington's sermon on weeping, the chief means of disciplining worship is also the instrument of stimulating the fancy and the senses: the ritual reception of communion toward which the sermon moves. With ceremony as with logic, geometry, and preaching, Lushington investigates the assets and liabilities of humanly devised intermediaries in matters of faith, for instance, in his sermon on Job 2:8, in which Job's sitting down "amonge ye ashes" instructs us in the movements and gestures of worship. In a sermon preached at St Mary's on 1625 in Romans 7:20 ("Sin taking occasion by ye Law deceiued

[49] Proclus, *The Elements of Theology: A Revised Text*, trans., intro., and commentary by E. R. Dodds (Oxford: Clarendon Press, 1933), 167.

[50] Leonard Hutton, "Antiquities of Oxford," in Charles Plummer, ed., *Elizabethan Oxford: Reprints of Rare Tracts* (Oxford: Clarendon Press, 1887), 100–1.

[51] Recorded by John Bayly in Bodleian MS Rawlinson E.95.

me"), Lushington faces head-on the skepticism about human knowledge that is entangled with his affection for Platonism and motivates his assiduous search for the best possible intermediaries between self and God. Far from having the necessary and demonstrable certainty of basic principles promised by syllogistic logic, we do not even possess a knowledge per se of the slightest phenomena in our mundane world. Proceeding to the point that true knowledge is a privilege of heavenly existence, Lushington clarifies that in the transient world, "we may haue some qualified notions & modified apprehensions but comprehend nothing, we know nothing as we out [i.e. ought], soe y^{n} we may haue some knowledge of ye truth but noe true knowledge especialy of y^{t} we should know" (13r).

Browne was clearly impressed by his tutor's vibrant investigations of the ways in which the modified, qualified, and accidental knowledge that we have both entails and compromises human accommodation of the divine. No matter what the instruments of mediation between human knowledge and divine truth, Lushington stresses, we must always concede the instability and limits of what we know, for "there is noe great hold to w[ha]t I my selfe conceiued for w[ha]t I believed yesterday I may doubt of today & to morrow find my selfe quite deceiued" (13r). This last point, one that clearly stayed with Browne in the *Religio*, makes the case that not only are we divided via circumstances from other people, but we are alienated via the fluxes of selfhood from ourselves. But Browne also learned from Lushington that the skeptics understood the basis of human deception, uncertainty, circumstantial knowledge, and fragmentation. In anticipation of Browne's *Religio* and *Pseudodoxia*, Lushington's critique of human knowledge focused on the rival claims of reason and experience, but also assailed our misguided reliance on authority as well as the various claims of authorities to infallibility.

In Oxford in the 1620s, Lushington's renown and infamy for wit, ingenuity, impersonation, and fancy corroborated his emphasis on the simultaneous frailty and necessity of the means by which we seek the divine and the true. His close relationship to Richard Corbett deepened this legacy and added to it the means of church ceremony, often assessed in the period as holy, regulated forms of fancy and impersonation.[52] Browne himself remembered Corbett as "a person of singular witt, and an eloquent preacher" (Keynes, 3.130). Serving in the 1620s first as Dean of Christ Church Cathedral then as bishop of Oxford before leaving with Lushington in tow to become, briefly, the bishop of Salisbury in 1631, then of Norwich in 1632, Corbett's legacy of wit, fancy, pranks, and impersonation included Lushington in his capacity as a sidekick.[53] In the 1620s, however, more was at stake in the puckish wit of Corbett than just the propriety of a prankster in the pulpit. In his assaults on zealous "distracted" Puritanism, and in the array of subjects that he valued—fairies, stained glass, obedience to authority, patronage, sport, ballads, "old abbies," "Ave Maryes," "Procession," British antiquarianism, and traditional

[52] Reid Barbour, *Literature and Religious Culture in Seventeenth-Century England* (Cambridge: Cambridge University Press, 2001), chapters 3–4.

[53] Richard Corbett, *Poems of Richard Corbett*, ed. J. A. W. Bennett and H. R. Trevor-Roper (Oxford: Clarendon Press, 1955), xxii–xxv.

social and ecclesiastical hierarchies—Corbett epitomized the love for Merry Old England, for the rites and ceremonies of the established church, for continuity with the customs of the English past, and for a reconciliation between the agricultural calendar of seasons or cycles and the church calendar of festivals.

The fact that Browne followed Lushington on the Corbett trail to Norwich is evidence that the author of the *Religio* was infected by the playful yet serious and skeptical wit of his tutor. Yet, if for Browne this legacy for the role of wit and humor in the performance of faith was formative, it would also prove a dissatisfying version of religious play, other instantiations of which Browne would experience on the Continent as well as invent in his *Religio*. Indeed Browne never conveys complete ease with or trust of a facetious wit: as he admits in the *Religio*, and as an early biographer confirmed, Browne was far more apt to be at least a little embarrassed by jocosity than he was to be boisterously productive of it. And he rarely if ever confused imaginative play with facetious insobriety.

Another bold, putatively "Arminian" thinker, taught at Pembroke for a brief period in the 1620s, one even more anticipatory than Lushington of the theological interests manifested in the *Religio*. According to Edmund Vaughan's seventeenth-century biography, Thomas Jackson "read a lecture of divinity in the college [Corpus Christi] every Sunday morning, and another day of the week at Pembroke College, (then newly erected,) by the instance of the master and fellows there."[54] While it is true that Jackson left his fellowship in early 1625 for a preferment in the north, he brought to his students a rich set of interests in Platonism, epistemology, and a critique of rigid Calvinism that harmonized with the innovative work of Lushington yet without duplicating it. Together, these two teachers provided Browne with complex models of what polemically minded critics called "Arminianism"—complex, because as Browne himself would be working out in the 1630s, reactions against Calvinism could be instigated by both liberating and persecutory motives. Given the elements of Calvinism still on display in *Religio Medici*, it cannot be argued that Browne simply took sides in Oxford theological debates, but his awareness that English orthodoxy needed reinvention began at Pembroke.

Among other tendencies, Jackson's preference for metaphor, imagination, and mystery over logic makes its way into Browne's *Religio*, though it is worth remembering at this point Lushington's Proclean interest in keeping Neoplatonic illumination rigorous and logical. Indeed despite Jackson's conviction that "ignorance of this Plotinical philosophy hath much perplexed some logicians" (*Works*, 5.69), his commentary on the Apostle's Creed is itself indebted to logical strategies of definition and division throughout.[55] At Browne's Pembroke, Lushington and Jackson alike worked in the same territory where a skeptical dissatisfaction with the conventional discourses and means of religious experience is too canny to posit that those conventions can simply be jettisoned rather than vigilantly reformed.

[54] *The Works of Thomas Jackson, D.D.*, 12 vols. (Oxford: Oxford University Press, 1844), 1. xlii–xliii.

[55] See for instance 5.16, point 4; 5.30–1, point 6.

As Jackson's protestation against polemic affirms, Browne's Oxford in the 1620s offered students a highly complex, disorienting but also exhilarating state of religious affairs.[56] On the one hand, in opposition to the triumph of Calvinism in the Low Countries, English divines developed an irenic discourse of common notions, self-deflating skepticism, limited free will, entente with the Catholic church, and a loving God who pays attention to faith wherever it is found. On the other, the tendency of such a discourse to be harnessed to the rise of powerful and persecutory officers of the monarchy and the state church meant that a staunchly Calvinist, sturdily anti-Papist contingent still prospered in Oxford. Clayton ranks among those who apparently got along with both sides in a culture that increasingly resorted to a hostile name-calling to which both "Puritans" and "Arminians" contributed. No wonder then that Jackson is keen to reassert the superiority of the Church of England in much the same way that Browne will in the *Religio*, for buried in the complex arguments of the treatise on divine attributes is a paean for that church's "middle course," success with "compromising connections," its commitment to "the extent of God's unspeakable love to mankind," and the author's belief that "no national council, though assembled for that purpose, could fit their doctrine more expressly to meet with all the late restrictions of God's love, than the church our mother, even from the beginning of reformation, hath done; as if she had then foreseen a necessity of declaring her judgment in this point, for preventing schisms or distraction in opinions amongst her sons" (5.148–9). This preference for love, mercy, and charity serves also as a reminder that Christians should pray for "all Jews, Turks, infidels, and heretics" (5.152). As Jackson is apt to remind his readers, the pagans in particular made up for their lack of scripture by their attention to the "great book of nature" in which they found the authorship and providence of God everywhere and readily apparent (5.223). It is a notion and a metaphor that play an enormous role in Browne's irenic version of his English faith in *Religio Medici*.

Browne's searching essay on the constituents of English orthodoxy in *Religio Medici* would reflect experiences and educations that he encountered in his travels on the Continent in the 1630s. But Oxford planted the seed—that the beliefs and practices of the home church could no longer be taken for granted. Given the complex state of religious learning in Browne's Oxford, it is not surprising that when asked by Aubrey to recall the writers produced by his college, Browne tended to remember authors in divinity. Of the divines that he recalled by name—Stamp, Dowdswell, and Bludworth—Browne summoned up fleeting memories of their lives (one perhaps a chaplain to the Queen of Bohemia, another a "learned man, lately prebend of Worcester") though nothing about what they had written or believed (Keynes, 4.376). Certainly some of the students at Pembroke during the 1620s were on a collision course with the Laudian authorities, an obvious case being George Hughes (MA Pembroke, 1625) who "was suspended by Laud in 1636, accused of stealing his neighbour's flock, of refusing to use the sign of the

[56] A good example can be glimpsed in Thomas Crosfield's diary, a transcription of which is Queens College, Oxford, MS 390; see for instance 14, 26, 32.

cross in baptism, and of not bowing to the altar."[57] At the same time, Lushington was perturbing (if also attracting) students such as Thomas Hall who would one day lambaste him for his Arminian poison. It was in the very year of Browne's MA, 1629, that the growing, highly factionalized tumult over English orthodoxy in Oxford came to a head, with "the Oxford Arminians" going "on to the offensive, by raising the question of the confessional basis of English Church teaching."[58] Given the view of Oxonians such as Robert Burton that the fights over the church might be partly remedied if discourse shifted toward medicine, one cannot help suspect that religious controversy—along with Clayton's model of the pious physician—redirected the course of Browne's vocation.[59] This Oxford tendency in the 1620s to be obsessed with religious dispute may have already been apparent in the student whom Browne remembered as "much my senior . . . in Oxford" (Keynes, 4.173), William Denton. Having taken his BA in 1624, Denton set about living and working with a physician named Henry Ashworth who, according to Wood, was "noted" in the Oxford area. Never taking his MA, Denton would receive both bachelor and doctorates in medicine in 1634, yet his several writings were exclusively concerned with the question of how to handle recusants living in a Protestant commonwealth.[60]

It is significant of Browne's turn to medicine that even though he was able to recall more religious writers from Broadgates and Pembroke than any other kind of author, he reserved his fondest memories for a man, suspected by some of atheism, who had taught him geography, natural philosophy, and mathematics, Robert Hues. In a 1678 letter to his son Edward, which is unfortunately damaged, Browne is ruminating on the differences among globes as well as Halley's "voyage for the observation of the stares about the south pole." Suddenly he is back "in Oxford" with his "old freind Mr H.," the author (he reminds Edward) of *De usu globi*. The sequence of memories about Hues is wide-ranging. First he was an adventurer who journeyed with Thomas Cavendish during his circumnavigation of the world in the 1580s. Second, these extraordinary travels had permitted Hues to offer cutting edge observations on "the state of . . . polarie starres" in the southern hemisphere, stars which (Hues had told Browne) were "dimmer comparatively to the north." Third, Hues was closely associated with Henry Percy, the ninth Earl of Northumberland, and his circle of intellectuals with brilliant credentials in the study of math and physics. Finally, perhaps most importantly, Hues was a good, warm, pious man, who "came to church constantly, the parish church, which was St. Aldates, commonly St. Owls" (Keynes, 4.83).

Each of these factors in Browne's memory of Robert Hues is more resonant than a thumbnail synopsis can capture. Hues had clearly taught math, geometry, cosmography, and natural philosophy to Browne (among others) in some informal capacity. Browne remembers that Hues "had read Euclide & Ptolemie very accurately, and

[57] *ODNB* article on George Hughes by Mary Wolffe.
[58] Tyacke, *Anti-Calvinists*, 78.
[59] Burton, *Anatomy*, 1.27.
[60] Wood, *Fasti*, 2.414, 474; 4.307f.

also Aristotle, whereof wee should often discourse." A close engagement with Euclidean geometry and Ptolemaic cosmography was something Hues shared with Henry Briggs and John Bainbridge, the Savilian professors of geometry and astronomy who in the inaugural years of their professorships had brought out editions of the two ancients' works. The frequent discussions of Aristotle, presumably his works on natural philosophy, are hardly surprising. Although Browne wrote a cautionary note about Aristotle's physics, the large, complex body of Aristotle's writings on the natural world still served as the most important foundation on which an Oxford student would build his education in natural philosophy. The Aristotelian foundation itself was uneven: some of it was held to be patently wrong, some enduringly right, and the logic and presuppositions of Aristotelian thought were so dynamically, flexibly, and thoroughly integrated into university instruction that a student might have an Aristotelian thought without even knowing it or identifying it as such. It is significant too that Hues is credited with actually having read Aristotle "very accurately," this reflective of his deep learning in Greek to which the translator of Homer, George Chapman, had long ago testified and which reflected Hues's humanist insistence on peeling away medieval scholastic accretions to wrangle with the great philosopher himself.[61] What Hues represented to his Oxford students was a lesson that Browne found reinforced in Padua: that Aristotle and his Renaissance commentators were not a lifeless, colorless tradition wholly resistant to innovation, experiential knowledge, or change, but rather a living, breathing, and changing phenomenon that voiced and embodied strong arguments for the value of direct experience.

It is true that Aristotelian writings on the natural world were held responsible, sometimes fairly, sometimes not, for stymieing the advancement of natural learning. In the *Physics*, one began to deploy the already mastered Aristotelian logic in the study of principles, causes, elements, and method. A student would learn that natural things are defined by motion, that the principal building blocks of the material world are limited in number, neither one nor innumerable, and that nature can best be understood by way of the logical categories and the distinction between "the primary underlying matter of things" and the "form" that renders matter a natural phenomenon per se.[62] One learned about the four causes—material, formal, efficient, and final—that shaped the analysis of every natural thing, as well as the proper way to assess chance, necessity, and monstrous errors in nature. Such principles as the one Browne attributed to the "schools"—"Nature is a principle of motion and change" (Aristotle, 342)—were to be had in abundance: "the science of nature is concerned with magnitudes and motion and time" (345); "there is no void existing separately" (365); "each of the simple bodies has a natural locomotion, e.g. fire upward and earth downward and towards the middle of the universe" (365); "there are three kinds of motion—qualitative, quantitative, and local" (381); "everything that is in motion must be moved by something" (407), yet there exists a "first mover... unmoved" (432). Moving from the general study of physics, the student of Aristotle encountered two strictly

[61] See Homer, *The Iliads of Homer Prince of Poets* (1611), translated by Chapman, A3v.

[62] *The Complete Works of Aristotle*, revised Oxford translation, ed. Jonathan Barnes, 1.315–30.

divided realms within nature. First there were the heavens, whose ethereal matter was "unaging and unalterable and unmodified," whose qualities include unity and eternity, and whose motions were always circular (450, 454, 461). Then there was the sub-celestial world of the four elements, of generation and decay, in which motion tended to be rectilinear. Throughout these texts the students would encounter again and again the basic features of the cosmos that had been reconciled, medically with the thought of Galen, cosmologically with the legacies of Pythagoras, Plato, and Ptolemy, politically with the hierarchical penchant of medieval and early modern societies, and spiritually with a Christian doctrine accommodating to both dualism and a redemptive interaction between heaven and earth. And one learned that all sensory information about the natural world could be stabilized by means of the belief that the accidental properties of things adhered as occult qualities to the substance of the things themselves.

In Hues, Browne had a teacher who thought it crucial to return again and again to the texts of Aristotle and to read them "accurately," which meant that Browne would learn critically to read these famous writings as *texts*, as complex and at times incommensurable discourses rather than as treasuries of inmost yet petrified wisdom. In Browne's Oxford intellectual culture, Francis Bacon's call in 1620 for the reform of natural philosophy—for its return to experience and methodized induction—did not entail a wholesale rejection of Aristotle or for that matter the belief that Aristotelian thought was any more monolithic or simplistic than work in magic, astrology, and alchemy.

As Browne makes clear in his recollection, Hues was not simply a good reader of Euclid, Aristotle, and Ptolemy; he was also, perhaps more notably, an Elizabethan with an extraordinarily exciting past. Here was a man who, with Thomas Cavendish, had sailed on brand new ships, the *Desire* and *Hugh Gallant*, together with the well-traveled *Free Pryson* and Ralegh's *Dorothy*, all the way to the South Sea, with "several of Drake's veterans" on board for good measure.[63] The cultural resonance of this heroic Elizabethan past was keenly felt in the 1620s. Critics of the Spanish Match, of noninvolvement on behalf of beleaguered Protestants throughout Europe, and of the suspect drift of contemporary royal policy toward reconciliation with popery all sought to elevate and enrich the heroic stature of the Elizabethan adventurers. By contrast, Henry Briggs's contribution to a publication on Virginia in the 1620s was an effort to initiate enthusiasm about discovering a northwest passage in the wake of the wretched massacre of (and internecine squabbles about) that colony. For Browne, the Armada of 1588 and the Gunpowder Plot of his birth year 1605 might share in a claim to providential protection; but for contemporaries in the 1620s, there was a difference between standing stoutly, even miraculously, against the Spanish menace and forcing God's hand to protect a Protestant people once the enemy had been mollycoddled. It is hardly surprising that Browne was fascinated by exotic travel right to the end of his life, and that his daughter Elizabeth read to him so many travel narratives (Keynes, 3.331–2).

[63] I follow (and quote) the *ODNB* article on Robert Hues by Susan M. Maxwell.

As Browne remembered him, Hues had pursued travel for the sake of advancing natural and mathematical knowledge, but Hues's affiliations with Ralegh, Northumberland, and the great mathematician Thomas Harriot entailed that his admirers work out whether the rumors of atheism and subversion surrounding these figures were true and, if so, to what extent and to what end. For Browne, Hues reconciled as much as any mortal could the potentially conflicting desiderata of natural philosophy in the 1620s. First was the premium on direct observation, which in turn produced a number of corollaries. To the observer in a culture of Baconian instauration and colonial exploration, the phenomena filling the world were noteworthy for their variation, singularity, and particularity. The more the wide world became accessible to European observers, the more they would have to reckon with the fact that their environment, flora, and fauna were not normative. For the accurate observer, monstrous aberrations were not to be ignored as trivial (if amusing) deviations but as the very stuff of nature whose relationship to divine providence was contingent on God's will rather than reflective of some neatly ordered and symmetrical plan. The fact that Hues found the stars in the southern hemisphere to be "dimmer" than those to the north exploded visions of geographic and cosmic symmetry as only direct observation could.[64]

If experience and the irregularities that it observed were crucial for Bacon's advancement of learning, early modern advancers such as Galileo and Kepler were equally committed to a belief in the mathematical and geometrical laws governing matter in motion. From Hues, Browne was learning that the mediation between observation and math was to be worked out through cartography, that is, through the imaginary and artificial fashioning of terrestrial and celestial space. That this mediation was not yet, perhaps never would or could be perfectly harmonious, is reflected in Browne's remark to his son Edward that "in the old & new globes there is some varietie" (Keynes, 4.83). But what makes Hues significant in Browne's development is that he worked most intensely in the intellectual space between abstraction and observation, in the area in which the artist sought reconciliation between soul and body.

At the same time in Oxford, Henry Briggs was working on logarithms in an attempt to make math more useful. As Browne makes clear in *Pseudodoxia*, Briggs was engaged in intellectual endeavors with a kindred spirit to Hues—recovering and criticizing the best of the classical sources, then uniting careful observation and mathematical rigor in order to make natural philosophy as true and as useful as possible (Robbins, ed., *Pseudodoxia Epidemica*, 1.93). For Browne, however, a globe was more resonant of the imagination's mediation between reason and sense than a tabular calculator. In his conversations with Hues, Browne encountered a learning that had everything: mathematical precision and sophistication; the feel, flavor, and prodigious unpredictability of world-wide experience (even longitude, after all, was notoriously difficult to stabilize); a discursive (Latin) brilliance and hieroglyphic (globular) beauty; a profoundly learned grounding in ancient and

[64] D. W. Waters, *The Art of Navigation in England in Elizabethan and Early Stuart Times* (New Haven, CT: Yale University Press, 1958), 192.

medieval literature; and a personal candor mixed in with a nearly mythical heroic past left over from the putatively nobler generation of the late Elizabethans. The *Tractatus* expresses this mixture of ingredients in simple ways: the final table offering longitudes and latitudes for an enormous range of rivers, gulfs, promontories, and other places around the globe surely provided an English undergraduate in the 1620s with both exactness and exoticism in its inclusion of both Oxford and Borneo.

As Browne recalled with particular emphasis, Hues had something else too: a steadfast devotion to the Church of England as its services were performed within the community of the parish church. The point of Hues's heartfelt and obedient piety was a significant one. As Browne's anecdote makes obvious, the great man's association with the "wizard" Earl of Northumberland and his coterie of brilliant mathematicians, physical theorists, and experimenters was a central part of his legacy. Given the Savilian and Sedleian lectureships, the publication in 1622 of Nathanael Carpenter's *Philosophia Libera*, and the advances engineered by Clayton in the study of medicine, interested parties in Oxford could be forgiven for thinking that they were prepared to press forward with the Harriot and Hues legacy of mathematical and scientific excellence.[65]

The question had to be the moral, political, and spiritual corollaries and costs, if any, of this legacy. In Browne's recollection of Hues persists a palpable sense of relief that the old Elizabethan navigator came to St Aldate's for his prayers. Lacking a college chapel of their own, the Pembroke scholars were allowed to make up the defect with a special aisle of their own in the parish church. Writing in 1625, Leonard Hutton explained further that the relatively new chapel inside St Aldate's "is peculier and propper to Broadgates, where they daily meete for the celebration of Divine Service."[66] There too, in the 1620s, Clayton had fused another connection between the college and the church by restoring the Broadgates, now Pembroke library in a chamber hired in the church for the purpose, a medieval practice that had fallen into disuse during the reign of Edward VI.[67] Its reconstituted library stocked with illuminated medical manuscripts from Clayton, its walls embossed with the "white fishes in a red circular feild" of a fishmonger and church patron named John Docklington, the church stayed in Browne's memory as the sacred space where Hues "constantly" proved that honesty, parish reverence, and a profound understanding of math and science were harmonious, perhaps (to believe all the rumors and proverbs) against the odds. To Browne's way of thinking, Hues had struck an idealized balance between colonial adventure and gentle, philosophical speculation and curiosity. In some measure, of course, this "balance" was illusory: as it is reported in Hakluyt, the Cavendish voyage around the world was replete with acts of violence, pillage, scorched-earth policy, and mutiny. Somehow Browne

[65] See Nicholas Tyacke, "Science and Religion at Oxford before the Civil War," in Donald Pennington and Keith Thomas, eds., *Puritans and Revolutionaries: Essays in Seventeenth-Century History Presented to Christopher Hill* (Oxford: Clarendon Press, 1978), 73–93.

[66] Hutton, *Antiquities of Oxford*, in Charles Plummer, ed., *Elizabethan Oxford: Reprints of Rare Tracts* (Oxford: Clarendon Press, 1887), 88–9.

[67] See Macleane, *History of Pembroke College*, 18.

managed to isolate Hues from the killing, maiming, and burning that the Cavendish party frequently perpetrated.[68]

In Browne's last year at Oxford, 1629, as his *Pseudodoxia* recalls, the Savilian professor of astronomy, John Bainbridge, "computed…that in the Horizon of Oxford the Dog-star arose not before the fifteenth of August; when in our Almanack accounts those daies are almost ended" (Robbins, ed., *Pseudodoxia Epidemica*, 1.356). In the summer of his graduation with an MA, Browne was on hand to witness the advanced accuracy or strictness with which Oxford mathematicians and natural philosophers were correcting the vulgar errors of almanac-makers, navigators, and all manner of folk. These errors were of the kind that Browne remembered with a smile in the *Religio*, when he quipped that "I know the names, and somewhat more, of all the constellations in my Horizon, yet I have seene a prating Mariner that could onely name the Poynters and the North Starre, out-talke mee, and conceit himselfe a whole Speare above mee" (Patrides, 147). Bainbridge and Briggs afforded young Browne with that "somewhat more," for while vulgar mariners might rely on eyeballing prominent stars to find their way, the Oxford vanguard in astronomy and math was deploying a far more precise knowledge in the service of devising extraordinary instruments for guiding action. Not that the experiential wisdom of living, breathing mariners was ridiculed and rejected: Browne's career in listening to them talk is not surprising, given the fact that a veteran seaman, Roger Fry, "had stayed intermittently with Bainbridge at Merton College from 1626."[69] Like Clayton, both Briggs and Bainbridge, together with the Sedleian professor of natural philosophy, Edward Lapworth, contributed updates on the advancement of learning as well as information on specific points for Hakewill's *Apology…of…Providence*. The very pursuit of consultation was redolent of that commitment to a collaborative, irenic republic of letters that Bacon had taken over from his humanist forefathers and helped transform into the invention of the early modern scientific society.

This emphasis on collaborative learning was integral to every scholarly enterprise that Browne ever undertook; the way in which Browne practiced collaboration was not reducible to his university training, but it was stimulated to growth by the cross-fertilization that he encountered in the 1620s. For Browne, a career that might well have centered in a parish church with the scholars at New College ended up on the Continent, in Halifax, and on horseback in Norwich visiting the sick. This is not to say that Browne abandoned theology, became secular, stopped thinking about scholastic metaphysical treatments of being, substance and accidents, the rational soul, angels, and the attributes of God.[70] Far from it, Browne's turn to medicine emulated the model of Clayton and Lushington in prizing a complex interweaving of the spiritual, philosophical, historical, and natural domains. And it was Clayton who, in the most immediate professional sense, showed Browne the way—the way to Montpellier but also to the religion of a physician.

[68] For the Cavendish journey taken from Richard Hakluyt, *Voyages and Discoveries*, ed. and intro. Jack Beeching (Baltimore, MD: Penguin, 1972), 275–97.

[69] Feingold, *Mathematicians' Apprenticeship*, 145.

[70] Typical list from Richard Crakanthorpe's *Introductio in metaphysicam*, 1619.

4. THE TURN TO MEDICINE

In the summer of 1629, Browne had more than an astronomical reason for considering that the dog days might arrive sooner than expected. Already in the late spring and early summer of his life, he had hurried his way through Oxford in six years, which meant that each time he supplicated for a degree, he was fined for being *defectus*, that is, short of the requisite number of semesters provided by the statutes (sixteen for a BA, twenty-eight for an MA).[71] Signing off on his inheritance in London on November 19, 1629, at twenty-four he was officially on his own recognizance;[72] money was not depleted—there would be enough for his travels on the Continent—but it was not in imperishable supply either.[73] (See Figure 3.1.) If the Thomas Browne who paid three shillings and fourpence to the Ewelme Hospital Foundation in 1629 is the newly graduated MA from Pembroke, then he was using a portion of his money to lease a cottage where, under the tuition of the Master of that hospital, Thomas Clayton, he might begin to learn the practice of medicine.[74]

Sometimes the seasons of life came upon one far more quickly than perhaps expected: Browne's fellow student at Pembroke, Nicholas Cruse, also short a term in 1626, would die in September 1629 just after Browne's graduation.[75] Answering a now anonymous query about the death of "T.M.," Browne recalled that the person in question died during the dog days, for Browne's own poem had beseeched that "if the Dogstarre up hath dranck | The streames that wash the Elyzian banck; | Wee'le waft him 'ore with teares, for sorrowe | Shall of our eyes a River borrowe" (Keynes, 3.234). This undated snippet in British Library Sloane MS 1869 refers to the death in question as "so long ago" that it is tempting to speculate on its beginnings in Browne's student days, a contribution to some communal expression of mourning for the death of a beloved and famous cultural hero, someone like the playwright Thomas Middleton whose death pressed the boundaries of the dog days in July 1627.[76]

[71] Oxford University Archives; SP/2, 37r and 39r; on each occasion, Michaelmas term 1626 and 1628, he paid 3*s.* 4*p.* for being defective one term. I am grateful to Simon Bailey, Keeper of the Archives at Oxford, for help with this term.

[72] LMA London Court of Aldermen Repertory 44, ff. 20v–21r.

[73] The fact that Browne's uncle Edward may have needed funds from his brother's estate in response to his nephew's failure to receive a scholarship may well have prompted further activity in the London Court of Aldermen. See LMA Repertory 36 ff. 101r and 122v; Repertory 38, f. 181r; and Repertory 40, f. 222b. See also Endicott, "Sir Thomas Browne as 'Orphan'" (187).

[74] MS D.D. Ewelme d.9 (EA 3). "Fine" meant an "entry fine" for a lease of land or a house from the foundation; thanks to John Goodall for help with this. According to Henry Alfred Napier, *Historical Notices of the Parishes of Swyncombe and Ewelme in the County of Oxford* (Oxford: James Wright, 1858), 213–14, the amount paid by Browne is about right for the leasing of a cottage in the area in the early seventeenth century. According to the personal name index in the Oxfordshire Record Office, only one Thomas Browne appears for the period of the 1620s, a gentleman from Wickham (near Banbury) involved in a financial transaction in 1624 (Oxfordshire Record Office, Dash/IX/i/19). But a baptism index yields two: one a son of a Richard of St Giles, Oxford, 1604; the other a son of John and Margett of Strandford/Val, 1605. The marriage index also yields two: one marrying in 1624, the other in Alderbury in 1627. The burial index has one Thomas Browne: buried at Woodstock in 1682. I am grateful to archivist Timothy Xu for this information.

[75] On Cruse's death, see the MS chronology of Oxford in the Bodleian, 126.

[76] It should be recalled that Browne owned a manuscript copy of Middleton's *Game at Chesse*.

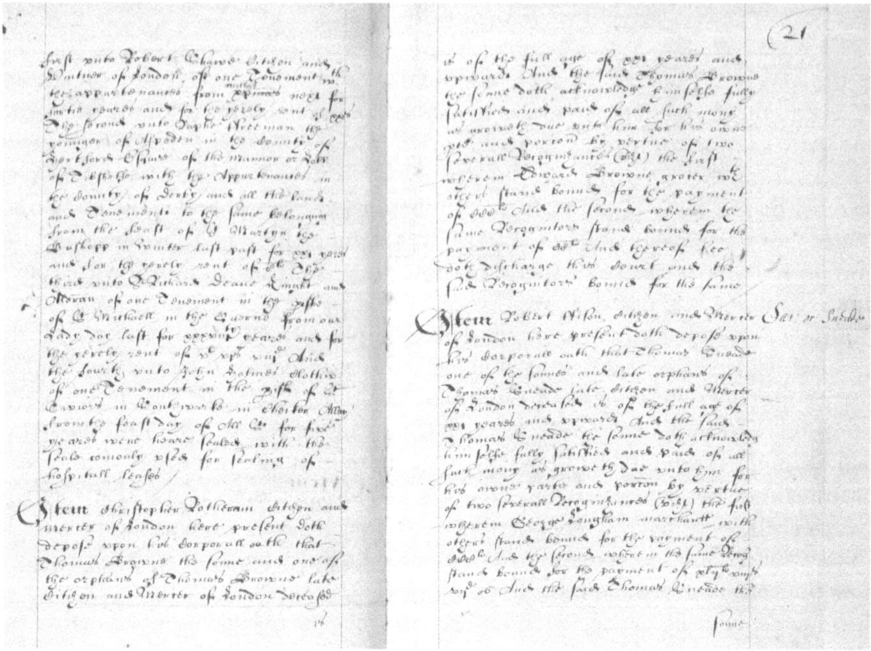

Figure 3.1 Browne signs off on his inheritance in 1629 (LMA Repertory 44, 20b–21). Reproduced with the permission of the London Metropolitan Archives.

In order to receive his two degrees, a BA on January 31, 1627, the MA on June 11, 1629,[77] Browne was required "to appear in hall either to present or to oppose a proposition approved in advance by Dr. Clayton, the master."[78] The format of these disputes was patently familiar to students by the time they reached this level. With a subject for debate posed in the form of a question, participants were then obliged to sharpen their wits by means of Aristotle's "dialectical procedures."[79] Among the lectures specified for scholars pursuing the BA, Greek had a strong and continuing role to play.[80] The three-year MA course required according to statue that bachelors "deliver a certain number of lectures for the benefit of undergraduates in arts"; attend lectures especially on moral, natural, and metaphysical philosophies; and continue to participate in disputations on appropriate subjects such as "the relationship between the heart and the brain and between melancholy and ability, whether the movement of the heavens was perpetual, whether sight was

[77] OUA register of congregation, 1622–30, 276r, 264v; he supplicated for his two degrees on January 22, 1627, and June 6, 1629, respectively.

[78] Huntley, *Sir Thomas Browne*, 37.

[79] See Lawrence D. Green, ed. and trans., *John Rainolds's Oxford Lectures on Aristotle's "Rhetoric"* (Newark: University of Delaware Press, 1986), 27.

[80] See Curtis, *Oxford and Cambridge in Transition*, 86; and Fletcher, "The Faculty of Arts," in McConica, ed., *The History of the University of Oxford: Volume III*, 196.

derived from internal or external forces, whether women should receive education, the good or bad nature of the appearance of comets, whether land should be inherited, the role of dreams," and so forth.[81] Finally, in keeping with concerns about cultivating excellent Latin speakers, candidates for the MA also delivered declamations on subjects such as "in praise of astronomy."[82] Browne's center of gravity for these performances was Pembroke.

The Acts at which Browne's graduation took place were enormous celebrations lasting several days; crowds could reach over two thousand.[83] The degree ceremony itself was held on the first Monday after July 7—in the case of Browne's MA on July 13—with a vespers coming the evening before. Lady and Sir Thomas Dutton may have attended the 1629 affair, since on July 19, the Privy Council granted Dutton "A Passe... to retourne into Ireland with his whole family and retinue."[84] In Crosfield's diary for the year 1627, an outline for the ceremony lists the various arts and faculties involved—philosophy (grammar, music, astronomy, geometry, physics, history, ethics), medicine, and theology (civil law is omitted); the location (the schools quadrangle of the university as well as the Church of St Mary's); the duration (four days from Saturday through Tuesday; the Act in 1629 started on Saturday July 11); and a hint of the various sermons (English and Latin), disputes, and orations with which the guests were greeted.[85] According to at least one anonymous satire, "A libel vppon ye Doctors of Oxon 1627," the unintentionally funny performances of scholars at the Acts were worthy of a dunciad.[86]

In beginning to study the medical care of more private bodies, however, Browne was on far less formalized ground and, with Clayton's help, had to devise his own curriculum in the same way that Henry Power learned to do from Browne in the 1640s. There was some help to be had from the requirements for medical degrees at Oxford according to the statutes of 1549 and 1564/5.[87] Surely Browne would have been prudent to attend the lectures given by the Regius Professor himself, as well as the disputations and praelectiones required of the medical students proper. These latter exercises might take up "topics dealing with popular medicine or the medical profession," such as that given by John Speed in 1628, in which the orator claimed that "that the whole man was the subject of medicine; not only could human life be extended by this art, but even the very day and hour of death might be predicted by the physician."[88] The very importance of such speeches reflected the belief that the physician needed to be rhetorically as well as medically gifted.

In assessing Browne's earliest medical learning in Oxford and anticipating the medical education that he would gain on the Continent, we are fortunate to have

[81] Fletcher, "Faculty of Arts," 195.

[82] Green, ed. and trans., *Rainolds's Oxford Lectures*, 28.

[83] Feingold, "The Humanities," in Tyacke, ed., *History of the University of Oxford*, 302.

[84] Papers of the Privy Council, National Archives, PC 2/39, f. 365.

[85] Transcription at Queen's College 390, 111.

[86] Bodleian MS Douce f. 5, 12v–13r.

[87] See Gillian Lewis, "The Faculty of Medicine," in James McConica, ed., *The History of the University of Oxford: Volume III* (Oxford: Clarendon Press, 1986), 218–19. Cf. Frank, "Medicine," in Tyacke, ed., *History of the University of Oxford: Volume IV*, 508.

[88] Frank, "Medicine," in Tyacke, ed., *History of the University of Oxford, Volume IV*, 527.

his own letter on this subject to Henry Power from 1646. While it certainly recommends a range of books for Power's reading, the letter clearly stresses the value of experience. Beginning with the quip that only a fool would hope to become a physician "out of book," Browne not only focuses on a handful of books that are especially useful guides in practice, but he urges the novice to gain experience of the *materia medicamentorum* "in gardens, [and] fields" for plants and herbs, in "Apothecaries' and Druggists' shops" for the making of medicines made from that flora as well as from "animals, and minerals," and in the laboratories of "Chymistators" (Keynes, 4.255). With the university botanical garden on hold in the late 1620s, Oxford students could still absorb knowledge of herbs and plants from the gardens, meadows, and fields in and around Oxford—with bulky assistance perhaps from "Theophrastus, Dioscorides, Mathiolus, Dodonæus, and our English Herbalists," or, more practically, Spigelius's introduction to herbs, a 1606 edition of which Browne owned and a text that he would encounter again in the context of Leiden's botanical garden in 1633. In the Bodleian, a printed copy of Rembert Dodoens's 1619 herbal contains manuscript notes indicating where the student has seen the various herbs in the Oxford area as well as in Padua. Oxford sites include ditches and meadows, the way from Oxford to Headington, the walk on the backside of Exeter College, the old town walls by New College near the gallows, St Bartholomew's well a mile's walk from the town, Woodstock park, various woods, the New College garden, and a meadow on the way to Aristotle's well "a flight shot from Madlin Bridge in a little close by ye riuer side."[89] At Browne's Pembroke, the 1620s may have been distinguished by the rapid rate of building construction, but the college was still fortunate in its possession of three rectangular gardens.

In addition to botanical experience, Oxford's anatomical reputation was enjoying a boom in the late 1620s, thanks not just to the Tomlins's lectureship but also to the publication, in 1628, of Oxonian William Harvey's discovery of the circulation of the blood. Browne refers to this knowledge as a "foundation" but also as "autopsia," direct experience. The various anatomical books mentioned by Browne, including those by Vesalius, Fallopius, and Aquapendente, are chosen for their service in the anatomy room; Clayton himself acted on this idea when, in 1633, he had Adriaan van den Spigel's guide to anatomy published for use by students. The excitement that Harvey's publication caused, even if its findings took a long time to find full acceptance, is still palpable in Browne's recommendation to Power that the young man "make [himself] master of Dr Harvey's piece De Circul. Sang.; which discovery I prefer to that of Columbus" (Keynes, 4.255). This comparison, obviously to Christopher the adventurer and not Realdo the anatomist, suggests that for Browne and his Oxford associates such as Edward Dawson, 1628 stood as a pivotal year in which the old Elizabethan model of the heroic navigator, still alive in the figure of Hues, shifted toward a more purely philosophical and intellectual model of the hero. Browne's one recollection of the room for medical instruction in the schools quadrangle clarifies, moreover, that his experience of the dissected

[89] This copy of Dodoens's *Herbal* is shelfmarked 50.d.25 in the Bodleian.

body stimulated his fascination with curiosities. In a letter to Edward in 1676, he recalled that "over fortie yeares agoe the tanned skinne of a man was hanged up in the physick schoole at Oxford" (Keynes, 4.72).[90] If examining an excoriated skin ranked in Browne's imagination with the inspection of rare instruments, plants, and animals, there was something especially provocative about this hanging human skin that stayed with Browne during the years in which he would write a dissertation on smallpox, wonder about the code of physiognomy, and take notes on the anatomy of skin. In addition, Browne was obliged by means of anatomical lessons to master each corporeal member's composition, complexion, substance, quantity, number, figure, operation, use, and diseases.[91]

For an ancient guide to modern experience, Browne singled out the Hippocratic aphorisms to "be conned for the frequent use which may be made of them." As his characterization of Hippocratic writing shows, Browne saw the Greek writer as especially helpful in dealing with the messy circumstances in which medicine was carried out: circumstances having to do with places, times, and the persons of the patients themselves. In short, Hippocratic medicine, newly revived in the Renaissance, "added impetus to an approach to knowledge through individual cases."[92] As a medical genre, consilia or casebooks were often to be found in the medical writings of authorities whom Browne admired, for instance, Lazare Rivière of Montpellier.

Everyone in medical training knew that the road of experience to knowledge was as long and complicated as it was unavoidable. For Browne the marriage of Hippocratic medicine to the humoral theory of Galen simplified matters considerably. Strongly theoretical as well as practical, making claims to necessary science as well as art and technique, learned medicine required a mastery of natural philosophy (part of the arts course) and of physiology, the certain knowledge from which was invaluable in applying logic (also part of the arts course) to the deciphering of symptoms and indications.[93] As Browne undertook to become a physician, however, the rules of interpretation, like the content of the course, were undergoing transformation in a complex and vibrant fashion. Just as men like Lushington, Sanderson, and Jackson felt compelled to rethink logic in the service of theology, so medical thinkers were faced with a situation in which "the particular uptake of medical discourse from the arts course is marked both by aspiration to rigour and

[90] As Jeremiah Finch points out, the skin was already in place when in 1630–31 visitors to the university made note of it (Finch, *Sir Thomas Browne*, 47). The room set apart for medical study was on the first floor of the southwest corner of the schools quadrangle (Frank, "Medicine," in Tyacke, ed., *History of the University of Oxford, Volume IV*, 541–2).

[91] List taken from Brian Twyne's seventeenth-century notes on anatomy, Corpus Christi College, Oxford, MS 263, 128r–29v.

[92] Ian Maclean, *Logic, Signs, and Nature in the Renaissance: The Case of Learned Medicine* (Cambridge: Cambridge University Press, 2002), 170.

[93] For the conviction through much of the seventeenth century that a liberal arts education was crucial for medical training, see Phyllis Allen, "Scientific Studies in the English Universities of the Seventeenth Century," *Journal of the History of Ideas* 10 (1949), 219–53; and Arnold Chaplin, "A History of Medical Education in the Universities of Oxford and Cambridge, 1500–1800," *Proceedings of the Royal Society of Medicine* 12 supplement (1920), 83–107.

certainty, and by the pursuit of more makeshift ways of weighing factors against each other, of reaching decisions about evidence and of justifying them" according to what Browne called judgment.[94] What is more, physicians felt a pressure that they deemed greater than that found in the logic of law by virtue of the fact that in medicine, one was accountable to the natural world as God had made it, not to some wholly artificial system of signs devised according to custom and over time by human agents to social ends; it made sense to argue both sides of an issue in law in a way that it did not in medicine or, for that matter, as Lushington points out, in theology.[95]

Indeed, with Bacon's Great Instauration, all savvy students of natural philosophy were charged with recalculating the relations between discourse and natural phenomena in a controversy over res and verba that stretched back to antiquity. For the Galenic physician, however, claims to science and demonstrable knowledge were intimately tied up with the conviction that "all errors in medicine arise from bad division," that is to say, from faulty logic.[96] The challenges to this logic were raised by several seventeenth-century factors: by the rise of skepticism, by changes in and debates about natural philosophy, by chemical or Paracelsian theories of the ontology of disease, but also by the prospect that in the case of diseases such as smallpox, nature might itself be undergoing change. There had always been debate over whether medicine was founded in science or art, in knowledge or opinion, in reason or experience, in the airy domain of philosophy or the gritty underworld of excrement, as a gentleman's dignified vocation or a tradesman's messy craft. Far from being submerged in the 1620s, these issues were prodded out into the open again by Bacon's powerful insistence that it was time at long last for the students of nature to get their hands dirty in the earthy labors of experiential learning.

Browne brings out the value of theoretical knowledge toward the end of his letter to Power when he insists that "in reading upon diseases satisfy yourself not so much with the remedies set down (although I would not have these altogether neglected) as with the true understanding the nature of the disease, its causes, and proper indications for cure. For by this knowledge, and that of the instruments you are to work by, the *Materia Medicamentorum*, you will often conquer with ease those difficulties, which books will not be able to bring you." This is Browne's tortuous attempt to weave together the value of book learning and experience; having tried to interrelate their offerings in this one sentence, he provides a mediator with a complex identity of its own: judgment. A faculty known in the language arts as the organizer of material so that it might be presented effectively, judgment links medical wisdom to logic; it is tinged with the moral authority of conscience (which is the faculty used for negotiating circumstances) but also with an experiential precision based on its tendency to prize distinctions over analogies and conflations. As an instrument of discourse, conscience, and experience, judgment provides

94 Quotations taken from Maclean, *Logic, Signs, and Nature*, 103.
95 Maclean, *Logic, Signs, and Nature*, 105.
96 Galen, *Ad Glauconem*, quoted in Maclean, *Logic, Signs, and Nature*, 123.

Browne with a single, packed term for the way in which the best physicians will translate back and forth between theory and the circumstances of experience. By calling it "secretum medicorum," he hints at the possibility that this mediatory agent in medical practice amounts to a divinely bestowed talent. No matter how much reading the injudicious novice might do, no matter how many flowers he might pick or patients that he might touch, he is never going to master the wisdom of Hippocrates, whose aphorisms formally embody this sense of enigma. If life is short while art is long, one had better have an extraordinary gift, indeed a Paracelsus's medical version of Origen's charisma.

The sort of book that Browne has most in mind for assisting the novice is the seventeenth-century compendium, from which genre he selects Daniel Sennert's *Institutes* for special recommendation. To be sure, there is still the challenge of translating basic medical notions into practice—into "reading upon diseases... in particular treatises, in counsels, and consultations" (Keynes, 4.256). But the advantage of Sennert is that he efficiently covers all the major parts of medical knowledge while accommodating and mediating the hotly debated rivalries among supporters of humoral, chemical, and mechanical medicine. In 1629, there remained "a coherent body of doctrine, with appropriate metaphysical and epistemological underpinning, which had evolved over the course of the preceding hundred years away from theory and towards practice, and still offered coherence and explanatory force to justify its existence."[97] But with Harvey's discovery in 1628, with Bacon's Great Instauration announced in 1620, and with the fuller emergence of atomism in the 1620s and 30s, Browne and his Oxford friends knew—Browne's letter to Power recreates this sense—that the ships for the America of new learning were ready to set sail, and that this state of affairs would be as perilous as it was thrilling.

From selected books both ancient and modern, Browne has the novice working his way through the five areas of basic medical wisdom: physiology ("the organization and functioning of the human body"), pathology, semiotics, therapy, and hygiene (having to do with keeping health intact).[98] In the course of these studies, prominent concepts include biological teleology (shared by Galen and Aristotle) and the naturals (the elements and humors, the members, spirits, faculties or strengths and operations of the various parts). The non-naturals involve six factors selected from the environment, the body, and the psyche as contingently conditioning health and including "air, exercise and rest, sleep and waking, food and drink, repletion and excretion, and the 'accidents of the soul,' or passions and emotions." Then there is complexion, understood as "a fundamental organizing principle of each individual human organism considered as a whole" and featuring the qualities of hot, cold, moist, and dry in a variety of combinations (Siraisi, 101–2, 79). Medical students also needed an understanding of the three main organs (brain, heart, liver, each with its own complexion, and each governing a system of operations via lesser organs); the three sets of roadways between them (nerves,

[97] Maclean, *Logic, Signs, and Nature*, 34–5.

[98] See Nancy G. Siraisi, *Medieval & Early Renaissance Medicine: An Introduction to Knowledge and Practice* (Chicago: University of Chicago Press, 1990), 78.

veins, arteries, each held to contain a distinctive material); and the three types or grades of spirit, a fiery-airy mixture thought by theologians to mediate between soul and body and responsible for effecting the operations of the body (animal, vital, natural). Most complicated by far was the role of circumstances in determining health and disease (place, time of year, time of life, sex, astral positions).

With regard to the diagnosis and prognosis of disease, the novice would need to accrue convenient resources such as humoral diagrams, recipe collections, and preferably indexed manuals comprising the essentials of the many afflictions. But he would also need to understand the nature of disease, which predictably divided into rubrics covering "congenital malformations…, complexional imbalance…, and trauma" or "a break in the body's continuity." With the first category amounting to the least prominent of the set, and with surgeons tending to handle the third, learned physicians would focus most of their attention on the imbalance of the humors. Cures were the product of opposition: that is, if the humors were erring on the side of one quality, the remedies had to restore balance by moving toward its opposite, with the physician always taking into account the complexion of the person in the given circumstances (season, age, sex, climate, region, dietary habits, and so forth) and the particular characteristics of the part affected. Some factors in dealing with disease would be learned from books: for example, fevers possessed certain narrative patterns featuring critical days that one either knew or did not. But diagnosis from symptoms and prognosis from indications involved a highly complex mixture of book learning and experience, especially with regard to interviewing the patient, inspecting his or her excrements, or feeling pulse and temperature. So too with cures, whether by bleeding, cupping, or purgative enemas, pills, syrups, and other (often elaborate) concoctions: neither book learning by itself nor experience on its own was going to maximize the chances for success. Sure, there were commonalities such as the three veins (cephalic, median, and basilica) from which blood was often drawn (Siraisi, 140). But the variety of medicaments was growing rapidly with the opening of the globe to exploration; even the well-known materials (mostly botanical, many from animal products, some from minerals (Siraisi, 148)) were highly various and complicated, promulgated by way of an unstable nomenclature; and disease could throw a curve at the system of curing by opposites, for instance in the case of smallpox which, once it had sufficiently advanced, was thought to require encouragement by way of increasing the already heightened heat of the body so that the disease might erupt. And physicians with a chemical or magical bent were concerned with far more than the human body or even the immediate circumstances in which it was living; for they believed that the microcosm was implicated in a cosmic network of correspondences that could be expressed by analogy but which operated across the various realms of the cosmos (celestial, elemental, human, animal, botanical, mineral) through a field of spiritual influences that could be managed only by mastering and intervening in the signatures of those correspondences as they were inscribed on all creation.

In addition to readings in standard texts such as Galen's *Ars parva*, Hippocrates's *Aphorisms*, and (perhaps) Avicenna's *Canon*, Browne's list for Henry Power makes the case for keeping up with more recent attempts to account for the etiology of disease in chemical studies but also in explorations of the nature of infection. But the novice's emerging sense of his profession would be powerfully shaped by the location in which he lived. For instance, specific diseases haunt generations in particular ways and diverse degrees, and in the 1620s, no disease could lay claim to the attention of the entrants into the English medical profession more than smallpox. In 1628, smallpox was dubbed by one Englishman the "popular disease" because it had become so widespread; its menace seemed to be rapidly on the rise, provoking concerns that its etiology and classification were not sufficiently understood by humoral means.[99]

As Browne moved from Oxford to the Continent, he was faced not just with learning medicine but with the challenges of modeling the medical profession. Coming from a business background in London, the social status of which was highly vexed, Browne faced the challenge of carving out a way of life and a professional identity whose position in the social order was unclear, not least because the learned physician's work was both highly intellectual and noxiously somatic. Setting out from the Oxford of Robert Burton and Thomas Clayton, Browne had every reason to concern himself with the need "to harmonise the idea of physic as a divine gift" celebrated in the Bible and in the figure of Jesus himself, "with the suspiciously pagan, not to say atheistic, implications of its overt veneration of ancient doctrine and tendency towards materialist explanations."[100] Being a good doctor would require the cultivation of spiritual purity and moral gravitas and honesty, for the spiritual and moral character of physicians was a topic on which Old Testament and New, Aristotle and Galen, medieval writers such as Chaucer, and the early humanists such as Thomas More had all weighed in. From Petrarch's *Invectiva contra medicum* (1355) to Francis Bacon's complaint in the year of Browne's birth that medical knowledge had been "more professed than laboured, and yet more laboured than advanced; the labour having been, in my judgment, rather in a circle than in progression,"[101] Browne embraced a future in which his education would have to concern his whole being over the course of his entire life. Among Oxford wits, moreover, his choice of medical studies over law and theology risked an association with the stereotypical vices attached to physicians: in the 1620s, John Earle's character studies circulated in Oxford with a satire of the "mere dull physician" who debased "speculation" in excrement; whose pompous show of learning concealed his actually meager reading; who tended to make patients less healthy but "his own purse... lusty and in flesh"; who gained employment from "ladies for wantonness, especially if he be a proper man"; who wasted leisure time with alchemy; and who showed a fundamental affinity with "man's corruption."[102]

[99] For smallpox and Browne see chapter 6 in this volume.

[100] Angus Gowland, *The Worlds of Renaissance Melancholy: Robert Burton in Context* (Cambridge: Cambridge University Press, 2006), 35.

[101] Quoted in Gowland, *Worlds of Renaissance Melancholy*, 103.

[102] John Earle, *Microcosmography*, ed. Harold Osborne (London: University Tutorial Press, 1933), 14–15.

With the medical curriculum at Oxford undergoing a renaissance in his time there, but also with exploratory teachers such as Lushington, Browne faced a life of learning in which he would never be able to lapse into complacency. Indeed discontent with one's understanding was part and parcel of what it meant to be Clayton's student at Oxford in the 1620s; for the Master of Pembroke was having Montpellier travel guides published for the simple reason that if Oxford scholars wanted to be good physicians, they had to travel abroad into the unknown, threatening world of a Europe torn apart by religious warfare. As Robert Frank argues, the period around 1630 was a watershed for the Oxford student on the medical trajectory, for this was the point at which it became no longer acceptable to lack drive and ambition.[103] Graduating from Oxford with Clayton as his medical mentor and the heroic Hues as his compass, Browne confronted a future in which a quiet and retiring complexion might prove seriously detrimental. If melancholy made Browne studious, at least it lacked phlegm's proneness to nod and agitated its patient into the ceaseless, never satisfied deciphering of the world.

Despite Browne's turn to medicine, the writing of verse remained a constant feature of his youth. In a manuscript compiling a various sampling of his youthful poetry, Browne collected a poem in which the love poetry of the Oxford manuscripts is cleansed of lust or sex and devoted to virtue, nature, and divinity. Unlike women, whose too-often idolized beauty is deformed by "age" and "scarre" (smallpox again?), nobler objects of love can be found in virtue's "lovely face," in the beauties of a "Tulip, rose, or marigold," in a companionate soul, and finally in God. If human rationality would only realize that roses and poppies have a "richer" color than any cosmetically altered face, it would also understand that human conventions of beauty are entirely relative ("This sweet vermillion wee adore | seemes ugly to the Jetty moore") and temporary in its quick progression toward a repellent and dusty decay (Keynes, 3.235). Having made his case for a nature-loving, rational, spiritual, and chaste love, Browne turns to the divine with a conceit that recalls Donne's eroticization of the sacred, and with an address ("great god") that directly links this poem to the verses on the storm: "There is no face so divine | wee all adore, great god, butt thine, | Bee thou my paramour: o lett mee | not looke on these butt gaze on thee."

Browne's other verses also suggest a young wit with one foot in the world of manuscript miscellanies and another directed toward the journey into medical and spiritual vocation. One set of couplets offers a botanically learned catalogue of plants: "The Almond fourisheth, the Birch trees flowe, | the sad Mezereon Cheerefully doth Blowe. | The flourie sonnes before their fathers seen, | and snayles beginne to Crop the Mandrake green. | The vernall sunne with Crocus gardens fills, | with Hyacinths, Anemones and Daffodills: | the Hazell Catskins now delate and fall, | and Paronychions peep upon each wall" (Keynes, 3.236). These are the verses of a young man beginning to read seriously the herbals and to see the world as written everywhere in a language of

[103] Frank, "Medicine," in Tyacke, ed., *History of the University of Oxford, Volume IV*, 546.

signatures that links humanity to flora in a network of analogies. Insofar as the "flourie sonnes" can be identified as the "*Filius ante Patrem*, the Mede-Saffron (Gerard) or Autumn Crocus, which produces leaves in February, seed in May, and flowers in September,"[104] the poem refigures father–son relations as wholly delightful, dependable, and fruitful; and the spontaneous burgeoning of nature is easily reconciled with and supportive of the artistry to be found in "gardens" or "upon each wall."

A shorter set of verses, comprising two couplets only, is unclear about whether it is eroticizing the divine or sublimating the erotic: "The courteous Sunne with dust & lowlie mire | Voutsafes to joyne his generative fire. | Disdaine not then my armes, scorne not to Joyne | thy heavenly substance to this earth of myne" (Keynes, 3.236). The stress on the quality of courtesy and on the capacity for generation suggests that Browne is playing an Oxford wit's part as love poet. Indeed, even such simple terms as "heavenly substance" reflect his student's learning of basic Aristotelian positions, in this case, the fundamental divide between *super*lunary and *sub*lunary natures. Of course the poem might well be in a fragmentary state, but as it exists, it might also be read in keeping with Browne's poem on the desirability of reorienting sexual desire toward the divine, with God as the only true "paramour" who can convert the muck of human nature into a generative vocation.

Only later in life would Browne leave record of his concern for the rites of passage undertaken in these years by other members of his extended family: the death of his maternal grandfather Paul Garraway in April 1620, for instance, the birth of two daughters (Elizabeth in 1622, Lucy in 1623) to his mother and stepfather, or the marriage of his eldest sister Anne to a London grocer named John Palmer at the church of St Martin Pomeroy, Ironmonger Lane, on December 30, 1628, of sister Mary (to Nevill Craddock on September 30, 1630) and of sister Jane in 1632 or 1633 to the future archbishop of Cashel, Thomas Price, a man from County Cavan in Ulster.[105] Browne has nothing on record about the lives of his mother and sister Ellen in the Irish plantation, either before or after the death of Dutton in 1634. As critics have often suggested, the *Religio* is stridently clear on the distance that Browne appears to have placed between his affections and his parents.[106] Yet Browne's experience of surrogate families at Winchester and Oxford was sufficiently uneven to ensure that he tried his best to establish the happiest of families when he and his wife made their own and when his *Pseudodoxia* sought to gather the republic of letters into its folds.

Browne's graduation and turn to medicine entailed that he was no longer an orphaned student responsible mainly for linguistic forms and arts but an adult persuing the vocation of a Christian physician with a responsibility for life, that of his patients to be sure, but also the value of his very own. Perhaps the awkwardness of his verses was owed in part to Browne's composing them in English, the

[104] See Keynes's note on 3.236.

[105] Hughes, "Childhood," 25, and Huntley, *Sir Thomas Browne*, 48.

[106] For instance, J.-J. Denonain, "Le reître et le jouvenceau," *Caliban*, n.s., 1 (1965), 7–20, largely based on the work of Endicott, "Sir Thomas Browne as 'Orphan,'" especially 201–3.

future language of his artful, exploratory discourse though not of his Winchester and Oxford past. A learned medicus would need his Greek and Latin always with him, of course, but a charitable and successful bedside physician would need a vernacular with its own healing charms. After his travels on the Continent, Browne would need a linguistic art that could help his neighbors with their most painful afflictions. He could not yet have realized that his English, in itself and once converted into Latin, would both heal and further afflict an early modern world of strife.

PART II

TRANSPLANT

4

Montpellier, 1631–1632

On February 11, 1631, probably in an effort to raise money for his impending travels, Thomas Browne, son of Thomas Browne late of London, mercer, co-signed with his uncle Edward a claim of arrears on an annuity of ten pounds regarding property in Cheshire.[1] Not long after that, probably in the spring or summer of 1631 in anticipation of the autumnal beginning of the school year, he set off for the Continent where he would spend the next three years of his life in pursuit of an advanced medical education in three centers of learning: Montpellier, Padua, and Leiden. The medical course at Montpellier was divided into two unequal semesters: a longer one extending from St Luke's Day (at the end of September or beginning of October) to Easter, the shorter one from Easter to St Luke's Day, with a major vacation lasting from July to St Luke's Day. How formally he approached the curriculum in Montpellier is unknown, since he never officially matriculated.[2] But Browne's later statements about medical education, as well as his own medical practice, place a high value on some of the professors, focuses, and vocational attitudes that he encountered in the south of France. And the distinctive culture of Languedoc impressed itself on Browne's imagination, not least on his ever-growing appreciation for the vitality of local habits, environments, and languages.

Even though Oxford was clearly making strides to advance its medical curriculum, the best education of the physician was still to be had on the Continent. Indeed, even had Oxford been far better in medicine than it was, travel abroad was deemed essential for a medical student as well as a gentleman. Despite the pervasive public image of travel abroad as conducive to atheism, apostasy, sedition, and immorality, such a journey was greeted among young English scholars as integral to their personal development, social and intellectual completeness, linguistic competence, and public service.[3] Even for the continental medical student, travel was especially advised. In 1674, Thomas Bartholin summarized this sentiment in *De peregrinatione medica* when he elaborated on Democritus's conviction that "the whole world is the native land of a powerful mind" and applied it to the modern physician:

[1] Cheshire and Chester Archives, Arderne Collection, ref. DAR/C/91/5.

[2] See Karen Meier Reeds, *Botany in Medieval and Renaissance Universities* (Thesis, Harvard University, 1975), 81–3. There is no mention of Browne's name in either the Liber congregationum (Montpellier medical school archives, MS S 10) or the Matricules (MS 20). In the city archives, a Jean Brune (but no Thomas) received medicine in the Livre des comptes de l'Hopital St Eloi, MS GG 95, 5r.

[3] For the perceived dangers, see Sara Warneke, *Images of the Educational Traveller in Early Modern England* (Leiden: Brill, 1995).

> In our age such great usefulness redounds to the physician from his travels that no one puts much faith in the authority of a physician who has not set foot outside his native land, and although each may have at home in abundance those things which are necessary for medical instruction, nevertheless they ought to be strengthened or increased by a comparison with things abroad.

Not just knowledge but also pleasure stood to be gained from such travel, for

> There is a vast delight and pleasure in gazing upon foreign lands and fields, mountains and rivers, observing the benignity of nature's variety everywhere, the different conditions of the sick in homes and in hospitals with their great number of beds, which can readily be seen here and there, examining the methods for treating the patients, enjoying the conversation of the learned men and calling forth their experiences, and visiting the laboratories, the furnaces of the chemists, the pharmacies and unguent shops.[4]

Bartholin explained that each environment offers instruction to the medical student, as does the widest range of medical professionals, including physicians, surgeons, apothecaries, chemists, gardeners, and "even the secrets of the gypsies by which they frequently make a fucus or satisfy the demands of the common people" (57). Bartholin also clarified that each medical school still bore its own strengths, with Padua famous for anatomy, Montpellier for botany, and the Low Countries for "the principles of the art." Each had its curricular bias, with the Paduans adhering to Galen, for instance, while in Montpellier "they boast themselves as the heirs of Arab doctrine carried to them by the disciples of Avicenna and Averroes who flourished for many centuries in the Academy of Cordoba through the diligence of the Moors" (58). In 1656, William Hammond summed up the special benefits of medical travel: "The Profession I have now undertaken, gathers like a Snowball in rowling; & tis apparent that our greatest Doctors in Physick, have been those, who by the advantage of Travelling, have view'd, compar'd, & digested the severall Practises of most of *th*e Europæan Physicians."[5]

1. NORTHERN TRAVELERS IN FRANCE

From his recollection of La Rochelle, it appears that, having crossed the Channel, Browne traveled to Montpellier over land instead of sailing direct to Marseilles.[6] Although Browne's memory of Toulouse could have derived from an excursion from Montpellier, it also lies on the course that he appears to have

[4] Thomas Bartholin, *De peregrinatione medical On Medical Travel*, trans. Charles D. O'Malley (Lawrence: University of Kansas Libraries, 1961), 45, 50–1.

[5] William Hammond, in Michael Brennan, ed., *The Origins of the Grand Tour: The Travels of Robert Montague, Lord Mandeville, 1649–1654; William Hammond, 1655–1658; Banaster Maynard, 1660–1663* (London: The Hakluyt Society, 2004), 201.

[6] For routes from England to France, see John Lough, *France Observed in the Seventeenth Century by British Travellers* (Boston: Oriel Press, 1985), 18.

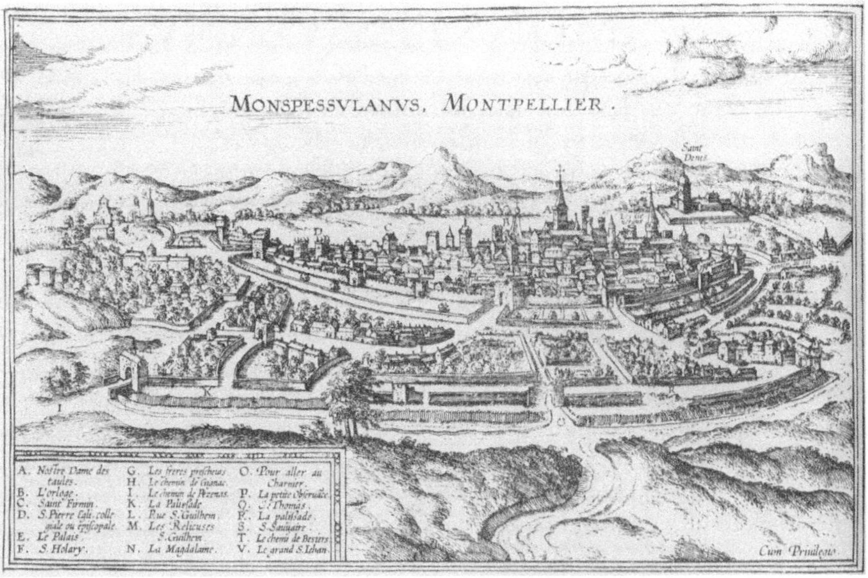

Figure 4.1 Montpellier, from Georg Braun and Frans Hogenberg, Civitates Orbis Terrarum, 1572–1618, with an introduction by R. A. Skelton, in six parts; volume 1, parts 1 and 2 (Amsterdam: Theatrvm Orbis Terrarvm Ltd., 1965), part one, section 8. Reproduced by the kind permission of Asher Rare Books, 't Goy-Houten (The Netherlands).

taken on his journey from England. The travel journal of Francis Mortoft follows the kind of trajectory that Browne is likely to have taken: from Dover to Calais, then Boulogne, Dieppe, Rouen, Paris, Orleans, the Loire region of Blois, Amboise, Tours, and Nantes, then southward to La Rochelle and Bordeaux, then along the Garonne to Toulouse before curving around eastward toward Narbonne, Beziers, and Montpellier.[7] (See Figure 4.1.) As for his destination, Montpellier, travel guides such as Théodore Turquet de Mayerne's *Sommaire Description de La France, Allemagne, Italie, et Espagne* (1604) not only encouraged tourists to anticipate the exceptional fertility, renowned medical school, and good governance in Montpellier and Languedoc; but they also provided practical information about roads, waterways, fairs, inns, distances, and costs.

It is not surprising that Browne headed to Montpellier first among his continental destinations, for as we learn from James Primerose's *Academia Monspeliensis* (1631), it was a destination to which Thomas Clayton was urging his students to travel. Having encouraged the Oxford student to expect that he will meet other English students at Montpellier, Primerose singles out certain alumni and professors for praise, including Jean de Lort (Regent professor, 1610–37) and the Scot,

[7] See Francis Mortoft, *Francis Mortoft: His Book*, ed. Malcolm Letts (London: Hakluyt Society, 1925), fold-out map.

George Scharpe (Regent professor, 1619–39), the latter, distinguished in philosophy as well as medicine. Other medical professors who taught at Montpellier in 1631 featured Lazare Rivière (professor of chirurgery and pharmacy 1622–55); the Chancellor François Ranchin (Regent professor of medicine, 1605–41); and Siméon Courtaud (Regent professor, 1620–64). The specialized professorships—of botany/anatomy and of surgery/pharmacy—had been added to the four Regents professorships in 1593 and 1597 respectively; in Browne's day, in addition to these six offices, two members of the medical faculty served as "agregatures," including Jacques Duranc (died 1652; Aggrégé from 1623 to 1639, when he took over Scharpe's professorship).[8] With the nurturing Clayton as his guarantor, Primerose makes the case that an Oxford undergraduate is bound to prosper in Montpellier as he makes his transition from homeland to foreign parts and from youth and study to adulthood and vocation.[9] Not only was Browne's Oxford master encouraging his students to commence their medical education in Montpellier, but Browne's 1628 copy of Hippocrates's *Aphorisms* presented that cornerstone of medical learning in a French translation.[10]

Browne's recollections of France from his travels there in 1631–2 are vivid both medically and culturally. In the Midi, so many of what would prove lifelong fascinations leaped into his field of experience for the first time. As John Stoye has remarked of young Thomas Wentworth, who was journeying to Montpellier in 1612, a traveler from Protestant England not only encountered ceremonial and ascetic Catholicism for the first time, but also found himself "in the heart of Roman France," where "apothecaries ... kept not only drugs and potions but ancient incinerary urns, lacrimals and little old lamps."[11] Here too was "the land of the chameleon, salamander and Jericho roses," among other specimens to which Browne would turn serious attention in *Pseudodoxia Epidemica* and to which he attached local colors and sounds—witness his remark about the praying mantis that it was called "by the Common people of Province, *Prega Dio*" (Robbins, ed., *Pseudodoxia Epidemica*, 1.292). As a testimony to the powerful sensory stimulation that English visitors to the Midi would experience, Browne noted in his tract "of Plants in Scripture" that the pleasing odor of vineyard flowers might prove "hard unto our Northern Nostrils, which discover not Odours, and smell them not in full Vineyards; whereas in hot Regions, and more spread and digested Flowers, a sweet savour may be allowed" (Keynes, 3.15).

The older Browne also recalled the temptations lurking among the French sensations. Having urged his son Thomas to see La Rochelle and the Isle of Rhe, he warns young Tom to "be warie, for Rochell was a place of too much good fellowship and a very drinking town, as I observed when I was there, more then other

[8] Louis Dulieu, *La Médecine à Montpellier*, vol. 3, part 1 (Avignon: Les Presses Universelles, 1983), 26–8; Jean Astruc, *Mémoires pour server a l'Histoire de Montpellier* (Paris, 1767), 258–9.

[9] James Primerose, *Academia Monspeliensis* (Oxford, 1631).

[10] Finch, ed., *A Catalogue of the Libraries of Sir Thomas Browne and Dr Edward Browne, His Son* (Leiden: E. J. Brill, 1986), 34.

[11] John Stoye, *English Travellers Abroad, 1604–1667: Their Influence in English Society and Politics* (revised ed., New Haven, CT: Yale University Press, 1989), 45.

Parts of France." In instructing Tom on whether to move on to Paris or to Nantes for the purposes of tourism, Browne adds a cautionary point: "I wish you had acquaintance with some Protestant of Nantes if you goe thither, or might be recommended, for there are English also" (Keynes, 4.12, 15). Yet if he worries about alcohol consumption in La Rochelle, Browne cherishes the festive exuberance and patois of Rabelais, Goudelin, and the everyday folk of Languedoc; embraces the eclectic, optimistic medicine of Montpellier professors such as Lazare Rivière; and sympathizes with a religious culture attempting to resurrect itself from the rubble of nearly a century of civil warfare. In 1630, the rebuilding of Montpellier's botanical garden and churches epitomized the resolve of a people intent on reanimating their physical and spiritual welfare as surely as its physicians and pharmacists were assuming the leadership in concocting robust medicaments from poisons but also a vital synthesis from the medical wars between Galenists and Paracelsians. In the early 1630s, the university was recovering from the plague of 1629, with thirty-three matriculations in 1630 an improvement over the seven from 1629.[12] But festivity, vitality, regeneration—sensations so pronounced in the early modern accounts of many northern Europeans in southern France—are entangled in Browne's memory with the perils of youth and with the intimacy that the brave spirit of life always shares with the macabre specter of death and gruesome decay.

In his anatomical notes, for instance, Browne linked together a wide range of examples in which the toughness of skin from dried bodies could produce exceptionally resilient glue, including the preserved corpses he had witnessed "in the vault of the Cordiliers at Tholouze." Relishing the juvenescent and carnivalesque langue d'oc of Rabelaisian humor as well as the amorous music of Languedoc, Browne found vitality in the traditional Midi. He encountered a professor, François Ranchin, who specialized in childhood health and had remarkably minimized the damage of a recent plague; yet he also remembered his bewilderment at those vermiculate or hirsute growths that crawled out of the flesh of Midi children afflicted by a disease called the "morgellons." In his tract "Of Plants in Scripture," Browne had recourse to another memory of Languedoc and Provence in his meditation on a parasitical growth known as "Worm" or "the Wormy Berry," and in the Midi as *manna rusticorum*. Adhering to an evergreen, the Ilex Coccigera "or dwarf and small kind of Oak," it produced "flies" and "powder" which could be made into a brilliant vermillion tincture. But the plant must not be gathered prematurely, Browne warned, lest it fail to produce its beautiful redness. Harvesters enlisted the sprinkling of vinegar in order to suppress the flies if their goal was "the fresh Pulp" from which "the confection of Alkermes" could be made according to the guidelines of Bellonius and Quinqueranus. "And the same we have beheld in Provence and Languedock, where it is plentifully gathered," its association with manna deriving "from the considerable profit which the Peasants make by gathering it" (Keynes, 3.34). Thus the most resplendent color and the means of vitality depended as much on worminess and flies as they did on evergreens and timely

[12] J. Trevor Hughes, "The Medical Education of Sir Thomas Browne," *Journal of Medical Biography* 9 (2001), 70–6; see 72.

maturation. The Midi abundance of yet another type of "worm," the silkworm, resonated in Browne's assertion that "Those strange and mysticall transmigrations that I have observed in Silkewormes, turn'd my Philosophy into Divinity" (Patrides, 110). In Browne's Midi memories, regeneration emerged out of corruption, but the two were usually inextricable from one another—as surely as they were in Browne's imagination when in 1658 he placed funeral urns and gardens next to one another in a single volume.

Years after his continental travels, in 1660, Browne advised his son Tom on things to see, to note, and to do on his travels to France in 1660–61: in Bordeaux, for instance, the ruined amphitheater; the country in which "Coynac wines" are produced, including those consumed by the Browne family during summers; opportunities to collect coins and urns; the salt works on the Isle of Rhe; and the production of oil, wine, and vinegar (Keynes, 4.3–16). But father Browne also cautioned his son that the key to prospering in France was paradoxical: the young traveler must grow up from provincialism into a cosmopolitan civility but somehow never lose his native province: his moral center and his English Protestantism. On the one hand he urged his son to make a strong Protestant connection so that his spiritual and cultural identity might be preserved. On the other, he stressed that French conversation was a necessary rung on a ladder leading to a maturation that put away rustic bashfulness for civility and sophistication: "put on a decent boldnes and avoid *pudor Rusticus*, not much known in France" (Keynes, 4.4). In remembering a French divine dismayed by Seneca's insistence on the mortality of the soul, the author of *Religio* betrayed the possible delusions of hope: he and his companions in France had failed to cure their friend of his melancholy atheism when "all our Antidotes, drawne from both Scripture and Philosophy, could not expell poyson of his errour" (Patrides, 87). In the *Religio*, this French divine, a "man of parts", keeps company with the Italian doctor whose reading of Galen produces a deadly atheism far more typical of the Paduan culture toward which Browne would move in 1632 than of the Midi in which heresy and oppression from within the Christian faith itself were the prominent dangers.

Despite the ravages of the civil wars, southern France often struck visitors from the north as the essence of vitality and fertility. Francis Mortoft's association of Languedoc with the essential ingredients of human vitality is typical of the way in which northerners travelling to the Midi responded: "the truth is all the ground in Languedoc beares nothing else but sweet herbes, where one may observe to grow together 3 of the Considerable things of man's life, that is, Corne, Wyne and oyle, the Olive trees being planted on that ground where the Corne growes, and close by are planted Vinyards, of which the Inhabitants make wyne in abundance."[13] Throughout Provence and Languedoc, a German traveler in the 1620s, the geographer Abraham Golnitz, also captured the intensity of the Northern experience of the Midi that responded alike to nature, antiquity, and local customs.[14] Clearly

[13] Mortoft, *Francis Mortoft: His Book*, 23, 25.

[14] See L. Malavialle, *Le Bas-Languedoc en 1626 d'après la description du géographie allemande Abraham Golnitz* (Montpellier: Sociéte Anonyme de L'Imprimerie Générale du Midi, 1909).

Golnizt was inspired by nature's fertility, variety, and beneficence, and by the fruitful agricultural and cottage industry that cheerfully cultivates natural bounty, all in the face of rampant, incessant military wreckage. For Golnitz, no less wonderful are the ancient monuments that, far from suggestive of ruin, are in such supply and often in such good repair that ancient Gaul itself seems resurrected from the dead—this is especially true, he remarks, of the Pont-du-Gard. In Montpellier Golnitz records just how filled the city is still with thousands of soldiers, lodging in residential homes and guarding the city in the name of the king. Despite this burden, he finds a pervasive and healthy good cheer among the artisans of the city as they whiten wax, produce verdigris, and craft knives, blue paint, woolens, and drinking vessels in their homes and shops. The drinking vessels are especially significant insofar as they figure centrally in the expulsion of melancholy. Of the famous medical school Golnitz has much to say regarding its original impetus from the influx of Arabs, its felicitous setting, healthy air, experienced medical professoriate, and herbal and floral plenty.

In basic ways, then, Languedoc struck northern visitors—Browne among them—as an irrepressible garden, one triumphant over the ravages of death, violence, and decay. Like Browne, Golnitz was also impressed by sights in the areas around Montpellier. Among their excursions, a trip to Marguelone, with its descendents from the Saracens, had the medically educative value of introducing the visitor to the roots of pharmacy. The Catelan family was the most recent in a long line of brilliant pharmacists in Montpellier; and their shop stocked the *materia medica* everywhere to be found in the local countryside. Indeed, Golnitz points out the grains of kermes mentioned by Browne. Exported for the purposes of dyeing, this material doubled as the antidote "Alkermes" used to remedy heart palpitations, anemia, fainting fits, and other ills. But in Catelan's shop, one found so many delightful local products, including oils, essences, and toothpicks.

2. MEDICINE IN MONTPELLIER

Montpellier and its medical school served as emblems of native toleration, amenity, and vitality.[15] Assisted by a belief in their healthy natural environment, physicians embraced the conviction that vitality, sociability, and comedy triumph over and even profit from death and decay; this proved a crucial feature of Browne's work as a physician and author. Students at the medical school often remarked on its basis in the experience of that environment. For one thing, there was the ample opportunity for botanizing trips. For another, the school placed a strong emphasis on clinical experience. In addition, trips to the local baths doubled as instruction and entertainment. Browne himself especially valued the opportunity to interact with apothecaries, urging his son to live with one while in France. In his visit to

[15] Elizabeth A. Williams, *A Cultural History of Medical Vitalism in Enlightenment Montpellier* (Burlington, VT: Ashgate, 2003), 16, 18–19. Cf. A. G. Chevalier, "Medical Teaching at Montpellier," *Ciba Symposia* 2 (1940), 408–11.

Montpellier, John Ray declared that "The number of Apothecaries in this little City is scarce credible, there being 130 shops, and yet all find something to do: their Cypres powder, sweet bags, Cassolets, Treacle, Confectio Alkermes, & Hyacintha having a name all over France."[16] As one walked through the streets of Montpellier in 1631, the smells—often noxious—of the apothecary's lab and shop were often to be met. In Browne's time, everyone visited the natural history museum of Laurent Catelan III, whose demonstration of his drugs was staged with great ceremony and music.[17] Even in the commercial industries of the area, apothecary procedures were everywhere in operation: in the making of dye, olive oil, or wax.[18]

In short, Browne's powerful appreciation for the materials of his trade, indeed of all the world, received extraordinary stimulation in Montpellier. A crucial figure in introducing students to the *materia medica* was Pierre Richer de Belleval, who died in 1632. As one student wrote in his journal, it was thanks to this professor that Montpellier was especially good about familiarizing students with the preparation of medicines.[19] The botanical garden, situated not far from the town walls, was designed to be both pleasant and useful. Its vaulted aquatic rooms—to which one gained access by the covered walkway with several twists and turns (the "labyrinth")—were singled out for their cool refreshment and repose. After 1601, their reverberant vaults were painted by Guillaume Baudoin with trompe l'oeil representing beautiful foliage and greenery, all strangely evocative, surreal, and tranquil.[20] Outside around the garden, golden inscriptions on the gates informed visitors where they might find "plants that grow in thickets or as spiny shrubs"; "plants that grow in sunny, stony, or sandy places"; or "plants that occur in shady places and woods."[21] For Browne, whose simpling thus far had included Cheapside, Winchester, and Oxford, Montpellier's extraordinary botanical resources would have been a revelation.

Montpellier's botanical garden was also known for the great size of its site among the fields and meadows next to the river Peyrou. There were several efforts at useful organization of course: the bifurcation of the garden into seminarium and herbarium (the former a nursery of interesting Languedoc plants, the latter inclusive of two areas for the *materia medica*); the species (1,332 in 1598) numbered and keyed to a visitor's guide; the endeavor to situate plants as much as possible in their natural habitats, including the construction of an artificial "mountain" with its

16 John Ray, quoted in John Lough, *France Observed in the Seventeenth Century by British Travellers* (Boston: Oriel Press, 1985), 67.

17 Louis Dulieu, *La Pharmacie à Montpellier: de ses origines à nos jours* (Avignon: Les Presses Universelles, 1973), 61–78.

18 Lough, *France Observed*, 67.

19 Thomas Platter, *Journal of a Younger Brother: The Life of Thomas Platter as a Medical Student in Montpellier at the Close of the Sixteenth Century*, trans. and intro. Seán Jennett (London: Frederick Muller, 1968), 38.

20 See Jean Nougaret, "Les Constructions du Jardin de Pierre Richer de Belleval," in Jean-Antoine Rioux, ed., *Le Jardin des Plantes de Montpellier: Quatre siècles d'histoire* (Grauhlet: Odyssée, 1994), 97–102; the labyrinth is discussed on 99–100.

21 Reeds, *Botany in Medieval and Renaissance Universities*, 110–11.

northward and southward faces reserved for plants with distinctive environmental needs; the vaulted subterranean room for aquatic plants; the buildings with a laboratory, conservatory, library, chapel, the custodial professor's house, and ambulatory; and the plant-beds raised to eye level with paths laid for easy circulation by the visitors. Yet the garden also had a penchant for Rabelaisian exaggeration, gaming, and unlimited multiplicity. The names of the so-called mountain and labyrinth struck some amused visitors as obvious overstatement and as intentionally humorous.[22] Others complained that the whole was too confused and perplexing.[23] Unlike the gardens that Browne would encounter in Leiden and Padua, the garden in Montpellier offered a sprawling, highly variegated experience, for all the method in its madness.[24] As *The Garden of Cyrus* shows, however, Browne was taken with the copiousness and multiplicity of plant life, even as he was tracing the geometrical and providential patterns in nature.

If Montpellier was in the vanguard of the chemical revolution in medicine, its legacy as the treasurehouse of botanical materials of medicine was equally integral to its reputation and identity. Montpellier was the center for antimony, but it was also a chief producer of extraordinary plant remedies such as the legendary and complicated theriac: produced with great ceremony, this medicine was associated with Mithidrates, described by Galen, revitalized by the medieval Arabs, and classed among opiates, a favorite with scholastic medicine until the end of the seventeenth century.[25] In the notes that he later took on plague and pestilence, Browne set down his appreciation for the value and complexity of this line of transmission, by means of which rare Hippocratic writings and commentaries were shepherded by "some Arabick writer, the Arabians being very carefull to preserve the workes of ancient Greekes wch they often translated, and sometimes fathered other works upon the best of them wch are now very rare or quite lost among us" (Keynes, 3.250). In these same notes, Browne purveyed an interest in theriac (3.251–2). But while Browne approached this medical history with a critical eye, his notes on pestilence also epitomize the hope that Montpellier medical training embodied: that the physician and his materials participated in and contributed to the astonishing resilence, resourcefulness, and exuberance of life.

The Montpellier faculty did not hide their light under a basket: unlike the professors whom Browne would encounter in Leiden, most of them published works both of a foundational and a controversial nature. And their students—chief among them, Théophraste Renaudot (1586–1653)—were taking strong stands against a Parisian medical establishment in making the case that a reformed chemical medicine could cure all the sicknesses of all the people. Sympathizers deemed

[22] See further Hubert Bonnet, "Pierre de Belleval et sa Dynastie," in Rioux, ed., *Le Jardin des Plantes de Montpellier: Quatre Siècles*, 25–33; and Jean-Antoine Rioux, *Le Jardin des Plantes de Montpellier: "Les leçons de l'histoire"* (Montpellier: Sauramps, 2003), 12–21.

[23] For instance, Claude Fabri de Peiresc in 1607: see Bonnet, in Rioux, 28. Cf. Guy de la Brosse's response in *Description du Jardin Royal des Plantes Medecinales* (Paris, 1636).

[24] Reeds, *Botany in Medieval and Renaissance Universities*, 117.

[25] Jean-Pierre Bénézet, "La Thériaque de Montpellier," in Rioux, ed., *Le Jardin des Plantes de Montpellier: Quatre Siècles*, 143–7.

Montpellier medicine to be progressive, optimistic, and charitable; critics read the same tendencies as recklessly interventionist in nature's own processes and naively empirical in violation of the ancient "science" of medicine. The Montpellier approach left "little room for hygiene, self-help, or leaving nature to cure herself." By contrast, Parisian rationalism "offered mankind the chance of controlling his medical destiny and turning his relations with the medical profession into an occasional event."[26] Browne's success as a practicing and consulting physician suggests that he gave his patients comfort and hope, and his fellow physicians a confidence in their vocation. If these qualities are traceable to the medical ethos at Montpellier, they are not the entire story of Browne's response to human affliction, which at times can prove far more committed to hygiene and nature's own way, and far more resigned to the afflictions dispensed by providence. Even so, training in Montpellier not only gave Browne a solid and eclectic introduction to medical principles, but it embodied an attitude toward the power, comedy, and resilience of the medically managed life that infused his vocational ethos and practice.

At the crux of their approach to medicine were two features of concern for Browne's professors such as Scharpe, Rivière, and Ranchin: that Galenic "science" would remain the foundation of instruction yet be softened to accommodate chemical and modern advances in a practical synthesis; and that a pessimism about the senescence of the world—about its increasing unhealthiness—could be offset by the physician's charitable and confident interventions in the processes of life from birth onward. Influenced by Jean Fernel's synthesis as "the first attempt since Galen's 'On the Usefulness of the Parts' to provide a systematic coverage of physiology,"[27] the Montpellier professors of Browne's time in the Midi were dedicated to an eclectic education of the physician who could aggressively rescue his patients from disease and suffering.

As a Scot, George Scharpe (*c.*1581–1637) provided some continuity with their homeland for British students coming to the Midi. (See Figure 4.2.) In his professional capacity, he embodied something of Montpellier's optimistic, philanthropic commitment to the amelioration of human suffering: he had served in l'Hotel-Dieu Saint-Eloi, a hospital serving the poor; he attended soldiers during the 1622 siege; and he was instrumental in assisting Ranchin during the plague of 1629–30 which, on the eve of Browne's arrival, more than anything else captured Montpellier's phoenix-like propensity to rise brilliantly from its own ashes. Scharpe's posthumous *Institutiones medicae*, based on his lectures at Montpellier, covers only the first two of the five major segments of medical learning: physiology and pathology.[28] These, the first two of the three purely theoretical subjects offer us a good picture of Scharpe's lectures. (The third is semiotics, for which the book includes

[26] L. Brockliss, "Seeing and Believing: Contrasting Attitudes towards Observational Autonomy among French Galenists in the First Half of the Seventeenth Century," in W. F. Bynum and Roy Porter, eds., *Medicine and the Five Senses* (New York: Cambridge University Press, 1993), 78.

[27] Brian Nance, *Turquet de Mayerne as Baroque Physician: The Art of Medical Portraiture* (New York: Rodopi, 2001), 45.

[28] All references to Scharpe's *Institutiones Medicae* (1638) are given parenthetically. For their source in his lectures, see Jean Astruc, *Mémoires pour server a l'Histoire de Montpellier* (Paris, 1767), 256.

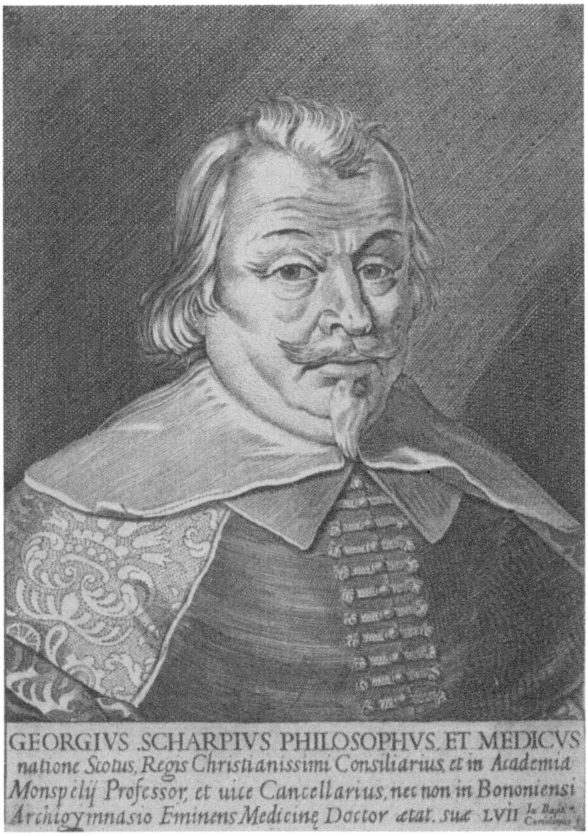

Figure 4.2 George Scharpe, from a line engraving by I. B. Coriolanus. Reproduced with the permission of the Wellcome Library, London.

only a preliminary chapter on indications and a few final chapters on symptoms; the practical subjects of regimen and therapy are amply covered by Rivière.) If this one publication is any indication, Scharpe was dedicated to cultivating clarity of thought and a strong foundation in initiates to the medical profession. Even Guy Patin, the nemesis of Montpellier, conceded that Scharpe had an acute logical mind.[29]

But Scharpe was not simply a rationalist in his medical thinking. For one thing, his lectures purvey a strong interest in the value and the variety of experience and are prefaced with a detailed analysis of experience. Grounding this account—as well as all the others—in Greek terminology, he moves quickly from that historical experience transmitted through writings to "autopsy," that is, to one's own experience (*Institutiones*, 12); so too, in advising Henry Power, Browne started with the

[29] J. Trevor Hughes, "George Scharpe, c.1581–1637: A Scots Doctor at Montpellier," *Scottish Medical Journal* 47 (2002), 40–3.

value of experience, remarking how "ridiculous are they who think out of book to become Physicians" (Keynes, 4.255). For Scharpe, direct, personal experience ranges widely: periptosis comprises conclusions that we draw from motions frequently elicited in nature but also from chance. The second type of autopsy, autochoedion, is more spontaneous, instinctive, and even surreal: if animals often reveal the instinct for remedies, human beings sometimes have access to a felicitous but mysterious event that produces theorems of the art. Whereas Scharpe's colleague Rivière limits his discussion of dreams to medical analysis,[30] Scharpe finds room in his medicine even for the prophetic power and truth of special dreams. On the spectrum between the two professors, Browne would later reflect on the problem of how far to take the meaning of dreams: in his tract on dreams, Browne himself would recall that "Wee owe unto dreames that Galen was a physitian" (Patrides, 477), while in *Letter to a Friend* he would carefully weigh the value of dreams in medical diagnosis and prognosis.[31] Mimesis, Scharpe's third type of direct experience, is built on the imitation or repetition of remedies found in spontaneous actions (*Institutiones*, 13). All in all, Scharpe's belief that experience is as crucial to the medical vocation as it is complex anticipates the layered construction of experience—variously textual, intellectual, and sensorily immediate, both patterned and unpredictable, even surreal—that constitutes Browne's method of interpretation in all his works and in his practice of medicine too.

The inclusion of dreams in his medical thinking leads to a second way in which Scharpe is not wholly a rationalist, namely, his allowance for the supernatural in medical discourse. As Laurence Brockliss has pointed out, Scharpe's 1617 Montpellier thesis concurred with the followers of Fernel in assigning "cures by fascination, incantation or the application to a wound of a dry piece of lint to the invisible power of devils."[32] But unlike Browne's experience of Padua, where supernatural and natural questions interacted in unsettling ways, his teachers in Montpellier, Scharpe especially, folded supernatural dimensions into an unruffled presentation of the essentials of learned medicine. Indeed Scharpe encouraged his students to believe not just that medicine is noble and necessary but that the ancient sectarian disputes over method have not prevented a clear consensus about and perfection of medical learning from developing by way of reason and experience. Scharpe is perhaps too much of a sophisticated philosopher to presuppose without question that the Galenic basis of his medical teaching is emphatically "scientific" (logically certain and necessary) rather than artistic—Rivière presupposes just such a state of affairs—but the Scottish professor affords his pupils ample reason to believe that their artistic training is not vulnerable to skeptical critique.

Scharpe's *Institutiones* ends with a short treatment of symptoms, including hurt actions, changed qualities, and (following from both) immoderate excrement. As with experience at the beginning, so too with pain at the end of Scharpe's lectures:

[30] Lester King, *The Road to Medical Enlightenment, 1650–1695* (New York: American Elsevier, 1970), 30.

[31] For the dream in medical history, see Emma J. Edelstein and Ludwig Edelstein, *Asclepius: A Collection and Interpretation of the Testimonies*, 2 vols. (Baltimore, MD: Johns Hopkins, 1945), 1.250.

[32] Brockliss, "Seeing and Believing," in *Medicine and the Five Senses*, 81.

his chapter "de dolore" develops a nuanced vocabulary designed to help the physician cope with what will prove his most overriding concern in maximizing human welfare (193–208). Not only would Browne retain this heightened sensitivity to the suffering of his patients, but he would also reflect in his letters Scharpe's attentiveness to the needs of differing age groups. Most striking is Browne's concern for cultivating the potential vitality of old age to which Scharpe directs his pupils. Having listed for his students the various stages of life, beginning with childhood (up to fourteen), puberty (14–18), adolescence (18–25), youth (25–35), and virility (35–50), Scharpe divides old age into three categories: "senectus viridis" or "green old age" (50–60), middle old age (60–70), and decrepitude (70–death). Whereas the relatively young can be subverted by weak natures, the older can prove quite robust so that a person in "middle" old age still appears "green." Doctors must always remember that life does not necessarily end with the demise of categorical "virility." Yet, given Browne's interest in pediatric medicine, it is also noteworthy that like several other Montpellier physicians, Scharpe lectured on the common childhood disease of scarlet fever.[33]

Nor was Scharpe alone among Montpellier authorities in encouraging Browne to consider the vitality hidden in old age. In his treatise on old age, François Ranchin rejects the Arabic and Paracelsian claim that gold can greatly extend longevity and even make immortality humanly possible—*Religio Medici*'s special attention to, but also its skepticism toward Paracelsus's more extraordinary claims resemble this assessment (Patrides, 99, 106). Even so, he offers several remedies involving gold of use to the health of the elderly as well as elixirs for their rejuvenation. The physician must proceed prudently as always and never overreach into the realm of natural immortality. But for the old as for the young, Ranchin's physician reveres life so ardently that he will marshal all his wits and experience in conserving strength, slowing down decay, and alleviating the difficulties and pains of the living. Chief among his medicaments for recreating the heart, enlivening the faculties, and repelling melancholy is Montpellier's own confection of alkermes, about which Browne would write in his tract on plants in Scripture, as well as prescribe in the case of a child's ague (Keynes, 3.34, 464).

Browne singled out Lazare Rivière of all the Montpellier professors as crucial for medical education. Predominantly Galenic in its framework, yet open to a synthesis between humoral and chemical medicine, Rivière's work on diseases could be recommended to Henry Power precisely because it skillfully taught "how Institutions are applicable to practice" (Keynes, 4.256; cf. 4.53). Not surprisingly, Browne's library included two editions of Rivière's *Medica Praxis* (1653, 1660) and one of his *Observationes medicæ* (1646). Rivière's *Institutionum Medicarum* was often reprinted, but the professor's fame depended on his *Medica Praxis*; based on his lectures, this lucid book described all the diseases together with "sensible and

[33] See p. 426 in this volume for Browne and pediatrics. A manuscript including twenty leaves of Scharpe's lecture "Tractatus de febre purpurata" is held in the Daniel and Eleanor Albert Collection in Memorial Library at the University of Wisconsin, Madison.

judicious" cures that have withstood the test of time. Contributing to a rising medical genre, Rivière added to these two works a set of case notes, the *Observationes Medicæ*, often responses to letters of consultation from other physicians. In 1631, moreover, Rivière's star was on the rise, for he had just cured Louis XIII himself of a serious disease.

Rivière's *Institutes* is a much more elaborate affair than Scharpe's, yet it strives for efficiency and clarity no less than his colleague's. Covering the complex theoretical subject of semiotics and the practical matters of regimen and therapy as well as physiology and pathology, Rivière also includes more detail in all five categories. Yet detail is not meant to be taken as an indication that medical learning is mired in the uncertainties of circumstance. More interested in productive synthesis than in argumentative problem-solving, he assures his pupils that medicine is a science rather than an art, and insists upon its certain, not conjectural, foundation whose indubitable axioms can be translated into practice as surely as those of math and geometry.[34] Rivière's students can rest assured that modern chemical changes, a Hippocratic involvement in circumstances, and Montpellier's strong emphasis on clinical interaction with individual patients would not erode the logical-cum-natural certitude of their theoretical framework and intellectual processes.

For Rivière as for Scharpe, medical beginners are supposed to be carefully *guided* by their teachers, not spiritually and philosophically vexed by them. For Browne, this resourceful, positive approach to medical care was instrumental in converting doubt into hope that the physician could nourish human welfare and cultivate vitality. Indeed, Browne's lifelong focus on generation was encouraged by Rivière, who devoted time and energy to questions of human sexuality such as whether female semen is fertile; predictably, Rivière sided with Galen and the physicians in claiming that it is (*Institutes*, 22).

No doubt because semiotics forms a critical bridge from medical theory to practice, Rivière's treatment of the third theoretical field is longer than the first two books combined. Indeed, as *Letter to a Friend* shows, Browne's own understanding of medical semiotics was a complex but essential dimension of his confident vocation.[35] At the outset, Rivière explains that a doctor must always proceed toward a cure in a legitimate and rational way (*Institutes*, 44): first, by investigating accurately the nature, causes and site of the disease; and second, by diligently inquiring whether we ought to hope for a cure to this disease. Semiotics is the key to both understanding and hope, for it comprises signs in general, as well as diagnostic, prognostic, and commemorative signs for the present, future, and past conditions of disease. For physicians, a sign signifies a latent condition by way of obvious sensory information; beyond this simple definition, signs can prove healthy, unhealthy, or neither; a necessary adherent to a disease or accidental (magnitude, for instance); they can signal the essence, cause, or effect of a disease. Following his introductory taxonomy of signs (44–5), Rivière provides the student with logically

[34] *Lazari Riverii... Opera Medica Universa* (1738), 1.

[35] Reid Barbour, "Thomas Browne's *A Letter to a Friend* and the Semiotics of Disease," *Renaissance Studies* 24 (2010), 407–19.

bifurcated tables of all the semiotic sources in the body, as well as tables analyzing signs of the parts affected, the magnitude, malignity, and duration of diseases (46, 50–3). The student learns how to track down a diagnosis: for instance, the diagnosis of an excessive humor considers material causes (such as food), efficient causes (such as heredity, age, or season), effects on actions (animal, vital, and natural), passions, excrements, and the habits of the body (skin, hair). Then he learns how to predict the outcome of the disease according to signs of essence, cause, and effect; the table of effects is by far the most elaborate, with considerations of animal, vital, and natural actions; of excrements, qualities (results of heat, cold, dryness, wetness, hardness, softness, color, odor, taste, sound), and other accidental factors. Students learn, among other things, to tell the difference between good sweat and bad; to read facial expressions and quotidian habits such as teeth-grinding, hunger or thirst, sputum, and sleep. They learn to pay special attention to the hypochondria, that is, to the whole region between the septum and umbilicus in which one finds the liver, spleen, and stomach (47–96).

In the final two books of his *Institutes*, Rivière explains regimen (the six non-naturals and the way in which their use or abuse creates health or disease) and therapy through animal, plant, and mineral medicaments (96–159). With the fifth book, on therapy, the *Institutes* leads the student through those indications according to which the method and means of healing are secured. Stressing that contrariety and balance are the keys to remedy, Rivière discusses the factors of administration such as how much, in what way, when, and where; of evacuation (blood, feces, vomit, sweat); of the patient's circumstances; and of the three remedial instruments (regimen, pharmacy, and chirurgery). In the final section, he focuses on pharmaceutical cures, both simple (nature alone) and composite (art added to nature). Throughout, Rivière marries moderns such as Sennert to ancients, especially Hippocrates, without any anxiety about their proving irreconcilable. What is more, his suggestions for remedies factor in chemical with more traditional cures—antimony and laudanum with tamarind and aloe—with only a slight show of controversy or anxiety. Conceding that chemical medicines can be very strong, that the unlearned should avoid them, and that he himself has been too timorous to make use of antimony to produce vomit, Rivière applauds the prudent employment of chemical means insofar as they can be extraordinarily effective in curing cases deemed hopeless by conventional medicine.

Whereas pathology offers a generalized account of disease, Rivière's *Praxeos Medicæ* focuses on the specific diseases of the body, moving part by part from the head down. Of the three main organic centers of the body, it is the head and the "animal faculties" that concern Rivière the most, the heart and its "vital faculties" the least.[36] Among the diseases of the head (160–95), Rivière discusses sleep disorders (such as apoplexy), epilepsy, vertigo, tremors, phrenitis (the inflammation of the brain and its membranes accompanied by delirium and fever), catarrh (the unnatural flow of excremental humors from the head to the parts below), and

[36] See Lester King, *The Road to Medical Enlightenment*, 26.

mania (furious melancholy, with delirium but not fever; modern advances have promoted antimony as a remedy). Regarding melancholy (187–9), Rivière warns that many patients appear joyous, laughing and singing for example, while others are so deluded as to believe that they are beasts. In this as in every case, he lays out the humoral and pneumatic causes, the diagnostic and prognostic signs (broken sleep, ear-ringing, dark coloration), and cures, reminding the student, however, that melancholy has especially eluded physicians.

Over the course of his vocational life, Browne showed an interest in, and a developing understanding of, the brain, its diseases, vulnerabilities, and anatomy (Keynes, 4.74, 92, 171, 187, 221). But if melancholy (for example) was fascinating to Browne, consumptive and congestive afflictions were more consistently worrisome in the workaday climate of Norwich. At Montpellier, he received his first instruction in how to assess and remedy diseases of the thorax. When he turns to the second major region of the body, the thorax, Rivière introduces the distinction between idiopathic and sympathetic diseases as he continues to discuss breathing problems en route to cardiac diseases (245). Chief afflictions include pleurisy (the inflammation of the membranes girdling the ribs or of the muscles amongst the ribs); on this subject, Rivière invokes anatomical experience in mediating the controversy of whether, how often, or how much the lung itself is affected by the disease (248–52). Rivière points out when a disease is relatively rare or difficult to diagnose; and he offers guidance on how the physician should examine the patient (for instance, on listening for water in the chest when the body is shaken by the shoulders or moved back and forth). When a disease is especially stubborn, Rivière proves even more ready to enlist and to praise chemical medicaments as a response to such recalcitrance (252–64).

Having moved through the heart, stomach, and intestines, Rivière covers the liver, the spleen, kidneys, and bladder among other lower sites, before turning to the diseases of women and ailments in the joints (316–420). Thus Rivière retains the most conventional of structures and trajectories, even as he gently promotes the bold optimism of the chemists. As he focuses in the final book on fever (421–66), he acknowledges that this subject is the most commonplace and the most controversial. In stressing practicality and necessity, Rivière insists, he has banished contentiousness and those dilatory debates which have obsessed school authors and produced no fruit. Offering a careful taxonomy of simple, putrid (continuous and intermittent), and pestilential fevers, he modestly criticizes ancient mistakes (for instance, their reliance on baths) but retains his spirit of synthesis on behalf of optimism, even when the danger is as grave as pestilence.

Throughout his long medical career, Browne would resourcefully and successfully follow this Montpellier master's lead in the essentials and instruments of his vocation. Passing this confidence along to Henry Power, Browne exhorted that if the medical student possessed "the true understanding [of] the nature of the disease, its cause, and proper indications for cure," then all he would need in addition would be a knowledge "of the instruments you are to work by, the *Materia Medicamentorum*" so that "you will often conquer with ease those difficulties, through which books will not be able to bring you" (Keynes, 4.256). Here in a nutshell was the Montpellier optimism that the physician could readily—even joyously—nurture and celebrate the extraordinary vitality that Browne found in the natural and cultural dimensions of the Midi.

If Rivière's installments in the first two medical genres (institutions and practica) are offered as comforting, easily digestible nourishment to his students, he reveals a more exciting side of Montpellier training in his contribution to the third genre, the "observations." In his *Observationum Medicarum*, Rivière joins the ranks of contemporary doctors who publish "centuries" of their case notes as a means of providing the type of circumstantial experience for which Hippocrates was the locus classicus. But unlike Hippocrates, whose cases very often end in death so that their value consists in the physician's proof of understanding rather than successful cure, Rivière offers his consulting services to failing doctors who turn to him for the key to victory. Even when he is summoned too late, he recalls successful remedies from the past. Some twenty-five years after his visit to Montpellier, Browne himself would experiment with this medical genre in *Letter to a Friend*. He would also include Rivière among the primary authors of what he told Henry Power was the exposition of diseases "in particular treatises, in counsels, and consultations, all of which are of singular benefit" (Keynes, 4.256).

As Rivière's observations clarify, Montpellier's commitment to the clinical dirtying of medical hands had discursive as well as practical ramifications for Browne, for the observation was neither a medieval consilium nor a Hippocratic case history. While the latter might depend on direct consultation with the patient, it often unfolded over an extended period of time with little sense of dramatic urgency or immediacy. With the observations more than with the Hippocratic historia, the drama of the consultation became an object of study together with the disease. As for the consilium, it "rarely involved any personal and direct contact between physician and patient" at all, but instead served as the scholastic means of reconciling theory and practice.[37] Clearly the consilium continued to survive as a form, including Browne's own work as a consulting physician, yet Browne's epistolary consultations normally involve a patient that at some point in time he has examined.

In his *Observationum*, Rivière covers a wide range of diseases from jaundice to syphilis, and including pleurisy, scarlet fever, indeed fevers of all kinds, arthritis, gonorrhea, childhood worms, consumption, as well as a sizable variety of pains and obstructions. His cases from 1631–32 include patients with asthma, heart palpitations (484), intestinal pain (484), headache, childhood fever (483), and bouts of bloody vomit (474–5). Rivière's fund of remedies is often conventional in its uses of cupping, bleeding, purging, injections (clysters), and herbal ingestions. But chemical medicaments such as mercury and sulfur appear among the cases also, especially when ancient remedies fail (561). All in all, the observations underscore medical success in Rivière's "remarkable cures." They portray the physician as attentive to a wide range of circumstances, from the patients' temperament and

[37] Nance, *Turquet de Mayerne*, 49.

profile to the season or climate to which they are exposed, and with a full understanding of the chronology of the disease. Even when—and this is very rare—the patient under treatment ends up dying, Rivière's account of the autopsy demonstrates the care and rigor with which he and his collaborators seek out the way to future success: such is the April 1632 case of an elderly widow who, having seemingly recovered from her respiratory and cardiac ailments, collapses and dies upon returning to her daily routine. In these dedicated, careful practices—both during and after the life of the patient—was born the widely acknowledged success of Browne's vocation.

Given Browne's later fascination with women's health, it is striking that from 1631–32, Rivière features the afflictions of various female patients in all stages of their lives. In April 1631, for example, a young widow suffers from a malignant fever (*Observationum*, 474). In October 1631, one wife requires cutting, clysters, and medical potions for help with her hysteria (473), a uterine disorder related to menstrual problems, an affliction that Browne discussed in letters, to be sure, but also in his testimony during a witch trial.[38] In a more elaborate report from August 1631, a 22-year-old wife suffering from the atrophy of her parts and a diminution of sensation in her left hand challenges Rivière's practical wisdom: dry, energetic, and irascible, the woman has been misjudged by other physicians as suffering from paralysis, or an obstruction of nerves and animal spirits. But Rivière precludes this diagnosis, since paralysis results in the abolition of motion rather than sensation alone. The key to success resides in countering her intemperately hot and dry liver by means of cool and wet foods, the avoidance of sorrow and anger, an abundance of rest, the liberation of the bowels, and a full spate of pharmaceutical remedies keyed to the various seasons and behaviors of the disease (481–3). During Browne's stay in Montpellier, Rivière is especially concerned about miscarriages, dealing carefully with three cases in January, March, and April of 1632. In one instance, he seeks to prevent a miscarriage in a patient who has already suffered three at various stages of pregnancy; for her, in addition to relieving a grievous pain, he lays out a full medical regimen for the whole of her parturition (483). In the second and third cases, a patient having suffered a miscarriage, Rivière vigilantly monitors the physical aftermath of the initial event, but also concerns himself with alleviating the woman's fear and sorrow (485). Just so, the letters reflecting Browne's medical tendencies in the later years of his life are filled with a high concern for the health and welfare of his female patients, especially those facing the enormous physical and emotional challenges of childbirth.

Among the diseases afflicting children—coughs, catarrhs, fevers, and worms—Rivière featured one that Browne remembered many years after his time in southern France. Calling the disease "Vlcus verminosum" or "wormy ulcer," Rivière included the case among those rare and challenging episodes about which he had read in books. It was a case whose physician was anonymous but brilliantly

[38] See Victoria Silver, "'Wonders of the Invisible World': The Trial of the Lowestoft Witches," in Reid Barbour and Claire Preston, eds., *Sir Thomas Browne: The World Proposed* (New York: Oxford University Press, 2008), 118–45, at 138–9.

successful. According to the document, a child of respectable parents was infested with strange tumors on his left tibia. The anonymous doctor admits that neither the cause nor the cure of this malignancy is clear to him until he suddenly remembers a herdsman's dog which was tortured by similar flesh-worms and responded well to the herb *eupatorius* (the plant agrimony named after Mithidrates Eupator). With an application of this herb, a crowd of the wormy ulcers swarmed together then fell off, prompting the physician to conclude that the case affords students with an excellent example of argument by analogy in the face of an unknown disease (*Observationum*, 591).

Even though he cannot fully understand why the strategy worked, its basis in reason, experiment, and analogy is especially useful for Rivière as an epitome of the good doctor's resourcefulness and persistence. A quarter of a century later, Browne vividly remembered how such strange infestations had taken on an immediate and alarming pertinence in the Midi. In *A Letter to A Friend*, Browne includes among diseased hairy growths an affliction he calls the morgellons: "'Hairs which have most amused mee…I long ago observed in that Endemial Distemper of little Children in *Languedock*, called the *Morgellons*, wherein they critically break out with harsh Hairs on their Backs, which takes off the unquiet Symptoms of the Disease, and delivers them from Coughs and Convulsions."[39] Although for the Rabelaisian spirit of the Midi, medical concerns are never far distant from laughter, Browne clearly means that he was "amused" in the sense of absorbed and perplexed.[40] As medical author Georg Welsch (1624–77) remarked in 1674, this disease was not mentioned by the ancients, discussed by a very few modern authorities, and in general misunderstood (as hairs rather than worms) or confounded with other diseases.[41] Browne's fascination with it is in keeping with his close attention to the emergence or evolution of diseases such as smallpox and rickets, and to the diseases that afflict children in particular. But as with smallpox, where an eruption was often believed to herald the advent of relief, the morgellons embodied for Browne a paradoxical relationship between hideous monstrosity and regeneration, a pairing that he would find once again, as we will see, in a crypt in southern France. The Languedoc children are relieved by the gruesome, fearsome monsters that according to other German and French authorities are threatening emaciation, epilepsy, and death. So it is with Rivière's account: in what proves a successful conclusion to a tough case, the disease is cured thanks to the assiduous and intelligent physician for whom analogy from animal to human ends up saving him the labor of plucking or shaving the worms.

The few authorities dealing with the disease which Browne called morgellons[42] agree that the disease is new and that it afflicts children so severely that they cannot

[39] Text taken from L. C. Martin, ed., *Sir Thomas Browne: "Religio Medici" and Other Works* (Oxford: Clarendon, 1964), 184.

[40] *OED Online*, "amused", †1 obs.

[41] Georg Welsch, *Exercitatio de vena medinensi, ad mentem Ebnsinae…Cui accedit altera, De vermiculis capillaribus infantium* (1674), 355–61.

[42] For the name itself, see C. E. Kellett, "Sir Thomas Browne and the Disease Called the Morgellons," *Annals of Medical History*, n.s., 7 (1935), 467–79.

sleep or eat and are tormented with heat, itching, and pain. As an especially gruesome version of the Brownean paradox according to which human beings consume themselves, the flesh of these children is severely emaciated by these outcroppings from within their skin. In dealing with the novelty of the disease, a few of the authorities resemble Rivière in having recourse to analogy, usually to pigs. But the medical writers disagree on what essentially the growths are. Among sixteenth-century and early seventeenth-century French writers such as Jerôme de Monteux de Merybel and Jacques Guillemeau, the disease is considered to produce hair, an understanding which Browne reflects. As Samuel X. Radbill has noted, it was the German authorities who insisted that the growths were in fact "parasites, little worms," which they named "zehr wurmen (consuming worms) because the children often wasted away."[43] But Browne was also an advocate of the work on skin by Samuel Hafenreffer (first published in 1630), in which the the disease appears variously as hairs ("*de cridonibus*") and "hair-worms" ("*Haar-wurm*"), a state of affairs suggestive of a strange hybridity between the hirsute and the vermiculate. Browne's library contained a few other books dealing with the morgellons, including Hucher's observation of worms on the backs of children called "masclons"; Guillemeau had spelled the disease "masquellon." Browne's version of these terms, "morgellons," evoked his experience of the disease in Languedoc, for his word is linked to terms such as "masquelons" and "masclous," the latter term "pure provencal" (Kellett, 474).

Browne's library contained a number of pediatric studies, and he included notes on children in his commonplace books (Keynes, 3.296–8). In fact, the topic of Browne's 1633 Leiden dissertation, smallpox, reflects the combination of two related concerns—generation and pediatric diseases—that were featured in the medical teachings at Monpellier. For Rivière's colleague François Ranchin, mothers and their children amounted to a chief area of specialization, and the need to attend to the afflictions of children was obvious.[44] Arguing that the subject of childhood diseases is highly useful but also difficult, Ranchin stresses that everyday experience shows just how vulnerable children are, not just before and during birth, but also after birth when the disparities in living conditions and the mutations of life itself can afflict children. The difficulties in pediatrics arise because children are helpless and inarticulate, often impatient and disobedient, but also because medical history has neglected their care. Ranchin goes so far as to claim that prior to his own work, only Geronimo Mercuriale has dealt with pediatrics and only briefly at that.[45] The point to stress is not the fact of Ranchin's originality

[43] Samuel X. Radbill, "Pediatrics," in *Medicine in Seventeenth-Century England*, ed. Allen G. Debus (Berkeley: University of California Press, 1974), 273–4.

[44] In the Montpellier medical manuscripts in the Daniel and Eleanor Albert Collection in Memorial Library at the University of Wisconsin, Madison, the longest work (ninety leaves) is a work on gynecology, "De virginum affectibus"; the work has no attribution yet it is still indicative of the faculty's interest in issues of motherhood, childbirth, and children.

[45] Ranchin may not have known about the work of Johann Stephan Strobelberger, whose *Brevissima manuductio ad curandos pueriles affectus* appeared in 1625. Some pediatric authors pointed out a treatment of children's diseases in the third book of Hippocrates's *Aphorisms*, but this section is quite short. He may also have intended to exclude vernacular works. Strictly speaking, though, Ranchin did

but the perception and advertisement that in Montpellier children and their diseases were of utmost concern.[46]

Ranchin makes the case for the vulnerability of childhood not from a vantage of helplessness or pessimism but in the interest of motivating his students to make a special commitment to protecting and preserving life in its earliest stages. The analysis of specific diseases takes up the bulk of the treatise. Ranchin's careful study of epilepsy as a specifically childhood disease evinces his typical optimism, for he protests against naysayers that the disease can and should be treated, not with magic or superstition but with the full slate of ancient and chemical medicaments available in the seventeenth century. Even the most squalid of human conditions—the odious affliction of lice and worms—should be met with this full medical arsenal. For Ranchin, the good physician will focus on children so that human bodies and lives might be freed from monstrous calamity as much as possible. On such a fundamental matter, medical students are exhorted to play no favorites with authorities old and new; they should feel free to analyze all the available evidence, weigh the pros and cons of theories and opinions, and contribute to the advancement of understanding on which human vitality depends. It is a matter of course that a book on childhood diseases include "variolae" (smallpox) and "morbilli" (measles), subjects to which Browne would be turning in his Leiden dissertation. All in all, Ranchin's intense dedication to the assistance of children in peril helps to make sense of Browne's memory of the morgellons, his dissertation on smallpox, his exchange with Henry Power about the new disease called the rickets, and his parental solicitude for the health of his own children.

For Ranchin as for Browne, a focus on pediatrics was linked with the careful study of women's health. In his treatise *De Morbis ante partum, in partu, & post partum*, a work published posthumously in 1645 and included in Browne's library, Ranchin includes the whole range of concerns about pregnancy, parturition, and post-natal care, and he helps the physician cope with moral, social, and theological problems such as whether pregnancy is natural, whether abortion is ever licit, whether the sin of Eve transformed maternity, whether pregnant women are obliged to observe Lent, and how cautious the physician should always be in deciding whether high-ranking women are pregnant. His book is filled with sensible advice, for instance, that the physician should care far more about the regimen of the mother than he does about predicting the sex of the fetus. Indeed everything about the mother's environment and habits—her air, food, sights, and sounds, clothing, sexual practices, moods, and excretions—is to be carefully controlled so

sell short contributions from the sixteenth century. See George Frederic Still, *The History of Paediatrics: The Progress of the Study of Diseases of Children up to the End of the XVIIIth Century* (Oxford: Oxford University Press, 1931); A. R. Colón, *Nurturing Children: A History of Pediatrics* (Westport, CT: Greenwood Press, 1999); and John Ruhräh, ed., *Pediatrics of the Past: An Anthology*, foreword by Fielding H. Garrison (New York: Paul B. Hoeber, 1925).

[46] No doubt it was under Ranchin's influence that James Primerose, that Oxford student who wrote the guidebook to Montpellier at Clayton's request, would end up dedicating a treatise to children's diseases, in which he complained that the ancients had neglected the category of childhood diseases; see James Primerose, *Partes duæ de morbis puerorum* (Rotterdam, 1658).

as to maximize her health and the baby's. On the matter of abortion, Ranchin argues that absolutely no circumstance justifies destroying the fetus: not an acute disease threatening the mother, an overabundance of children in the family, or the preservation of honor and heredity. Rejecting the analogy between a ship with its cargo and a mother with her child, Ranchin exhorts the physician to enlist the full force of his art to save both lives.[47] For Ranchin, this absolute stand against abortion was consistent with a physician's preparedness to rescue life from the grip of death when patients faced dire threats such as poison, suffocation, or gangrene.[48]

Browne's own references to abortion illustrate his belief that physicians were to work hard in opposing their accidental occurrence and that women who aborted fetuses on purpose were immoral. In his commonplace books, he made note of an amazing remedy against abortion found in the writings of Julius Caesar Baricellus, then added "the wearing of a girdle of sea horse lether, & the Æglestone" as tried and true preventatives of his own (Keynes, 3.299). Of herbal aborticants, he remarked in *Pseudodoxia* that "[i]t were a strange effect, and whores would forsake the experiment of Savine, if that were a truth which hee delivereth of Brake or femall fearne, that only treading over it, it causeth an abortion" (Robbins, ed., *Pseudodoxia Epidemica*, 1.48). As John M. Riddle has shown, the history of herbally induced abortions was rich and ancient, though early modern herbalists had a tendency to deal with this dimension of herbal properties obliquely. Yet Ranchin's—and Browne's—repugnance for the immorality of abortion was strengthened by the typical contemporary interpretation of the warning in the Hippocratic oath against the physician's administration of abortifacients. Although the text of that oath is now understood to have referred only to the use of pessaries, early modern editions of the oath tended to phrase the warning so that it prohibited all manner of drugs productive of abortion.[49]

Browne also followed Ranchin in the more positive corollary to the discrediting of abortion, namely, the all-out effort to relieve the pain and danger of the mother in labor. Although his mantra is prudence and caution, Ranchin includes among the instruments of his art the modern as well as the ancient remedies that help produce a happy and easy birth in the fullness of time. Citing "elegant" Galen's *De usu partium*, he heralds the giving of birth as an anatomical miracle and a great wonder in whose presence we are forced simply to marvel at nature's wisdom and power. As a testimony to this miracle, the physician is to surround himself with

[47] See Audrey Eccles, *Obstetrics and Gynaecology in Tudor and Stuart England* (Kent, OH: Kent State University Press, 1982), 69. Among the Montpellier medical faculty, Ranchin was not alone in his opposition to abortive and contraceptive prescriptions. In 1617, for instance, Jacques Duranc argued that "it is not permitted for a physician to prescribe…abortives or anti-conception medicaments." Paul Delmas, *Sept Siècles D'Obstétrique à la Faculté de Médecine de Montpellier* (Montpellier: Librairie Coulet, 1927), 27: "Il n'est pas permis au médecin de prescrire…des abortifs ou des medicaments anticonceptionnels."

[48] Ranchin left a manuscript treatise *De Morbis ac symptomatis acutissmis*, in the Daniel and Eleanor Albert Collection, Memorial Library, University of Wisconsin, Madison.

[49] John M. Riddle, *Eve's Herbs: A History of Contraception and Abortion in the West* (Cambridge, MA: Harvard University Press, 1997), and *Contraception and Abortion from the Ancient World to the Renaissance* (Cambridge, MA: Harvard University Press, 1992).

midwives who are cheerful, patient, strong, skillful, and diligent; and with assistants as well as a matron whose office features cheerleading: exhorting the mother to bear up patiently, to work more strenuously, and above all to have good hope. It is a point to which Ranchin returns: during birth, mothers require emotional support and above all hope. In the same vein, Ranchin supports sexual activity for pregnant women because it is healthy for and pleasurable to them. Ranchin's belief in the power of the mother's hope is an extension of his optimism about the beneficence of medicine.[50] What is more, his insistence on the learned physician's intervention in matters of birth extends his authority into domains often overseen by surgeons or midwives: an extension that might be understood both as unusually controlling and as charitable or democratic, with the learned physician eager to be directly involved in the somatic processes.[51]

There is clear evidence that Browne also devoted serious attention to the prenatal care of the mother. In letters to his son Edward, he elaborated on remedies for "woemen of hard labour or much griped in labour" (Keynes, 4.87), and, on a personal note, he and his wife Dorothy expressed both hope for family members' easy labor and grief in the face of disaster (4.88). Other letters purveyed his serious concern for cases of uterine disorder and his up-to-date scholarship on issues of women's health (Keynes, 4.123, 165). Browne's overall success as a practising physician, however, reflects a strong commitment that Ranchin shared with Scharpe and Rivière, that is, to fashioning physicians from the ground up. For instance, Ranchin derives from the Hippocratic oath a moral profile of the physician who is free from stain, pure in habits, wary of encouraging suspicion that he lusts after members of the families he visits, whether parents, children, or servants. Ironically, Ranchin discourages sexual activity among his physicians with the same conviction that he encourages it in the non-medical family—perhaps a contributing factor to Browne's insistence on his inexperience with women in *Religio Medici*. Indeed, he is apt to compare the physician to a priestly confessor who must keep silent about the ailments with which he is entrusted. The physician's emblem, Ranchin remarks, should depict a finger held to his lips. In short, Ranchin was preparing students such as Browne to succeed as trustworthy attending physicians. It is significant, then, that Browne owned a 1627 edition of Ranchin's *Opuscula Medica*, in all likelihood one of the first medical books that he had acquired as an Oxford undergraduate realizing his life's destiny.

Browne adopted with conviction the high value that Ranchin placed on wise and fruitful consultation with other doctors. Defending collaboration as a wise course in justice, government, military strategy, and the very elements themselves,

[50] See Mireille Laget, *Naissance et Conscience de la Vie: Procréation, Enfantement, Obstétrique en Languedoc aux XVIIe et XVIIIe Siècles* (Thesis, Sorbonne, 1980), 501, regarding Ranchin's awareness "de l'état psychique de la femme, et de son économie physique"; and his "idée que l'espoir conditionne un bon accouchement.…Mais la plus grande partie des discours sur l'accouchement privilège les interventions extérieures, rarement les attitudes et la volonté de la femme elle-même."

[51] For general backgrounds that do not discuss Ranchin, see Rolande Graves, *Born to Procreate: Women and Childbirth in France from the Middle Ages to the Eighteenth Century* (New York: Peter Lang, 2001); and Lianne McTavish, *Childbirth and the Display of Authority in Early Modern France* (Burlington, VT: Ashgate, 2005).

Ranchin argues that collective thinking is even more essential to medicine, and he answers questions regarding how many others to consult, in which language, in which cases, at which point in a case, and according to which criteria. The proper consultant will have a range of virtues, but piety toward God and charity toward neighbors are especially valued, since all human endeavors require God's grace and support, and since God is the supreme physician, author of life, and governor over health. Indeed, Ranchin helps the consulting physician confront the possibility that all his efforts will fail. In cases where the impediments are simply too great, the physician must accomplish more than just understanding of the disease: he must console the patient, mitigate the pain, and offer palliatives. Ranchin's physician is always needed and useful: even if the disease is lethal, he will mitigate its ferocity. The Christian doctor never just abandons his patient to a desperate prognosis, for charity will not allow this. He plays a part in helping friends and family: explaining to them, consoling them, and invoking divine grace that it might restore nature in a manner beyond the reach of the physician.

The Montpellier approach was that health depended on the medical profession's fullest control over the processes of life. But in the decade leading up to Browne's arrival, Ranchin had witnessed the armies of the king and of the rebel Huguenots as they did their level best to destroy Montpellier and its Rabelaisian mythos of festive, exuberant living no matter what humanity's deformities and vanities. The significance of Ranchin as civil and university leader in the 1620s and early 1630s is that his public service came to symbolize the resurgence of a town, a medical school, and a people after a tragic civil war and an epidemic. For Ranchin and his colleagues, indeed for the Thomas Browne who remembered the morgellons, there was simply no pretending that poverty, corruption, violence, hatred, and calamity were negligible factors of their lives. Browne had witnessed firsthand graphic testaments to the Languedoc captured in Emmanuel Le Roy Ladurie's scholarship: a world in which the peasantry suffered from "brutal and tragic" poverty and disease, a world in which the "naïve visions of happiness" purveyed by visitors such as Felix Platter ended up interweaving "[i]nnocent gaiety" with "cruel pleasures, money, sadism, luxury" from within "the enchanted circle of leading families" without concern for "the precarious situation of the rustics: a diet of chestnuts, sour wine, and black bread; goatherds living on bread crusts; ignorant peasants dressed like the devil himself; raging fevers that killed many people."[52] In the more macabre Midi imagination, human fertility was always threatened by folkloric preoccupations with castration, the bewitchment of the marriage bed, and those popular myths "inseparable from the obsession of impotence on the husband's part and, in certain cases, of frigidity on the part of the wife."[53] In many respects—religious, social, linguistic, political, economic, as well as medical—the 1620s and 30s were decades in which the difficulties of Languedoc doubled as a provincial pride that took one last hapless stand against the forces of cultural homogenization, political centralization, religious uniformity,

[52] Emmanuel Le Roy Ladurie, *The Peasants of Languedoc*, trans. John Day (Urbana: University of Illinois, 1974), 108, 152–5, 205, 215. Cf. Lough, *France Observed*, 34.

[53] Le Roy Ladurie, *The Peasants of Languedoc*, 108, 152–5, 205, 215.

and medical privilege. If Browne remembered the local disease, itself so symptomatic of poverty, he also cherished the local language and indeed the very notion of dialect and patois.

The siege of 1622 brought out the best in the proactive Ranchin's commitment to the vitality and the beauty of his university.[54] But Ranchin's noblest efforts on behalf of the health of Montpellier came in 1629–30, when, with medical insight, decisive actions and efficient quarantine policies, he brilliantly minimized the suffering caused by plague and oversaw the careful, systematic fumigation of the town in April–May 1630.[55] The grievous toll taken by the pestilence was expressed by celebrated Occitan poet, Daniel Le Sage (1567–1642), whose collection of poems (*Las Foulies da Sage de Mounpelis*) was in the library of Browne's grandson, Owen Brigstock, and probably originally in Browne's.[56] In Ranchin's amazing response to crisis, however, not just minimal damage but even the resilience of beauty seemed possible. In making use of ancient baths as a means of disinfection, he even concerned himself with the restoration of their beautiful rooms.[57] When Browne arrived just after the plague in 1631, this heroism in defense of public health in Montpellier was obviously on everyone's minds, and Ranchin himself made sure that a careful record of their success was left for posterity. In the decades prior to the 1640s, the Montpellier medical school was not yet unsettled and embarrassed by the Parisian critiques and polemics of the so-called antimony wars. No doubt part of Browne's rejection of the limitations of Laurent Joubert's *Popular Errors*[58] in the *Pseudodoxia* derived from a growing sense in the 1640s that Montpellier was not sufficiently free of the folkloric. But Browne's own training there, and his affection for the people and customs of the Midi, helped to ensure that his academic learning would always have room for the lore of common folk and for the eccentric vitality of the local.

3. RELIGION AND CULTURE IN THE MIDI

As Browne's fond memories of the lyricism of everyday speech in the Midi suggest, a journey to Montpellier from afar involved for the young student an introduction to a way and philosophy of life as well as a solid foundation in the medical arts. For Browne, as for so many other visitors to Montpellier, the figure who integrated

[54] For background, see Jean Baumel, *Montpellier au Cours des XVIe et XVIIe Siècles: Les Guerres de Religion, 1510–1685* (Montpellier: Causse et la Grande Revue, 1976), 175–204; and 255–80.

[55] See Ranchin's *Traité de la Peste* (Lyon, 1637).

[56] See André Berry, *Anthologie de la poésie occitane* (Paris: Stock, 1961), 131, quoted in Philippe Wolff, ed., *Documents de l'Histoire du Languedoc* (Toulouse: Édouard Privat, 1969), 181–3. For Brigstock's book, see N. J. Endicott, "Sir Thomas Browne, Montpellier, and the Tract 'Of Languages,'" *TLS* August 24, 1962, 645.

[57] Charles D'Aigrefeuille, *Histoire de la Ville de Montpellier depuis son origine jusqu'à notre temps* (Marseille: Laffitte Reprints, 1976), vol. 2, 106–7.

[58] Joubert (1529–82) published *Les Erreurs populaires* in two parts (published together in the 1587 Micard edition, ed. and trans. Gregory David de Rocher in two volumes (Tuscaloosa: University of Alabama Press, 1989, 1995).

medical study with the comic vitality and festive exuberance of the mythos surrounding the Midi was of course Rabelais, whose doctoral robe was regarded with awe in the seventeenth century.[59] Side by side with awe sat farce, for visitors to the medical school were also greeted with funny tales of how Rabelais himself, "going up the stares to the seat" at a ceremony, "voluntary fell downe with his nose upon the stare, arising kepte a snorting; the reason asked, saide he felt the smel of many an asse that had gone thear before him."[60]

Medically, Browne was connected to Rabelais in his use of the Frenchman's Latin translation of Hippocrates's seminal *Aphorisms*.[61] Culturally and literarily, Rabelais's appeal to Browne was more complex if also formative. In his tract "On Languages," Browne insisted on the significance of Rabelais's langue d'oc, for it was "not understood in a petty corner or between a few mountains, but in parts of early civility, in Languedoc, Provence, and Catalonia, which put together will make little less than England" (Keynes, 3.81). So many people spoke this patois—indeed many civilized people—and it had been used in the widest possible range of discursive enterprises, from official documents to a treatise on falconry, "a pleasant Dialogue of Love," a narrative poem about "the Holy War, and taking of Constantinople," as well as the festive works of Rabelais and Goudelin. Although the dialect attracted Browne in part for its antiquarian value—"by this the French themselves are fain to make out that preserved relique of old French, containing the League between Charles and Lewis and the Sons of Lodovicus Pius"—its resonances were still very much alive in Browne's imagination. The patois's "esteem" drew poets from distant parts "about a hundred years ago... many Italian Wits flocked into Provence; and the famous Petrarcha wrote many of his Poems in Vaucluse in that Country." This spirited, amorous, evocative language, Browne recalls, continued to connect past to present as it permeated the everyday usage of the Midi people: "and the people in these parts being very poeticall I was often delighted with their songs & poems in that speech while I lived in their country." In one manuscript version of this account, he noted that this was the dialect "spoaken about Montpellier and Thoulouze."

One clear motivation to understand langue d'oc for Browne was a desire to comprehend and enjoy Rabelais as fully as possible. In an anti-clerical, anti-scholastic moment in the *Religio*, Browne dismisses that "bundle of curiosities, not onely in Philosophy but in Divinity, proposed and discussed by men of most supposed abilities, which indeed are not worthy our vacant houres, much lesse our serious studies; Pieces onely fit to be placed in *Pantagruels* Library, or bound up with

[59] For the robe as relic, see Mortoft, *Francis Mortoft: His Book*, 26n.

[60] Thomas Wentworth in 1612, quoted by Lough, *France Observed*, 301.

[61] N. J. Endicott pointed out Browne's ownership of this book in "Sir Thomas Browne, Montpellier, and the Tract 'Of Languages,'" 645, but offered no documentation for the claim. None of the editions of Hippocrates in Browne's library catalogue is connected to Rabelais. But in *Pseudodoxia Epidemica*, Browne twice quotes Aphorism iv. 5 in a Latin version that is virtually identical to Rabelais's, differing only in the final word, where Browne has substituted *purgationes* for *medicationes*, a natural slip given the context. As Robbins points out in his commentary, James Primerose used the same translation but with *medicationes* (Robbins, ed. *Pseudodoxia*, 2.943; for the two quotations, 1.361, 499); in the 1532 edition of Rabelais's Hippocrates see p. 37.

Tartaretus de modo Cacandi" (Patrides, 88). From the vantage of a Montpellier satirist, it is apt that Rabelais's Library of Saint-Victor is in Paris. From a library inclusive of hyper-serious treatises on such concerns as legal balderdash, black puddings, and jingle-bells, Browne selects one of the many scatological entries, "on the method of shitting," as his example. And he was so taken by this Rabelaisian critique of abstruse scholarship that he eventually devised his own version of the library in *Musaeum Clausum*. In opposition to the langue d'oui of Paris, langue d'oc integrates wit with the passions, the body, and the dirt under our feet; for Browne as for Rabelais, it punctures the ridiculously sober and oppressive tendencies of inquisitorial scholasticism; and it draws the reader or auditor into a creed of happiness that has far more to do with laughter, generosity, inversion, and festivity than it does with censorship, asceticism, hierarchy, and contempus mundi.

As Rabelais's great fiction is apt to remind its reader, it is the physician in particular who must choose between competing philosophies of happiness. The first oath of the Pantagruelian doctor is that joy is the best medicine.[62] The best way to deal with human misery is to remember that "the practice of medicine is aptly compared by Hippocrates to a combat and farce played by three personae: the patient, the doctor, and the illness." As in a tilt, the doctor must proceed strenuously and methodically; as in a farce, he must somehow convert the haphazard and crude materials of human existence into a healing laughter. In *Pantagruel*, Montpellier is associated with a comedy in which Rabelais himself played (*Complete Works*, 361); with every medical graduate privileged to don the robe of Rabelais himself, it is easy to see the basis for Ranchin's emphasis on the hopefulness of the often tragic and bloody scene of childbirth. The legacy of Pantagruelism for the Montpellier medical student also intensified the naturalist's attention to flora and fauna. If Browne's imitation of Rabelais in the tract on languages delights in nonsense—"though the words be plain and genuine, yet the sense may afford some trouble unto the apprehension"—the medical, moral, and spiritual dimension of Pantagruelism extended from the Rabelaisian conviction that, as Harold J. Cook has summarized it, "the world was not built by the human mind and could not be known by reason alone. Rabelais therefore located truth in the simple and strange in all its variety rather than in its supposedly hidden and unitary meanings."[63]

In the year after his period in Montpellier, Browne would confront the Paduan intellectual legacies of Pomponazzi, Cremonini, and Liceti, which would question such vitalism and variety with a highly charged skepticism and complex neo-scholasticism. The life-affirming paradoxes of Rabelais would come up against the more unsettling, if still highly playful, theater of Venetian carnival. It is striking, then, that while Rabelais's library at St Victor is outrageously satirical, Browne's imitation in *Musaeum Clausum* purveys a longing for what has been lost—for books that exist only in the lovely, happy dreams of the waking melancholic.

[62] *The Complete Works of François Rabelais*, trans. Donald Frame (Berkeley: University of California Press, 1991), 419, 421.

[63] Harold J. Cook, *Matters of Exchange: Commerce, Medicine, and Science in the Dutch Golden Age* (New Haven, CT: Yale University Press, 2007), 23.

In the tract on languages, Browne also mentions Pierre Goudelin (1579–1649) as a poet whose language will elude those readers unequipped with langue d'oc. Indeed, the compilers of the auction catalogue mistook Goudelin's dialect for Spanish. Not only was Goudelin the unofficial poet laureate of the Midi during Browne's visit there, but he accentuated the spirit of the patois by featuring a number of poems on the occasion of Mardi Gras. With a chorus that proclaims that we must "drink as long as we can, for as long as we drink, we live," Goudelin chided Lent as a time when "fish galls our throats," and embraced the "galliardize" which, according to the *Religio*, was foreign to Browne's melancholy nature until he was transformed in the experience of dreaming (Patrides, 154).[64]

In the early 1630s, the most immediate evidence that Montpellier was a place committed to rejuvenation was for Browne the most complicated cultural factor of all: that resurgence of Catholic spirituality under the aegis of Louis XIII and Cardinal Richelieu.[65] One of Browne's most vivid memories of the Midi centered on the miraculous capacity of medieval religious institutions to generate new life. On testimonials concerning the resilience of skin, "Wee had a like experience in a body wh. had been buried some hundreds of yeares in St Pauls, as I have observed in the vault of the Cordiliers at Tholouze." This memory hardly ennobles the famous cadavers in Toulouse, for they are likened to a dead rat and to sows as well as to Egyptian mummies similar to "the bark of a tree." For Protestant visitors to the Toulouse vault, claims about the bodies sometimes were mocked as an example of superstition and credulousness.[66] But in Toulouse itself, the cadavers counted as evidence of the miraculous power of certain spaces in the church, even if, curiously, those spaces have lay rather than clerical associations. For Browne, the site marked an early, if not his very first, encounter with the dilemma of how to experience Catholicism, a problem that, in *Religio Medici*, appears with intensity in Browne's response to processions and to Jesuit claims on miraculous conversions. Moreover, a dismissal of strictly spiritual explanations of phenomena rarely prompted mockery; instead, Browne sought medical or natural explanations. Thus the cadavers belonged in his imagination with the morgellons: with morgellons, skin threatened to consume the vitality of Midi children, but somehow its horrific eruptions might save them; in the Toulouse crypt, skin could make even cadavers seem to live, though as specters arrested forever in their final expressions or poses.

Guillaume Catel's *Mémoires de l'histoire du Languedoc curieusement et fidèlement recueillis de divers auteurs* (Toulouse, 1633) captures the experience of visiting the highly touristed Franciscan house in the early 1630s. As one of the biggest and most beautiful convents in Toulouse, one closely located to the cathedral, a wide variety

[64] See Christian Anatole, ed. *Pèire Godolin 1580–1649: Actes du Colloque international Université de Toulouse-Le Mirail, 8–10 mai 1980* (Toulouse: Service des publications de l'Université, 1983), 229–33.

[65] For an overview, see Louise Guiraud, *Études sur la réforme à Montpellier* (Montpellier: Louis Valat, 1918).

[66] See for instance Henry Oldenburg, *The Correspondence of Henry Oldenburg*, ed. A. Rupert Hall and Marie Boas Hall (Madison: University of Wisconsin Press, 1966), 3.134. I owe this reference to Claire Preston.

of colleges and monasteries, and the famous university, it featured frescos of the life of St Francis and colorful flowers in the courtyard.[67] Select tombs from the church played an integral part in the fame of the famous vault, in which were preserved a great number of dried corpses which were believed to owe their triumph over physical decay to the miraculous power of their original tombs upstairs. Reached from the street, the vault was a small subterranean chapel shaped like an oval, with its dimensions reported at 18 x 12 x 6.5 feet. Tourists approached the vault through a corridor of the same length and height but only 5 feet wide, having first descended down a narrow spiral staircase built from stone. In the vault proper, breathing was known to be difficult, not least because the odor was so disagreeable. The vault was attributed with no special ability to preserve bodies from decay for it was only a depository or ossuary to which mummified bodies were brought once they had received the privilege of perpetuity from special burial spots in the cloister and church above. Dried after their removal from entombment in the church tower, the bodies were then situated about the walls of the vault for inspection by tourists. We are told that these bodies had belonged to citizens rather than clergy, that they included both sexes, and that their bony structures and skin were so perfectly retained that the cadavers could support their own weight. At one end of the vault one saw a large pile of debris, which time and accidents had created from severed limbs and heads, all perfectly preserved if no longer intact.[68] Some of the bodies had identities with stories. One had belonged to a student who, dying from a sword cut received in single combat, had instinctively reached his hand to the wound, in which position the hand could still be seen. Visitors could displace the hand with considerable effort but it always resumed its resting place, the last living gesture of a dying man. Another body belonged to a rare beauty, Paule de Viguier, or "beautiful Paule." On all the mummies, one saw the expressions which they showed during the instant at which their souls departed their bodies, including faces of despair, sorrow, calm, fear, confidence, and hope, some tranquil, others tormented. Unlike the skeletons which Browne would see in Leiden, simple evocations of mortality, the preserved cadavers in the vault of the Cordeliers fused the macabre with the vital in the strangest fashion. At once, the cadavers testified to the life-giving dispensation of the Catholic Church and to the ability of ordinary citizens to assert their beauty, vitality, and idiosyncratic inner life even within the oppressive framework of that church, this in a city famous for the Dominican Inquisition that had hounded heretics from the medieval Albigensians to Giulio Cesare Vanini (d. 1619).

Whether Browne visited Toulouse on his journey south from England or during a vacation, he would have encountered the University buildings, including the theological faculty, which were directly adjacent to the Cordeliers church.[69] No

[67] My account derives from Alexandre du Mège, *Histoire des institutions religieuses, politiques, judiciares et littéraires de la ville de Toulouse*, 4 vols. (Toulouse: Larent Chapelle, 1844–1846), 4.615–17.

[68] See Michael Brennan, ed., *The Origins of the Grand Tour*, 46.

[69] It is possible on this occasion that a youthful Browne participated in the scholastic exercise on a passage from the Acts of the Apostles which he recalls in the *Religio*, the one with a Franciscan respondent who denied the legitimacy of Browne's interpretation on the meaning of angels. But he spent more time in the vicinity of Franciscans in Padua at the hospital where medical students did their clinical work. See chapter 5 in this volume.

doubt here too he encountered for the first time those macabre and elaborate processions of penitents that, according to *Religio Medici*, prompted his friends to mock but Browne himself to weep in sympathy. In Montpellier as in Toulouse, penitent fraternities were on the rise as part of a general resurgence of Catholic spirituality in the 1620s and 30s.[70] In Montpellier, Browne experienced a culture striving for unity in ceremonial orthodoxy against the backdrop of a fierce and fearless resistance to persecution that was inextricable from the proud local genius of Rabelais, of botanical plenitude, and of Huguenot spirituality. The recovery of Catholic spiritual institutions and practices was as hopeful to a city wearied by years of warfare and siege mentality as it was threatening to robust localism and anti-clericalism.[71] Whatever the complex effects of Browne's European travels on *Religio Medici*, his first extensive encounter with Catholic culture in 1632 was one in which that culture was triumphant after years of strife, for better or worse.

This is not to say that the provincial spirit of Languedoc was dead. Far from it; the controversy over the *élus* (royal officers for the levy of the *taille* accused of usurping local privileges) reached from 1628 to 1632, and epitomized the region's insistence on its autonomy and its resistance to royal intervention in the crucial matter of tax assessments.[72] For the university in Montpellier itself, however, the most significant reform brought about in the 1620s was the re-installation of the Jesuits in June 1629, for this brotherhood was to be assigned an integral role in the future of humanities and theological education in the city.[73] In all likelihood, his dispute with a Jesuit priest took place in Languedoc, either in Montpellier or in Toulouse where in 1616 the order had no fewer than ten colleges.[74] By contrast, the expulsion of

[70] Cf. Kurt Brenner, *Montpellier*, trans. Phillp Mattson (Heidelberg: HVA, 1990), 74; and Jules Delalain, *Les pénitents blancs et les pénitents bleus de la ville de Montpellier: leur origines, leur histoire, leur reglès* (Montpellier: Jean Martel Ainé, 1874). Cf. John Charles Dawson, *Toulouse in the Renaissance* (New York: Columbia University Press, 1923); and Cyril Eugene Smith, *The University of Toulouse in the Middle Ages: Its Origins and Growth to 1500 A.D.* (Milwaukee, WI: Marquette University Press, 1958).

[71] See Robin Briggs, *Early Modern France 1560–1715* (Oxford: Oxford University Press, 1977), 93. See also Emmanuel Le Roy Ladurie, *The Ancien Régime: A History of France, 1610–1774*, trans. Mark Greengrass (Oxford: Blackwell, 1996), 45–6; and Victor-L. Tapié, *France in the Age of Louis XIII and Richelieu*, trans. and ed. D. Mc.N. Lockie (New York: Praeger, 1975), 243.

[72] See William Beik, *Absolutism and Society in Seventeenth-Century France: State Power and Provincial Aristocracy in Languedoc* (Cambridge: Cambridge University Press, 1985), 39; Ladurie, *The Ancien Régime*, 52; and Dom. Cl. de Vic and Dom J. Vaissete, *Histoire Generale de Languedoc* (reprinted Osnabruck: Otto Zeller, 1973), vol. 11, 1049–53.

[73] See Simonne Guenée, *Les Universités Françaises des origines à la révolution* (Paris: Picard, 1982), 93; Michel Péronnet, "La théologie á Montpellier durant l'époque moderne," in *L'Université de Montpellier: ses maîtres et ses étudiants depuis sept siècles, 1289–1989* (Montpellier: La Fédération, 1995), 59–70, see 64; and A. Germain, *La Faculté de Théologie de Montpellier* (Montpellier: Boehm et Fils, 1883), 36. Other famous orders were restored in the city proper as well: the Capuchins in 1624 and the Dominicans in 1627, for instance. According to André Delort, on September 11, 1631, the Franciscans took possession of their ancient house, which they instantly began to rebuild under the direction of their leader Antoine Chrestien. See Gérard Cholvy, ed., *Historie de Montpellier* (Toulouse: Privat, 1984), 189; André Delort, *Mémoires inédits d'André Delort sur la ville de Montpellier au XVIIe siècle* (Marseille: J Martel, 1876–78), 66.

[74] Martin P. Harney, S.J., *The Jesuits in History: The Society of Jesus through Four Centuries* (New York: The America Press, 1941), 186. The Jesuits had an excellent pharmacy as well, one celebrated in a variety of books in the 1620s and 30s, including *Apothicairerie du Collège des Jésuites de Toulouse* (1630).

the Jesuits from the Venetian Republic was strictly enforced in Browne's time in Padua.[75] It is noteworthy of Midi optimism, then, that in the case of the Jesuit, Browne's initially contentious critique of a sermon ends in a friendship between the English foreigner and his national and religious "other." In the process, a melancholy piece of erroneous teaching is remedied.

The episode as it appears in the Pembroke manuscript is evocative of Browne's complex relationship to his experiences abroad:

> That Judas hanged himselfe, t'is an absurdity, and an affirmative that is not expressed in the text, but quite contrarie to the words and their externall construction. With this paradoxe I remember I netled an angrie Jesuite who had that day let this fall in his sermon, who afterwards, upon a serious perusall of the text, confessed my opinion, and proved a courteous friend to mee, a stranger, and noe enemy.[76]

On the one hand, Browne's combativeness is symptomatic of his own status as a foreigner or "stranger"; on the other, his paradoxical intimidation of a Jesuit is in keeping with the larger history of arguing for rigorous philosophical interpretation in the face of ecclesiastical pressure. Yet the passage, for all its bravura, also purveys Browne's openness to the kindness of the Jesuit, and though this recounting has Browne reshaping the foreign, it portrays him in extended and finally amicable dialogue with the cultural other. Indeed the bravura might be construed as an English Protestant's combination of scriptural rigor, honed by Robinson in Winchester and emboldened by Lushington, with the gusto for debate developed at Oxford, yet profiting from interaction with a quite distant point of view. Yet somehow the angry Jesuit and the nettlesome Englishman find courtesy and friendship. Indeed, not only did Browne remove the bravado regarding the Jesuit from all but the Pembroke manuscript, but his return to the question of Judas's death in the *Pseudodoxia* clearly sounds a retreat from provocative paradox (Robbins, ed., *Pseudodoxia Epidemica*, 1.569). What matters, Browne concludes in this chapter of the *Pseudodoxia*, is that when the Bible presents ambiguities, "worthy Divines and Preachers doe often draw" the passage in question "into wholesome and sober uses" (1.570). From this vantage, the Jesuit would have been justified in carefully moralizing the passage, and attempts to nettle him would all be in vain: "with industry we decline such paradoxies, and peaceably submit unto their received acceptions."

As Browne argues elsewhere in the *Pseudodoxia*, the ways in which narrators handle tragedies such as Judas's usually reflect their own "hopes" in the face of the ironic and incommensurable workings of justice and redemption in the world. If

[75] The crucial point about Browne's account is that the Jesuit was preaching. Whilst Jesuits might be living secretly or privately in Padua, it is virtually impossible to suppose that one would have been preaching in some public or official capacity. (I am indebted to correspondence from Professors Paul Grendler and Edward Muir for clarification of this point.) There were some "Jesuit 'hidden churches' " in the United Provinces (see Jeffrey Muller, "Jesuit Uses of Art in the Province of Flanders," in *The Jesuits II: Cultures, Sciences, and the Arts, 1540–1773*, ed. John W. O'Malley et al. (Toronto: University of Toronto Press, 2006), 113–56, especially 139–41); but the odds are clearly in favor of southern France for Browne's experience. There is an outside chance that Browne is using the term "Jesuit" in a vague polemical fashion, but he tends to be specific in his denomination of clerical orders.

[76] Jean-Jacques Denonain, *Une Version Primitive de "Religio Medici" par Thomas Browne* (Publications de la Faculté d'Alger 36 (1958), 43).

"sad and Tragicall stories are seldome drawne within the circle of their verities; but as their Relators doe either intend the hatred or pitty of the persons," the crimes of Judas are bound to be, and have in fact been, exaggerated (Robbins, ed., *Pseudodoxia Epidemica*, 1.593–4). Browne's encounter with the Jesuit concerned more than just his youthful posturing in recounting a traveler's experience of the foreign; it captured a sense of how Browne's interaction with cultural estrangement provoked him to come to grips with what at times seemed his own slippery hold on the truth in faith, hope, and charity. In Padua, where Browne would find new forms of toleration and liberty in philosophizing, there was nonetheless no pretending that English Protestants, let alone philosophizing physicians, could work out their salvation with immature jokes and brave paradoxes. Accordingly, debates with the Catholic clergy there are not remembered as concluding in friendship. But in Languedoc, despite the powerful anti-clericalism of Rabelais, Browne was encouraged to believe that the worst possible ailments afflicting European religious culture in the first half of the seventeenth century might somehow be healed.

The assessments of Montpellier as a smallish, relatively non-urbanized city were always inseparable from the impression purveyed by travelers that its environs were somehow more innocent, uncorrupted, and protected than the world outside the Midi garden. Indeed, Browne's perplexity about "How to make good the account of Benjamin Tudelensis the Jew concerning Montpellier" centers on the latter's claim that the city is the mercantile and linguistic confluence of the world: Browne has trouble agreeing with this characterization, "since [Montpellier] hath no port nor any considerable river & Marseilles not far of hath caryed a mayne trade as the same Author delivers" (Keynes, 3.312). The very geography of the place captures the paradox of a region at once vital and provincial, for its land is at once amazingly fertile but decidedly rocky and rude.

In the *Religio*, Browne recalls that he had been happy to eat "dishes of frogges, snailes, and toadstools" with the French (Patrides, 133). His other French recollection in that memorial to himself was less pleasant and hopeful: "I was familiarly acquainted in France [with] a Divine and man of singular parts, that on the same point"—the immortality of the soul—"was so plunged and gravelled with three lines of *Seneca*, that all our Antidotes, drawne from both Scripture and Philosophy, could not expel the poyson of his errour" (Patrides, 87). In this one passage, the essential optimism of Montpellier medicine—that any affliction can be healed with the compassionate and energetic dedication of a community of healers—gives way to the somber realization that some diseases are just too powerful and entrenched to be eradicated. Instead of finding virtue in a poisonous material, the French divine has discovered Epicurean poison lurking in a virtuous writer, in his *Troades*, according to which "There is nothing after death, and death itself is nothing. Death is indivisible, destructive to the body and unsparing to the soul... We die wholly, and no part of us remains."[77] It is significant that this

[77] Passage given in Latin in Browne's margin; translation in Patrides, 87.

recollection follows just after the memory of a physician in Italy "who could not perfectly believe the immortality of the soule, because *Galen* seemed to make a doubt thereof."[78]

In the *Pseudodoxia*, the critique of Laurent Joubert as Montpellier's premiere exposer of "popular errors" is revealing of Browne's complex understanding of his training in the Midi. Joubert was famous for, among other things, his treatise on laughter, which included a panegyric to the human face in all its irreducible variety. This fascination with the singularity of each human face made its mark on the *Religio*, as did Joubert's paradox that man's most wonderful and distinctive gift from God, laughter, often took its prompt from what "is ugly, deformed, improper, indecent, unfitting, and indecorous... provided we are not moved to compassion."[79] As with the morgellons and the cadavers in the crypt, in Joubert as in Rabelais, the humor in the Midi integrated celebration and monstrosity, vitality and decay, the regenerative and the gruesome. Like Browne, Joubert shied away from criticizing too harshly the customs and proverbs of the Languedoc locals, preferring instead to "interpret" some kernel of wisdom buried within those vestiges of superstition and folklore. But Joubert's quotation of a saying about how there are "so many fools in the outskirts of Montpellier" captured a widespread assumption that Midi folk were more than a little slow, incorrigibly doltish if also quaint.[80] In the *Pseudodoxia*, Browne distanced himself from those childish ways by complaining that his expectations for a rigorous, epistemologically sophisticated critique in Joubert had been sorely disappointed in his "thoughts of great releef" (Robbins, ed., *Pseudodoxia Epidemica*, 1.3). The panacea offered from the

[78] One tantalizing candidate for the French acquaintance of "singular parts" is Adam Abrenethy. As a Scot who was from a good family, was an accomplished and published humanist, taught in Montpellier's medical school, and was sometimes characterized as a theologian, Abrenethy is especially attractive for the role insofar as Thomas Dempster once lamented his "infelici sorte philosophiam." A pertinent sense of what this unhappiness might involve derives from Abrenethy's "Theses Philosophica e Physica" in a work entitled *Quæstiones IV Cardinales*, a predominantly medical dissertation presented to the university faculty and published in Montpellier in 1609. In his final theses, Abrenethy asserted that "the rational soul has a physical form and nature," that "it is ridiculous to aver that the rational soul does not participate in the mass of elements," that its very subjection to temporal processes proves its materiality, and that, even if we have no desire for our forms and qualities to perish altogether in the mixture of elements, we can take some solace in the fact that they do not so much perish as persist latently in a remote level of existence. See *Quæstiones IV Cardinales* (Montpellier, 1609), 22. The key thesis is phrased: "*Anima rationalis est forma, naturaque physica*." Dempster also attributed to him a work entitled *Psychologia Medica et Philosophica* which smacks of a non-theological approach to the human soul, but so far there is no trace of this work. More defensively, but in keeping with his astuteness about how we dread complete annihilation, Abrenethy devoted one of his Latin poems to shoring up the ways in which he had conquered the fear of death. Having been expelled from his directorship of the College of Arts in Nimes in 1627, in part because he let lapse "des exercises de piete," he continued to practice medicine until his death sometime in the 1650s, and his previous habitation in Montpellier makes it a good probability that he spent his last years there. What is more, his Scottish heritage would help explain a friendship with Browne, since early modern compatriots often stuck together in their travels abroad. See Thomas Dempster, *Historia ecclesiastica gentis Scotorum, sive, de scriptoribus Scotis* (Edinburgh: Andreas Balfour, 1829), vol. 1, 61–2.

[79] Laurent Joubert, *Treatise on Laughter*, trans. and ed. Gregory David de Rocher (Tuscaloosa: University of Alabama Press, 1980), 20, 65.

[80] Laurent Joubert, *The Second Part of the Popular Errors* (Tuscaloosa: University of Alabama, 1995), 137; the word in question is "bauch" or "bauc."

Montpellier tradition had proved an empty fantasy from which Browne would have to grow up. But in mentioning the "Discourse of vulgar Errors in Physick" written by Primerose, that former Montpellier scholar, author of Clayton's guidebook, and also a critic of Joubert, Browne implicitly recorded the debt to Montpellier owed by those mature moderns with a strong desire to alleviate human error and suffering.[81]

It is tempting to see Browne's affection for the "why" of final causes, in tandem with his love of natural hieroglyphs and the rites and festivals of Merry Old England, as essentially a childlike response to "cultural despair."[82] One can only speculate about whether Browne's proposed dialogue between two twins in their mother's womb "concerning the world they were to come into" would have proved on balance an expression of hope or anxiety. On a few striking occasions, Browne associates irreparable loss with France. In the *Musaeum*, one fantasy of regret invokes "Some Pieces of Julius Scaliger, which he complains to have been stoln from him, sold to the Bishop of Mende in Languedock, and afterward taken away and sold in the Civil Wars under the Duke of Rohan" (Keynes, 3.111). In the same text, he catalogues an item lost in the vault of the Cordeliers for all the earthly immortality of its residents: "*Mummia Tholosana*; or, The complete Head and Body of Father Crispin, buried long ago in the Vault of the Cordeliers at Tholouse, where the Skins of the dead so drie and parch up without corruption that their persons may be known very long after" (Keynes, 3.117). But Browne is rarely simplistically nostalgic, and his contemporary biographer remarked that he was disinclined to be excessively mirthful (John Whitefoot, "Some Minutes," in Browne, *Posthumous Works*, xxx). Indeed, Browne urged his own son to grow up in France, to shed the naïveté of provinciality. But the transition between boyhood and manhood was neither simply defined—whence Browne's remark in the commonplace books about "A way to know men from boys, or boyish men and manly boys, deducible from the character in Homer"—nor absolutely good.

Among medical travelers, particular places had their educational limits: William Hammond generalized

> that a French Physician is made up of a little reading & a very great deal of Experience; their Usuall Study goes noe farther than having been at Courses of the severall Parts of Physick, as a Course of Chyrurgery, a Course of Herbalizing, Physiology, & Courses of all Apothecarys Businesses: by the means of which they get a thorow Superficiall Knowledge of all things Necessary to Physick, & afterwards perfect it by running to publick Hospitalls, & many private Operations, that they may help one another to.[83]

[81] For the debt, see de Rocher's introduction in Joubert, *Popular Errors*, xvi.

[82] Leah Sinanoglou Marcus, *Childhood and Cultural Despair: A Theme and Variations in Seventeenth-Century Literature* (Pittsburgh: University of Pittsburgh Press, 1978), 92–3.

[83] Brennan, ed., *The Origins of the Grand Tour*, 198.

In the same letter, Hammond told his father that some English friends are bound now for Padua, and that he longs to join them. Even Primerose, in writing his guidebook for Clayton, conceded that while the faculty at Montpellier is more indulgent to foreigners seeking degrees without much fuss, Padua in particular offers more serious and scrupulous education.[84]

In moving to Padua in 1632, Browne chose cosmopolitan over provincial, Venice over village. For young man Browne, the culture and learning of Padua were more sophisticated, liberated, and expansive than Montpellier's, but they were also more dangerously skeptical, libertine, and foreign. In a *Letter to a Friend*, Browne means only to make a point about humoral medicine when he remarks that it does not pay for people of an "infirm Head" to live in Venice or Paris. In Montpellier, a soul might be lost to atheism; but Padua was a world in which one expected souls thus to be lost; for all the Venetian republic's autonomy from the Pope, the English traveler's umbilical connection to Protestantism would be severely strained there, if not entirely cut. If in Montpellier one delighted in the festivity of the locals, in Padua one encountered a world of masquerade in which the stability of identity was breathtakingly subverted. Nonetheless, as the *Religio* declares, God demanded more from speculative students of nature than "a grosse rusticity." If, in Padua, philosophical wits found ample opportunity for the liberty of philosophizing, their challenge was to convert speculation into what Browne called "the duty of a devout and learned admiration" (Patrides, 75).

[84] Primerose, *Academia Monspeliensis*, A4r–A4v.

5

Padua, 1632–1633

The journals of Giovanni Vincenzo Imperiale from 1622 offer an account of how a traveler proceeded most directly from Marseilles to the Venetian Republic: having taken a boat to Genoa (or to Leghorn), the traveler then rode on a carriage to Pavia, from which a boat traveling on the Po carried passengers across the peninsula past, among other towns, Piacenza, Cremona, Mantua, and Ferrara before they made their way north into Venice.[1] Browne may be remembering this course from first-hand experience when he pondered whether it is legitimate to include humor in epitaphs: "Whether Jocular & ænigmaticall epitaphs be allowable, what to thinck of epitaphs upon Brutes as that upon Boristhenes the horse of Adrian & that upon Roldano prince Doria's dogge, still to bee seen & reade in his garden at Genoa" (Keynes, 3.226). It was also possible to travel over land from Montpellier to Genoa, as Francis Mortoft did; but no matter which way travelers came to Italy, the experience of passing across the peninsula was fragmented by the parceling of republics and duchies, including the Republic of Genoa, the Duchy of Parma, the Duchy of Milan, and the Republic of Venice.[2] For English Protestants moving from west to east, the transformation of the world could be profound and troubling, on the order of taking a voyage "to the Antipodes."[3]

For Browne the move from Montpellier to Padua involved a transition from innocence to experience and to a Paduan tradition of skeptical, open-minded, libertine, and "honest" thought.[4] In Toulouse the dangerous thinker Vanini had been persecuted by the Inquisition; in Montpellier, the Jesuits were returning to oversee culture and education. In Padua, by contrast, Venetian autonomy helped ensure that the libertine honesty of Pietro Pomponazzi persisted. In Padua, Browne found an environment far less immediately afflicted by religious warfare, far less overshadowed by the church and the recently expelled Jesuit brotherhood, more tolerant of philosophical liberty, yet shocked anew into self-reflection by the

[1] Giovanni Vincenzo Imperiale, *Viaggi*, ed., Anton Guilio Barrili (Genoa: Società ligure di storia patria, 1898), 139–42.

[2] See the map in Mortoft, *Francis Mortoft: His Book*, facing p. 38. For more on routes, see Sir George Newman, *A Century of Medicine at Padua* (London: British Periodicals, 1922), 15–16; A. Lytton Sells, *The Paradise of Travellers: The Italian Influence on Englishmen in the Seventeenth Century* (Bloomington: Indiana University Press, 1964), and chapter 6 in this volume.

[3] The words of William Hammond in Brennan, ed., *The Origins of the Grand Tour*, 218.

[4] J.-J. Denonain, "Les Problèmes de L'Honnête Homme vers 1635: *Religio Medici* et les *Conférences* du Bureau d'Adresse," *Études Anglaises* 18 (1965), 235–47.

Galilean challenge to conventional wisdom, by the unsettling affront to philosophical liberty unleashed by Galileo's difficulties with the Inquisition, by the creeping threats of materialism and skepticism, and by the university's own continuing association with atheism. It is worth remembering that Galileo's *Dialogo sopra i due massimi sistemi del mondo* was published in the very year in which Browne arrived in Italy. In 1632, Padua was sometimes more restrictive in medical learning than Montpellier. But in Padua, Browne confronted an intellectual culture with a penchant for testing the limits of acceptability, newly under duress with Galileo, and consequently both brilliant and anxious. In their deep commitment to Aristotelianism, moreover, Paduan professors offered a crucial hybrid for young man Browne: an intensely innovative conservatism.[5]

The "generall scandal" of medicine and the sinister potential for impiety in natural philosophy; the anxiety produced by powerful arguments in support of the soul's mortality; conflicts in the works of Galen between a stress on final cause and a penchant to materialize the soul; the threat of monstrosity to a belief in divine providence; the philosophical strengths and weaknesses of disputation, syllogism, and definition; vexations among scholastics, humanists, and skeptics over the criteria of philosophical discourse; the hieroglyphics of nature and the geometry of providence; the strange kinship between anatomy theaters and botanical gardens; the danger of neglecting charity toward Jews; the contrast between pity and scorn in the presence of a Catholic "solemn procession"; and the theatricality of civil life: in all these concerns, Thomas Browne's works resonate with its author's period of life and study in Padua. But Padua offered more than a wide range of specific points of curiosity; more than either Montpellier or Leiden, it authorized Browne to exercise his speculative fancy and bold skepticism. Indeed, both speculation and skepticism are captured in Browne's recollection of "an old Italian long ago" whose attempt to convince Browne of the moon's role in human mortality both dissatisfied his "Curiosity" and provoked him to meditate on the celestial influences affecting life and death.[6]

Browne's engagement with what for him was a provocatively unusual place worked in at least two dimensions. As the *Religio* but also Browne's later works clarify, the memory of Padua enlarged the author's capacity for tolerance—for learning that monsters might not be ugly, or that Jews might not stink; this uncommon place disrupted his provincial sense of identity, provoked wonder and curiosity about natural philosophy but also anxiety about the insinuative power of atheism. In turn, by way of memory's penchant for transforming what it digests,

[5] Early biographers and Browne himself make it clear that Browne spent part of his medical education in Padua. But there is no archival trace of his time there. As Sells summarizes the problem (*The Paradise of Travellers*, 114), "the records of British students and visitors are scattered and incomplete," with the fullest record published by Horatio Brown for 1618–1762. But by no means all the students were in this register. In the Centro per la storia dell'Università di Padova, Browne does not appear in matriculation records, in the records having to do with the various "nations," or in those containing students promoted at the medical college in Venice.

[6] See *Letter to a Friend*, in Patrides, 394.

Browne transported Paduan culture to an English audience facing a heightened cultural divisiveness and antagonism of its own. This domestication of Padua can be glimpsed in a letter in the Hartlib papers, addressed September 27, 1658, from John Beale to Samuel Hartlib. Beale has been worried about the immortality of his soul, he admits, not because his Christian faith is weak but rather because he has read Pomponazzi, the Socinians, and some Schoolmen who have been influenced by an Arabian heresy and "allso weakened" by "some principles of naturall philosophy."[7] Not only does Beale take comfort from the fact that Dr Browne has struggled with the same problem, but he is encouraged, like Browne, "with all candor & ingenuity to examine the first Christian writers" in an effort to test religious controversies by the standard of his own conscience.

1. PLAGUE AND ATHEISM

Evidence points to the second half of 1632 through early 1633 as the period during which Browne lived and studied in Padua. Two natural disasters made travel from Montpellier to Venice virtually impossible just prior to this time. In December 1631, an eruption of Vesuvius "sprinked ashes as far as Venice," prompting classically minded natural historians to remember the ultimate sacrifice paid by Pliny the Elder.[8] More prohibitively, by the time Browne reached Padua, the famous university town and its medical school were reeling in the aftermath of the 1630–31 plague.[9] In the second half of 1630 Padua began to experience cases of plague, but less so than in Venice itself and the countryside where already the fear, flight, and mortality were rampant: from the Jewish ghetto in Venice, one rabbi lamented the "great panic in the various congregations," the economic havoc

[7] Beale's letter can be accessed in the *Hartlib Papers: A Complete Text and Image Database of the Papers of Samuel Hartlib (c. 1600–1662) Held in Sheffield University Library* (Sheffield: Humanities Research Institute, 2002).

[8] For a brief account of Vesuvius's eruption, see Bartholin, *On Medical Travel*, 69.

[9] As part of the Republic, Padua lost some 19,000 of its 32,000 residents in the years 1630–31. See George Childs Kohn, ed., *Encyclopedia of Plague and Pestilence from Ancient Times to the Present*, rev. ed. (New York: Facts on File, 2001). Scholarship on this plague includes Carlo M. Cipolla, *Fighting the Plague in Seventeenth-Century Italy* (Madison: University of Wisconsin Press, 1981); *Venezia e la Peste 1348/1797*, preface by Paolo Peruzza, Comune di Venezia (Venice: Marsilio Editori, 1979); Ciro Ferrari, *L'Ufficio della Sanità di Padova nella Prima Meta del Sec. XVII* (Venice: A Spese della Società, 1910); and Franco Bertolli and Umberto Colombo, *La Peste del 1630 a Busto Arsizio* (Busto Arsizio: Bramante Editrice, 1999). For the university and its medical school, see Hilde de Ridder-Symoens, ed., *A History of the University in Europe*, vol. 2 (Cambridge: Cambridge University Press, 1996); Jerome J. Bylebyl, "The School of Padua: Humanistic Medicine in the Sixteenth Century," in Charles Webster, ed., *Health, Medicine, and Mortality in the Sixteenth Century* (Cambridge: Cambridge University Press, 1979), pp. 335–70; J. P. Tomasini, *Gymnasium Patavinum* (Udine, 1654); Lucia Rossetti, *The University of Padua: An Outline of Its History* (Trieste: LINT, 1983); Jonathan Woolfson, *Padua and the Tudors: English Students in Italy, 1485–1603* (Toronto: University of Toronto Press, 1998); Arturo Castiglioni, "The Medical School at Padua and the Renaissance of Medicine," *Annals of Medical History*, n.s., 7 (1935), 214–27; and Paul F. Grendler, *The Universities of the Italian Renaissance* (Baltimore, MD: Johns Hopkins University Press, 2002).

wreaked by the disease, and the ubiquitous death. The same source tells us that it was impossible to travel into the Republic at this time, "for all passes leading from the cities were closed because of the pestilence."[10] By May of 1631, the Paduan rate of death was also soaring.[11] The university itself was so badly hit that at the outset of 1632, the professoriate was significantly reduced in size, and many positions remained unfilled.[12] Even setting aside the famous philosopher Cesare Cremonini's death in 1631—insofar as it resulted from causes separate from plague—Jacob Philip Tomasino's *Gymnasium Patavinum* (1654) clarifies how devastating for the academy the recent plague had proved.[13] The medical school especially suffered from its lack of an anatomist in 1632.

At the outset of 1632, then, the University of Padua not only *housed* a theater of death; it very much *was* one itself. In response to the wretchedness that the plague cast over a city, the epidemic instilled in the Venetian Republic a heightened atmosphere of Marian piety, supplication, and contrition.[14] For Browne, the pathos of religious ceremony played a vital part in transforming his sensibilities and loyalties. The plague also heightened Paduan anger toward visitors, for instance in the paranoia directed against two French alchemists who were suspected of intentionally spreading the disease; in order to placate popular unrest over foreign visitors, the Venetian government passed an ordinance requiring that they register with the authorities. By October 1631, the Venetian leaders were once again encouraging and soliciting a new influx of immigrants.[15]

More complexly, the plague prompted various writers to offer their accounts of its history, causes, and effects. Medical or natural explanations alone varied in their focus on the role of air, poison, and contagion. Sometimes such natural explanations were interwoven with the attribution of the plague to divine punishment.[16] But taken together, these explanations were liable to conflict with those moral and religious explanations that accentuated the means of divine castigation for the sins and impieties of the people.[17] As early as the 1630s, Browne revealed that his time in Padua was instrumental in provoking a shocking but also exhilarating confrontation with the dangers lurking in his own intellect. In *Religio Medici*, he criticizes

[10] Leon Modena, *The Autobiography of a Seventeenth-Century Venetian Rabbi: Leon Modena's 'Life of Judah,'* trans. and ed. Mark R. Cohen (Princeton, NJ: Princeton University Press, 1988), 135–6.

[11] Paolo Ulvioni, *Il Gran Castigo di Dio: Carestia ed epidemie a Venezia e nella Terraferma 1628–1632* (Milan: Franco Angeli, 1989), 200–1. Randolph Starn, foreword to Giulia Calvi, *Histories of a Plague Year: The Social and the Imaginary in Baroque Florence*, trans. Dario Biocca and Bryant T. Ragan, Jr. (Berkeley: University of California Press, 1989), ix.

[12] See *Acta Nationis Germanicae Artistarum (1616–1636)*, ed. Lucia Rossetti (Padua: Editrice Antenore, 1967), 310–13.

[13] Tomasino, *Gymnasium Patavinum*, 240–453.

[14] Most famously in the construction of the Church of Santa Maria della Salute in Venice. For a number of images capturing this atmosphere, see *Venezia e la Peste*, 260–70.

[15] *Venezia e la Peste 1348/1797*; see Paolo Preto, "Le grandi pesti dell'età moderna: 1575–77 e 1630–31," 145–7. For the heightened piety, in the same volume see Antonio Niero, "I temple del Redentore e della Salute: motivazioni teologiche," 294–328.

[16] See Bartolomeo Barbato, *Il Contagio di Padova nell'Anno M. DC. XXXI* (Rovigo, 1640).

[17] *Venezia e la Peste*, 61, 145, 306.

those weak Christians whose faith can be subverted by a satanic rhetoric of naturalism, such heads as can be "carried off with the wind and breath of such motives." Then he recalls, "I remember a Doctor in Physick of Italy, who could not perfectly believe the immortality of the soule, because *Galen* seemed to make a doubt thereof" (Patrides, 87). In other passages, however, Browne is less confident: he is both puzzled and relieved by the anatomist's inability to locate an organ and a history for the soul's residence; he acknowledges how vulnerable he has been to naturalistic explanations of miracles or to the heresy of mortalism; and he speaks of how bodily temperaments can match the humors of the mind. His admission that the death of the soul is a tenet "which faith, not Philosophy hath yet throughly disproved" (Patrides, 67) replicates the infamous position of Pomponazzi,[18] and his meditations on the organic status of the soul can be subtle and involved when he concedes that "for the performance of her ordinary actions, is required not onely a symmetry and proper disposition of Organs, but a Crasis and temper correspondent to its operations" (Patrides, 106–7).

Who was the physician befuddled by Galen? And how did his doubts fit into Browne's complex and intricate response to Paduan culture? Of the several contemporary accounts of the 1630–31 plague, one author confronts the problem of competing authorities by daringly having recourse to Galen's argument that the soul relies on the temperament of the body. This is Giovanni Imperiale, whose *Pestis Anni MDCXXX Historico-Medica* (Vicenza, 1631) and *Musæum Historicum et Physicum* (Venice, 1640) elaborate the position that Imperiale derived from a single work by Galen: that the soul follows the body in its humoral and organic characteristics.[19] Browne owned the latter, more famous, work; more importantly, Imperiale lived and practiced medicine in nearby Vicenza and was trained by and friendly with the faculty of the university in Padua where at least one modern authority claims that he was also a medical professor.[20] Throughout his writings, Imperiale is a perfect match for Browne's memory of an Italian "physician" who struggled between Galen's view on temperament and the orthodox Christian rebuke of the same. For Browne, moreover, such a struggle was complicated by the fact that Galen himself is not monolithic; as the *Religio* makes plain, Browne applauded the powerful argument for divine providence in Galen's *De usu partium*.

Describing himself (like a typical Paduan medical professor) as both a philosopher and a physician, Imperiale sets out in the plague treatise to detail the beginnings, progress, and habits of the epidemic. The discussion of the plague's final cause or ultimate purpose is said to be double, first, the divine punishment of evil (as in several books of the Old Testament, where God punishes idolatry and

[18] See Brooke Conti, "*Religio Medici*'s Profession of Faith," in Reid Barbour and Claire Preston, eds., *Sir Thomas Browne: The World Proposed* (Oxford: Oxford University Press, 2008), 158.

[19] All references are made parenthetically to these editions; translations are my own. This medical writer Giovanni Imperiale is not to be confused with the Giovanni Vincenzo Imperiale cited in note 1 of this chapter.

[20] Anton Sebastian, *A Dictionary of the History of Medicine* (New York: Parthenon, 1999), 416.

disobedience), and, second, nature's perpetual cycles between generation and corruption. The remainder of the causal analysis is unsurprisingly medical: the disease is formally a contagious poison; its material cause resides in the humors; its preference for certain victims is determined by "non-natural" or circumstantial factors such as age and diet. Regarding the spread of plague via contact, however, something new enters into the discussion: the very conflict between church and medical authorities that pervaded regions of Italy in these years.[21]

In his treatise on the plague, Imperiale cites a number of texts by Galen, including *De usu partium* which Browne celebrates as an essentially pious account of providential purpose in the human body. But a strikingly different Galen emerges when Imperiale turns to discuss the last of the non-natural considerations, the "animi accidentia" or "accidents of the soul."[22] At first he offers commonplaces heralding the soul's wonderful double duty as master of organic processes and guarantor of human immortality. Then, with one provocative question to the reader, Imperiale enters into the dangerous territory for which Padua had been infamous ever since Pomponazzi in the early sixteenth century. "Truly who can possibly not know," he queries either defensively or audaciously, "how much communion there is between body and soul? Galen shows this quite plainly in his book [that the habits of the soul follow the temperament of the body] in which he teaches from most certain experiments that from the disposition of one [the body] it is necessary for the other [the soul] to be affected" (38–9). In an effort to make things better for Galen—by invoking the support of Aristotle—Imperiale well may be making things better for Paduan neo-scholasticism: "The first philosopher of physiognomy agrees, where, for an entire treatise he takes it as fundamental, that souls follow bodies and in turn bodies are altered by the passions of souls, which he explains with clear examples." This formulation has the merit of orthodoxy in at least allowing the influence to be bilateral—soul on body as well as body on soul. But it is the threat of materialism from the argument that the soul is a disposition or temperament that obviously prompts such modifications.

In fact, Imperiale's sudden foray into the relations between body and soul spirals deeper and deeper into what appears to be an unintended ambiguity. We are reminded that the soul itself comprises three organic sites, the brain, heart, and liver, and that the central role played by the so-called innate heat of the body or the spirits throughout the body is a notoriously difficult problem from Aristotle through Fernel.[23] But no matter how complicated or standard his analysis of

[21] See Carlo M. Cipolla, *Faith, Reason, and the Plague in Seventeenth-Century Tuscany*, trans. Muriel Kittel (Ithaca, NY: Cornell University Press, 1979), 4–6.

[22] Imperiale, *Pestis*, 38–9.

[23] Jean Fernel, *The Physiologia of Jean Fernel (1567)*, trans. John M. Forrester (Philadelphia: American Philosophical Society, 2003), 276–95; Aristotle, *Generation of Animals*, in *The Complete Works*, ed. Barnes, 1.1143–4; Cesare Cremonini, *De calido innato* (Leiden, 1634); Everett Mendelsohn, *Heat and Life: The Development of the Theory of Animal Heat* (Cambridge, MA: Harvard University Press, 1964), 8–66; Dennis Des Chene, *Life's Form: Late Aristotelian Conceptions of the Soul* (Ithaca, NY: Cornell University Press, 2000), 65; Thomas S. Hall, *Ideas of Life and Matter: Studies in the History of General Physiology, 600 B.C.–1900 A.D.*, vol. 1 (Chicago: University of Chicago Press, 1969); Martin L. Pine,

disposition becomes in the course of these pages, the boldest, strangest moment in this text is the rhetorical question prompted by that text of Galen least amenable to Christian orthodoxy: "The Soul's Dependence on the Body." Whatever the complexities, flexibilities, and ambiguities of Galen's position on psyche and pneuma, however, "The soul's dependence on the body" clearly advances a materialist, "specifically *humoral* definition of the soul," for it maintains that "the characteristics of the soul are derived purely from the particular 'mixture' of the relevant substance of the body."[24] In declaring essentially that only a fool doesn't know about and agree with Galen's position in this particular text, Imperiale converts his treatise on plague into a provocation to the orthodox, then he quickly and rather confusingly beats a retreat to what is at least vaguely safer ground.

If Browne's report of the Italian Galenist claims immunity from the latter's disease, *Religio Medici* betrays a more painful truth: that Browne frets his own naturalizing tendency toward a Paduan legacy deriving from Pomponazzi in the sixteenth century through Cremonini in the seventeenth. When Browne was in residence in the Venetian Republic, Paduan philosophers were infamous for asserting that the soul's immortality could not be proved by the light of nature or philosophy and that only strict obedience to and faith in church doctrine could establish this key tenet. Gabriel Naudé stressed that Cremonini's motto, "intus ut libet; foris ut moris est" ("inwardly as you like; outwardly as the custom is"), epitomized his private regard for philosophical liberty as well as his membership in a legacy of materialists stretching through Pomponazzi back to Lucretius and Epicurus.[25] Indeed, a key corollary to the Pomponazzi affair was that the notorious philosopher had actually triumphed on behalf of a liberty of philosophizing. What is more, he offered a prototype of the kind of double truth toward which Browne gestures in the *Religio* when he divides between submission to the church, on the one hand, and philosophical paradox on the other. By contrast, Imperiale comes across as willing neither to think what he suspects in private nor to conform to what he should in public. Galen is especially significant for physicians, and to a large extent adrift from the Aristotelian debates of the early sixteenth century. For a religious physician, that is, Galen allows less room for error and more room for uncertainty than Aristotle.

The struggle over Galen's material soul is clarified further in Imperiale's study of character, *Musæum Historicum et Physicum* (Venice, 1640). As Imperiale prepares to launch into his study of the various dispositions—regional, urban, philosophical, legal, oratorical, poetic, medical, theological, military, mathematical, artistic, and magical—he pauses to explain what Galen's humoral soul has meant to his

Pietro Pomponazzi: Radical Philosopher of the Renaissance (Padua: Antenore, 1986); Heinrich C. Kuhn, *Venetischer Aristotelismus im Ende der Aristotelischen Welt: Aspekte der Welt und des Denkens des Cesare Cremonini (1550–1631)* (New York: Peter Lang, 1996); Linda Allen Dear, *Academic Theories of Generation in the Renaissance: The Contemporaries and Successors of Jean Fernel (1497–1558)*, PhD thesis, Warburg Institute, London, 1990.

24 Galen, *Selected Works*, trans. and intro. P. N. Singer (New York: Oxford University Press, 1997), xxxvi–xxxvii.

25 Gabriel Naudé, *Gabrielis Navdæi... Epistolæ* (Geneva, 1667), 27–8.

endeavor, namely, a heightened anxiety and labor over the body–soul problem: "So that we might sweat more actively in this battle, we have chosen Galen as the leader, his book on how the habits of the soul follow the temperament of the body." In the recent past, Imperiale had been obsessed with the book, and its wider implications have prompted this very work, he tells us: on it, "we strove to offer commentaries a short time ago, but as the field of discussion stretched out to us more broadly, our purpose became to explore the issue more variously [than in a commentary]."[26] His military metaphor leaves it unclear whether Galen's leadership exercises Imperiale's troops from their own side or from the enemy position, that is, whether this study is a kind of exercise of a critical intellect, or far more dangerously a spiritual battle in its own right. The dusty field of contest might be an arena or a battlefield.

As he works through the dangers of Galen, with Aristotle as his chief assistant, Imperiale draws a comparison of striking import for Browne: physicians, he emphasizes, find their humoral likeness in poets, for both vocations must mediate between theory and practice, the contemplative soul and the body in action.[27] For a young physician such as Browne with a penchant for flights of fancy and a strong sense of humoral identity, this connection between medicine and poetry afforded potent stimulus for an inventive exploration of world, vocation, and self. But it was also perilous. After all, Imperiale was not ahead of the curve in Paduan intellectual culture; far from it, his significance lies, first, in demonstrating that a longstanding legacy of atheism still haunted the university and, second, that the danger pertained in particular to medical learning. Even if Pomponazzi was not a practicing physician, he had been trained in medicine and, with his lively, candid commentaries on Aristotle circulating both in print and in manuscript, was the cultural hero behind Imperiale's anxious inheritance: that Paduans investigating the relations between the body and mind or soul implicated medical education in the philosophical problem of whether truth is unified or "double-faced," to give Browne's own term for it (Patrides, 66).[28]

In Padua, young Thomas Browne discovered that putatively familiar and safe authorities—Galen and Aristotle—had accrued a largely unfamiliar danger. In the *Religio*, however, Browne also recorded his gratitude to a Paduan liberty of philosophizing when he embraced a motto very similar to Cremonini's: "I have therefore on[e] common and authentick Philosophy I learned in the Schooles, whereby I discourse and satisfie the reason of other men, another more reserved and drawne from experience, whereby I content mine owne" (Patrides, 148).[29] But as entrenched

[26] Imperiale, *Musæum Historicum et Physicum*, 3–5, my translation.

[27] In a later work, *Le Notti Beriche* (Venice, 1663), Imperiale revisited the question of the intellectual soul's immortality. He clearly longs for the soul's immortality; he also recognizes that Aristotle can be very obscure on the matter, and that Galen's humoral basis for the soul pressures the philosopher-physician with powerful arguments for materialism.

[28] On Pomponazzi, philosophy, medicine, and heterodoxy, see Ian Maclean, "Heterodoxy in Natural Philosophy and Medicine: Pietro Pomponazzi, Guglielmo Gratarolo, Girolamo Cardano," in John Brooke and Ian Maclean, eds., *Heterodoxy in Early Modern Science and Religion* (Oxford: Oxford University Press, 2005), 4, 8–10, 17, 28.

[29] For this legacy see Emily Michael, "The Nature and Influence of Late Renaissance Paduan Psychology," *History of Universities* 12 (1993), 65–94; quotation on 68.

and pervasive as the reputation for Paduan atheism might be in 1632, equally strenuous and far more prominent were philosophical endeavors to confront and overthrow godlessness in its most persuasive forms—and to secure this triumph on behalf of Aristotle. Whereas Browne grappled with the dangerous heritage of Pomponazzi, he owed a more pervasive and less potentially embarrassing debt to those prominent Paduans who concocted antidotes to homebred atheism. Their arguments for divine providence assumed the forms of an elaborate dialogue between Plato and Aristotle in the work of Fortunio Liceti; of the hieroglyphically circular theaters of anatomy and botany; and of one gifted professor's analogies between the ashes of death and the burgeoning of life.

2. MONSTERS AND MYSTERIES

By the time Browne reached Padua in 1632, the premiere Aristotelian defending the orthodoxy of his ancient master was Fortunio Liceti (1577–1657), who sought "to demonstrate that each individual human mind is a separate incorporeal substance," that each "is created and infused in the body by God," and that, "because the human mind is incorporeal, it must also be immortal."[30] What makes Liceti so valuable for an understanding of Browne's own complex relation to Aristotelianism, however, was that the prolific professor's habits of thought were undergoing an inventive make-over in style and scope during the period of Browne's visit. *Religio* clarifies how Liceti's intellectual obsessions were so often Browne's own; *Pseudodoxia* and Browne's library catalogue reveal that Liceti ranked among Browne's favorite polymaths. As we will see, it is even possible that Browne recalled a conversation with the great Paduan professor. More than anything else, however, Liceti modeled for Browne an Aristotelian way of thinking that was flexibly open to revision and expansion and also inventive in its modes and styles of expression.

As the several references in the *Pseudodoxia Epidemica* make plain, Browne admired Liceti as an excellent source on phenomena such as the chameleon, and as a keen analyst of scholastic-cum-medical problems such as the body's alimentary requirements. Browne looked to Liceti for help with the question of whether Aristotle had converted to Judaism.[31] But no problem united Liceti and Browne more than their mutual fascination with the significance of monstrosity. Liceti's treatise on monsters makes the case that in devising monstrosities, the artistry of nature overcomes imperfect material conditions and cleverly fashions "another form still more admirable."[32] For his part, Browne's meditations on the soul are accompanied by his complex considerations of monsters. Having insisted in the *Religio* on the maxim (indebted to both Aristotle and Galen) that nature never does anything in

[30] Michael, "Nature and Influence," 78–9.

[31] See Robbins, ed., *Pseudodoxia Epidemica*, source index, 2.1189, for the pervasive use of Liceti in *Pseudodoxia*.

[32] Lorraine Daston and Katharine Park, *Wonders and the Order of Nature, 1150–1750* (New York: Zone Books, 1998), 200.

vain, and on the natural theology on display in the "common Hieroglyphicks" of nature, he tests his belief in "a generall beauty in the works of God" by three types of evidence apparently to the contrary. Aside from the putatively "ugly" animals such as "a Toad, a Beare, or an Elephant," and the "Chaos" from which God is thought to have created the forms of all things, there is the "deformity" to be seen "in monstrosity."

For a medical student in Padua, thinking about monsters in the 1630s entailed an engagement with Liceti's work. In a larger sense, what rendered Liceti especially important for an understanding of Browne is that in lectures and in print, the great Paduan professor was committed to the problems facing European intellectual culture: to debating yet also befriending innovative philosophers such as Galileo;[33] to reassuring his students and readers of the unimpeachable piety of both Aristotle and Galen on questions of immortality, vitality, and heat; to rethinking what it means to write disputatious scholastic philosophy in a world after the humanist revival of dialogue and of the hieroglyphic tendencies in Platonic and Hermetic philosophies; and to devising a synthesis of Christian providentialism, Aristotelian scholasticism, Galenic medicine, and Platonic hieroglyphics with a focus on human generation. What this emphasis on synthesis and comprehensiveness overlooks is the persistence with which Liceti strenuously sought to reinvent both the style and the substance of his own unwavering commitment to a pious Aristotle.[34]

In the 1620s and 30s, the theological and philosophical significance of the old Aristotelian concern with monsters was newly prominent and unstable. With the revival of ancient atomism taking hold in these decades, concessions to the imperfection of the universe carried also the prospect of a critique of divine providence in the manner of the Greek and Roman Epicureans. On a more positive note, the value of monstrosity was heightened by virtue of the experimental scientist's new appreciation for nature under duress, nature beside or unlike her normal self, singular, eccentric, and abnormal. Experiment was no longer exclusively aimed, in an Aristotelian fashion, at demonstrating how nature usually or normatively behaves, but at how phenomena behaved in a particular case at a particular moment.[35]

Until recently, scholarship has often presupposed that early modern Aristotelianism was static and reactionary, adding "nothing of importance to the intellectual changes unfolding in the early modern period."[36] But following the lead of Charles Schmitt, scholars have demonstrated "that the Aristotelianism of the later period was far from being static or inflexible with regard to its medieval inheritance," and

[33] Pietro Redondi, *Galileo Heretic* (Princeton, NJ: Princeton University Press, 1987), 20–6.

[34] Charles B. Schmitt is the scholar mainly responsible for teaching us to see Renaissance Aristotelianism as a complex, dynamic, plural, and flexible legacy. See, for instance, *The Aristotelian Tradition and Renaissance Universities* (London: Variorum, 1984); and *Aristotle and the Renaissance* (Cambridge, MA: Harvard University Press, 1983). For Liceti as commentator on Aristotle, see Charles H. Lohr, *Latin Aristotle Commentaries, Vol. 2, Renaissance Authors* (Florence: Leo S. Olschki, 1988), 222–3.

[35] For experiment, see Peter Dear, *Discipline and Experience: The Mathematical Way in the Scientific Revolution* (Chicago: University of Chicago Press, 1995), 13–14.

[36] Christia Mercer, "The Vitality and Importance of Early Modern Aristotelianism," in Tom Sorell, ed., *The Rise of Modern Philosophy: The Tension between the New and Traditional Philosophies from Machiavelli to Leibniz* (Oxford: Clarendon Press, 1993), 38.

that it folded into its framework seemingly alien philosophical legacies such as Hermeticism and Platonism.[37] It could even engage new natural discoveries at odds with Aristotelian cosmology or astronomy. Above all, dynamism, eclecticism, and flexibility meant that even if scholasticism had always molded Aristotelian philosophy to Christian dogma, early modern versions of Aristotelianism had "a wider diversity of ideas from a more varied group of sources which could be combined with the philosophy of the ancient."[38]

Given the admiration with which he is invoked in the *Pseudodoxia Epidemica*, it is clear that Liceti contributed to the formation of Browne's own more skeptical but complex response to Aristotle and Aristotelianism. In Padua, Browne discovered an Aristotelianism that could be inclusive and eclectic, but that was shadowed by a legacy of materialism and heresy that shocked his nascent sense of what it meant to be a Peripatetic. In this context, Browne's apparent surprise that the Italian physician had so much trouble with the Galenic text makes more sense: Paduan intellectual culture had a way of intensifying the hidden dangers of those authorities that were so widely and complacently taken for granted.

For Liceti, the dividing line between monsters and marvels was not always clear, and he devoted enormous energy to developing an Aristotelianism that could encompass or co-exist with both marvels and monsters as well as hieroglyphs transmitting mysterious wisdom. Many of Liceti's books in the 1630s show vivid signs of accommodating mystery; but his most famous book, on monsters, reconsiders phenomena potentially subversive of natural providence. For some Renaissance scholastics such as the Spanish Jesuit Francisco de Toledo Herrara (1532–96), monstrosity involved "a mistake of nature acting on account of some end, from which it is frustrated by some corrupt principle."[39] What Liceti aimed to show in his treatise on monsters, however, was that nature triumphs no matter what her frustrations. It was precisely this apology for an inventively and heroically purposeful nature that Browne emulated in *Religio Medici.*

Liceti's *De Monstrorum natura, caussis, et differentiis*, like many of those works dealing with his focal problems, underwent revision over several decades. The 1634 edition was the second, with a new cover featuring a gymnastic pyramid of monsters in their various stages of deformity. (See Figure 5.1.) The cover announces that far from impugning the providential wonder, variety, orderliness, or beauty of nature, monsters somehow reinforce those qualities. And indeed from start to finish, Liceti's treatise proceeds along Aristotelian lines by presupposing that nature always works purposefully, that monsters need to be carefully and properly defined in contradistinction to the many vulgar uses of the term, and that an analysis of the four causes as well as the distinction between substance and accidents or between

[37] The words are Stuart Clark's in *Thinking with Demons: The Idea of Witchcraft in Early Modern Europe* (Oxford: Oxford University Press, 1997), 225. See also Eckhard Kessler, "The Transformation of Aristotelianism during the Renaissance," in John Henry and Sarah Hutton, eds., *New Perspectives on Renaissance Thought* (London: Duckworth, 1990), 137–47.

[38] Mercer, "The Vitality and Importance of Early Modern Aristotelianism," 44.

[39] Quoted and translated thus in Dennis Des Chene, *Life's Form,* 32.

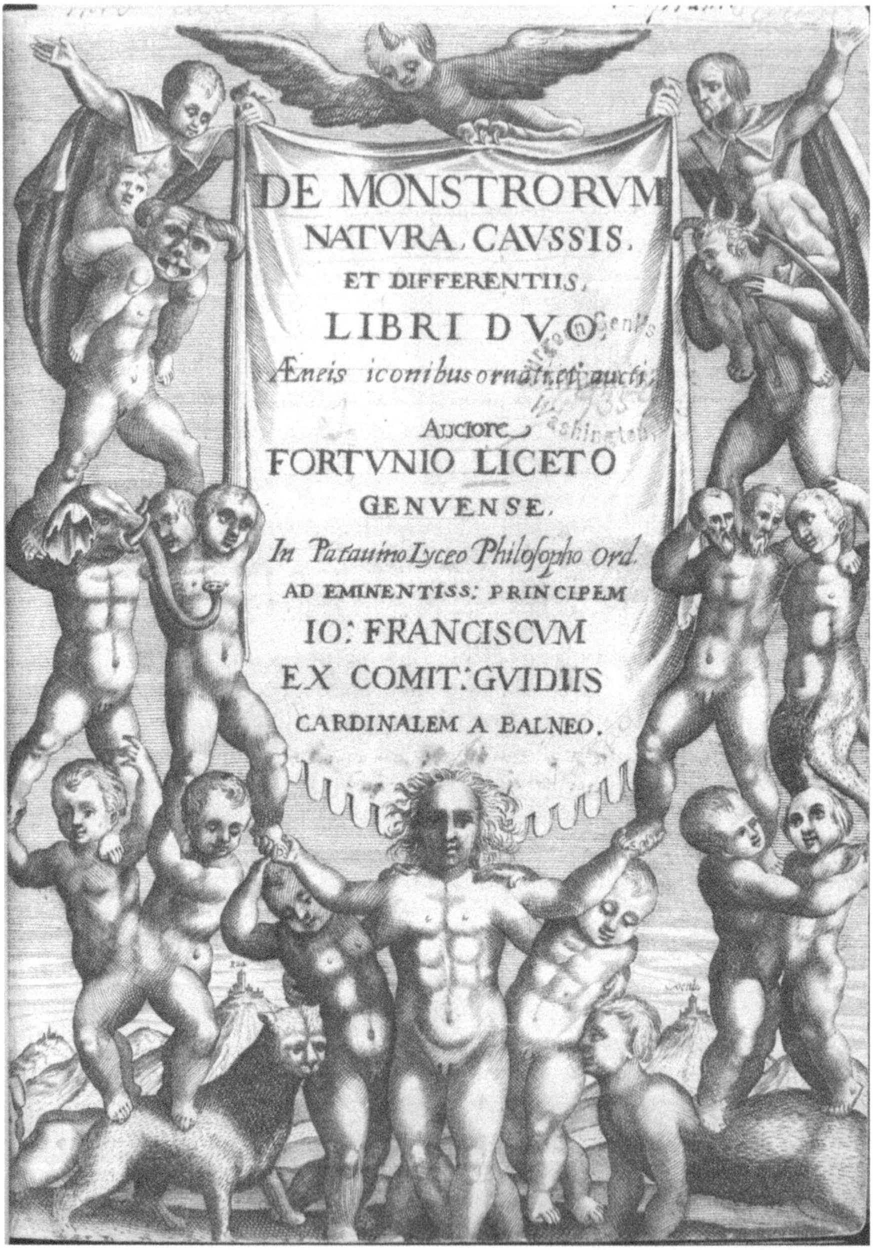

Figure 5.1 Frontispiece of Fortunio Liceti's *De Monstrorum natura* (1634). National Library of Medicine.

matter and form supports a providential cosmology. What is more, the 1634 edition invokes recent examples of monstrosity from the Paduan area itself, as ocular proof supporting a predominantly axiomatic argument. Liceti recalls a monster exhibited recently in Padua for dissection, a male infant six months old, with his head in his thorax; or in 1629 in the countryside, a herdsman's wife who has given birth to a cat, from whose buttocks extended human buttocks and legs, a monster thrown into the river where it sank. In one instance from 1624, a Paduan servant preparing a bird for cooking found five toes on each foot, each with its distinctive nail. But many of the examples are taken from books, ancient, medieval, and early modern. Given these records, it is no wonder that Browne could speak of the experience of monsters as though it were a matter of course.

Why, Liceti must ask, would nature produce monsters? Does this mean that nature makes mistakes? To be sure, monstrosity has a purpose in appealing to the human penchant for and exultation in the strange or astonishing. When we see a monster, Liceti says, we cannot rest until we share it with others. And his book is replete with images of deformity, for instance, a man without arms next to the cards, dice, and tools that he can manipulate with his feet; a child with one hand and two heads; a man with an infant protruding from his chest; and a wide variety of humans with too few, too many, or simply misshapen parts, together with many crossovers between animals and humans, but also between one beast and another. But in some measure it must be admitted, and Liceti does concede, that in the case of monsters nature has made some type of mistake.

The challenge, then, is to locate and explain that error so as to control the damage to nature's reputation. For one thing, nature is more apt to make mistakes in beasts and humans than in plants, since the first two are more complicated than the third. Liceti moves closer toward the identity of the mistake when he turns to the Aristotelian four causes, material, formal, efficient, and final. Unlike arts such as medicine, which are defined by what they do, nature always pursues forms; so monsters will involve form as well as matter, and they will need a producer—the efficient cause—as well as a final cause, a purpose, according to Aristotle's notion that nature never does anything in vain.

It was this, the final cause that Browne celebrated as most valuable in *Religio Medici*—as the cause most supportive of a Christian belief in divine providence and as the lesson that, at their best, Aristotle and Galen were excellent at teaching. For Liceti, final cause in the case of monsters tends to prove nature not just purposeful but heroic. Nature finds herself working in less than perfect conditions as she pursues her main goal of conserving all species. With monsters, then, the accidents might be perverted or the parts badly arranged, but nature has done the best with what she has to conserve a reality far more essential than arms and legs. Monsters possess what nature values most, substance or essence, while errors tend to arise in the process of organization after nature has already animated matter with form. Given Browne's fascination with generation, it is significant that for Liceti monsters can result from deficiencies in the procreative materials of the parents: too much semen or not enough, a uterus too small, or a seminal spirit donated from a mutilated parent. In certain very limited instances, the mother's passions or imagination might conduct deformity into her embryo. For Liceti as for Browne, the problem of monsters is linked to the controversy over how human beings receive their intellectual souls and, as a corollary, the question of whether those souls are purely non-corporeal or intricately caught up in the workings of bodies, fantasies, and organs. Like Browne, Liceti is clearly concerned with the question of whether the seminal characteristics of one parent will tend to dominate those of the other in cases of human copulation with beasts; he considers very carefully an incisive critique from a doubter who argues that bestiality can never produce a virtually pure version of man or beast. Liceti disagrees by maintaining that nature can manage a virtually pure essence even in these unnatural circumstances. So a child of cow and man might be essentially human, only with a propensity to chew the cud.

From the very beginning of the century, Liceti was prolific in producing major works that dealt with one of Browne's most lingering and absorbing fascinations, namely, human generation, with its ramifications for thinking about the nature of innate heat, spirit, and vitality. Browne's library included some of the most important of this series.[40] At the center of all these sophisticated works was a matter of great intrigue to Browne, namely, the tireless effort to establish the communion between the intellectual soul and its bodily residence and instrument. As the 1620s came to an end and the 1630s began, Liceti showed no signs of letting up with these concerns, not least because Padua was dominated by a professor very much in the legacy of Pomponazzi, Cesare Cremonini. In 1629, Liceti published one of a very many works in which he explains how the intellectual soul is at once immortal and disposed to organs and bodily processes. This text, *De animarum rationalium immortalitate: Aristotelis opinionem diligenter explicantes*, confidently opposes the various versions of the argument that the intellectual soul is mortal, not least given its generation, motion, inseparability from the body, and its means of knowing by phantasms. Not only is Aristotle his chief defense attorney for the soul's immortality, but Liceti endeavors to extricate the Greek philosopher from the charge that he is ambiguous on the question. But Aristotle offers something more, he avers, namely, a more meditative manner of argument that reinforces non-Aristotelian resources in Liceti's text such as allegories of Homer or emphases such as the human capacity for wonder. Throughout, the negotiation between medicine and contemplation is especially hard for Liceti to get right, and to the end of *De animarum*, he is adjusting their relationship, insisting on the high regard in which the ancients held medicine, on the commonplace notion that medicine is grounded in philosophy, on the recommendation that Aristotle made of medical knowledge even to kings, and on the equal esteem in which wise ancients held medicine and philosophy.

Liceti found room in his Aristotelianism for a philosophical and religious discourse that cannot be reduced to definitions, terms, and syllogisms, even if these latter persist as the solid grounding for hieroglyphically oriented flights of fancy. When, a few years after his departure from Padua, Browne worked out his views of the relationship between logic and fancy in *Religio*, he illuminated just how

[40] See Finch, ed., *Catalogue of the Libraries*, p. 19, items 85 and 86.

powerful this model was for his intellectual growth. At stake in this adaptation of Aristotelianism to hieroglyphic and oracular wisdom is an enriched way of saving medicine from the materialistic impiety that Liceti worries is threatening once again to corrupt Paduan intellectual culture. In the peroration of *De animarum*, he likens this creeping atheism to a pestilence.

Liceti's emerging affection for Platonic, allegorical, and hieroglyphic thinking can be gleaned from many works ranging from *Allegoria Peripatetica* (1630) to the *Hieroglyphica* (1653). Such studies concern a wide range of vestiges from the past, including enigmatic monuments, altar inscriptions, jeweled rings, and shape poems, and not surprisingly Browne's dual fascination with hieroglyphs and antiquities meant that several of these works would be included in his library.[41] But all of these works in their own way also seek to reconcile Aristotle to Plato, and to build on the legacy reported by Diogenes Laertius that Aristotle himself wrote one book of allegories and another of proverbs. In the peroration of *Allegoria Peripatetica*, Liceti apologizes for the text as an exercise of wit in a short term of idleness from the business of university teaching. Such "recreation," he contends, assuages the mind from its more severe, more difficult studies.[42] But despite this treatment of allegory as holiday relaxation, Liceti is beginning to expand and reinvent his scholastic Aristotelianism with the enigmatic fancies of mystical and analogical hieroglyphics.

For Browne, the model of the philosopher involved in serious playfulness was of seminal force. One further trend corroborating Liceti's appeal to Browne in the 1630s was the Paduan professor's heightened affection for analogical thinking. Indeed, not long after Browne's departure from Padua, in a work featuring analogies between macrocosm and microcosm, Liceti would reach out to English intellectual culture: his *De Mundi, & Hominis Analogia* was dedicated to English philosopher Lord Herbert of Cherbury in 1635, and profiled Liceti's strong commitment to reconciling Plato and Aristotle. In this work were so many foci also found in *Religio Medici*: the hieroglyphics of divine providence, forays into Christian allegories of the soul as an epitome of the trinity, the stress on both man and the macrocosm as made in the image and as the temple of God, emblematic evidence drawn from Egyptian and Greek mythology, and ocular evidence drawn from anatomy in support of the shape of the circle to be found in man and the world alike. Beyond these shared concerns, however, Browne obviously gravitated toward Liceti's seemingly endless curiosity about theological, ethical, and physical fields of knowledge and toward the professor's desire to find civil forms—dialogue and epistle—in which to convey Aristotelian notions to the republic of letters.[43] This latter point about genre offers one impetus motivating Browne in *Religio Medici* to transplant high, often scholastic, philosophy, grafted as it was onto Platonic mysteries and Egyptian hieroglyphs, into a series of informal essays addressed to a friend.

[41] See Finch, ed., *Catalogue of the Libraries*, p. 6, item 39; p. 8, item 96; p. 22, item 112.

[42] Liceti, *Allegoria Peripatetica* (1630), 321.

[43] Browne's library included not just focused works by Liceti—his treatise on the motion of comets, for instance (catalogue, p. 29, item 19)—but also an edition of *De Quæsitis* (1640) in two volumes.

Crucially for Browne, Liceti did not abandon his scholastic Aristotelianism in the dialogues; during the 1630s the Paduan professor was civilizing, mythologizing, and spiritualizing its contentious and torturous terms, its rigorous definitions of what is real, and its syllogisms aimed at resolving knotty problems such as the nature of innate heat, the meaning of the prime mover, the body's alimentary needs, and the soul's propensity to the body.[44] Browne's career both in print and in manuscript involved his own version of the flexing, testing, and transforming of Aristotelian philosophy. The very settings of Liceti's dialogues—gardens and grottoes—lend themselves to courtesy and allegory alike, for instance, on the spiritual and moral meanings of metamorphosis. All in all, Liceti showed Browne how a physician-philosopher's Aristotelianism might metamorphose in order to counter atheism, intellectual discord, and skepticism with ancient hieroglyphics, Christian mysteries, and civility.

In complex ways, Browne's *Religio* is haunted by the attractions and liabilities of an obsession with Aristotelian authority and argumentation. It too speaks to the dire need for a transformation, though not an abandonment, of scholastic terms, methods, and problems. The *Religio*'s opposition to dispute is obvious; its affection for evocative Platonic metaphors and mysteries at the expense of rigid definitions and abstruse "niceties" easy to show. It takes Aristotle but also Suárez to task for botching their explorations of final cause. But it still confesses the theological power of the syllogism; captures Browne's exegetical dispute with a "young Divine" and his "Franciscan Opponent," lingers on "scruple[s]" about infusion and traduction (while protesting that they are not "wrung from speculations and subtleties"); and with Liceti distinguishes the naturalness with which souls outlive their bodies from the miracle that reunites them. Browne characterizes scholastic rationality as "solid" and "demonstrative"; he also deems it woefully inadequate in the pursuit of faith, mystery, and natural hieroglyphics. The "contemplative and schoole Philosopher" requires assistance from the "sensible Artist" or he will mistake mystical signatures for substance and accidents, form and matter. Aristotelian rules must often be suspended; they cannot be jettisoned but must be metamorphosed, if only within the leisure of intellectual recreation. While "acute and singular," Aristotle tends to omit those "mysticall sciences" to which the Egyptians tended, though the Egyptians (Browne continues) have a capacity for "vagabond and counterfeit" pretenses that one would never find in Aristotle, "who understood the uncertainty of knowledge." But then Aristotle "is too severe," too disputatious with Platonic Ideas, and not thorough enough in his singular study of the spiritual liberation found in dreams.[45]

[44] For Paduan philosophy's obsession with method and logic, see John Herman Randall, *The School of Padua and the Emergence of Modern Science* (Padua: Antenore, 1961); Neal W. Gilbert, *Renaissance Concepts of Method* (New York: Columbia University Press, 1960); and Nicholas Jardine, "Keeping Order in the School of Padua: Jacopo Zabarella and Francesco Piccolomini on the Offices of Philosophy," in Daniel A. Di Liscia et al., eds., *Method and Order in Renaissance Philosophy of Nature: The Aristotle Commentary Tradition* (Burlington, VT: Ashgate, 1997), 183–210.

[45] Patrides, 63–4, 69–71, 77, 69, 90–1, 106, 158, 155.

Strikingly, Liceti and Browne appeared side by side in the musings of Guy Patin.[46] In *A Letter to a Friend*, Browne recounts one memory suggesting that he enjoyed conversing—if not to Liceti himself—then to someone very much like him. Speaking of the circumstances under which the patient discussed in the letter has died, Browne remarks that while astrology has not really entered into his thinking on the case, he "could not but take notice that he died when the Moon was in motion from the Meridian; at which time, an old *Italian* long ago would persuade me, that the greatest part of Men died" (Patrides, 394). In 1632–33, Liceti was in his mid-fifties, enough to qualify him as "old." More importantly, his works are simply filled with meditations on how the moon influences life and death on earth.[47] Whether Liceti himself was the Italian in question, Browne speaks of the conversation with fondness and, if with a critical distance from the old man's beliefs, then also with a testimony to how the discussion has stayed with him for decades after.

3. HOSPITALS, ANATOMY THEATERS, AND GARDENS

In seventeenth-century Padua, medical students were in an especially good position to enjoy the city's rich intellectual culture, with its vital sites including "the back rooms of the pharmacies and bookstores, where professors and rich gentlemen met informally to talk about their common concerns."[48] Beyond these informal settings, Padua offered the medical student more directly experienced means of assessing the relationship between divinity and medicine, featuring the paired circular hieroglyphs in the theaters set aside for anatomy and botany. Perhaps most extraordinary was the city's revolutionary hospital clinic which, in addition to its fame for an "exclusive focus on the sick poor," participated in the Catholic pursuit for the unified health of soul and body in the service of Christ.[49]

Browne's Paduan education extended outside the walls of the university building, the Palazzo del Bo, into the streets and the culture of the city itself. This extracurricular training was of course not radically divorced from university life; the two

[46] Guy Patin, *Naudæana et Patiniana*, with *Patiniana* (Paris, 1701), separately paginated, 11–12.

[47] See for instance *De natura & efficientia luminis* (1640), 173–206; and *De lunae subobscura luce prope coniunctiones* (1642). Liceti considers the hieroglyphic significance of the moon in *Hieroglyphica* (1653), 433, 438.

[48] Eric Cochrane, "The Renaissance Academies in their Italian and European Setting," in *The Fairest Flower: The Emergence of Linguistic National Consciousness in Renaissance Europe* (Florence: Firenze presso l'Accademia, 1985), 21–40, see 28; this is based on Michela L. Nichetti Spanio, "Accademie Padovane nel Dei e nel Settecento," in *Accademie e Cultura: Aspetti Storici tra Sei e Settecento* (Florence: Leo S. Olschki, 1979), 211–21; see 211. For pharmacies as Venetian gathering places, see also Filippo de Vivo, "Pharmacies as Centres of Communication in Early Modern Venice," *Renaissance Studies* 21 (2007), 505–21.

[49] Richard Palmer, "'Ad Una Sancta Perfettione': Health Care and Poor Relief in the Republic of Venice in the Era of the Counter-Reformation," in Ole Peter Grell and Andrew Cunningham, eds., *Health Care and Poor Relief in Counter-Reformation Europe* (New York: Routledge, 1999), 87–101, see 89–90.

arenas of learning were interactive, for instance, in the clinical medical program for which Padua was famous. Padua's offer of experiential learning in the hospital of San Francisco was one of the medical school's chief attractions. Foreign students, especially, insisted on clinical practice as their reason for being in Padua, with one remarking in 1624 that he "did not miss the occasion of going around mid-day to the Hospital of St. Francis."[50] Three key components made up clinical education: "daily hospital rounds with formal discussion of major cases, systematic teaching of urines (and pulses), and autopsies of fatal cases."[51] Browne had already had the opportunity to go on medical rounds in Montpellier, but his expertise as a case-by-case, hands-on physician clearly stood to profit from the program in Padua.

In 1632, the program was overseen by two physicians whose excellent reputations as both teachers and practicing physicians have come down to us in abundant evidence: Giovanni Domenico Sala (1579–1644) and Benedictus Silvaticus (1575–1658). And although the learned and successful physician, Johan Rode, had thus far refused any official post in the university, he too was on hand to assist students with their medical training as well as with their scholarly interests in ancients such as Celsus. Born in Copenhagen, Rode (1587–1659) had been elevated to *lector, ostensor simplicium*, and prefect of the botanical garden in 1631 but he quickly abandoned these positions even before the year was complete. Even so, he was a central figure in the intellectual life of the medical school in the early 1630s, not least because he welcomed students to his house but also because he was a polymath with an extraordinary library of books and manuscripts, including "an illuminated manuscript copy of Dioscorides."[52] His major scholarship, which Browne owned, specialized in editions of and commentaries on ancient medical writers such as Scribonius and Celsus.

As a marvelous explicator of practical medicine, Sala allured his auditors with the dignity and eloquence of his words and actions, and they in turn hung on his every phrase. Silvaticus, by contrast to Sala, was remarkable for the incisive authority with which he affirmed and secured doctrine of a seemingly ambiguous nature and freed medical ideas from corruptions and barbarity. Sala emerges from contemporary reports as more aphoristic and enigmatic in the Hippocratic sense; Silvaticus spoke more copiously like Galen but also more lucidly. Above all, both men were impressive in their sway with the powerful leaders of church and state; they were indeed very busy men, whose concern for the private as well as the public tuition of their students was undeniable, but whose schedules sometimes impeded the activation of their wishes to teach. Thus the university's German students, whose patron Silvaticus became in 1632, were awed by his concern for them and by the excellence of instruction—not just public but also private, the latter established by Silvaticus in November 1632.[53]

[50] Jerome J. Bylebyl, "Commentary on Loris Premuda's Influence of the Nineteenth-Century Vienna School on Italian Medicine: The Roles of Padua and Trieste," in Lloyd G. Stevenson, ed., *A Celebration of Medical History* (Baltimore, MD: Johns Hopkins University Press, 1981), 200–11, see 201–2, 207.

[51] Bylebyl, "The School of Padua: Humanistic Medicine," 350–1.

[52] Paola Mariani, "Johann Rhode," in Alessandro Minelli, ed., *The Botanical Garden of Padua, 1545–1995* (Venice: Marsilio, 1995), 71–2.

[53] Lucia Rossetti, ed., *Acta Nationis Germanicae Artistarum*, 321.

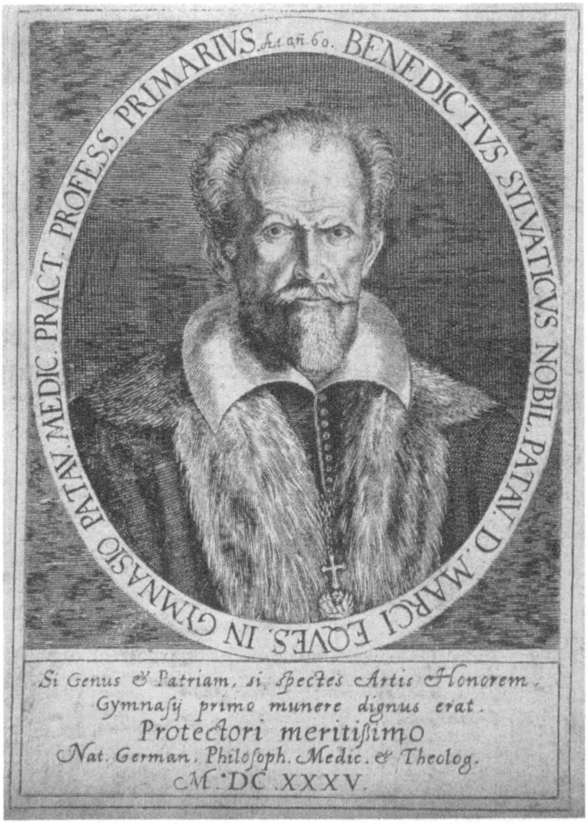

Figure 5.2 Benedictus Silvaticus, from a line engraving (1635): reproduced with the permission of the Wellcome Library, London.

For Browne, a physician such as Silvaticus epitomized the medical man as a significant man of affairs, a visible public figure who carried weight in his society and who brilliantly fused civic prominence, professorial skill, and vocational success. (See Figure 5.2.) Years later, Browne reflected his appreciation of such public stature in a letter to his son Edward regarding the Harveian Orations, in which he noted that Dr George Rogers had orated at Padua when taking his medical degree in 1646, "*Benedicto Sylvatico præside, Fortunio Liceti promotore*" (Keynes, 4.227). Both Sala and Silvaticus made a point of publishing explanations of their medical theory and practice as part of the civic duty to the Venetian Republic.[54] And both were distinguished as practitioners and clinical educators as well. Silvaticus's clinical expertise was highly renowned; of Sala Thomas Bartholin recalled "three years of visiting the sick of Padua" during which Sala proved himself an "outstanding"

[54] For an introduction, see Giuseppe Vedova, *Biografia degli Scrittori Padovani* (Padua,1836), 2.190–3, 200.

guide, a "great physician, renowned in years, merits, teaching and experience. I shall remember him to the end of my life."[55]

In Sala's case, we have chiefly an introductory textbook entitled *Ars Medica* (1620, but used in his lectures in the 1630s), comprising the five parts of medicine (physiology, pathology, semiotics, therapy, and hygiene), strongly Galenic, and committed to the unity of medical knowledge via reason, experience, and analogy, decidedly in that order of preference. In Silvaticus's case we are even more fortunate, for there is a record of four hundred actual cases, including an appendix on his method of consultation. In the great tradition of Paduan professors such as Giacomo Zabarella and Galileo, he is keen to fashion the messy circumstances of consultation into the clarity and stability of logic (for instance, the resolutive method according to which the physician proceeds from conclusions and effects to precedent causes). Throughout Silvaticus's cases, however, circumstantial experience does throw curves at reason whenever the consultant confronts conditions in which theology and medicine cross paths. In Padua, Browne could not move between religion and medicine with the ease that apparently Thomas Clayton had done so in Oxford. Offering not just a case but a medico-philosophical meditation, Silvaticus writes in a letter to a fellow physician about the notoriously difficult problem of the nature of innate heat. Along the way, Silvaticus introduces not just the categorical instability of the innate heat itself but the pertinence of this instability to the way in which we speak of the human mind as eternal and immortal, then in the final part of the discussion, he repeats that the innate heat is not identical to the human essence or form, the incorporeal and immortal soul. For the incisive practical physician, then, logic and semiotics cross paths, however briefly, with theology.

Theology and medicine abut one another in the further case of a young nun named Cypriana, whose deficiencies in mathematics have led her order to consult Silvaticus. Closely linked to her problems with numbers is the girl's trouble with spiritual understanding, as a consequence of which her physician introduces into his thinking about the case those hieroglyphic and transcendent values placed on numbers by ancients such as the Pythagoreans, as well as by sacred divines. The dilemma is this: rational human beings are supposed to have the capacity to work with numbers and, *a fortiori*, spiritually gifted persons should be especially attuned to the proportions and ratios so beautifully revealing of the divine mind. What does it mean, then, if a nun cannot cipher? A key question in this matter is whether such ineptitude with numbers is simply and naturally human in the fallen world, congenital in this specific case, or acquired from her environment or from some external affliction, and whether anything can be done to correct the difficulty. Theologians as well as physicians have devoted their energies to this case, we learn, and Silvaticus deems it a difficult one.[56] One can readily imagine how the Paduan mediation between medicine and theology could leave Browne still worried about

[55] For Sala, see Bartholin, *On Medical Travel,* trans. O'Malley, 83–4.

[56] Silvaticus, *Medicinalium Centuriæ Quatuor* (Geneva, 1662), 56.

the devil's delight in those wits with tendencies to naturalize all phenomena.[57] What makes the case of the numberless nun so striking is its exploration of the gray area between supernatural and natural. In *Religio Medici*, Browne insisted that a sensitivity to mathematics together with musical harmony was an integral part of one's understanding of divine providence, not just a human art or logic. That he did so reflected the Paduan desire to overcome a naturalizing atheism from within, a prospect made all the more feasible for Browne in the context of the ceremonialism in which his Paduan experiences were framed.

In the clinical rounds led by Silvaticus for his students, puzzles on the threshold between divinity and medicine were underscored by the very setting of the hospital, for the sickrooms and medical offices adjoined a Franciscan church and cloisters as part of a large complex; the Sala family palazzo was apparently very close by.[58] Upon entering the complex, a visitor encountered an elegant outside staircase leading to the first story with its two large rooms, including the Aula Magna for assemblies of the medical and law faculties, with an altar nearby, its ornament depicting the Assumption of the Virgin, and probably an imposing library owned by Carmelites. On its east side, the hospital abutted the wall of the church apse and the convent. Evidence suggests that the church was plain and darkish, with a wooden crucifix and four windows, a clear contrast with the more elegant and elaborate chambers of the medical professors. Dated 1628, one inscription captured the tension between medical and ascetic goals; of a physician dead at thirty-three, it declared that neither youth nor strength nor medicine could conquer his mortal fate. This *memento mori* was a far cry from the inscription that greeted students as they poured into the Palazzo del Bo itself, which urged them to exit everyday in a more learned state than when they entered.

As John Henderson has explained, "the idea of Christus Medicus and the relationship between the divine physician and the mortal physician" were at the very crux of the Renaissance hospital[59]; in Padua, this relationship was all the more valuable by virtue of the fact that it could not be taken for granted. Far from neglecting the tension between a resignation to death and a commitment to activity, learning, and life, the Paduan medical establishment reconstituted their harmony in stressing the parallels between the anatomy theater (within Palazzo del Bo) and the botanical garden situated on the outskirts of the city between Padua's two most extraordinary and ornamental churches. These features of the cityscape made an indelible impression on the ways in which Browne juxtaposed nature and

[57] See also David Gentilcore, *Healers and Healing in Early Modern Italy* (New York: Manchester University Press, 1998), 178, 187–9.

[58] See L. Premuda and B. Bertolaso, "La Prima Sede dell'Insegnamento Clinico nel Mondo: L'Ospedale di S. Francesco Grande in Padova," *Acta Medicae Historiae Patavina* 7 (1960–61), 61–92; and Francesco Pellegrini, *La Clinica Medica Padovana Attraverso I Secoli* (Verona: La Tipographia Veronese, 1939). See also Caspar Bartholin, *De studio medico inchoando, continuando et absolvendo consilium breve atque extemporaneum* (1628); and Gerardo Zelante, *S. Francesco Grande di Padova* (Padua: Messaggero, 1921).

[59] John Henderson, *The Renaissance Hospital: Healing the Body and Healing the Soul* (New Haven, CT: Yale University Press, 2006), 113.

religion. With his own version of the combination between ringing church bells and the geometry of nature, Browne carved out a discursive space in which to test out dangerous speculations and to overcome their capacity for evil. And in the pairing of urns and gardens in his 1658 volume, he recreated Padua's evocative connection between anatomy and botany.

Writing in 1624, a German student, Otto Sperling, listed the clinical program, the anatomy lectures, and the botanical demonstrations as the three premiere attractions of the Paduan medical education. At the bedsides in San Francisco, students learned to examine a patient's carriage, facial expression, skin color, breath, pulse, and heartbeat, to interview the patients, to order and administer medicines, and to appreciate the wonders of the profession, for Sperling testifies to the marvelous cures of seemingly desperate cases that he witnessed.[60] But the bedside was also the scene of misery, helplessness, and death. The intimacy between life and death so basic to medical practice was underscored in Padua in a hieroglyphic way, for both the anatomy theater and the botanical garden enclosed the spectator in profoundly symbolic circles.

The great value placed on these interactive circles of death and life was underscored by the university's German nation in 1632, when in the wake of the plague and of the difficulty securing professors, the school year ending in early June concluded without either the customary anatomical demonstration in January–February or the botanical exhibitions of the spring. The academic year beginning in early November 1632 got off to a rocky start inasmuch as even the customary roster of classes was not published: so many professors had died or left the city without returning that the university was on shaky ground. There was the usual opening-day celebration with Latin oration on the 14th, and professors such as Silvaticus did their best to supplement public instruction with private lessons at their homes, but it was a bitter winter, both from the cold and from the shadow of the plague over Padua.

Then, in January 1633 the university struck gold. Just before and throughout 1632, a German named Johann Vesling had been luring students to Venice with his excellent anatomical lectures.[61] Vesling's appointment to the anatomy chair in Padua in December 1632 was especially welcome, given the vacancy of the chair for the two years prior to that date. On January 17, St Anthony's Day, he enthralled the university audience with a brilliant lecture; on the 22nd, he commenced the anatomy of a human body and carried it out with dexterous hand, elegant speech, and perspicuous mind, far surpassing the already high expectations for his abilities. Vesling's anatomy lesson lasted all the way until early March, even after the rest of the university—which generally took a holiday from normal activities both for festival and anatomy—had returned to work on February 10. So pleased were the German students by Vesling's performance that they presented him with a

[60] Gerhard Fichtner, "Padova e Tübingen: La Formazione Medica nei Secoli XVI e XVII," *Acta Medicae Historiae Patavina* 19 (1972–73), 43–62.

[61] Minelli, ed., *The Botanical Garden*, 74–5.

congratulatory poem in the anatomy theater itself, and interceded with the university authorities to ensure that Vesling was in the Palazzo del Bo for good.[62]

The famous Paduan anatomical theater in which Vesling performed was decidedly cramped and gloomy, with auditors stacked on one another in a high, narrow space—six levels formed into a funnel—and dimly lit by its fourteen candles and scarcely effective windows. The demonstration space itself was tiny: if the total capacity might reach 250 participants, this was thanks to their willingness to pack live bodies into the elliptical space surrounding the dead one. But as we learn from Tomasino, the anatomy (begun just after St Anthony's Day on January 17) was carried out with a solemn mood and in ceremonial fashion, with doorways crowned in laurel and music welcoming the comers to the theater, which itself was beautified with vermiculate decorations. After the completion of the anatomy, the bones were carried off to a church, escorted by a priest, presbyters, and the whole university, transported in a magnificent bier, and buried according to the rites of the church with a noble funeral oration.

Vesling was also fascinating to students such as Browne for his recent travels with the Venetian embassy in Palestine and Egypt, where he had undertaken serious botanical study of the local flora as well as direct experience of that most hieroglyphic of all ancient cultures, the Egyptian. Not only did he carry on Prospero Alpini's work of importing plants from Egypt as well as the Indies, but "he himself went collecting in Egypt" in the 1620s, and published *De plantis Aegyptiis observationes* in 1638. Vesling's far-reaching expertise in flora was in keeping with the Venetian Republic's especially rich opportunities for pharmaceutical study.[63] Nor were local botanical offerings in short supply: the traveler from the west entered the city through an herbal largesse for which the Euganean Hills were chief sources. In Padua, plant life was wonderfully local but also as global as the lines of trade, and Browne could experience a fascination with Egypt that would be seconded by the collections in Leiden.

When Vesling took over as botany professor a few years later in 1638, he reminded his students of the complementary relation that the anatomy theater had developed to the botanical garden in the Paduan medical program. Publishing work in both areas of medical expertise,[64] he emphasized in his anatomy textbook (designed to emulate the experience of the theater) that the human body shows the workmanship of God; that the ancients were both too secretive and complicated in their handling of its make-up, and that the anatomy theater is no place for controversy: the body needs to be studied there, not contended over. His anatomy textbook was meant to simplify the analysis of the body for students, but also to remind them of those admirable purposes bestowed by a wise Creator, indeed even of its hieroglyphs, for instance in the wrinkles on the forehead, palms, and soles. In his botanical

[62] Rossetti, ed., *Acta Nationis Germanicae Artistarum*, 324–7.

[63] Richard Palmer, "Pharmacy in the Republic of Venice in the Sixteenth Century," in A. Wear et al., eds., *The Medical Renaissance of the Sixteenth Century* (New York: Cambridge University Press, 1985), 100–17; see 101.

[64] Johann Vesling, *De plantis Aegyptiis observationes et notae ad Prosperum Alpinum* (1638); and *Syntagma Anatomicum* (1647).

lectures, he especially reinforced the intersection between the circles of life and death, spring and winter, light in the garden and shadows in the theater, generation in the flower and decay in the cadaver. For whatever the variation between anatomy and botany, he argues, there is no contrariety but only harmony in medicine. Also appealing to Browne was Vesling's analogical thinking. In addressing the university, Vesling points to Homer as the key source of an analogy between men and plants; and just as philosophers agree (he continues) on the divine origin and orientation of the human mind, so too ancients believed that many flowers derived their sap from the immortal gods. Analogous in their general beauty but also in the distribution of their parts, human beings and plants are also alike in having marvelously wise modes of generation. Perhaps most evocatively for the occasion, they resemble one another in their fragility. As with Liceti's hieroglyphic recreations, Vesling's playful analogies are aimed at healing the stubborn wound in the Paduan embodiment of the Christian physician.

This is very much the same Vesling who challenged Cremonini's critique of purpose in the diverse materials of generation. With one exasperated "O Cremonini," Vesling summarizes his and Liceti's attempts to save Paduan medical learning from atheism. In all, Vesling perpetuates a specifically Paduan tradition of founding anatomy in a natural philosophy committed to "natural order and purposeful design," only now with the promise of moving anatomical learning in the direction of hands-on experience.[65] And Vesling's pupils clearly grasped his stress on divine providence: the poet Edmund Waller praised Vesling, among other things, for going beyond an explanation of the body: "For not the inventory, we alone | Of every Nerve, Vein, Artery and Bone, | Receive from thence, but are instructed too | What the wise Maker has design'd them to: | The great importance of the slendrest string, | And use of every (seeming useless) thing."[66] Moreover, the ceremonial theater of Paduan anatomy was not lost on British visitors. In the early seventeenth century, for instance, Arthur Johnston composed two epigrams on the superiority of the anatomical spectacle there to the more vulgar entertainment to be had in ancient amphitheatres.[67] Medically inflected theater featured another civic festival, the annual concoction of theriac or treacle which involved, as Evelyn remarked, an "extraordinary ceremony... extremely pompous and worth seeing."[68]

[65] I quote Cynthia Klestinec on the sixteenth-century tradition; see *Theaters of Anatomy: Students, Teachers, and Traditions of Dissection in Renaissance Venice* (Baltimore, MD: Johns Hopkins University Press, 2011), 9. Klestinec has shown that the Paduan tradition should not be conflated with the carnivalesque anatomical performances in Bologna; she also notes that while in the sixteenth century the public performance of anatomy was distinctly separate from the private lessons that offered students hands-on experience of the cadaver, this private–public separation was overridden with the arrival of Vesling (*Theaters of Anatomy*, passim). See also Cynthia Klestinec, "Civility, Comportment, and the Anatomy Theater: Girolamo Fabrici and His Medical Students in Renaissance Padua," *Renaissance Quarterly* 60 (2007), 434–63; and Klestinec, "A History of Anatomy Theaters in Sixteenth-Century Padua," *Journal of the History of Medicine and Allied Sciences* 59 (2004), 375–412.

[66] E. S. De Beer, "An Uncollected Poem by Waller," *Review of English Studies* 8 (1932), 203–5.

[67] See Arthur Johnston, *Musa Latina Aberdonensis*, ed. Sir William Duguid Geddes, 3 vols. (Aberdeen: New Spalding Club, 1895), 2.59–60.

[68] Quoted in Gilbert Watson, *Theriac and Mithridatium: A Study in Therapeutics* (London: The Wellcome Historical Medical Library, 1966), 104.

What all this amounts to for the education of Browne is that the Paduan professors teaching during his residence made ceremonial assertions of providence in full view of the materialist legacy that always threatened to subvert Paduan intellectual culture from within.

As Vesling points out to his students, the very construction of the botanical garden speaks of paradise and perfection, even as it resonates with the death and darkness of the anatomy theater. (See Figure 5.3.) For the most striking feature of the garden is its circular frame. Situated between the great churches of St Giustina and St Antonio, surrounded by groves, lesser gardens, a labyrinth and open fields,

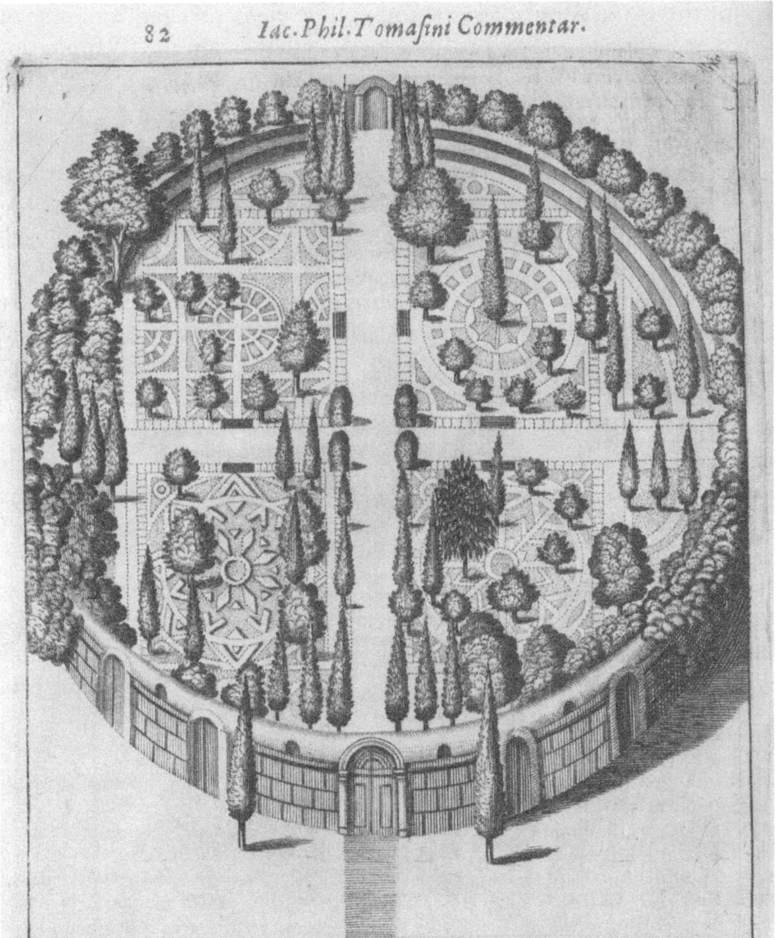

Figure 5.3 Padua's botanical garden, from Tomasino's *Gymnasium Patavinum* (1654). University of Toronto Rare Book Library.

and edged by a refreshing river, the circle comprised within its circumference a square, itself divided into four squares, with each containing elaborate geometrical patterns, interlacements, and tracery. Seemingly all the plants of the world filled the carefully apportioned and manifold beds in this geometrical hieroglyph. The shapes were not just symbolic, with circle, squares, triangles, star patterns, and quincunxes: they were useful in ensuring that no land in the complex was wasted in the display of nature's variety. The garden was not just a little world: it was a paradise on earth, with the circle a symbol of divinity, perfection, divine justice, divine infinitude, simplicity, uniformity, strength, capaciousness, the planetary orbs in whose region there could be no opposition or disharmony (compare the star shapes in the garden), and the very cosmos itself; the square an emblem of the world's four corners, continents, elements, and humors, and the other shapes having their part to play in a Pythagorean and Platonic imagery emblematic of a cosmos governed, harmonized, filled, employed, and beautified by divine providence.[69]

Contemporary discussions of the circular garden readily identify its emblematic resonance as a microcosm as well as the sublime and magical codes of math and geometry.[70] For Browne, the congregation of geometry, Egypt, and the hieroglyphs of nature, all framed by two of Padua's most magnificent churches with their own combination of rounded and triangular towers, translated in the *Religio* into the very distillation of divine providence in a cosmos laced together by correspondences. Indeed, in a 1633 work, a commentator explained how the round garden of Padua served "as a microcosm of the world."[71] In the garden's stress on how contrariety might be converted into an ensemble harmony, visitors were known also to politicize the lesson that the garden taught: that the Venetian Republic—when compared to Germany across the Alps, to France in the west, to Milan and the Papal States nearer to home, and to the Dutch Republic's ongoing war with Spain—was itself a paradise of tolerance, peace, and even piety: one would hear bells and see the towers of the two great churches as one strolled among and learned from the diverse flower beds in the perfect circle. Indeed, despite the fame of St Anthony's, visitors to Padua were always awed by its partner Santa Giustina.[72] Church, nature, and artifice embedded one in the bosom of providence. In a letter to Petrus Servius, Vesling enthused that the garden was Padua's most beautiful place, far

[69] Margherita Azzi Visentini, "Il giardino dei semplici di Padova: Un prodotto della cultura del Rinascimento," *Comunità* 34 (1980), 259–338; Girolamo Porro, *L'Horti de I Semplici di Padoua* (Venice, 1591); and Dennis E. Rhodes, "The Botanical Garden of Padua: The First Hundred Years," *Journal of Garden History* 4 (1984), 327–31. See also Claudia Lazzaro, *The Italian Renaissance Garden: From the Conventions of Planting, Design, and Ornament to the Grand Gardens of Sixteenth-Century Central Italy* (New Haven, CT: Yale University Press, 1990). For the significance of geometry, see S. K. Heninger, Jr., *Touches of Sweet Harmony: Pythagorean Cosmology and Renaissance Poetics* (San Marino, CA: Huntington Library, 1974). The key classical source is Plato's *Timaeus*.

[70] Peter Davidson, "The Jesuit Garden," in O'Malley, ed., *The Jesuits II*, 86–107; see 101; and Cook, *Matters of Exchange*, 27.

[71] Giovanni Battista Ferrari, *De florum cultura* (Rome, 1633); see Davidson, "The Jesuit Garden," in *The Jesuits II*, 101.

[72] Sells, *The Paradise of Travellers*, 201.

from the city tumult, between two august churches, and next to the waters of the Brenta. "To the North," he commented, "I see Alps, which represent to me the boundaries between our country and the German funeral in lingering war."[73] From the garden, Padua struck Vesling as perfect, for all the city's noise: with ample courts and palaces, with Minerva's treasure chest in the university and its anatomy theater; to the east, fertile fields and the Adriatic, to the west, the beautiful and medicinal Euganean hills; beneath his window, the garden itself, with its flowers from all over Italy and the world, and its geometrical shapes: the circle, its squares, and even those stars intended as a monument to the priests of Apollo. In all, the garden offered sanctuary, Vesling believed, from all that is sordid or vile in the world.

The role that political peace played in the effect that Padua had on northern students must be stressed in the case of Thomas Browne, whose partnership between church ceremony and natural hieroglyphs in *Religio Medici* was invented in support of peace. With great Paduan churches to frame the whole experience, the enclosed garden in particular, together with its flowers, inspired the Christian sage to meditate on the mysteries of the faith, "a kind of surrogate Bible" and a supplementary church.[74] In this setting, Browne's sensible artist heard Ave Marie bells from within the gardener's imitation of providential geometry. The garden's circles and quincunxes—those shapes that would linger in Browne's imagination and permeate his artistry—structured a space whose beauty, tranquility, and mystery were also charitably and medically purposeful in the hospital back in the city.

The medical student visiting the garden was obliged to remember that the university itself and the physician's vocation summoned the philosopher back to the wilderness of the city. The place of the wilderness in Christian thought always challenged and subverted the garden as the chief location for achieving wisdom, virtue, and salvation. As a city with its academy, Padua offered students a decidedly fallen education, filled with conflict, violence, labor, anxiety, motion, intolerance, disease, impiety, and monstrous vice. In the wilderness, Prest notes, one fed on locusts not on delicious fruit; one experienced trial and temptation, not rest and sublimation (*The Garden of Eden*, 24). In the city, human beings strove to assert order, to harmonize community, to apprehend the scattered or decaying vestiges of nature's final causes, and to live in the ways of God against all pressures to the contrary. In the Jewish ghetto and in the ongoing customs, problems, and pageantry of city life, students found, not an escape from a war-faring Europe but a struggle to minimize the damage of its intellectual crisis, religious persecution, political hostility, and human malice. In this environment, Browne would have a bold encounter with the realities of toleration and intolerance that would have a decisive impact on his sense of national, cultural, and religious identity.

[73] Vesling's letter appears in Tomasini, *Gymnasium Patavinum*, 86–9.

[74] See John Prest, *The Garden of Eden: The Botanic Garden and the Re-Creation of Paradise* (New Haven, CT: Yale University Press, 1981), 23.

4. THE GHETTO AND THE CITY

When Browne arrived in Padua in 1632, the city's Jewish ghetto was a newly established space.[75] Like the ghettoes in Venice, it afforded the Jews a certain measure of autonomy in their lives, worship, and even governance, and protection from the violence of prejudice; in bringing Jews together from all over Europe (especially Spain and Portugal, Germany, and Italy itself), it also accentuated the cultural variety and intense energy within Judaism itself. But with its overcrowding and guarded, lockable gates, the ghetto also reinforced prejudice, as though the Jews were diseased animals that needed to be quarantined. Not surprisingly, some of the richest Jews attempted to live outside the walls of the narrow, dark, dirty ghetto in nicer, larger houses; contemporary documents contrasted the claustrophobic ghetto with the spacious, green, courtyard-laden city outside.[76] For their part, city officials were keen to prevent inappropriate, especially sexual, liaisons between Jews and Christians. Most obviously, they made the Jews wear a distinguishing badge (at first a patch of yellow material, later in Browne's time a yellow beret, later still a red beret); and they exhorted Christian women to refrain from entering the ghetto. Jewish physicians were permitted to wear a black beret, and other Jews managed to evade the rules about wearing the Jewish badge; in turn, Venetian officials saw the badges as key measures of social order and they persisted in urging Paduan officials to enforce them.

Because the Jews traded in clothes, furniture, utensils, candles, books, and other secondhand goods, students had practical reasons—in addition to their curiosity—for visiting this space. Students living in a lodging-house (as they often did) could live pretty cheaply in Padua,[77] and the Jewish markets helped make this possible. In 1615, 74 shops were opened with great appeal to the student body seeking both a gentlemanly and scholarly life at discount prices. Records show that the students treated their Jewish suppliers in conflicting ways, bullying them but also defending them in lawsuits with the city guilds. Student violence against the Jews was a perennial problem for city officials; in 1621 for instance, preachers admonished their auditors not to use violent language against the Jews and not to incite violence against them. Officials also lamented the fact that the church's solemn processions sometimes had to pass alongside the ghetto walls; on these occasions, Jews were made to stay at home in the ghetto, both to prevent harm against them and to protect the sacramental march from contamination. On the last days of carnival and on the first day of snowfall (during which students extorted money or goods in exchange for "protection" against assault), Jews were so vulnerable to violent attacks on their persons, not least from the students themselves, that the

[75] Antonio Ciscato, *Gli Ebrei in Padova (1300–1800)* (orig. Padua, 1901; reprinted, Bologna: Forni, 2004). For a recent discussion of the Jews in Venice in the context of the history of toleration, see Benjamin J. Kaplan, *Divided by Faith: Religious Conflict and the Practice of Toleration in Early Modern Europe* (Cambridge, MA: Harvard University Press, 2007), 294–300.

[76] Antonio Ciscato, *Gli Ebrei in Padova (1300–1800)*, 74.

[77] See Sells, *The Paradise of Travellers*, 114–15.

officials suspended rules requiring them to wear a beret. The holiday violence of the first snowfall became so irksome to the Jews that in January 1633, while Browne was in residence, the Senate abolished the custom altogether. One ongoing source of tension was the students' penchant for stealing cadavers from Jewish funerals for the purposes of anatomy; indeed the Jews had a secret place in the ghetto to preserve the bodies against theft until burial. In 1624, led by the assistant to the anatomy professor, students halted a Jewish funeral in order to pilfer a body, and only the intervention of citizens appalled at the sacrilege impeded the students from succeeding at the theft (Ciscato, 73–91; 107–17; 165–9).

Christian medical students did not have to visit the ghetto or a synagogue to mingle with Jews; for there was a strong tradition of Jewish students enrolled at the medical school, though they could not receive their degrees in the normal ceremony presided over by the bishop.[78] Despite the admission of Jewish medical students to the university, Christian physicians did their best to prevent Jewish physicians from practicing outside the ghetto; indeed the church threatened to excommunicate Christians who employed Jewish doctors, while Catholic doctors beseeched the Senate to preserve their exclusive rights in the trade.

Whatever the tensions between students and Jews, and even setting aside their business relations, students like other tourists visiting Padua were often eager to see the ghetto and especially the synagogues. The synagogue built in 1548 was rich and majestic on the inside, with an elegant altar, black and white marble columns, a door of sculpted wood, a beautiful pulpit, and walls covered in gold. Another house of worship was opened in 1617. Travel accounts by Fynes Morison, Thomas Coryate, William Bedell, John Evelyn, and others are filled with reports of religious services among the Jews. During one Jewish festival in 1628, the Venetian ghetto was kept open into the evening so that Christians might witness the goings-on and hear the "'solemn music that lasted several hours into the night,'" a sign that whereas Jews were prevented from exiting the ghetto during evening hours, gentlefolk would be accommodated in their desire to enter if their touring agenda required it.[79] Evaluations ranged widely: the Jews were, by turns, uncommonly pious, appropriately iconoclastic, sorely in need of Christ and the New Testament, more instructive than the Catholics, ritualistic like the Catholics, lacking in apt gestures of reverence such as removing their hats, obnoxious to the ear with their "exceeding loud yaling, undecent roaring, and as it were... beastly bellowing" of the law, "goodly and proper men" contrary to the stereotype of the deformed, frantic, and discontented Jew, the women especially beautiful and ornamented in their separate area of the synagogue, strict sabbatarians, tedious babblers, genuinely committed to their ancient festivals, and strangely loath to convert. In one respect at least, the Protestants and Jews in the Venetian Republic were protected

[78] Riccardo Calimani, *The Ghetto of Venice*, trans. Katherine Silberblatt Wolfthal (New York: M. Evans, 1987), 140.

[79] Benjamin Ravid, "Curfew Time in the Ghetto of Venice," reprinted in *Studies on the Jews of Venice, 1382–1797* (Burlington, VT: Ashgate, 2003), separately paginated 237–75, quotation on 251.

from the Roman church by the government's famous assertion of its autonomy at the outset of the seventeenth century.[80]

Just prior to and during Browne's visit to Padua, the years 1631–32 drove home both the commonality and the alienation experienced between Jews and Christians in the Venetian Republic. On the one hand there was the plague: despite Rabbi Leon Modena's hope that the Jews might escape its wrath within the ghetto,[81] this was not to prove the case, and thousands of Jews died from the same contagion that killed the Christians beyond its borders (Cohen, 135–6). On the other hand, in May 1631, a major conflict arose between the Venetian government and the Jewish community over whether the Jews ought to resolve their internal conflicts among themselves, without any recourse to Venetian courts and laws. In particular, a question arose about whether Jewish rabbis should excommunicate those Jews who failed to keep their controversies within the community; such uncertainty had arisen about this legal matter that Leon Modena had consulted the so-called Great Book of collected laws and customs. In September 1631, the Venetian Senate required that this book governing daily life in the ghetto be translated into Italian; the stakes of the translation and of the resulting interpretations of Jewish law were very high, with even the possible expulsion of the Jews from the Republic on the table. By December 1632 this translation was finished and the tension over the question of Jewish autonomy was at its height.[82] Clearly, Browne's Padua was a setting in which Jewish–Christian relations were newly contentious, sometimes violent, sometimes uncommonly tolerant, and exceedingly complex.[83]

Despite the plague, Jewish life was thriving so fully in the Republic that in 1633, a new ghetto was undertaken in order to alleviate crowding in the old. But hostilities and suspicions were also high, at the most mundane level (throwing snowballs) and at the most abstract and pervasive (on the question of Jewish autonomy). *Religio Medici* reflects this state of affairs, with Browne decrying a lack of charity toward Jews; expressing dismay but also envy at their refusal to convert, not least in the face of enormous persecution, "a bad and indirect way to plant Religion"; and recalling his willingness when among the Jews to dine on those "Locusts and Grasse-hoppers" that, according to his teacher Sala, were eaten quite commonly in the vein of Leviticus 11.21–2 and of John the Baptist.[84] More extensively,

[80] See William J. Bouwsma, *Venice and the Defense of Republican Liberty: Renaissance Values in the Age of the Counter Reformation* (Berkeley: University of California Press, 1968); David Wootton, *Paolo Sarpi: Between Renaissance and Enlightenment* (Cambridge: Cambridge University Press, 1983); Frederic C. Lane, *Venice: A Maritime Republic* (Baltimore, MD: Johns Hopkins University Press, 1973); and David Chambers and Brian Pullan, eds., *Venice: A Documentary History, 1450–1630* (Toronto: University of Toronto Press, 2001).

[81] Leon Modena, *The Autobiography of a Seventeenth-Century Venetian Rabbi*, 135–6.

[82] Simone Luzzatto, *Discorso circa il Stato de Gl'Hebrei et in particolar... Venezia*, intro. Riccardo Bachi (facsimile of the 1638 edition, first published 1946, reprinted, Bologna: Forni, 1976). See David Joshua Malkiel, *A Separate Republic: The Mechanics and Dynamics of Venetian Jewish Self-Government, 1607–1624* (Jerusalem: Magnes, 1991).

[83] For other conflicts between Jews and Christians, see Brian Pullan, *The Jews of Europe and the Inquisition of Venice, 1550–1670* (Oxford: Blackwell, 1983), 305–7.

[84] Sala, *De Alimentis et eorum recta administratione* (Padua, 1628), 8. Patrides, 61, 93, 133.

Pseudodoxia Epidemica not only studies the nature of locusts and grasshoppers, but revisits in order to reject the "received opinion" that "Jews stinck naturally" (Robbins, ed., *Pseudodoxia Epidemica*, 1.61). But the ghetto took the question of toleration into a realm quite distinctive from curious vulgar errors or even the enlightened claims for a liberty of philosophizing and a fundamental unity of all world religions. For the Jews and the Venetian government in Padua were more immediately grappling with matters of law, in fact with competing codes of law and their positions on the civic status of a religious and cultural subgroup. When, in *Pseudodoxia*, Browne turned to dispute the "received opinion" that "Jews stinck naturally," he summoned a careful study of their history and customs, together with a direct experience of "their Synagogues," of "their commerce or conversation," in teaching his English readers that it might prove "a dangerous point to annex a constant property unto any Nation, and much more this unto the Jews" (Robbins, ed., *Pseudodoxia Epidemica*, 1.324–29). "For," he observes, "this offensive odor is in no way discoverable in their Synagogues where many are, and by reason of their number could not be concealed; nor is the same discernible in commerce or conversation with such as are cleanly in apparel, and decent in their houses." In *Urne-Buriall*, Browne shifted into present tense in his appreciation of the ceremonies of Jewish burials: "he that observeth their funerall Feasts, their Lamentations at the grave, their musick, and weeping mourners; how they closed the eyes of their friends, how they washed, anointed, and kissed the dead; may easily conclude these were not meere Pagan-Civilities" (Patrides, 273).

One major conflict among the Jews themselves was the extent to which they should participate in the pervasive theater, music, and ornamentation of the sophisticated culture outside the ghetto walls.[85] English Protestants also had a mixed attitude to the pageantry of the Venetian Republic, but they were rarely indifferent to it. In typical fashion, one early modern traveler reported that " 'the Ceremonyes of State and Processions of Religion...are frequent and performed with great pompe, in both of which they passe all States not only of Italy, but of the whole Worlde' " (Horowitz, 232). In defending both state and religious ceremonies, Browne laments that his companions have made arguments, sometimes rudely, to the contrary. "At a solemne Procession I have wept abundantly," he divulges, "while my consorts, blinde with opposition and prejudice, have fallen into an accesse of scorne and laughter" (Patrides, 63). His argument on behalf of state ritual prompts a casuistic analysis rather than a passion: "The Duke of *Venice*, that weds himselfe unto the Sea, by a ring of Gold, I will not argue of prodigality, because it is a solemnity of good use and consequence in the State. But the Philosopher that threw his money into the Sea to avoyd avarice, was a notorious prodigal" (Patrides, 128). Indeed, Browne's transformation of a highly celebrated and jingoistic Venetian triumph—the 1571 triumph of the Catholic League, featuring the

[85] Elliott Horowitz, "Processions, Piety, and Jewish Confraternities," in Robert C. Davis and Benjamin Ravid, eds., *The Jews of Early Modern Venice*, (Baltimore, MD: Johns Hopkins University Press, 2001), 231–47.

Venetian Republic, over the Ottoman Empire in the battle of Lepanto (Patrides, 145)—into a spiritual battle between his faith, reason, and passion embodies what in the *Religio* affords the key to all Italianate ceremonial experience: the viewer's response must actively and flexibly internalize as metaphor the outward signs of hubris, excess, and superstition.[86]

Browne, of course, had grown up among the London guilds with their elaborate urban pageantry. In Padua, however, state ritual was given new meaning and danger for Protestant visitors by its close proximity in sight and significance to the continual solemnities of saints' days and church processions. Held after Mass, the annual rite of the Venetian wedding with the sea staged the Doge wrapped in regal mantle, accompanied by thirty cardinals, embarking in a richly engraved, gold-covered vessel, with an array of soldiers and musicians on board, and with all manner of galleys and gondolas joining in the procession to the Lido where, with a salute of the artillery, the Patriarch poured holy water into the Adriatic and the Doge cast a gold ring into the same, pledging his troth to the mistress over whom he exerted "universal and perpetual domination." The very circularity of the ring was symbolic, an emblem of "joining, continuity, eternity, and fertility," even as the huge rowdy crowds threatened to undo "communal stability." The ring carried the significance of harmony between opposites, a unity in the face of division, even as it pitted man against the terrifying and often unknowable forces of nature and, by the 1630s, asserted Venetian domination over a world economy in which it was very clearly losing ground.[87]

It was, however, the extraordinary carnival season of winter that served as the climax of a year filled with theatrical piety. From Padua, Evelyn exclaimed on Shrovetide, February 13, 1646, that "all the world repaire[s] to Venice to see the folly & madnesse of the Carnevall."[88] With Carnival, religious celebration was topsy-turvy, paradoxical, and impromptu to the same extent that processions were solemn, measured, and prescriptive. And at the intersection between decorum and masquerade was the morally ambiguous fashioning of the Italian gentleman, a troubled code of behavior that Browne had criticized in his poem on dueling. As in the life of the mind, so too in the social habits of the young gentleman, Padua was at once exceptionally exhilarating and undeniably threatening.[89] Many students went about armed; some were involved in high crimes such as murder and rape; dueling over precedence in the street was not uncommon. If the life of the scholar-cum-gentleman could be barbarous in Padua—violent, debauched, nocturnally wild—it was also stylized, sophisticated, and elegant.[90] Writing of the late 1620s, Gabriel Naudé captured both sides of university life, mocking the many

[86] On this point, see Ingo Berensmeyer, "Rhetoric, Religion and Politics in Sir Thomas Browne's *Religio Medici*," *SEL* 46 (2006), 113–32, at 124.

[87] Imperiale, *Viaggi*, ed. Barrili, 214; Edward Muir, *Civic Ritual in Renaissance Venice* (Princeton, NJ: Princeton University Press, 1981), 120–5, 131–4.

[88] Evelyn, *The Diary*, ed. E. S. De Beer, 6 vols. (Oxford: Oxford University Press, 1955), 2.474–5. One seventeenth-century traveler noted that on a clear day one could see Venice from Padua (Newberry MS Case G. 35, f. 182).

[89] Evelyn, *The Diary*, 472–3.

[90] Coryate quotes Emperor Constantine Paleologus to this effect; see Sells, *The Paradise of Travellers*, 116.

rowdy students who cared nothing whatsoever for scholarship, then stressing that opportunities to master riding, music, and fencing were uncommonly good in Padua.[91] The city itself and the Euganean Hills nearby had their fair share of cultural heroes, from Livy in antiquity to Petrarch in more recent times. Despite ongoing concerns in the seventeenth century about a decline in the Republic and its university,[92] Padua still was fortunate in manifestations of the Muses. Everywhere there were plays (both religious and secular) and operas to be taken in; a wide variety of scenic representations and allegories; a strong tradition of comedy; the survival of olden barriers, jousts, tourneys, and other mock-battles underway;[93] imposing palaces with their elaborate gardens, immense and decorative rooms, and prominent family arms; stunning sartorial fashions; frescoed churches such as the famous Arena chapel;[94] monumental allegorical extravaganzas such as the ancient heroic figures painted on walls of the "Room of the Giants" in the Carrara palace;[95] stately funerals; masquerades and balls, academies of a cultural, intellectual, or military orientation, costly weddings; dances; everywhere music to be heard. In carnival, February 1632, a Padua recovering from the plague enjoyed a "bacchanalia of solemn entertainments, comedies and many other forms of mirth."[96] But during that same year, there was also an exceptional display of humility, repentance, and charity, in response to a wrathful God's scourging in epidemic proportions.

Within the various echelons of Venetian culture, theatricality was promoted and expected virtually everywhere.[97] But as carnival became increasingly a tourist attraction in the seventeenth century, the Venetian penchant for theater was heightened by the sense that countless outsiders had come to observe (as much as to participate in) this exciting, permissive suspension of the normal markers of rank and identity.[98] With emphasis on what for young intellectuals such as Browne was the category of "the seriously playful," "the carnival seasons of the 1630s and 1640s" promoted "theatrical experimentation on an unprecedented scale."[99] Both literally and metaphorically, Browne would summon up this pageantry in what might be considered his own version of carnival in which selfhood might be tested, disguised, refashioned, and perhaps lost.

[91] Naudé, *Gabrielis Navdæi... Epistolæ*, 62–3.

[92] Lionello Puppi and Mario Universo, *Le citta nella storia d'Italia: Padova* (Rome: Laterza, 1982), 165.

[93] See M. Borgherini-Scarabellin, "La Vita Privata a Padova nel secolo XVII," *R. Deputazione veneta di storia patria, Miscellanea*, 3rd series, 12, 1917.

[94] It needs to be said however that travel writers rarely mention Giotto's famous works or this chapel; Sells, *The Paradise of Travellers*, 165.

[95] Theodor E. Mommsen, *Medieval and Renaissance Studies*, ed. Eugene F. Rice, Jr. (Ithaca, NY: Cornell University Press, 1959), 130–74.

[96] Anton-Bonaventura Sberti, *Degli Spettacoli e delle Feste che si facevano in Padova* (Padua, 1818), 147.

[97] Peter Burke, *Venice and Amsterdam: A Study of Seventeenth-Century Élites* (London: Temple Smith, 1974), 63–4.

[98] Peter Burke, *The Historical Anthropology of Early Modern Italy: Essays on Perception and Communication* (New York: Cambridge University Press, 1987), 185.

[99] See Edward Muir, *The Culture Wars of the Late Renaissance: Skeptics, Libertines, and Opera* (Cambridge, MA: Harvard University Press, 2007), 1–59, 124–5, 131.

From a philosophical vantage, Paduan skepticism promoted the free trying-on of ideas, but it also necessitated the masking concealment or mitigation of that freedom. The posthumous sway that Cremonini continued to exert through the 1630s on the students at the university had more to do with "his sense of playful intellectual gamesmanship... than any particular philosophical or theological position";[100] and Liceti offered a safer version of the philosophical theater with his turn to the dialogue in his writings. In many ways, then, Paduan intellectual culture served as what Muir has characterized as an incubator for Venetian theater.[101] But visitors to Padua also remarked that all the city was a theater, even if they differed strikingly on whether it was predominantly comic or tragic in the stage play world of everyday life. In the theater of the city, visitors could learn further lessons in civility, it is true, but they also encountered forms of theater that destabilized, threatened, and liberated identity. In *Letter to a Friend*, Browne warned that people with an "infirm Head" should never spend time in Venice.[102] But *Religio Medici* demonstrates that Browne discovered exhilarating possibilities for selfhood in a culture where one could also become badly lost. As Margaret Doody has observed, in Venice visitors often anxiously lost a sense of self in the very moment of discovering an identity far more "free floating" and wondrously strange than the one they had presupposed.[103] For Browne, Paduan intellectual culture and the Venetian Republic proved equally disconcerting and liberating.

Browne's fellow English visitors often registered their bemusement over carnival. In early 1634 Thomas Raymond wrote that the season embodied "sober debaucherie," that men and women alike could wear "any sort of habitt and maske—any sort except religious, and those are forbidden." He continued that in this time of serious mirth, you could "put your selfe into what shape you please." A man could be a woman for instance, and folks could "play all the ridiculous tricks [they] could imagine."[104] For visitors such as Raymond, carnival embodied a stage-play world in which fancy knows no limit, in which the unimaginable is suddenly possible and even tangible. But, if these observers made note of the liberation of the moment, they also capture its attendant dangers: its desperation, violence, madness, and even malignity. Both the exhilaration and the anxiety of skeptical improvisation made an impact on *Religio Medici*, written by the intellectually adventurous yet melancholy Thomas Browne for whom the legacy of Pomponazzi found a complex reworking in the culture of Liceti.[105]

In Padua, the young Thomas Browne was invited to put on many cultural, intellectual, spiritual, social, and moral personae. In the spirit of carnival, this delight

[100] Muir, *The Culture Wars*, 56.

[101] Muir, *The Culture Wars*, 131.

[102] Patrides, 393; Browne includes Paris with Venice.

[103] Margaret Doody, *Tropic of Venice* (Philadelphia: University of Pennsylvania Press, 2007), 259, 262, 290–1.

[104] Thomas Raymond, *Autobiography of Thomas Raymond*, ed. G. Davies (London: Camden Society, 1917), 54–6. Cf. Robert Belgrave, *The Travel Diary of Robert Bargrave, Levant Merchant (1647–1656)*, ed. Michael G. Brennan (London: The Hakluyt Society, 1999), 236–7.

[105] Belgrave, *Travel Diary of Robert Bargrave*, 236–7.

in improvisation was at once playful and serious, evocative of excess, illegality, and indecorum, yet framed by sacred ritual and formulaic ceremony. Some roles suited him, others made him feel deformed, but all together they helped to transform him from a decidedly English student from Winchester and Oxford into a civil, speculative, imaginative writer whose first book—always something of an embarrassment to the older, settled, mature Thomas Browne—enraptured, horrified, and unsettled continental intellectuals as a singular microcosm of their own throes in a critical, skeptical phase of reinvention. Perhaps Browne learned more medicine in Montpellier; and Leiden—in which he may have lived for a relatively brief time—offered fewer distractions for the tourist as well as greater familiarity for an English visitor. In Leiden, Browne would find less leisure to philosophize, a greater emphasis on practical training and moral habits, and no invitation to pretend to be anything other than what he essentially was. By contrast, in part by default of a depleted faculty, Padua enticed its visitors to participate in a seventeenth-century liberty of philosophizing that was as monstrous to Browne's thinking as it was uplifting and transformative. If we are to credit one of Browne's friends and earliest biographers, the Venetian world of sophisticated civility somehow lingered in the physician of Norfolk: in another life, in different circumstances, John Whitefoot tells us, Sir Thomas might have proved another Paolo Sarpi, his brilliance channeled into a wisdom penetrating the political vagaries of the world ("Some Minutes," xxxvi–xxxvii). Far more than Montpellier or Leiden, the Venetian Republic rendered him more inclusively human but also more skeptical and savvy than he was upon arrival in a city reeling in the aftermath of plague.

As an episode in the *Religio* maintains, the liberty of philosophizing on offer in Padua appears to have reinforced Browne's already established tendency to engage in theological disputation with members of clerical orders. Recalling his bold participation in an academic dispute carried out between a young theology student and his Franciscan opponent, Browne explains that while "The Church of Rome confidently proves the opinion of Tutelary Angels, from that answer when *Peter* knockt at the doore, '*Tis not he but his Angel*," a careful reader of the Bible might conclude that "angel" here meant Peter's "Messenger, or some body from him; for so the Originall signifies; and is as likely to be the doubtfull Families meaning. This exposition I once suggested to a young Divine, that answered upon this point, to which I remember the *Franciscan* Opponent replyed no more, but, That it was a new and no authentick interpretation." In all likelihood this dispute took place in Padua, either between a Dominican and a Franciscan at the university itself or between Franciscans training in the excellent academy in San Francesco Grande, the same convent complex that housed the hospital at which medical students did their clinical work. As a small but vibrant center of learning, the convent held public disputations, the texts of which were distributed to clergy and laity alike.[106]

It is of course impossible to reconstruct how closely, if at all, this account comes to what in fact happened. As related, however, Browne's intervention is both sloppy

[106] For *Religio*, see Patrides, 90–1. See Zelante, *S. Francesco Grande di Padova*, especially 86–91.

and audacious. In Acts 12, Peter is freed from prison by an angel of the Lord whose appearance to Peter is so miraculous as to bemuse the apostle himself (he wonders whether the angel might be a dream vision). If Browne tried to argue that this angel is just a human messenger, then his is clearly "no authentick interpretation." Instead, at least in hindsight, he focuses the thrust of his suggestion on the point at which Peter's knock at "the house of Mary, the mother of John Mark, where a large company was at prayer," is received by a maid, Rhoda, who is so excited by Peter's voice that she rushes back to the company to tell them the news without even opening the door. "You are crazy," they reproach her, "but she insisted that it was so. Then they said, 'It must be his guardian angel.'"

The doubting company is of course wrong; it is not Peter's angel in any sense but rather Peter recently saved by an angel in the heavenly sense. The passage is frequently invoked in treatises on angels as a key litmus test on the question of guardian angels. Catholic writers and many Protestants as well acknowledge that "angelos" can mean simply "messenger," but they side with the weight of Greek and Latin patristic authority in making the case for tutelary angels in Acts 12. What is more, some early modern commentators identify general skepticism about angels with the Epicurean, Sadducee, and specifically Paduan Aristotelian penchant for materialist atheism (with Pomponazzi the chief of the third legacy).[107] By contrast, however, Protestants also acknowledge—and attempt to heed—Calvin's warning that the Bible is obscure on the question of guardian angels, that it is dangerous to speculate about their existence, that with the spread of the Gospel their mission on earth becomes far less necessary, and that a lingering desire to rely on angels smacks of popery. Browne's interjection in the disputation bears a paradoxical relation to Paduan culture: bound to offend or confuse the clergy, it also owes its audacity to the liberty of philosophizing of which Cremonini was only the most recent embodiment.

In the *Religio*, Browne himself uses this memory as an example of the type of doubt, based in critical readings of the Bible, that proves of "no consequence," only "the conclusions, and fallible discourses of man upon the word of God" (Patrides, 90–1). The Acts passage prompts Calvin himself to conclude that "it is not worthwhile anxiously to investigate what it does not much concern us to know."[108] The dismissal of his doubting intervention in the disputation is a key factor of Browne's fashioning of his faith in the *Religio*, but so too is the penchant to doubt, to challenge conventional wisdom, and to try on the habits of heretics and libertines. Strikingly, the encounter with the Franciscan ends less happily than that with the Jesuit which in all likelihood took place in Languedoc.[109]

[107] Pierre le Loyer, *A Treatise of Specters* (1605); cf. John Salkeld, *A Treatise of Angels* (1613), chapters 44–5; Urbanus Rhegius, *An Homely or Sermon of Good and Euill Angels* (1590), 30r–30v; John Mayer, *A Commentarie vpon the New Testament* (1631), 578–9; and Henry Ainsworth, *The Communion of Saincts* (1607), 302–14.

[108] *Institutes of the Christian Religion*, ed. John T. McNeill, trans. Ford Lewis Battles, 2 vols. (Philadelphia: Westminster Press, 1960), vol. 1, I. XIV. 7, p. 167.

[109] See chapter 4 in this volume.

Years later, in traveling from Venice to Vienna, Edward Browne would speak of the journey as productive of an unusual quiet and calm, his response to what travelers often found to be "the sometimes oppressive vitality of Italy."[110] In a letter home from Lyons, William Hammond told his father that while he was indifferent to his choices among Montpellier, Padua, and Leiden, "this Advantage I may hope for in Holland, above that of France or Italy, that being a Country more like our Fenns, I may at spare times get there a more pertinent & Usefull knowledge concerning their husbandry or Improvement of their lands" (Brennan, ed., 191). For these English travelers, Leiden was more familiar and practical—less distracting and dangerous—than Venice.[111] In Leiden Browne would write up and present his dissertation on smallpox in a hurry, then return home to England for good.

110 Antoni Mączak, *Travel in Early Modern Europe* (Cambridge: Cambridge University Press, 1995), 111.
111 Brennan, ed., *The Origins of the Grand Tour*, 293.

6

Leiden, 1633–1634

1. TOURISTS AND STUDENTS IN LEIDEN

For two reasons, the trip from Padua to Leiden in 1633 was the most challenging that Browne made on his European tour. For one thing, despite the resurgence of insurrection in France in 1632, and even with the German fields of battle sufficiently far removed from his course, it was this trip that brought him closer to the most active arenas of war, especially in the border region between the United Provinces and the Spanish Netherlands. More critically for Browne, autumn 1632 had yielded a truce in the Netherlands issuing in thirteen months of peace talks lasting through 1633, a momentous year in the history of the longstanding war between north and south in the Low Countries. In 1633, the borders between France, the Spanish Netherlands, and the United Provinces were highly militarized and especially tense. Albeit a little later, Evelyn's account captured the prospect of imprisonment one might encounter at border crossings where Protestantism was synonymous with rebellion and heresy.[1]

The second challenge for Browne's trip from Padua to Leiden was the necessity of crossing the Alps. In all likelihood Browne traveled to Leiden after the Alpine thaw in the spring of 1633. Like William Hammond on April 20, 1654, he may have gathered with his companions in Geneva for their crossing of the Alps "in a Caravan"; after all, most travelers opted for the Simplon pass, the principal route from Geneva. But as John Stoye points out, the pass that a traveler took—Great and Little St Bernard, St Gotthard, the Grisons—was affected by "various considerations, war, diplomacy and public health.... Local quarantine regulations narrowed the possibilities still further."[2] In passing between the Adriatic coast and France, moreover, travelers varied their routes according to sights that they wished to see. Browne's ownership of a 1622 print catalogue for Francesco Calceolari's collection of curiosities in Verona suggests one of the many sights in which he would have taken interest in a journey across Italy.[3] Fynes Moryson makes plain one key consideration for all travelers through the Alps no matter where: the necessity of the best possible horse, one both strong and calm. But there were many other dangers both real and imagined. Moryson's decision to avoid the Alpine

[1] Mączak, *Travel in Early Modern Europe*, 114.

[2] See Brennan, ed., *The Origins of the Grand Tour*, 165; and Stoye, *English Travellers Abroad*, 94, 132.

[3] For this suggestion, see Brent Nelson, "The Browne Family's Culture of Curiosity," in Barbour and Preston, eds., *Sir Thomas Browne: The World Proposed*, 83.

pass to Geneva was determined by a fear of robbers, not least because he was traveling alone.[4] Having crossed the Simplon pass in 1646, Evelyn remembered "strange, horrid and fearfull crags and tracts," the presence of "beares, wolves, and wild goates," the poor visibility, the deafening noise of "melted snow and other waters," the extremes of heat and cold, and the treacherous bridges.[5] A Protestant traveler would have to worry about having unorthodox reading matter in his luggage when searched; it was commonplace, moreover, for travelers—for instance in the Habsburg domain of Milan—to feign a national identity quite different from their own.[6]

Having exited the pass, a westward traveler toward Leiden would move along the Loire from Lyons to Paris before turning north to face the potentially hostile border encounters of the Spanish Netherlands.[7] Despite the lack of conclusive evidence, it is likely that Browne passed through Paris on the road to the Netherlands as well as on his journey south to Montpellier. As Robbins notes, Browne had at the ready a number of travel books with information about tourist attractions.[8] Yet his references to Parisian sights sometimes resonate as vivid memories: in *Pseudodoxia*, Saint Christopher is said to loom "Colossus like in the entrance of Nostre Dame in Paris" (Robbins, ed. *Pseudodoxia Epidemica*, 1.409), while the "famous" unicorn's horn "preserved at S. Dennis neere Paris, hath wreathy spires, and cochleary turnings about it" (1.257). From start to finish, Browne's trip from Padua to Leiden might well involve all the early modern vehicles of travel: horses, donkeys, and mules, boats, litters, wagons (without suspension, imperfectly covered), and foot. As he approached Leiden, however, transportation would have been more uniform and convenient, since the Dutch were developing a new and improved canal service in the early 1630s, "with unimaginable success."[9]

On December 3, 1633, Browne matriculated at the University of Leiden as a 29-year-old medical student from London whose residence in the Netherlands was the home of Richard Monck on the Sonneveltsteeg. On this occasion, he would begin to receive the benefits of exemption from certain taxes on wine and beer, plus freedom from Dutch tolls on the transport of books, clothes, and furniture. As part of the university's attempt to preserve order while encouraging an international student body, he would have sworn obedience "to the statutes and university authorities."[10] Writing a little later in August 1641, the diarist John Evelyn filled out the scene of a Leiden matriculation for a foreigner:

[4] Moryson, *The Itinerary*, 4 vols. (Glasgow: James MacLehose and Sons, 1907), 1.375–82.

[5] Quoted in Mączak, *Travel in Early Modern Europe*, 6.

[6] See Mączak, *Travel in Early Modern Europe*, 108, 134.

[7] Mączak, *Travel in Early Modern Europe*, 242–7.

[8] Robbins, ed., *Pseudodoxia Epidemica*, 409, 980; cf. Albert Favre, "Sir Thomas Browne, *Pseudodoxia Epidemica*: Revelation d'une Personnalité? Le Livre V," *Études Anglaises* 42 (1989), 140–50, see 148.

[9] Mączak, *Travel in Early Modern Europe*, 19.

[10] Edward G. Ruestow, *Physics at Seventeenth and Eighteenth-Century Leiden: Philosophy and the New Science in the University* (The Hague: Martinus Nijhoff, 1973), 4; theology students had to swear fidelity to orthodox Calvinism, though the University had been founded for the sake of religious liberty among Protestants (see Cook, *Matters of Exchange*, 104–6).

> Matriculated by the then Magnificus Proffessor who first in Latine demanded of me where my Lod(g)ing in the Towne was; my Name, Age, birth; & to what faculty I addicted my selfe; then recording my Answers in a Booke, he adminstred an Oath to me; that I should observe the Statutes, & Orders of the University, whiles I stay'd, and then deliver'd me a ticket, by virtue whereof I was made Excise-free; for all which worthy Priveleges, and the paines of Writing, he accepted of a Rix-dollar.[11]

On December 21, 1633, Browne received his MD from Professor Adolph Vorstius (1597–1665). It is possible, then, that Browne was in Leiden for just a month.[12] "A small Time and less Learning will suffice to make one a Graduate," James Howell scoffed of Leiden in 1619, "nor are those Formalities of Habits, and other Decencies here, as with you [in Oxford], much less those Exhibitions and Supports for Scholars, with other Encouragements."[13] James Primerose boasted that the composition of his Leiden theses required only "a matter of hours."[14] It is far more likely, however, that having resided and studied in Leiden for a substantial portion of 1633, Browne matriculated only once he was prepared to pay the fee for official status on the way to receiving his degree.[15] He had time to make friends that he remembered over forty years later: in 1679, Browne sent his regards via Edward to Sir John Hinton who entered the university in April, 1633: "tis a long time agoe since I had the honour to knowe him beyond the sea" (Keynes, 4.141).[16] The two men were essentially the same age, and both from London; they were, superficially at least, the mirror image of one another in a strange land.[17] At least one student registered for the Leiden medical curriculum would have a significant role to play in Browne's later life: the son of Separatist John Robinson, also John, would respond in print to the *Pseudodoxia Epidemica* of his "Fellow citizen and fellow student." It is worth noting, given the major influence of George Hakewill on *Pseudodoxia Epidemica*, that John Jonston had already published a treatise on the constancy of nature—one extremely indebted to, even plagiarized from Hakewill's apology for providence—when he was a Leiden medical student from 1632 to 1634.

[11] Evelyn, *The Diary*, 2.52–3.

[12] For the varying length of stays by English students in Leiden at this time, see Harm Beukers, "Studying Medicine in Leiden in the 1630s," in Kathryn Murphy and Richard Todd, eds., *"A man very well studyed": New Contexts for Thomas Browne* (Leiden: Brill, 2008), 49–64, at 52, 60, 63.

[13] Quoted in Anthony Grafton, *Athenae Batavae: The Research Imperative at Leiden, 1575–1650* (Leiden: Primavera Pers, 2003), 5.

[14] For a list, see Beukers, "Studying Medicine," 63. For the case of one student, John Buggs, see A. H. T. Robb-Smith, "Cambridge Medicine," in Allen G. Debus, ed., *Medicine in Seventeenth Century England* (Berkeley: University of California Press, 1974), 327–69, at 331; for Primerose, see Roger French, "Harvey in Holland: Circulation and the Calvinists," in Roger French and Andrew Wear, eds., *The Medical Revolution of the Seventeenth Century* (New York: Cambridge University Press, 1989), 46–86, at 67.

[15] There is no evidence to support the speculation by Saumaise in 1648 that Browne had lived in The Hague. See Constantijn Huygens, *De Briefwisseling van Constantijn Huygens, 1608–1697*, ed. J. A. Worp, 5 vols. (The Hague: M. Nijhoff, 1911–1917), 4.456; and Keynes, *Bibliography*, 178.

[16] Cf. Cornelis W. Schoneveld, "Sir Thomas Browne and Leiden University in 1633," in *English Language Notes* 19 (1982), 337; the essay is reworked in Schoneveld, *Sea-Changes: Studies in Three Centuries of Anglo-Dutch Cultural Transmission* (Amsterdam: Rodopi, 1996), 1–30.

[17] The number of English students during the year February 1633–February 1634 was relatively high at 30 (Beukers, "Studying Medicine," 58).

Like many travelers, Browne probably continued on in Leiden until the Dutch thaw in the next April, a decision which also would have assured that he witnessed an anatomy in the theater. Indeed, his matriculation and graduation took place during a severely cold spell; university records tell us that classes had to be delayed because of the excessive cold. The traveler Sir William Brereton noted that the winter of 1633–34 was especially harsh, recalling also that in and around Dort, there was "a terrible flood last winter, which put this town and all the inhabitants of the country in great fear. It overflowed their banks, which are twelve yards high... It drowned abundance of cattle in the country... it came also into the streets of Rotterdam, and into the houses a yard deep."[18] Even so, the relative brevity of Browne's residence in Leiden would have been induced by the fact that the city was expensive for students as well as for everyone else, even with the exemptions that the students received. Students commonly complained about the costs of living and tuition, the biggest cost being for accommodation.[19] Contact with landlords was largely businesslike, cordial to be sure, but students did not receive the key. A student had to purchase heating and, if so inclined, tobacco.[20]

Browne's residence with Monck on the Sonneveltsteeg is unsurprising: many students lived in this neighborhood near the Pieterskirk and the university and, while some lived with professors or at home with their parents, archives suggest that merchants such as Monck rented simple rooms to students on a regular basis. Monck's students were always Englishmen, including one John Grey, a 30-year-old language student who was residing with Monck when he registered on October 8, 1633.[21] Monck was a man who took the honest reputation of his household seriously; in 1624, he pursued the prosecution of three men, fellow tobacco merchants, who allegedly had slandered and intimidated his maid-servant Lysbeth, claiming that her children were products of an adulterous liaison with Monck, and making "obscene gestures to Lysbeth" that prompted "a riot outside." Although she was still in London, Monck's wife experienced "much distress" from the allegations.[22]

Like so many of his fellow travelers, Browne responded to Dutch mores in potent, if complex, ways. Even those observers who were apt to admire the Dutch for their frugality and industry were equally likely to dislike them for their indecorum and even "mutiny."[23] The well-known writer of character sketches, Sir Thomas Overbury, summarized the difficulty of assessing the balance between Dutch virtue and vice:

[18] William Brereton, *Travels in Holland, the United Provinces, England, Scotland, and Ireland, M.DC.XXXVI-M.DC.XXXV* ed. Edward Hawkins, *Remains Historical & Literary... of Lancaster and Chester* (Chetham Society, 1844), 14.

[19] Willem Otterspeer, *Groepsportret met Dame, I: Het bolwerk van de vrijheid de Leidse universiteit 1575–1672* (Amsterdam: Bert Bakker, 2000), 262.

[20] Otterspeer, *Groepsportret met Dame, I*, 262–3.

[21] Volumina Inscriptionum, ASF 9, Leiden University.

[22] MS 231/ONA293 no. 89/8-6-1624, Leiden University.

[23] See Donne's "Satire 3" for the "mutinous Dutch."

> They are neither much devout, nor much wicked; given all to drink, and eminently to no other vice; hard in bargaining, but just; surly and respectless, as in all democracies; thirsty, industrious, and cleanly; disheartened upon the least ill success, and insolent upon good; inventive in manufactures, and cunning in traffick.[24]

An observer as resistant to simplistic national stereotypes as Browne would note the complexities and paradoxes in this characterization, for "cunning in traffick" could produce the type of wildly risky practices that produced the topsy-turvy culture of "tulipmania" in the mid-1630s, a far cry from a country for "stable wits."[25]

In transit, travelers called attention to the dogged industry and efforts at improvement that they witnessed on the sides of the canals—indeed, a ceaseless battle against the recalcitrance of nature—and they commented on the delightful neatness of the houses and gardens along the way. But the landscape itself struck them as monotonous, especially in winter, when land and water became hard to distinguish, and the native Dutch as singularly lacking in ceremony or even decorum.[26] For Browne, such an ethos stood in marked contrast to the highly formal and decorous civility of Padua, as surely as Dutch practicality differed from Paduan metaphysical speculation. For Browne as for so many other travelers, there was a special regard for Dutch neatness, frugality, and industry; for an unceremonious simplicity in everything from table manners to funeral rites; and for a strong sense of justice and equality. This latter leveling tendency was especially manifested in habits of dress, for "in the beginning of the century, there was reportedly 'no difference of habit between a burgomaster and an ordinary man.' Both were plainly dressed in dark clothes with little lace but with fine linen."[27] This does not mean, however, that honor and hierarchy were unimportant in Dutch culture; more precisely, the resistance to ornament was part and parcel of a culture for which the honor in one's trustworthiness was crucial.[28] Theirs was a style of dress that Browne emulated throughout his adult life; as his friend John Whitefoot tells us, Browne dressed with "an Aversion to all Finery, and affected Plainness, both in Fashion and Ornaments."[29]

In *Religio Medici* the Dutch figured centrally in Browne's analysis of the part that providence might play in national destinies. As Browne well knew, it was widely believed that the supposed humoral deficiencies of the Dutch constitution—so much like those attributed to the English—only rendered the miracle

[24] Thomas Overbury, "Sir Thomas Overbury's Observations in his Travels, upon the State of the Seventeen Provinces, as they stood Anno Domini, 1609 (published 1626)," in *The Harleian Miscellany* (London: Robert Dutton, 1809), 3.97–100; quotation on 100.

[25] For tulipmania, see Anne Goldgar, *Tulipmania: Money, Honor, and Knowledge in the Dutch Golden Age* (Chicago: University of Chicago Press, 2007). For risk, see 220–1.

[26] C. D. van Strien, *British Travellers in Holland During the Stuart Period: Edward Browne and John Locke as Tourists in the United Provinces* (New York: Brill, 1993), 73, 87–8.

[27] van Strien, *British Travellers in Holland*, 212–13, 216.

[28] Goldgar, *Tulipmania*, 276–7, 304.

[29] Whitefoot, "Some Minutes," xxviii.

as well as the industry of their victory over the hostilities of nature and the Spanish all the more extraordinary.[30] Behind all the foreign admiration for Dutch industry was the visitors' awe for the wonder that was recent history in the United Provinces, and Browne's *Religio Medici* demonstrates that he was no exception. Browne's experience in Leiden drove home the value of a minimalist, utilitarian, duty-bound approach to his profession—and his life—that stayed with him all his years after. Yet his direct references to the Dutch or to Leiden in his later writings reflect a somewhat ambivalent concession to their practicality. In *Religio Medici*, Browne reduced the "pety Province" of Holland to a capacity to accomplish much with little that he attributes at once "to the mercy of God" behind their "thriving Genius" and to their "ingenuity and industry" (Patrides, 82). Later, in letters to Edward, he remarked on how the Dutch "make defences agaynst sea inundations" (Keynes, 4.31) and also on the fact that they, "though a drincking nation, yet managed their warre [more] carefully and advantageously then the English" (4.141). Given Leiden's amazing survival of the Spanish siege in 1574, an event celebrated every October, the city was the young country's poster child for a synthesis of divine redemption and sturdy human discipline. Dutch common sense went hand in hand with their faith in a miraculous God: on the pavement in front of the State House on the Breede-Straat—a building just a block or two from Browne's residence with Monck—was engraved "Niet zonder God" ("nothing without God"), a motto that anticipates the inscription at the start of one manuscript copy of *Religio Medici*, *syn theo* (with God's help).[31]

In the seventeenth century, Dutch cleanliness and discipline were understood to mount a constant contest against the unpredictable tides of the surrounding waters, and the Dutch "unrefined literalness" embodied their constant efforts to keep souls, bodies, and social spaces purified in the face of what hostile critics joked was the "amphibious baseness" of the fenny world in which the Dutch lived.[32] For Browne, a metaphorical concern with amphibian man would be featured in *Religio Medici* but a more literal sense of the notion would follow him throughout the bulk of his adult life in Norfolk, where dwelling on the threshold between land and water was as intellectually stimulating as it was a matter for technological concern. In the 1620s and 30s, the Dutch resistance to the liabilities of prosperity was manifested in a wide range of cultural phenomena, from the flourishing of still life (in which the plain was rendered artistic) to the "ample but not opulent" diet, prescribed for Leiden students in 1632 and epitomized by a stew called the *hutspot*. With its "fairly generous proportions of fish and meat," its specifications for weekly beer, bread, cheese, butter, and (on Sunday) a roast, the Leiden University diet

[30] For the traveler reports, see van Strien, *British Travellers in Holland*, 211–15; for the impression of the Dutch as miraculous, see K. W. Swart, *The Miracle of the Dutch Republic as Seen in the Seventeenth Century* (London: H. K. Lewis, 1969), 6–7.

[31] Henry Martyn Dexter and Morton Dexter, *The England and Holland of the Pilgrims* (New York: Houghton, Mifflin and Company, 1905), 491–2. Cf. the discussion of the Lansdowne MS on p. 237 below.

[32] Simon Schama, *The Embarrassment of Riches: An Interpretation of Dutch Culture in the Golden Age* (London: Harper, 1987), 7, 24, 44, 265, 384.

afforded its charges with what the Dutch considered a "daily sufficiency."[33] Such practices of restraint in prosperity would resonate throughout Browne's letters to his children and in some of his personal habits as well. Yet, paradoxically, the intellectual and commercial tendencies of Dutch culture also encouraged Browne to care intensely about the things of this world, the streaks of a tulip, sea shells, exotic medicaments, and infinite variety of natural and artistic collectibles that would stuff Browne's house in the last decades of his life and would sometimes obscure the boundary between an ethos of "scholarly courtesy and exchange and the commercial negotiations of capitalism."[34]

For Browne, Leiden had some obviously appealing qualities. For instance, it was a town of books: Browne lived around the corner from the famous medieval residence, the Temple of Solomon, where a significant holding of legal books had been in residence for hundreds of years.[35] Just to the right of the entrance to the Academy Building was the internationally renowned Elzevier Press. Located in the Beguines chapel together with the anatomy theater, the university library was divided into two rows of bookcases for folios (cases for smaller volumes can be seen in the back), with math, philosophy, literature, and theology on the left, and history, medicine, and law on the right. Each row of books had a table at which readers might stand in order to study a chained volume. Also on the right was the cabinet holding Scaliger's gift of 208 manuscripts—Hebraic, Chaldaic, Arabic, Ethiopian, Latin, Greek, Russian, and Syriac.[36] In an extant engraving of the early seventeenth-century library, the early seventeenth-century would-be tourist to Leiden found the library's rows of chained folios, its portraits of Willem and Maurits of Orange, a picture of Constantinople, portraits of Erasmus and Janus Secundus, the Scaliger cabinet, two men closely examining a globe, and visitors courteously greeting and conversing with one another—all this in an architectural space redolent of Christian devotion. Here was an image of the ideal synopsis: all useful learning, framed by a sacred-civic patriotism, international in intellectual and economic breadth, but nationalistic in its agenda, polite and irenic yet also assiduous and sober.

These very qualities of irenicism, vocational purpose, and sobriety were fundamental ingredients of the medical ethos that Browne would cultivate. The world of Leiden in 1633 underscored the ways in which industrious sobriety might frame curiosity and stabilize indeterminacy without ever quite threatening to quash them. Modifying his more playful, speculative, and fanciful wit, Browne's Leiden provenance encapsulated a vocational utility and moral discipline that stayed with him and affected how he dressed, parented, dealt with emotion, and flourished in the watery regions of Norfolk. The lessons learned in Leiden had much to do with

[33] Schama, *The Embarrassment of Riches*, 160, 174–7.

[34] See Goldgar, *Tulipmania*, 196–7.

[35] See H. A. van Oerle, *Leiden binnen en buiten de stadvesten* (Leiden: Brill, 1975), 80, 110.

[36] See Joannes Meursius, *Athenae Batavae* (Leiden, 1625); and the essay by Elfriede Hulshoff Pol in Th. H. Lunsingh Scheurleer and G. H. M. Posthumus Meyjes, eds., *Leiden University in the Seventeenth Century: An Exchange of Learning* (Leiden: Brill, 1975), 395–459.

avoiding distraction and needlessly convoluted self-reflection; the mottoes inscribed on the anatomy theater provoked the visitor to remember fragility and mortality.

If Padua offered a world in which medical knowledge and practice were implicated in exploratory and unorthodox thought and sophisticated masquerades of self-fashioning, Leiden offered medicine as a highly practical course of study in the context of a young Protestant nation with a strong need for physicians, lawyers, and preachers. The extraordinary collection of curiosities displayed in the anatomy theater exhorted the medical student to confront life and death with gusto to be sure, but also with utmost practicality, a strong sense of duty, and economy. It should also never be forgotten that the essential mission of the university was the production of professionals to support the welfare of an emerging Protestant nation. It served Browne in precisely this fashion—from the lectures that the faculty gave on practical medicine, to the design of the botanical garden and anatomy theater, and including the focus of dissertations on a single disease such as we now know Browne to have authored. Vocation was the crux of the Leiden experience, for Browne as for his Dutch colleagues.

2. A MORAL AND PRACTICAL MEDICINE

It is not known whether Browne took medical classes, either formally on Mondays, Tuesdays, Thursdays, and Fridays in the small upstairs auditorium (now the Senate Chamber) of the main Academy Building (formerly St Barbaraklooster or the cloister of the White Nuns), or under private tuition in a professor's home on Wednesdays and Saturdays. But he was certainly indebted to the Leiden medical ethos that sought to discipline minds and bodies alike. More than anything else, the university in Leiden insisted on the practicalities—vocational, commercial, moral, spiritual, and national—of a medical education.[37] As Harold Cook has shown, the Dutch natural historian's experiential and accurate knowledge of the materials of the entire world was inextricable from the commercial and colonial "discovery of the world—its geography, peoples, plants and animals, and astrological and alchemical associations; the accumulation of specimens of it, the cataloging of its variety, and the detailing of its structure."[38] For Browne, the scion of a London merchant, this intimacy between the desiderata of physicians or naturalists and the goals of "the hard-headed merchant" (Cook, 81) established a pattern of livelihood that he pursued for the rest of his life, one in which the responsible and assiduous fulfillment of a medical living coincided with a heightened curiosity for and attention to the materials of the world.

[37] Frank Huisman, "Medicine and Health Care in the Netherlands, 1500–1800," in Klaas van Berkel et al., eds., *A History of Science in the Netherlands* (Leiden: Brill, 1999), 239–78, see 241; and Harm Beukers, "Clinical Teaching in Leiden from Its Beginning until the End of the Eighteenth Century," in H. Beukers and J. Moll, eds., *Clinical Teaching, Past and Present* (Amsterdam: Rodopi, 1989), 139–52; see 139.

[38] Cook, *Matters of Exchange*, 41, 81.

Such a program framed the medical emphasis on regimen that Johannes Walaeus (1604–49) was touting during the year in which Browne arrived. With its stress on the non-naturals or lifestyle choices, Walaeus's approach set a standard for assessing and advising patients that is abundantly in evidence in Browne's extant letters of consultation. In December 1632, Walaeus gave an oration (published in 1633) which epitomized the university's highly practical approach to medical instruction.[39] Warning against the kind of study that shows a false face of erudition, the kind that pursues only that knowledge which is remote from human understanding, Walaeus exhorted his auditors to attend to the easily understood sapience to be found at their very feet. According to his warning, scholars who neglected the immediate and readily mastered ingredients of health were vainly seeking only an admirable reputation that depended on the ignorance of others; they cared nothing for the excellent utility of their knowledge and rejected the substantial food of useful knowledge for the mere seasoning of esotericism (7–8). By contrast, Walaeus announced, he and the Leiden medical professoriate would offer solid knowledge rather than splendor and cleverness—in short, the art comprising the means to prevent disease and preserve health. In his inaugural speech, Walaeus concluded his oration by announcing that he planned to take this practical, preventative approach to medicine in his lessons over the course of the next school year, with major emphasis on nutrition (30–1).[40] Browne's own strongly practical approach to medicine reflects Walaeus's signature teachings from the latter's first years in the university.[41] Yet *Religio Medici*'s intricate speculations on so many potentially perilous questions—the role of providence, the significance of monstrosity, the nature and activity of angels, the mysterious relations between body and soul—also testify to Browne's lingering dissatisfaction with a curriculum that reduced wisdom to praxis.

If Walaeus embodied the practical spirit of medical learning at Leiden, he also captured its cautious receptivity to new ideas, especially to William Harvey's discovery of the circulation of the blood (published in 1628) which Browne would soon praise so highly. For even if he at first opposed the circulation in his lectures on Wednesday and Saturday, it was Walaeus, together with Franciscus de la Boe Sylvius, who over the course of the 1630s would urge a greater openness on the part of the medical professoriate to Harvey's circulation. During Browne's days in Leiden, the professoriate remained prudent about disturbing the foundations of medical theory, even as the anatomy theater and the botanical garden reflected the modernization of medical learning associated with Renaissance humanism. In 1680, Browne recalled that discussions of the circulation commenced immediately after its publication in 1628, and Leiden was clearly a place in which the conversation had vitality. To put this another way, the situation in the Leiden of 1633 was less open than, say, the controversial welcome offered to chemical medicine in

[39] Johannes Walaeus, *Iohannis Walæi Oratio Inavgvralis* (Leiden, 1633).
[40] Jacob Schouten, *Johannes Walaeus* (Assen: Van Gorcum, 1972), 142.
[41] Cf. Schoneveld, "Sir Thomas Browne and Leiden University in 1633," 349.

Montpellier, but new ideas—especially about the circulation—were not completely or rigidly suppressed.[42]

Aside from Walaeus, the medical professoriate at Leiden in 1633 included Otto Heurnius (1577–1652, basic medicine and anatomy); Ewaldus Schrevelius (1575–1647, practical medicine); Adolphus Vorstius (1597–1663, basic medicine and botany); and Adrianus Falcoburgius (1581–1650, anatomy and surgery).[43] None of these professors left an abundance of published writings, in keeping with their commitment to the practical production of physicians rather than the speculative vagaries of philosophy.[44] Whatever the narrow scope of their reputations, these professors could model for Browne a civically minded vocation—Heurnius committed his energies in the 1630s to helping the poor with their medical needs[45]—but also an impressive and wide-ranging learning. For instance, Heurnius was deeply interested in Babylonian, Indian, and especially Egyptian history and culture; in print as well as the museum collection of artifacts included in the anatomy theater, he testified to a belief that Adam's original wisdom might be traced by careful attention to the extremely ancient wisdom of the Egyptian Hermes, the Chaldeans, and Zoroaster.[46] Indeed Vorstius studied obscure as well as famous medical writers and was committed to the value of foreign languages such as Arabic.[47]

Falcoburgius was known to be quiet—indeed eventually because of hardness of hearing—and traditional in his teaching.[48] But in *Beschrijvinge der Stadt Leyden*, the seventeenth-century historian J. J. Orlers filled in a biographical picture that offered a model for Browne's developing understanding of his vocation. As Orlers tells the story, Falcoburgius was resolutely on his way to a degree and career in divinity when his pious and impartial devotion to the vocation was subverted by the fierce storm of contention that arose between the Gomarists and Arminians. With no end to this controversy in sight, Falcoburgius found a more peaceful way to serve his God in medicine. A medical career for him, then, was a deeply spiritual decision, one on which the peace of the body politic depended as surely as the welfare of body private.[49]

The rotational scheme of the medical program at Leiden meant that it was Vorstius from whom Browne actually received his degree. He was often characterized as cautious or prudent, advising against headlong zeal in pursuit of novelty or in

[42] A good example is the development of clinical medicine just after Browne left. For the clinical program, see J. E. Kroon, *Bijdragen tot de Geschiedenis van het Geneeskundig Onderwijs aan de Leidsche Universiteit 1575–1625* (Leiden: S. C. Van Doesburgh, 1911), 45.

[43] See Beukers, "Studying Medicine," 57; and G. A. Lindeboom, *Dutch Medical Biography* (Amsterdam: Rodopi, 1984).

[44] For information about faculty personalities, see J. A. J. Barge, *De Oudste Inventaris der Oudste Academische Anatomie in Nederland* (Leiden: H. E. Stenfert Kroese's Uitgevers, 1934), 25. Otterspeer, *Groepsportret met Dame, I*, 230.

[45] Otterspeer, *Groepsportret met Dame, I*, 203.

[46] Tim Huisman, *The Finger of God: Anatomical Practice in Seventeenth-Century Leiden* (Leiden: Primavera Pers, 2009), 64–5, 73.

[47] Beukers, "Studying Medicine," 56.

[48] Otterspeer, *Groepsportret met Dame, I*, 288.

[49] J. J. Orlers, *Beschrijvinge der Stadt Leyden* (1641), 349–50.

addiction to controversy yet not tyrannically closed minded.[50] In the 1620s and 30s, he was responsible for botanical as well as medical instruction, adding the 1633 appendix of plants in the Leiden garden to Adrian van den Spigel's *Isagoges in rem herbarum libri duo* (Leiden, 1633). His other publications were devoted to the explication of Hippocrates, in one of which—a tiny pocket book—he stressed the Hippocratic tendency to pack an abundance of medical wisdom into a small space.[51] Browne's conviction that the aphorisms of Hippocrates were especially valuable to the physician would have been strengthened by his encounter with Vorstius.[52] Similarly, with Browne's dissertation on smallpox, the candidate himself was required to distill the best available wisdom concerning a particular and controversial disease into the narrow room of a small pamphlet.

The prominence of the *hortus botanicus* and the anatomy theater for medical education at the young Protestant university was obviously indebted to—and established clear continuity with—the medical curriculum at Padua. But the Leiden garden (situated behind the main Academy building on the south side of the Rapenburg) and anatomy theater (situated in the chapel of the former Beguinehof on the north side) also exemplified habits of study, collection, and moralization that corroborated the university's practical mission in a world of wonderful variety and grim adversity. It is true that the anatomy theater in Leiden anticipated the possible conflict in Browne's habits of thought between a collector's comfort in disorder and a magician's penchant for cosmic analogies, hierarchies, and encircling patterns.[53] Nonetheless, with strong commitments to the study of worldwide natural history as well as to medical vocation, the medical curriculum promoted the anatomy theater and botanical garden as integral parts of a "resolutely practical and descriptive" program that adhered to a Hippocratic emphasis on "careful observation and a reluctance to jump to conclusions about the causes of diseases," the very reverse of the emphasis often promoted in Padua. The requirement that doctoral candidates "be examined on two of the Hippocratic aphorisms" was a key part of this "practical and observational orientation" which "also encouraged the development of natural history as a part of medical study at Leiden."[54] Especially in the simultaneously allegorical and practical anatomy theater of Leiden, medical training concentrated one's intellectual, spiritual, and physical faculties on the practical disciplining of vigorous curiosity in the ever-present face of laxity, vanity, and strife. For Browne, this combination struck a sympathetic chord, one heard in his lifelong commitment to the knowledge-yielding collection of natural and artificial curiosities, in his wonderment at "Why Tulips of one colour produce some of another, and running through almost all, should still escape a blew?" (Robbins, ed.,

[50] J. Banga, *Geschiedenis van de Geneeskunde... in Nederland* (Leeuwarden: W. Eekhoff, 1868), 322–3.

[51] A. Vorstius, *Aphorismi Hippocratis* (1628), *2r.

[52] Schoneveld, "Sir Thomas Browne and Leiden University in 1633," 353.

[53] For this conflict in Leiden, and its relevance to the writings of the English magical author Robert Fludd, see Huisman, *The Finger of God*, 75.

[54] Cook, *Matters of Exchange*, 110–11.

Pseudodoxia Epidemica, 1.508); but perhaps above all in the moralizing that came to dominate the fifth chapter of *Hydriotaphia*, the ending of *A Letter to a Friend*, and the whole of the *Christian Morals*.

The design and ornamentation of the *hortus* and its gallery aimed to delight the visitor with its neat symmetries, classical porticoes, and phenomenal variety. But early commentators—and scholars ever since—have remarked on its simplicity in comparison to the elaborately hieroglyphic design of Padua or the mazy adventurous sprawl of Montpellier.[55] The designers of the garden wanted to maximize the botanical knowledge of the observer who would encounter plants from the Middle East and America alike. With the College of Theology bordering the garden and the garden's own simple geometry, the Leiden botanical experience was supposed to evoke a moral and providential framework for the study of nature.[56] But neither the moral-cum-theological framework nor the delight that one might take in the beds or in the collections of the ambulatory was supposed to work at cross-purposes with the strongly practical aims of the university or indeed of the United Provinces.[57] Theology, morality, natural studies, and pleasure: praxis as against speculative vagaries and mazes held them all together for the Leiden medical student, who joined the city's public in the garden's cultivation of civic virtue.[58] Browne's exhortation that Edward pay special attention to the flora in the Netherlands and his statement of familiarity with the plant life in the countries bordering England suggest that he may have arrived in time to go simpling in the countryside with his fellow students.[59]

Both the garden and anatomy theater included a museum comprising an astonishing range of things, far more than just the "charts and maps.... strange animals and plants" to which Orlers referred in 1614.[60] In each, the visitor encountered natural, ethnographic, artificial, and textual material of that extraordinary variety found in contemporary cabinets of curiosity. (See Figure 6.1.) Indeed, Brereton's list of favorites from the anatomy theater—an "Egyptian king," human skins, "the anatomy of a woman executed for murdering her bastard child, and the child anatomized in her arms," human ribs, whale teeth, an Egyptian princess, many anatomized animals, "a very great Roman urn," and so forth—is interwoven with his lists of curiosities from the garden.[61] In 1634, Brereton recorded that "in the physic-garden," he saw "an eagle fifty years old, white head and white train; another was here (now dead) which was a hundred years old; this inscription over her:

[55] Leslie Tjon Sie Fat, "Clusius' garden: a reconstruction" in L. Tjon Sie Fat and E. de Jong, eds., *The Authentic Garden: A Symposium on Gardens* (Leiden: Clusius Foundation, 1991), 3.

[56] Florence Hopper, "Clusius' World: The Meeting of Science and Art," in *The Authentic Garden: A Symposium on Gardens*, ed. L. Tjon Sie Fat and E. de Jong, 15.

[57] Hopper, "Clusius' World," 18.

[58] Erik de Jong, "Nature and Art," 47. Cf. Paula Findlen, "Sites of Anatomy, Botany, and Natural History," in Katharine Park and Lorraine Daston, eds., *Cambridge History of Science: Volume 3: Early Modern Science* (New York: Cambridge University Press, 2006), 283; and H. Veendorp and L. G. M. Baas Becking, *Hortvs Academicvs Lvgdvno-Batavvs 1587–1937* (Harlaam: Enschedaiana, 1938), 36.

[59] Schoneveld, "Sir Thomas Browne and Leiden University in 1633," 351–2.

[60] Erik de Jong, "Nature and Art," 40–6.

[61] Brereton, "My Travels into Holland," 41–2.

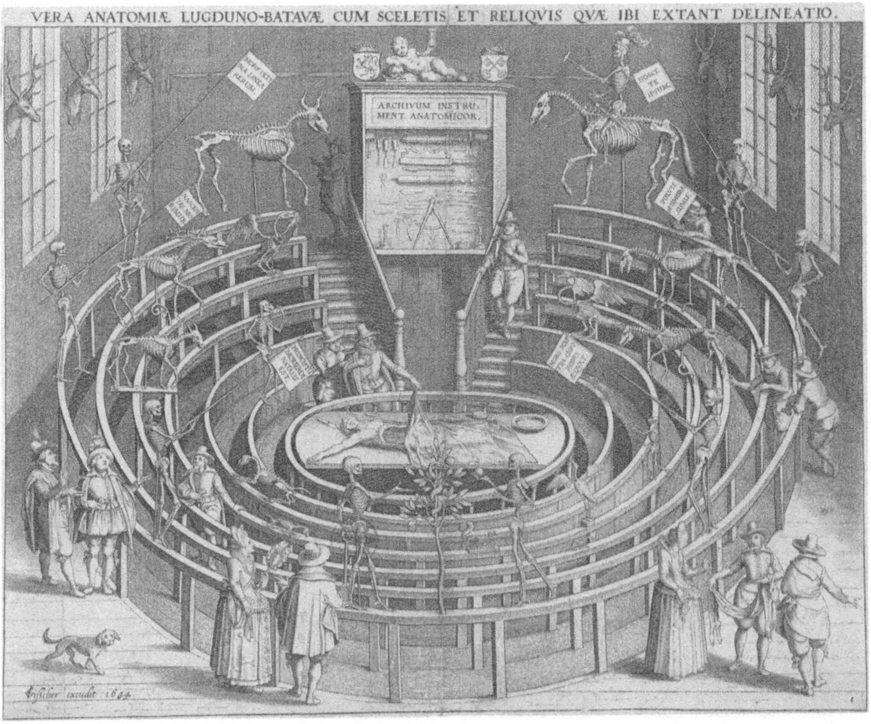

Figure 6.1 Anatomy theater, Leiden, from an engraving by Willem Swanenburgh after Jan Cornelisz, published by Andries Clouck (1610). Leiden University Libraries, COLLBN Port 315-III N19.

'Sum celebris pennis, oculis, clangore, senecta; | Spectator caveas pande, beabis, ave.'"[62] With the help of David le Leu de Wilhelm, Heurnius extended the ethnographic scope of the collection to Egypt, and he introduced a chastening Christian morality into the experience of anatomy—all this in an effort to make the anatomy theater a "centre where as many as possible building blocks necessary for knowledge of people and the world were concentrated" and in which spectators could "contemplate on the relation between God, His creation and the place of man within this."[63] The theater was, moreover, in the eastern section of the former chapel, its eastern boundary curved as a reminder to those so inclined in their devotions that this space had been considered by the lay sisterhood who worshiped there the most sacred area in their world. Here as in so many ways, the Leiden theater stressed the criterion that physicians be religious. With intellectual curiosity

[62] Brereton, "My Travels into Holland," 42.

[63] Tim Huisman, *A Theatre for Anatomy: The Leiden Theatrum Anatomicum, 1594–1821* (Leiden: Museum Boerhaave, 2002), 13. See also Barge, *De Oudste Inventaris der Oudste Academische Anatomie in Nederland* (Leiden: H. E. Stenfert Kroese's Uitgevers, 1934).

on the one hand and sober discipline on the other, these developments epitomized the scholarly balance that Browne would pursue over the rest of his life. But just as formatively, Leiden provided Browne with a premiere example of the kind of menagerie and collection into which he would convert his living space in Norwich, each an epitome of the world's boundless variety rendered accessible by international commerce.

Side by side in the anatomy theater with the remains of skeletons, organs, and skins lay the ethnographic marvels from which the bodily pieces were not clearly or categorically distinguished: the half-arm of a mummy as well as stone idols found buried in Egypt. Among the more impressive Egyptian artifacts, there was a large mummy whose lid featured a representation of Isis; statuettes of Isis and Osiris with hieroglyphics; and vases for storing intestines, complete with the head of a god formed into lids. From Moscovia there were a vest and underpants; from China, certain red and white scrolls; from Java medical simples; skates from Norway and Finland; a Roman urn; and a variety of other Japanese, Chinese, and Indian (east and west) things, including drinking vessels, puppets, depilatories, and musical instruments. Under the instrument case affixed above the entrance on the western side of the room—itself an impressive display of surgical devices—one found, framed with black margins, those verses from Statius in which we are exhorted: "Ut tibi mors felix contingat, vivere disce | Ut felix possis vivere, disce mori" (So that a happy death comes to you, learn to live; so that you can live happily, learn to die).[64] Thus natural, artificial, and textual phenomena cohered, even as they abounded; in the theater complex, which included those rooms beneath the first floor on which the theater's foundation rested, one circulated through an encyclopedia at once various and cohesive, in which Biblical, classical Greco-Roman, Egyptian, Asian, and Near Eastern cultures came together in a synthesis of nature, art, spirituality, and moral discipline.[65]

The emblematic messages developed by Heurnius in the wake of Pauw's original scheme were twofold: "all humans are mortal, and the glory of God could be seen in the extraordinarily complex handiwork of his creation." This combination of dark and light memorials was aimed at creating an urgency as well as a discipline in exerting oneself in the pursuit of a learned vocation. As Browne experienced it, the anatomy theater taught a lesson of personal agency that served two distinct purposes. One was a message of religious liberty and peace that had informed the original foundation of the university in the sixteenth century.[66] The other was that

[64] Barge, *De Oudste Inventaris*, 40–3.

[65] Barge, *De Oudste Inventaris*, 54–61.

[66] Cook emphasizes this point in order to correct the commonplace view that the university was founded primarily to provide strictly orthodox Calvinist ministers, though the original stress on liberty did change over the decades that followed; *Matters of Exchange*, 104–6.

the combination of life's brevity and divinely created, microcosmic, and "wonderful collaboration of organs and faculties" in the human fabric necessitated that no moment, resource, or effort be wasted in the fulfillment or exertion of vocation.[67] For Browne, one obvious benefit of this dedication to moral discipline was that it was reconcilable with the excitement and fulfillment of curiosity.

After their visits to the anatomy theater, tourists testified to the awesome ways in which, for instance, the animal and human skeletons chastised human sin and vanity: one cow bore a thief or (according to an alternative theory) its ravisher.[68] Overseeing the whole skeletal array were two human frames positioned in a tableau evocative of Adam and Eve at the tree of the knowledge of good and evil, the source of all human vanity. Together with the mottos, the many engravings and paintings of a morally and spiritually disciplined nature, and the former chapel of the Beguines in which the theater was housed, the experience of anatomy in Leiden left no doubt that spectators were to learn to anatomize their own sins as surely as they were to learn the physiology of the bodies that they might cure. To the latter, medical end, of course, the bones of the many skeletons were equally useful, as was the amount of light—superior to that in Padua—that the theater afforded for the business of anatomy.[69] All in all, Browne received his medical degree within the living embodiment of what would become his signature adult orientations: toward sober moral analysis, vocational discipline, providential wonder, and intellectual curiosity.[70]

On the banners held by the skeletons, one read that "death is the end of all things," that we are merely "dust and shadows," that life is short, man a bubble, that death should be remembered, and that self-knowledge should be our priority. Among the engravings, visitors encountered: the three Fates spinning and cutting the thread of life; a child making bubbles next to a flower and a smoking vessel, commonplace emblems of fragility and vanity; a powerful king side by side with a peasant, and both reduced to skeletal remains in death. They read quotations from Seneca, Statius, and the Bible stressing the fragility and precariousness of life, the omnipresence of death, and the complete control that providence possesses over both life and death in human affairs. The lesson to be garnered from the theater underscored redemption as well as demise: the images collected by Heurnius included the childhood of Christ (the circumcision and the visit of the Magi), for instance, as well as one of Christ on the Mount of Olives and another (based on Michelangelo's depiction in the Sistine Chapel) of Christ's apotheosis on Judgment Day, while the theater itself included the words of a prayer to the Savior.

This iconography would permeate not just Browne's explicitly didactic works (such as *Christian Morals*) but also his experimental notes on physical phenomena such as bubbles.[71] Indeed Browne grew increasingly favorable of the moral discipline

[67] See Cook, *Matters of Exchange*, 166, 168.

[68] van Strien, *British Travellers in Holland*, 126.

[69] Th. H. Lunsingh Scheurleer, "Un amphithéâtre d'anatomie moralisée," in Scheurleer and G. H. M. Posthumus Meyjes, eds., *Leiden University in the Seventeenth Century*, 217–78.

[70] A. J. F. Gogelein and R. E. O. Ekkart, *Leidse universiteit 400* (Amsterdam: Rijksmuseum, 1975), 104–8.

[71] See Keynes, 3.438–40.

urged by the Leiden anatomy theater, for instance, in its depiction of eight virtuous Roman heroes, including Horatius Cocles, Marcus Curtius, Mucius Scaevola, among others, all suggestive of the lesson that virtue alone resists mortality in this world. A very muscular Hercules, depicted with his club and surrounded by his labors, encapsulated the merits of reason, wisdom, constancy, honesty, and moral valor. Equally impressive were the engravings with cautionary tales against vice: the four falling personae known as the "somersaulters" (Tantalus, Icarus, Phaeton, and Ixion, with warnings about arrogance, excess, presumption, and ambition); an allegory of the World, Flesh, and Devil in combat with the Christian soldier; images of the progressive decay of the ages from Golden to Bronze; a juxtaposition of Esau with Jacob, the former a personification of fleshly pride. This sort of proverbial wisdom not only informed the very essence of Browne's *Christian Morals*, but also contributed to his prose specific, compelling images such as the meditation on Icarus in the poem added to section 13 of the 1643 edition of *Religio Medici*.[72] No doubt the tumbler saved by God's hand on the frontispiece of the unauthorized *Religio Medici* in 1642 offered Browne an impressive reason for retaining its publisher.

3. BROWNE'S DISSERTATION

The botanical garden and anatomy theater offered Browne uncontroversial lessons in the fragility of human life, in the responsibilities of vocation, and in the need to frame curiosity within religious and moral boundaries. But Leiden's greatest value for Browne derived from the fact that the university awarded him an MD in 1633. In a surviving image of a seventeenth-century doctoral procession emerging from the Academy Building, the graduate is surrounded by professors and beadles while nearby alongside the canal, a woman holds a baby, women and men pause to chat, a child holds a hoop, and two dogs scrounge on a summer's day. Less gaily, a tabletop survives in the "Sweating Room" where students wait for the results of their exams, its earliest of many inscriptions deriving from the 1630s and 40s.[73]

In Browne's day, Leiden offered each candidate two levels of ceremonial in the promotion and subsequent fete provided for the professors and associates: one elaborate and expensive, the other scaled down and inexpensive. In the first instance, the student graduated in the theological auditorium in which all such major university events were held—this in front of a large audience inclusive of other students—and he splurged on a feast as well as exam-money and a gratuity. In the second instance, the graduation took place privately in the smaller senatorial chamber before faculty alone, and entailed less supernumerary expense. Indeed, one visitor commented on the conferral of the doctorate as happening "without

[72] Patrides, 76.

[73] For these images, see R. E. O. Ekkart, *Athenae Batavae: De Leidse Universiteit, 1575–1975* (Leiden: University of Leiden, 1975), 32.

that pomp and extravagant expense in practice in England."[74] The lesser cost of the private promotions meant that they were frequently chosen, but also that those who opted for the more extravagant affair often did their best to make them appealing, with music and decorations.[75]

To reach this celebration, the doctoral candidate passed through the three trials preliminary to his promotion: a secret (private) exam covering the fundamentals of the whole of medicine and especially the methods of curing which (if passed) was followed on the next day at 5:00 p.m. by a defense of two selected Hippocratic aphorisms against objections posed by members of the faculty. After these two stages, the candidate publicly presented his thesis (in which he usually explained the cure of a disease according to the methods of Galen and Hippocrates), and answered objections to his argument, all in Latin.[76] According to the 1631 statutes this promotion could take place on Wednesday or Saturday as well as on the normal workdays. In general, the university community in attendance wore full regalia and the candidate also wore a gown, according to the 1631 statutes a robe of black damask; after delivering his thesis, the new doctor received a book, a gold ring for scholarly excellence, and a velvet cap. He gave a short oration, then joined a procession to a church or to some other "honest" house for a worship service, after which there was a feast. According to the curators of the university, the doctoral recipient had to be at least twenty-eight years old; Browne had just recently turned twenty-nine.[77] A contemporary described the theology faculty's version of this event as follows:

> At the school gates stood a beadle without a gown, having a silver staff, where he stayed for the coming of the professor, who was in his gown, and the respondent, who was in his cloak; then the beadle ushered them into the school, where the professor took his seat and the respondent his under the professor. The printed theses were some of them dispersed the night before at the printing house, and now by the respondent, who distributed them in his seat. After that he made a Latin prayer and read the beginning of his theses. Immediately an opponent, first craving leave of the professor, argued against them.

Eventually three opponents would dispute the theses, with thanks to the professor, all of which was concluded with another prayer from the candidate.[78]

Many of the medical dissertations from the period of Browne's matriculation are lost from the Leiden records, thanks to the negligence of Daniel Heinsius whose charge it was to retain them. But enough survive to give us a good sense of what the typical medical dissertation involved. Joannes Le Clerc published his Leiden dissertation or "disputatio medica inauguralis" on melancholy in 1633. Divided

[74] See van Strien, *British Travellers in Holland*, 200–1.

[75] For costs, see Otterspeer, *Groepsportret met Dame, I*, 266–7.

[76] Otterspeer, *Groepsportret met Dame, I*, 240–1; and J. E. Kroon, *Bijdragen tot de Geschiedenis van het Geneeskundig Onderwijs aan de Leidsche Universiteit 1575–1625* (Leiden: S. C. Van Doesburgh, 1911), 15–16.

[77] Otterspeer, *Groepsportret met Dame, I*, 240–2.

[78] For these accounts, see van Strien, *British Travellers in Holland*, 200–1.

into two sections, one for theses and the other for corollaries, the paper includes among its seventeen theses a standard set of concerns: the different names for and types of the disease; its symptoms, causes, and definition; its humoral or complexional varieties; diagnostic signs; prognosis; indications (the semiotics of the cure); and curative methods and materials. The dissertation's chief authorities—Galen, Aretus, Aristotle, Averroes, and Hippocrates—are not at all surprising. There is none of the anxiety, let alone the speculative elaboration, of Paduan discourse: the potential for unorthodoxy in notions of body–soul relations is simply nullified within the limited and rigid framework of the doctoral disputation.[79] The defense of the thesis tended to be brief.[80]

As early as the 1640s, French physician and author Guy Patin (1601–72) claimed that the author of *Religio Medici* was a capable English doctor who had written on the subject of syphilis, a statement that has prompted scholars to ponder whether Patin had information about Browne's doctoral dissertation.[81] Early in the eighteenth century, medical biographer Jean Astruc maintained that Patin had been wrong and that no such thesis by Browne had ever existed. In 1642, it turns out, "a young Englishman named Robert Wright... had defended his thesis *De Lue Venerea* with such brilliance that Professor Vorstius wrote to [Baldwin Hamey] about it," so it is possible that Patin was confusing Browne with this other English medical student.[82] Scholars unwilling to accept Patin's view sometimes offered alternatives of their own, as did Huntley in speculating that "[i]f Browne's thesis still exists, a good place to look for it might be among works on generation."[83] Huntley was on the right track insofar as in the centuries leading up to the seventeenth, the dominant theory of its actual topic—smallpox—was the Arabic view that fetuses contracted the disease from the menstrual blood of their mothers (Robbins, ed., *Pseudodoxia Epidemica*, 1.327).

In the Oxford University Archives, a document, shelved in the archives as OUA NEP/supra/Reg Q, comprises the certificate authorizing Browne's incorporation on July 10, 1637 of his Leiden MD into Oxford University. Divided into two sections, the certificate begins with a testimonial from Browne's Oxford supporters—Richard Baily (Vice Chancellor of the university), Thomas Clayton (Regius Professor of Medicine and head of Browne's own Broadgates Hall and Pembroke College), John Bainbridge (Savilian Professor of Astronomy as well as MD), Daniel Lawford (senior proctor), and John Glisson (junior proctor). Attached to this brief testimonial is a longer one from Leiden University itself, dated December 21, 1633, and signed by Antonius Thysius (*Rector Magnificus*), Daniel Heinsius (secretary of the Senate), and Otto Heurnius (Professor of Practical Medicine, Anatomy, and Chirurgery). In the course of this formulaic witness to Browne's

[79] Joannes Le Clerc, *Disputatio Medica Inauguralis, De Melancholia* (1633).
[80] Beukers, "Studying Medicine," 51.
[81] Guy Patin, *Naudæana et Patiniana* (Paris, 1701), separately paginated, 25.
[82] Huntley, *Sir Thomas Browne*, 68.
[83] Huntley, *Sir Thomas Browne*, 68.

successful completion of his medical degree, his Leiden professors note that he has defended his dissertation "*de variolis*", that is, on smallpox (161v).[84]

Whether Browne chose his particular disease or was assigned it by his professors, his topic was clearly framed by the highly practical tendencies of the Leiden medical program. Nonetheless, an interest in skin and in the diseases that afflict it appears elsewhere in his writings: in his memory of the "morgellons" among the children in southern France; in his anatomical observations; in letters on medical and anatomical subjects; and in his fearful, prayerful account of a virulent strain of smallpox ravaging Norwich in the final year of his life.[85] Smallpox was especially troubling in its monstrous scarring of the human hieroglyph whose face, Browne believed, ought to manifest the divine Creator, not the pocked legacy of corrupt generation.[86] Yet given *Religio Medici*'s plea for spontaneous, botanical generation among human beings, young Browne at times found himself demoting sexual mingling to a vulgar error.[87] What is more, the virulent strain of smallpox appeared to have arisen suddenly and shockingly in the very years at Oxford during which Browne was resolving to study medicine. In the years just before and after Browne's thesis, England suffered from two in a series of smallpox epidemics, with 531 perishing in 1632, and 1,354 in 1634. From the New World, reports in 1634 indicated in graphic detail that smallpox was a horrible factor in the colonies, though one that could be interpreted as favoring the divine protection of the colonists.[88] Despite those few English medical writers who persisted in deeming smallpox among the mild diseases, most were intensely aware of the fact that, as of the 1620s, it was replacing plague as the most hideous and lethal.[89] On the Continent where Browne was traveling, a fear of smallpox was just as powerful: indeed, in 1635 a French physician maintained "that smallpox was caused by the fear of smallpox."[90]

[84] See Reid Barbour, "The Topic of Sir Thomas Browne's Dissertation," *Notes & Queries* 54 (2007), 38–9.

[85] Keynes, ed., *The Works of Sir Thomas Browne*, 1.106, 3.338–40; 4.69–74, 241–4, 4.200, 202, 218.

[86] See Reid Barbour, "The Hieroglyphics of Skin," in Barbour and Claire Preston, eds., *Sir Thomas Browne: The World Proposed*, 279–95. For skin and skin diseases, see also Luke Demaitre, *Leprosy in Premodern Medicine: A Malady of the Whole Body* (Baltimore, MD: Johns Hopkins University Press, 2007), 83–4, 115, 188; and Elizabeth D. Harvey, "The Touching Organ: Allegory, Anatomy, and the Renaissance Skin Envelope," in Harvey, ed., *Sensible Flesh: On Touch in Early Modern Culture* (Philadelphia: University of Pennsylvania Press, 2003), 81–102.

[87] For Browne and spontaneous generation, see Marjorie Swann, "'Procreate like Trees': Generation and Society in Thomas Browne's *Religio Medici*," in Barbara Hanawalt and Lisa Kiser, eds., *Nature in the Middle Ages and Renaissance* (Notre Dame, IN: University of Notre Dame Press, 2008), 137–54.

[88] John Aberth, *The First Horseman: Disease in Human History* (Upper Saddle River, NJ: Prentice Hall, 2007), 67.

[89] See Tobias Whitaker, *An Elenchus of Opinions Concerning the Cure of the Small Pox* (London: 1661); Anonymous, *Hactenus Inaudita* (London, 1663); Anthony Westwood, *De Variolis & Morbillis* (London, 1656); and Marchamont Nedham, *Medela Medicinæ* (London: 1665), 52–5; for lingering views on mildness, see the discussion of Walter Harris in A. W. Sloan, *English Medicine in the Seventeenth Century* (Durham: Durham Academic Press, 1996), 159.

[90] The physician was Marc Duncan: see Joel N. Shurkin, *The Invisible Fire: The Story of Mankind's Victory Over the Ancient Scourge of Smallpox* (New York: G. P. Putnam's Sons, 1979), 60.

Smallpox was proving all the more fearsome in the 1620s and 30s because orthodoxies about its nature and treatment were being challenged, with the implication that either the disease had never been properly understood or, perhaps worse, it was evolving into a monster far more lethal than the seemingly benign, even natural version discussed by medieval authorities. Over the course of the sixteenth century, medical authorities on smallpox proved strongly indebted to the standard Arabic explanations of the disease, but in part because medicine was changing, in part because the disease appeared to be mutating, those medieval accounts were called into question by, among others, a favorite writer of Browne's, Girolamo Mercuriale.

The explanations offered by Rhazes and Avicenna—that childhood smallpox involves the natural fermentation and ebullition of the blood, and that children derived the disease from the impure menstrual blood of their mothers—located the disease within matters of generation, no doubt another reason for Browne's interest in it. But Mercuriale criticized these theses on numerous grounds in his study of the diseases of children, *De morbis puerorum tractatus locupletissimi*.[91] For Mercuriale, smallpox and measles were diseases of the whole external body. Moving according to medical custom from nomenclature to definition, causes, diagnosis, prognosis, and cures, he argued (contrary to Arab authorities) that smallpox was not known among the ancients, that its occurrence in human beings but not in beasts helped to rule out menstrual blood, and that smallpox could be differentiated from measles by the nature of its pustules as well as by the havoc that it wreaked in the body. Challenging the isolation of smallpox as a disease of the skin, he nonetheless offered an analysis of the skin in relation to the question of whether it was a proper part of the body.[92]

Extending his argument that smallpox, like the great pox or syphilis, was a relatively new disease into an argument for causation, Mercuriale turned to the one medieval authority, Avenzoar, who in his estimation had managed to break free of the grip held by Avicenna and Rhazes. The critical cause was to be found in the environment, in vitiated air, though he is not entirely clear whether this source is, as in the work of Jean Fernel, a celestial one or some type of mundane miasma.[93] All the same, Mercuriale criticized Fernel for focusing exclusively on the air, for this cause must unite with heredity, an aptitude that disposes certain children to the diseases of their family. This explanation was not the same as menstrual blood, which Mercuriale rejected, but it kept smallpox in the category of diseases having to do with generation.[94]

Mercuriale accentuated the questions raised by the new, or newly virulent, disease. Between Mercuriale and other authorities on smallpox, the list of questions was large and often Brownean in its focuses. Was it mainly a disease for children?

[91] On Girolamo Mercuriale, see *Sixteenth Century Physician and His Methods: Mercurialis on Diseases of the Skin*, trans. and ed. Richard L. Sutton (Kansas City, MO: Lowell Press, 1986).

[92] Mercuriale, *De morbis puerorum* (Venice, 1588), 2v–16v.

[93] See *Jean Fernel's On the Hidden Causes of Things*, trans. and ed. John M. Forrester, introduction and notes by John Henry and John M. Forrester (Boston: Brill, 2005), 586–95 on celestial cause.

[94] Mercuriale, *De morbis puerorum*, 8v–9v.

Was its virulence among adults a new twist in its history? Why was it nearly impossible to evade? Could it be attributed to contagion, as by physician and poet Hieronymous Fracastoro?[95] Was it to be classed with fevers or with skin diseases, as Giovanni Minadoi argued in *De variolis et morbillis liber unicus*, and as Hafenreffer claimed in his *Pandocheion* of 1630?[96] Was the smallpox a humoral condition like all the other diseases or, according to newer theories of disease, was it an ontological entity? Was skin disease the provenance of the surgeon or the physician, or both? Might the disease be located in ancient history, perhaps in the Athenian plague described by Thucydides? Was it a disease that developed among certain peoples in specific circumstances at particular times, owing as much to custom as to nature? Why did some people get it more than once? Did a cure involve heating further what nature was already boiling, and how might traditional methods of bleeding and purging be challenged by the habits of smallpox? Why did it seem to pick on the royalty and aristocracy? Was it a "Northern" disease? Why were there both benign and lethal versions of the same disease? Why was smallpox so savage in its pocking or blemishing of humanity's God-given beauty? Was this ironically nature's way of using the less noble periphery to save the nobler parts of the body, or was it a token of corruption at the human core?[97]

Browne's contemporaries were shocked by the brutality of smallpox on the face and skin. Alice Thornton, a medical practitioner and a mother, not only recorded the "violent and extreme pain" of her children as they suffered with smallpox, "such scrikes and torments that [one] was deprived of reason," but she also lamented how a daughter had "lost by this sickness her fair hair on her head, and that beautiful complexion God had given."[98] In Browne's Oxford, leading wits such as Richard Corbett and William Strode grappled with the deformity that the disease wrought.[99] Corbett had lost his wife to smallpox in 1628 while Browne was in residence in Oxford. In "An Elegie upon the death of the Lady Haddington who dyed of the small Pox," Corbett decried "thou deform'd unwoeman-like Disease, | That plowest up flesh and bloud, & there sow'st pease, | And leav'st such printes on

[95] Hieronymus Fracastoro, *Contagion, Contagious Diseases and Their Treatment*, ed. and trans. Wilmer Cave Wright (New York: G. P. Putnam's Sons, 1930), 72–5.

[96] Minadoi, *De variolis et morbillis liber unicus* (Padua, 1603); and Hafenreffer, *Pandocheion aiolodermon* (1630); on Hafenreffer, see Peter Lyncker, *Samuel Hafenreffer (1587–1660): Leben, Werk, seine Bedeutung für die Dermatologie* (Dissertation, Eberhard-Karls University, Tübingen, 1966).

[97] For these questions, histories of smallpox include Donald R. Hopkins, *Princes and Peasants: Smallpox in History* (Chicago: University of Chicago Press, 1983); Hopkins, *The Greatest Killer: Smallpox in History* (Chicago: University of Chicago Press, 2002), with a new introduction; J. R. Smith, *The Speckled Monster: Smallpox in England, 1670–1970, with particular reference to Essex* (Chelmsford: Essex Record Office, 1987); Ian Glynn and Jenifer Glynn, *The Life and Death of Smallpox* (London: Profile, 2004); C. W. Dixon, *Smallpox* (London: J & A Churchill, 1962); Genevieve Miller, *The Adoption of Inoculation for Smallpox in England and France* (Philadelphia: University of Pennsylvania Press, 1957); James Moore, *The History of the Small Pox* (London: Longmans, 1815); Edward J. Edwards, *A Concise History of Small-Pox and Vaccination in Europe* (London: H. K. Lewis, 1902); and Charles Creighton, *A History of Epidemics in Britain* (London: Frank Cass, 1965), 2.434–59.

[98] On Alice Thornton, see Lucinda McCray Beier, *Sufferers & Healers: The Experience of Illness in Seventeenth-Century England* (New York: Routledge & Kegan Paul, 1987), 228–30.

[99] See Raymond Anselment, "Smallpox in Seventeenth-Century English Literature: Reality and the Metamorphosis of Wit," *Medical History* 33 (1989), 72–95.

Beauty, that dost come | As *clouted shon* do on a floore of lome."[100] Strode's poem on the death of Sir Thomas Savile offered a similar conceit in bemoaning how the smallpox "by a thousand stroakes... made one wound" of Savill's body, an occasion for Strode's wit to counter "hatefull spots" with his subject's "virtuous gemmes" and to convert his "every scar" into stars "when death itselfe is dead."[101] In 1633, however, Oxford poets found a special reason to respond in verses against smallpox: King Charles had recently recovered from it. To this collection, *Musarum Oxoniensium Pro Rege Svo Soteria* (Oxford, 1633), Thomas Clayton contributed a poem in which he acknowledged the disease's power over that vast majority of human beings who lacked the king's strong temperament and healthy mind.

From the considerable body of smallpox poetry, a triple motivation for Browne's focus on smallpox becomes clearer. For one thing, the disease repelled contemporaries with its unprecedented virulence.[102] For another, like any new disease, the smallpox confronted the physician with his helplessness and ignorance. Perhaps above all, its ability to render hideous the most beautiful, youthful face wreaked havoc on a fanciful hieroglyphic thinker such as Browne for whom the visible was understood as a manifestation, if an "equivocal" or imperfect one, of the invisible world of proportion, order, and beauty. More than any other in the seventeenth century, smallpox disturbed a hieroglyphic imagination.

These dilemmas produced the kind of "strained, often questionable wit" with which Browne himself often responded to monstrosity's mockery of the hieroglyphs of providence.[103] As much as one might turn to dualism as a way of coping with the hideous body, the wit produced by smallpox was more apt to reinforce the "inextricable relationship between appearance and identity";[104] this question of whether visage was wrapped up with identity concerned Browne throughout his adult life, from the *Religio*'s digression on physiognomy to the extensive notes that he took on the anatomy of skin, the discussion of pigmentation in the *Pseudodoxia*, and his meditations on the meaning of skin in *The Garden of Cyrus*. As the smallpox poetry shows, the disease complicated in "ironic, albeit grotesque" ways the power of wit to metamorphose the graphic realities of disease into spiritual, moral, and social assets.[105]

A collection of twenty-six Leiden medical theses from 1639–40 corroborates that Browne's focus on smallpox was typical of contemporary Leiden dissertations in its concentration on a particular disease, with apoplexy, epilepsy, pleurisy, syphilis, heart palpitations, and arthritis included in the series of topics.[106] One of these

[100] For Corbett's poem, see *The Poems*, ed. Bennett and Trevor-Roper, 59–62.

[101] William Strode, *The Poetical Works*, ed. Bertram Dobell (London: B. Dobell, 1907), 86–7.

[102] Chamberlain's letter quoted in Anselment, "Smallpox in Seventeenth-Century English Literature," 77.

[103] Anselment, "Smallpox in Seventeenth-Century English Literature," 73–4.

[104] Anselment, "Smallpox in Seventeenth-Century English Literature," 90.

[105] For the Browne texts, see Patrides, 135–7; Keynes, 3.338; Robbins, ed., *Pseudodoxia Epidemica*, 1.508–22; Patrides, 356. For wit and metamorphosis, see Anselment, "Smallpox in Seventeenth-Century English Literature," 94.

[106] The collection is found in St John's College, Oxford, where it is shelved as HB.415.6.4.5.

theses treats smallpox and, therefore, offers us strong evidence of what was expected from Browne's own. Submitted in 1640 by one Franciscus Nansius, and comprising twenty-nine theses, the document begins with a declaration of the ubiquity of smallpox which follows (without citing) a formulation in the work of Montpellier's Lazare Rivière, namely, that among thousands of men and women, scarcely one will have escaped the disease. The paper does not yet explain the Arabic theories for this state of affairs, one deriving the contagion from the impure menstrual blood of the mother, the other naturalizing the smallpox as an outgrowth of the inevitable maturation and desiccation of the blood. Instead, it moves on in conventional fashion to establish the ancient terms for the disease. Here, however, an early modern dissertation on smallpox is bound to encounter questions, not least because the disease appeared to be mutating in the seventeenth century.

The theory of humors at the basis of Galenic medicine was ill equipped to deal with the possibility of new diseases, and smallpox accentuated this problem by virtue of its apparent universality. Although the Arab theories of Rhazes and Avicenna differed in their explanations, they agreed in crediting the inevitability of the smallpox. For Rhazes, the affliction—if it could be called that—arose rather benignly from the maturation of the child's blood, like the fermentation of wine; for Avicenna, every fetus derived impurity from its mother's blood. The two theories were commonly conflated in the seventeenth century, then framed—sometimes uncomfortably—within the ancient medical theories of the humors. If, however, Nansius establishes knowledge of smallpox amongst the ancients, it is nonetheless the case that the ancients did not discuss the disease extensively, nor was their distinction between smallpox and measles sufficiently clear or consistent to prevent ongoing disagreement among authorities about just this matter. The struggle over the antiquity and universality of smallpox increased in the first quarter of the seventeenth century with the growing suspicion that the highly virulent smallpox experienced by early modern patients might in fact prove radically different from a relatively benign medieval version.[107] As Browne himself would later express in *Letter to a Friend*, early modern medical authorities were faced with the prospect that even if the smallpox was not entirely new, at the very least its contemporary strain was increasingly deadly (Keynes, 1.107). Not surprisingly, medical notebooks from the period are sometimes unsure about how to categorize the smallpox: as a skin disease, a pediatric matter, a fever, a "common disease," a contagious one, or an acute disease for instance.[108] Walaeus opted for the febrile explanation.[109]

Because it required full knowledge of the ancients yet openness to new ideas, smallpox was a perfect litmus test for the Leiden approach to medical vocation.

[107] See Ann G. Carmichael and Arthur M. Silverstein, "Smallpox in Europe before the Seventeenth Century: Virulent Killer or Benign Disease?" *Journal of the History of Medicine and Allied Sciences* 42 (1987), 147–68, see 160.

[108] See for instance Cambridge University Library MSS Dd.2.41, Dd.2.34, Dd.3.21, and Dd.3.10.

[109] Johannes Walaeus, *Medica Omnia* (1660), 126–7.

Accordingly, over the course of his life, Browne proved scrupulously up-to-date in his assessment of work regarding dermatology and pediatrics, categories under which smallpox was often filed. In writing to his son Edward years later, Browne singled out two authorities whose works appeared in the years just before his medical training: Girolamo Mercuriale and Samuel Hafenreffer. In *Pseudodoxia Epidemica*, he outlined the medical orthodoxy according to which "in the purest and most faire conceptions, learned men derive the cause of Pox and Meazels, from the principles of that nature, that is, the menstruous impurities in the mothers blood, and virulent tinctures contracted by the Infant, in the nutriment of the wombe." Yet his familiarity with Mercuriale's work on children's diseases—on a par with the special focus of Browne's Montpellier professors—also showed how well he knew that this orthodox etiology had been contested.[110]

The conventions of the dissertation dictated that, like Nansius, Browne move efficiently to a definition. Thus, Nansius asserts that among the extant views, physicians speak of smallpox proper as those more prominent pustules which suppurate from an abundance of malignant humors. By contrast, the measles are smaller red bumps responsive to the malignancy of attenuated humors. Moving from definition to cause, Nansius divides between early, internal and eventual, external causes. The former involve the corruption absorbed in the mother's womb into the fetus where it lurks until some impulsive cause discharges its lively fermentation into the whole mass of the blood. At this point in the maturation of the human being, the blood effervesces and boils. External causes, some univocal but others equivocal, are most clearly illustrated by corrupted and contagious air; according to Nansius, experience has not yet proven that food and drink can play a role in causing smallpox but, he notes, it is not improbably the case.

In an effort to differentiate smallpox from measles more carefully, Nansius examines in good Aristotelian fashion their respective substances, qualities, and quantities. In theses XVII–XVIII, Nansius follows the standard practice of rendering the signs of the disease, beginning with those symptoms that precede the pustules: problems with natural functions (surrounding the liver, stomach, and groin areas) such as nausea; with vital functions (heart and thorax) including heart palpitations; and with animal functions (head, brain, external senses) including headache, delirium, nightmares, difficult respiration, cough, and lethargy. Other signs feature excrement (an overflow of tears), red eyes, and the entire body's painful sensitivity to touch. Nansius's further attempts to define and distinguish smallpox from measles include a classification of both as acute, but with the measles working themselves out in seven days, the smallpox in fourteen.

Adhering further to medical convention, Nansius turns next to prognosis as a means of reading the body's "indications" so as to determine whether a cure is possible and, if so, what the best of the several approaches to cure will be in the circumstances. In this section, he adheres exceedingly closely to two sources of which Browne himself was very fond, the work of Rivière and the standard,

[110] Robbins, ed., *Pseudodoxia Epidemica*, 1.327.

synthesizing textbook of Daniel Sennert. Two factors made the cure of smallpox especially problematic. For one thing, rather than counterbalance the heat of fever with a regimen of coolness, the physician attempted to facilitate nature's endeavor to expel the corruption by doing everything in his power to keep the patient hot. For another, many victims of smallpox were small children, a factor which excluded the bleeding thought necessary to ease nature's burden with expulsion of the corrupt humors as too potent. As for medicines, stronger purges were never used with the smallpox, lest nature find herself impeded in her endeavor to expel the humors or subverted by a dangerous fluidity within the body's beleaguered economy. Thesis XXV offers the recipe for a bland purgative, but thesis XXVI persists in a Hippocratic warning against the overuse of medication in subversion of nature's own course.

From this point on, however, Nansius follows convention in offering recipes for curative medicines (in this case, one productive of sweat), as well as medicaments for protecting the eyes, nose, and internal parts from the harm that smallpox can leave behind its ordinary course. As he turns to regimen and the so-called six non-naturals, Nansius again factors in the young age of many smallpox patients, maintaining (again with Rivière and Sennert) that children can be allowed to eat more than adult patients since the younger the patient, the more his or her innate heat. With smallpox, Nansius knows, the final consideration is both crucial and cosmetic: the prevention of scarring. To this end, physicians must assess the size, color, number, consistency, and conjuncture of the pustules and decide what instrument, if any, to apply to them. One persistent question concerns whether a gold or a silver probe should be deployed, but the conciseness of a dissertation prevents Nansius from saying much about the horror—the ravages left by the pox—that is everywhere to be found in everyday experience and commentary. As one contemporary pundit claimed, "I hardly knowe that there is any disease whereof weomen are more carefull then of the comlines of their faces that they be disfigured or blemished wth the hollow pitts or markes of the Small pox."[111]

Over the final fifty years of his life, Browne continued to worry about smallpox. Having generalized in *Religio* that fetuses are "subject to . . . the malice of diseases in that other world, the truest Microcosme, the wombe of our mother," he was more specific in *Pseudodoxia* on the causes of smallpox. In *Letter to a Friend* he observed that like rickets and the king's evil, smallpox "grows more pernicious than the Great." He jotted down queries about "whether anyone suffers from smallpox and pestilence simultaneously" ("*An quis variolis et peste simul laborat*"). In the *Musæum Clausum*'s desire for the survival of "A Commentary of Galen upon the Plague of Athens described by Thucydides," he may have been longing for ancient insight into the new menace.[112] Browne was certainly anxious about smallpox in letters to his children on the devastating epidemic in Norwich from autumn 1681 through early 1682, a bout so intense and pervasive that Browne left it "to Gods mercy

[111] Cambridge UL MS Dd 2.41, f. 63.

[112] *Religio Medici*, ed. Patrides, 109; *Pseudodoxia*, ed. Robbins, 507–30; *Letter*, ed. Martin, 185; and *Works*, ed. Keynes, 3.326.

when he pleaseth to abate or Cease it, for the last run of the small Pox lasted much longer then this has yet dun" (Keynes, 4.200). Browne's experiences in Leiden reinforced the practical demands of preserving and recovering health, but they also pointed the way toward patience in the face of human vanity and fragility. First and last, the medical education in Leiden was a moral and religious one.

4. PEACE, CONFLICT, AND RELIGION AFTER DORT

Chief among the fascinations for travellers such as Browne was Dutch religious culture. In Leiden and the surrounding areas, Browne would have had the opportunity to advance his Paduan experience of Jewish culture. Browne's son Edward would later note how during his Dutch travels he "met a Jewish doctor and was present at a circumcision in a private house."[113] Tourists often commented on Dutch religious laxity, for better and worse, whether it violated the Sabbath or devolved into a hurly burly distribution of church seating among the social groups. Visitors differed on the value of the Dutch toleration of different religions or sects: Evelyn was eager to live among the sectaries while the Laudian Peter Heylyn found in the Dutch religious medley a modern-day Babel.[114] Travelers were moved by the obvious fact that Leiden was a haven for refugees fleeing religious oppression and hopeful for a better life. When, two years after his graduation from Leiden, Browne turned to write down his thoughts on religious persecution and toleration, his experience of the complex Dutch religious dynamics was still vivid in his mind.

Theological controversies preoccupied both the city and the University of Leiden.[115] In the longer history of religious sectarianism and toleration in the Netherlands, 1633, the year in which Browne took his doctorate, was particularly fraught. A few years after he returned from the Continent, Browne would write in *Religio Medici* that he refused to subscribe to the extremes of religious dogma epitomized by the Council at Trent and the Synod at Dort. In 1633, just over a decade after the triumph of Calvinism at Dort, the Netherlands into which Browne traveled was experiencing an intense struggle—military, cultural, and religious—to recover its sense of direction and purpose after the internecine conflicts leading to, and emerging from, that famous meeting.

As a medical student, Browne had an opportunity to observe Dutch confessional dynamics in the very building in which he worked. For Browne's developing sense of religious flexibility and tolerance, it was important that the university may have rented out space in the chapel to congregations seeking a place to worship, at

[113] See van Strien, *British Travellers in Holland*, 209–11.

[114] van Strien, *British Travellers in Holland*, 201–3; Evelyn's *The Diary*, 2.46.

[115] There is no way to know whether in locating sustained debate about the origins of the soul in "*Germane* auditories" (Patrides, 106), Browne intended to single out Dutch lecture halls in *Religio Medici*. But his German commentator in the Latin translation suggested a Dutch context in citing the philosopher Franco Burgersdijck (1590–1635), *Collegium physicum, disputationibus XXXII absolutum* (first published 1632 as a set of dissertations in philosophy), dispute 29, pp. 313–23.

a time when two main religious groups—Dutch Reformed and Walloon—dominated the three principal churches of the city but did not exclude Scottish or English Reformed, English Separatist, Lutheran, Arminian, Mennonite, Jewish, and Catholic groups from worshiping as they saw fit within the city. In 1633, the prudent harmony of the churches in Leiden was in many ways more important than the cautious, synoptic mediation between traditional and newfangled medicine, and in so many ways much harder to achieve and sustain. The levels of openness with which the several churches could worship varied considerably. For instance, the Remonstrants were treated relatively harshly; the Mennonites might be frowned upon as Anabaptists yet they were largely left alone; the peaceful, poor, and Calvinist Walloons were welcomed "as brethren of the public church," and worshiped in the third largest church in the city, the Lieve Vrowe or Marie Kirk (third after the Pieterskirk and St Pancras or Hooglansche Kerk, both Dutch Reformed); both the English congregations were largely ignored by the magistracy, and even the Catholics were left to their own private devices.[116] In *Religio Medici* but also in *Pseudodoxia Epidemica* and *Repertorium*, Browne would weigh in on the motives of iconoclasts, so it was clearly of concern to him as a visitor to Leiden that the city's reformed churches varied in their degree of iconoclasm.[117] While the drawings of Pieter Saenredam illustrate how some of the greatest Dutch churches were whitewashed of ornament,[118] the Pieterskerk around the corner from Browne's residence in Leiden retained images and its organ.

By the time Browne reached Leiden in 1633, the city's position on religious toleration and conformity was at once clear and complicated. After the Synod at Dort, the Calvinist victors had purged the university of its Arminian leaders and scholars, and the town citizenry was strongly Counter Remonstrant in emphasis, though the university magistracy remained beholden to no church in particular. It was a typical remark from a traveler to Leiden that "every Sunday here there is open preaching in three Dutch, one French, one English, one Lutheran and about three Mennonite churches."[119] By the 1630s, moreover, there was something of a thaw in the suppression of the Remonstrants, as well as a lessening or at least a destabilizing of the political corollaries of the debate, though it is also true that the regents of the States of Holland refused to let the exiled Grotius return in 1632.[120] In 1633, religious controversy among the Dutch came to a new head in response to recent events in the longstanding war with Spain. The war with Spain had first nationalized then powerfully consolidated Dutch religious identity, of course, but

[116] Christine Kooi, *Liberty and Religion: Church and State in Leiden's Reformation,* 1572–1620 (Boston: Brill, 2000), 163–81.

[117] On Browne and iconoclasm, see Kevin Killeen's and Jonathan Post's essays in Barbour and Preston, eds., *Sir Thomas Browne: The World Proposed,* respectively 188–205 and 258–75.

[118] See Gary Schwartz and Marten Jan Bok, *Pieter Saenredam: The Painter and His Time* (New York: Abbeville, 1989).

[119] Quoted in Kooi, *Liberty and Religion*, 162.

[120] See Jonathan Israel, *The Dutch Republic 1477–1806: Its Rise, Greatness, and Fall* (Oxford: Oxford University Press, 1995), 513.

in 1633 the United Provinces found themselves at a major point of contention between those who desired ongoing war with a diminished Spanish power and those who sought détente. During the autumn of 1633, the internecine debate over what to do with the Spanish came to a climax, with political conflict between those Arminians subversive of the authority of the Stadholder and the Calvinists with whom he was once again aligned. 1633 has been called "the great watershed in the stadholderate of Frederick Henry," the year in which he changed sides, came to support war and Calvinism, contributed to the reemergence of the Arminian political party, and undercut the basis of his own authority. As Israel summarizes, "[t]he year 1633 was thus one of the key turning-points of the Dutch Golden Age,"[121] and as such, it placed Browne in a crucible in which all the ingredients of early modern religious politics were activated and tested.

At the same time, Leiden was leading the way in the Dutch efforts to stabilize doctrinal orthodoxy. Whereas Holland was renowned among tourists for its tolerance of sectarian Protestants and Jews, the theology faculty in Leiden—Johannes Polyander, Antonius Walaeus, Antonius Thysius, and (until 1632) Andreas Rivetus—so strongly believed in religious unity or at least harmony in Dutch Reform that they tended to present a united front rather than diversity or debate in their theological declarations. Making use of the different strengths that each possessed,[122] they ensured that their differences added up to a synthesis or "synopsis"—as in their 1625 *Synopsis Purioris Theologiae*, a handbook of fifty-two disputations with an aim toward stabilizing and consolidating Dutch orthodoxy.[123] In this respect, the theology faculty epitomized what for Browne would be one dispensation in which harmony could subsume differing religious tendencies in what historians have characterized as the Dutch culture of discussion and arbitration.[124]

With a greater capacity for disharmony than the Leiden theological faculty, Thomas Browne's English associates in Leiden suggest a situation in which divided groups—Scottish and English Reformed and Separatists—found themselves caught between their strong commitment to a vision of religious truth and their resistance to the persecution that such commitments can yield. In 1633, Hugh Goodyear was the pastor of the English Reformed Church, which worshiped in the Jerusalem Chapel not far from the university building and on the southwest side of the Cellebroeders Canal (now Keizerstraat). Situated within the Jerusalem Hofje—the hofje "was a square block of twelve housing units built around an interior courtyard" according to the paradigm of the late medieval lay communities[125]—the chapel was known for having a representation of the holy sepulcher in

[121] Israel, *The Dutch Republic*, 523–4.

[122] Walaeus was gifted in philosophy, Thysius in languages, especially Hebrew; Thysius and Rivetus had wider erudition in theology, while Walaeus and Polyander were more solid. Thysius and Walaeus were more fervent while Rivetus was calmer and Polyander the calmest of all. See H. Bavinck, ed., *Synopsis Purioris Theologiae* (Leiden, 1881).

[123] Peter T. van Rooden, *Theology, Biblical Scholarship and Rabbinical Studies in the Seventeenth Century: Constantijn L'Empereur (1591–1648), Professor of Hebrew and Theology at Leiden* (New York: Brill, 1989), 54.

[124] See Goldgar, *Tulipmania*, 17.

[125] Kooi, *Liberty and Religion*, 182.

Jerusalem, evidence of its past associations with pilgrims to that holy shrine.[126] Brereton recorded his impressions of a service there on June 8, 1634: "We stayed the Sabbath at Leyden . . . and heard Mr. Goodier (a worthy, honest man) in the English church, a little (yet neat) place, and not fully furnished with hearers. Hither also to this church we went in afternoon: came thither before two, yet sermon begun. After sermon, all of that congregation desired to stay: we departed." Having left the church, the group proceeded to observe the goings-on in the Pieterskirk, where Brereton remarked that the bread and wine were distributed among the men and women without "such decency and reverence as in England."[127] That decency might be harmonized with Dutch Protestantism was a stimulating lesson for Browne's efforts in *Religio Medici* to work out his own version of the merger. By 1633, not only Goodyear's congregation but also the Dutch Reformed Church itself had absorbed many of the Separatists with whom Goodyear had always had good relations. But in a manner that anticipated Browne's own ecumenicalism and independence, Goodyear's relation to contemporary English and Dutch religious alternatives resisted neat classification: as Jeremy Bangs explains, Goodyear "never fully supported congregationalism," but he "clearly did not consider the office of bishops to be important" either.[128] So too in the various stages of revising *Religio Medici*, Browne would find himself torn over whether to blame presbyters or prelates for corrupting the good work of the Reformation.

While in Leiden, Browne had connections to the Separatists: he was joined in medical school by the son of their late spiritual leader John Robinson, and the tobacconist Richard Monck, with whom Browne lodged, was affiliated with Separatists such as John Lee. These Separatists were prepared radically to change their lives for the sake of their beliefs but their leader, Robinson, had argued late in his life for the legitimacy of their hearing preachers from the Church of England.[129] The Leiden Separatists often mitigated the starkness of those beliefs in an effort to get along with the other churches in Leiden. Browne's encounter with a Separatist community was thus facilitated by their flexible, generous relations with the university, with Calvinism, and with the Dutch and English Reformed churches into which they were folded. What Browne encountered in this religious community was a living version of the *Synopsis*: the imperfect but deeply felt commitment to reconciling truth with peace within a workable community.[130]

In 1633, however, peace and harmony in Leiden could not be taken for granted. If Goodyear was on predominantly good relations with the Separatists, cases of severe dissatisfaction arose in his congregation, threatened to drag the English Reformed Church into scandal, and introduced Browne to the level of polemical discord awaiting

[126] Orlers, 143–4. Cf. van Oerle, *Leiden binnen en buiten de stadvesten*, 202.

[127] Brereton, *Travels in Holland*, 45–6.

[128] J. D. Bangs, ed. and intro., *The Auction Catalogue of the Library of Hugh Goodyear, English Reformed Minister at Leiden* (Utrecht: HES Publishers, 1985), 5–6.

[129] For Robinson, see *The Works of John Robinson, Pastor of the Pilgrim Fathers*, ed. Robert Ashton (London: John Snow, 1851), 3.343–78.

[130] Contrast the situation in Amsterdam: Keith L. Sprunger, *Dutch Puritanism: A History of English and Scottish Churches of the Netherlands in the Sixteenth and Seventeenth Centuries* (Leiden: Brill, 1982), 124.

him at home in England. As Sprunger has shown, Goodyear was a stern and persistent regulator of his congregants' faith and manners, an unintended effect of which was that his church tended to be more isolated than he would have liked. The Laudian, Stephen Goffe, who matriculated at the university in February 1633, joked that while Goodyear "refuseth to be of the English Classis," his application to join the Leiden Classis "is refused here among the Dutch: The reason is, because they conceive him to be of a disagreing disposition in generall; and in particular that he would governe his owne church with a more rigid discipline then is used or thought fitt by the Dutch Classis."[131] Furthermore, there is evidence from the early 1630s that Goodyear, unhappy with the Presbyterian structure, was moving in the direction of an autonomous congregation, in keeping with his conviction that "orthodox words do not necessarily prove faith for membership or baptism. 'Every assent is not faith.'"[132]

Already in Leiden, then, Browne was privy to the debate over Laudian and Caroline religious culture in the England to which he would soon return, even as he was experiencing firsthand a culture in which liberal Arminianism had been persecuted. With the coming of 1633 and the reign of Archbishop Laud, the strict disciplinarian Goodyear expressed displeasure about the likes of Goffe in his world, and was unsettled by the vocal congregants who were urging him to adopt the English prayer book and other Anglican ceremonies. In 1632, Goodyear had struggled to relieve his church of what he considered its tragic isolation from other legitimately Reformed churches. This proved difficult: on July 1, 1633, Goodyear complained in a letter to Ralph Smith that

> the Lord hath placed me over a congregacion wch injoyeth the use of the ordinances, but wanteth [i.e. lacks] that power of godliness wch is in those rare Christians in Manchestre and there abut: some without the licencie of the English Churches here seek to bring us under the command of the service book in England and I hear that the cheife in England wil bring it in some congregacion, but cannot so easily bring it in ours.[133]

Goodyear himself was pretending to play along with the Caroline prescriptions by devising a catechism in these years—Charles and Laud were eager to minimize the centrality of sermons by emphasizing the gain in conformity to be had through afternoon catechisms. But Goodyear clearly disliked the famous Hugo Grotius's affection for the Church of England, and he complained bitterly in 1633 about those members of his congregation who were pushing for more ceremonial, liturgical, and conformist services. In this context, Browne's own commitment to the Church of England was newly tested on the eve of his return to England.[134]

Given Browne's interest in relations between Christian and Jew, it is noteworthy that in Leiden, another embodiment of the post-Dort tension between toleration and orthodoxy, between peace and truth-claims, and between comprehension and divisiveness, emerged from the Judaic scholarship for which Constantijn L'Empereur

[131] Quoted in Sprunger, *Dutch Puritanism*, 130.

[132] Sprunger, *Dutch Puritanism*, 131.

[133] D. Plooij, *The Pilgrim Fathers from a Dutch Point of View* (New York: New York University Press, 1932), 107.

[134] For more on Goffe, see Sprunger, *Dutch Puritanism* 132–4.

became renowned. For him, for Daniel Heinsius, and for the other theological scholars of Leiden University, 1633 was a critical year for a number of reasons. On December 29, 1633, L'Empereur was authorized to write in an official capacity against the Jews.[135] But how he arrived at this polemical position in the month of Browne's matriculation and graduation involved a development of a sophisticated hermeneutics in the context of the world-class Biblical scholarship that included Daniel Heinsius and the newly arrived Claude Saumaise. As Peter T. van Rooden has explained, the thrust of L'Empereur's scholarship, most of which was produced in the years 1627–34, reflected the scholar's staunch Calvinism in its campaign against unorthodoxy (Arminianism, Socinianism) and undue tolerance (especially toward Judaism).[136]

1633 was an especially noteworthy year for Dutch–Jewish relations. In March of that year, the first Jew took his doctorate from the medical faculty in Leiden and the Senate confronted the problem of what to do about the religious aspect of the graduation ceremony.[137] In September a controversy over attempts made by Menasseh Ben Israel to reconcile Jews and Christians came to a head when, encouraged by G. J. Vossius, Menasseh had his Spanish work, *Conciliador*, translated into Latin and the book was sent by the States to the theological faculty for their judgment. The book attempted to reconcile apparent contradictions in the Old Testament for the benefit predominantly of new converts to Judaism, and Menasseh sought legitimacy in the form of permission to dedicate the Latin translation of the work to the States General.[138]

L'Empereur epitomized what in 1633 was the university's divided identity: on the one hand, strongly confessional and Dutch, on the other a key node in a network of interconfessional, non-polemical scholarly exchange in the republic of letters. For Browne, the significance of Leiden's position in the republic of letters was powerful—and rewarding once the Dutch led the way in Browne's own reception into that republic with the Latin translation of *Religio Medici* in 1644. Even a cursory reading of *Pseudodoxia Epidemica* reveals how prominent the Scaliger family legacy was in Browne's scholarship, and Leiden University's reputation had been established by a past professoriate including Josephus Justus Scaliger, who was buried in the city and whose amazing manuscript collection was housed in a special cabinet in the library. While Browne was in Leiden, students felt the continuing presence of the morally suspect but brilliant teacher and scholar, Daniel Heinsius, but they were also excited by the coaxing in 1631 of the great Claude Saumaise (1588–1653) to the university by means of a high salary, full and private access to the library, the suspension of all teaching duties, and what Saumaise himself called "Surtout la liberté"—in short, a set of privileges on which Saumaise proudly insisted and to which he tried to add.[139] Browne's library contained a slew of works

[135] *Bronnen tot de geschiedenis der Leidsche Universiteit*, ed. Molhuysen.

[136] van Rooden, *Constantijn L'Empereur*, 56–7, 90.

[137] Acta Senatus Academici Rectore, ASF 260, Leiden University.

[138] van Rooden, *Constantijn L'Empereur*, 164–5.

[139] Paul R. Sellin, *Daniel Heinsius and Stuart England* (Leiden: Leiden University Press, 1968), 39–40.

by Heinsius and Saumaise alike, some of them probable purchases during Browne's visit.[140]

Browne's fascination with biblical scholarship, developed at Winchester and Oxford, would have been stimulated further by events in 1633 Leiden. Heinsius's analysis of the New Testament involved an elaborate set of criteria that comprised the clarification of hard passages, the careful consideration of patristic exegesis and of comparable texts from early Christian, Jewish, and pagan literature; a juxtaposition of New with Old Testament; the introduction of philological information about the "Hellenistic idiom"; an insistence on the historical or literal sense at the expense of allegory; and a resistance to controversy.[141] Indeed Heinsius's chief contribution to Leiden religious scholarship was his production of the "textus receptus" of the New Testament, an edition brought out by the Elzeviers in 1624 and 1633.[142] In 1633, Heinsius declared himself a protector of the New Testament from all contamination; he also informed his reader that the desideratum of his edition—and the "meticulous care" involved in executing it so well—were matters of wide consensus among those who care about religion.[143]

Of all the members of the Leiden faculty who sought a stable union of truth and peace in orthodoxy, the most exemplary for Browne is Johannes Polyander. It has been speculated that in the 1640s, Browne wrote a panegyric for this theologian and churchman on the occasion of his death. Although the attribution is highly doubtful at best,[144] Polyander figured prominently in 1633 as Leiden's hero for irenic religion.[145] In his views of salvation, Polyander was a moderate, an infralapsarian who believed that election took place after the Fall. The prevailing view of Polyander in comparison to the other members of the theology faculty was that he was less scholarly but more practical, calm, tactful, elegant, and adaptable to

[140] For instance, Heinsius's edition of Clement of Alexandria (1629); his *Aristarchus* (1627), and editions of Hesiod (1603), Greek pastoral poets (1604), and Theophrastus (1613). For Salmasius, a commentary on Julius Solinus (1629) praised by Browne as excellent (see Finch, ed., *Catalogue of the Libraries*, 86, p. 5, note 11), and an edition of *Historiae Augustae Scriptores* (1620). Browne continued to collect their works for years to come.

[141] H. J. de Jonge, "The Study of the New Testament," in Scheurleer and G. H. M. Posthumus Meyjes, eds., *Leiden University in the Seventeenth Century*, 94.

[142] H. J. de Jonge, *Daniel Heinsius and the Textus Receptus of the New Testament* (Leiden: Brill, 1971), 1.

[143] Grafton, *Athenae Batavae*, 10.

[144] The verses appear in a manuscript called *The Letter Book of Philip Stanhope, Earl of Chesterfield, 1657–1712*, found in BL Additional MS 19253, printed in Keynes in 3.237–38. It shows up in the writings that are found upside down and in reverse order (back to front) on the versos of the letters. In "A catalogue of some freinds and acquaintance of mine who killed them selves," the first on the list is Polyander's son, "intimate friend and bed-fellow" of the writer, and a suicide by stabbing whose body "was found some dayes after his death in a heap of Nettels" (211v). Born in 1633, the author of these words was seven when his mother married an ambassador from the Prince of Orange to Charles I, after which he moved to Holland to live at court in Buren. Then we learn that "I boarded with a learned and reverend Divine named Monsieur Poliander," that Polyander was in full possession of his senses at his pious death, and that he "well deserued this folloing [*sic*] Epitaph, made by Doctor Broun a fine Poet." In all likelihood this was Mathias Browne, who was a medical student at Leiden in the 1640s.

[145] This entire paragraph is based on A. J. Lamping, *Johannes Polyander: Een dienaar van Kerk en Universiteit* (Leiden: Brill, 1980), 1–63.

exigencies, a faithful Calvinist holding to the notion that understanding should be subordinated to piety. Polyander's opposition to dispute and emphasis on adoration were features of his thought that would soon reverberate in Browne's *Religio Medici.*

1633 was a big year for Polyander, not least because he commenced a major dispute with what he considered the worst heresy afflicting the church—Socinianism—a tendency toward which he himself had been suspected of when the Curators were deciding whether to bring him into the faculty.[146] Whatever his anxieties in 1633, Polyander believed that he lived in a paradise on earth.[147] Even if Thomas Browne wrote no verses for Polyander, it is unlikely that he would have left Leiden in 1633 without a strong sense of what this theologian meant to the university and indeed to Christendom as a hero for irenic religion. In 1633, Polyander was organizing student disputes against the Socinians and doing his best to prevent egregious heresy from infiltrating Dutch Reform. But he was also the most prudent and peaceful of the Leiden divines, his motto "pie et prudenter." Schoneveld suggests, rightly, that Polyander would have represented to Browne the urgent need to purge those heretical tendencies of which *Religio Medici* included an honest account,[148] and to ground his faith in orthodox authorities. To the medical student seeking the religion of a physician, Polyander and Johannes Walaeus presented a united front.

In a passage included in both *Letter to a Friend* and *Christian Morals,* Browne urged upon his reader practical moral advice,

> Consider where about thou art in Cebes's Table, or that old Philosophical Pinax of the Life of Man: whether thou art yet in the Road of uncertainties; whether thou has entred the narrow Gate, got up the Hill and asperous way, which leadeth unto the House of Sanity, or taken that purifying Potion from the hand of sincere Erudition, which may send Thee clear and pure away unto a virtuous and happy Life. (Patrides, 417)

Hanging in the anatomy theater in Leiden was a detailed, elaborate engraving of this well-known allegory of the road of life, attributed to Cebes, a friend of Socrates. The engraving depicts at its outmost circle a group of children gathered around an elderly teacher—Genius—outside the Gates of Life and attended by Seduction. Curving upward past Lady Fortuna, those maturing travelers who make it past her distractions and beyond the wavering uncertainties of opinions, appetites, and companionships come in the second ring of the circular path to the study of the liberal arts. Those—far fewer—who persist still further make it to the tiny portal and the steep hill climbing upward to the abode of health. Only there do they find modesty, liberality, temperance, sincere erudition, truth, and persuasion.[149] Having

[146] Lamping, *Johannes Polyander*, 93–5.

[147] Quoted in Edward Arber, *The Story of the Pilgrim Fathers, 1606–1623 A. D.: As Told by Themselves, Their Friends, and Their Enemies* (Boston: Houghton, Mifflin, 1897), 143.

[148] Schoneveld, "Sir Thomas Browne and Leiden University in 1633," 358.

[149] Scheurleer, "Un amphithéâtre d'anatomie moralisée," in Scheurleer and G. H. M. Posthumus Meyjes, eds., *Leiden University in the Seventeenth Century*, 255–9.

traveled from Montpellier to Padua, then over the Alps in search of his doctorate in medicine, Browne graduated into his professional life from a university that exhorted him always to take stock of where he was in the way of life on the road to both physical and spiritual health. Once back in England, he wrote a stock-taking account of his development thus far, and settled down into a vocation that he was to serve wisely and well.

PART III

FRUITION

7

Halifax, 1634–1637

Having returned from the Continent in 1634, Browne confidently declared in *Religio Medici* that "I have not onely seene severall Countries, beheld the nature of their climes, the Chorography of their Provinces, Topography of their Cities, but understood their severall Lawes, Customes and Policies" (Patrides, 147). Resisting uncharitable national stereotypes (Patrides, 139), he also stressed that plurality existed not just between the "Countries" that he had experienced but also within them. What he "understood" about these places continued to grow and deepen in Browne's imagination even as the physical domain of his life narrowed, first to provincial Halifax from 1634 to 1637, then to urban Norwich for the rest of his life. Even as his fascination with the far reaches of the world intensified by way of correspondence, the travels of his children, and his extensive reading about faraway places, Browne came to appreciate the richness and layered depth, naturally and historically, of the local. With Halifax as with Norwich, Browne's personal and vocational maturation had as much to do with social context and contacts as it did with ideas and education.

The England to which Thomas Browne returned from the Continent in 1634 was much changed over the years since Browne's Oxford graduation in 1629. From one vantage, that of King Charles, Bishop then Archbishop William Laud, and their supporters, England was more prosperous, peaceful, and orderly than it had been at the end of the 1620s, years of contentious parliaments, of failed wars with both Spain and France, of the assassination of Buckingham, and of roils over "Arminianism" and royal prerogative. By contrast, in the early 1630s, there were no Parliaments, no wars, a loving royal marriage with Henrietta Maria at the center of court life, and a full-scale program of enriching English religion with physical refurbishment and of ensuring uniformity to the prayer book, continuity with a festive past, and the "beauty of holiness." From another vantage, however, the so-called Puritan one, the early 1630s might be outwardly placid, but this calm reflected the suppression of healthy parliamentary collaboration in governance, the inquisitorial quashing of true spirituality, the embarrassment of noninvolvement in the apocalyptic battle against the Antichrist, the flight of the godly from oppression to America, and the profanity of a dominant culture infatuated with popery and masques. Browne returned to an England in which seemingly innocuous or otherwise obviously valued concepts—recreation, charity, peace, unity, and sociability—might serve as litmus tests for one's deepest values. This context, filtered through the particular concerns of a local West Yorkshire culture, interacted with Browne's continental and earlier British experiences in the composition of *Religio Medici* and in the formation of his vocational, authorial, and social identity.

Because he could not yet officially operate as a physician in England until he had converted his Leiden degree into an incorporated doctorate from Oxford or Cambridge, Browne expended approximately three years in a provincial town in West Yorkshire, Halifax, a place appropriately obscure for the purposes of exercising his medical learning and far ruder than the sites of learning he had visited en route through Europe—in fact, he apologizes in the published preface to *Religio Medici*'s readers, "a place ... with such disadvantage, that ... I had not the assistance of any good booke, whereby to promote my invention or relieve my memory" (Patrides, 60). But Halifax would prove far more significant for Browne's development than simply as a training ground for a young physician en route to the obligatory fourteen years between his Oxford matriculation in 1623 and the Oxford incorporation of his Leiden medical degree in 1637. For in this remote region of England, Browne discovered a supportive coterie of friends as well as an environment in which the relationship between faith and charity was explored and enacted in vivid, complex ways; and with his continental experiences in tow, Browne converted this unofficial apprenticeship for a medical practice into *Religio Medici*.

Far from providing Browne with a bland or neutral setting for the composition of *Religio*, the town offered him experiments in charity, a model for reconciling Laudian and Puritan strains in contemporary culture, and a threshold between the intellectually transformative Continent and the practical life of vocation and family matters. It also afforded him profound friendship and a sympathetic audience for his manuscript. In this remote place without books, Browne took stock of a singular mind with its modes of both skeptical melancholy and playful expatiation, and of a self at once intensely private and immensely sociable. What is more, Browne found in West Yorkshire a mode of virtually utopian reform that challenged the playful experimentation of his intellect with a differently inverted commitment to reforming contemporary customs and habits. In dynamic and uneven ways, the disadvantageous place in which the *Religio* was first conceived worked in Browne's imagination as a provocation to investigate how his philosophical explorations—of such matters as hieroglyphs, heresy, and atheism—pertained to the seemingly more mundane but still vexing issues of charity, poverty, vocation, and social discipline. The fact *that* Browne explored relations between faith and charity is not surprising, given the religious culture of the 1630s; what his residence in Halifax and friendship with the Powers, Mitchells, and Waterhouses help to explain are the intensity with which he envisioned charity as an extension of faith, and the complexity with which he subjected charity to analysis.

1. HALIFAX AND SHIBDEN HALL

Despite F. L. Huntley's influential resistance to the evidence in its favor, there is little if any question that Browne wrote *Religio Medici* in Halifax.[1] The legend that

[1] Patrides, *The Major Works*, 97; for an example of influence, see 60 n.5.

he had done so began as early as 1708, when Samuel Midgley inserted into his book on the town's famous "Gibbet-law" this aside: "I cannot forbear adding the learned Dr. Brown . . . because in his Juvinal Years, he fixed himself in the Populous, and rich Trading Place, wherein to shew his Skill, and gain Respect in the World: And that during his Residence amongst us, and in his vacant Hours he writ his admired Peice, called by him *Religio Medici*." As Trevor Hughes points out, Midgley's birth around 1630 indicates that "he was recollecting events in Halifax, when he was a child."[2] Just a few years later in 1712, the Reverend Thomas Wright confirmed Midgley's claim and added a key piece of information about Browne's residence in Halifax: "Neither must I omit in this Place Sir Thomas Browne, Doctor of Physick, who, tho' born in London, October 19, 1605, yet practis'd here as a Physician in his younger Years. About the year 1630, he lived in Shibden Hall, nigh Halifax, at which time he wrote that excellent Piece, intitled *Religio Medici*."[3] Browne himself dated the composition of the *Religio* to the years around 1634–35, so Wright's approximation of the date—"about the year"—is accurate. The striking piece of added information is the identification of Shibden Hall as the house in which Browne lived. (See Figure 7.1.)

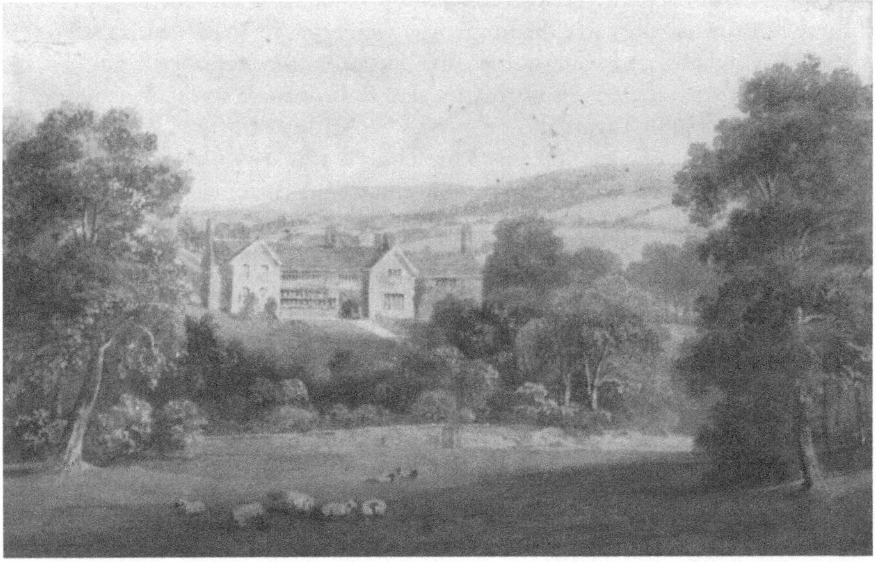

Figure 7.1 Shibden Hall, by John Horner. Reproduced with the permission of the Calderdale MBC Museums, Halifax, West Yorkshire.

[2] Samuel Midgley, *Halifax and its Gibbet-Law Placed in a True Light* (London, 1708), 88–9. J. Trevor Hughes's essay, "Sir Thomas Browne, Shibden Dale and the Writing of *Religio Medici*," was first published in *Yorkshire History Quarterly* 5 (2000), 89–94; now it is included in J. Trevor Hughes, *Essays in Medical Biography* (Oxford: Rimes House, 2008), 40–50. See also Bryan Dale, "Shibden Dale and Sir Thomas Browne's *Religio Medici*," *Bradford Antiquary* 1 (1896), 45–57.

[3] Thomas Wright, *The Antiquities of the Town of Halifax in Yorkshire* (Leeds, 1738), 132.

The most conclusive evidence for Browne's residence in Halifax derives, however, from Browne himself. Not only was he the cultural hero and vocational model for Henry Power, a Halifax adolescent during the years of Browne's stay; but in the letters passed between Power and Browne from 1646 through 1659, the two men certify that Browne was friendly with several Halifax families whose collective acquaintance he had no other way of making aside from residence in their town. "Our Towne can furnish you with very small news," Power wrote in June 1646, "only the death of some of your acquaintance, vz. Mr Waterhouse & Mr Sam. Mitchell." In the same letter, Power enclosed a note from his father-in-law, that is, his stepfather, Anthony Foxcroft; in a letter from 1648, Power added that "My Father Foxcroft & Mother in their last to Cambridge forgott not to tender their best respects to you." In 1658, Henry Power sent to Browne "3 old Spanish Bookes I have found of my Fathers," with this reason noted concerning Henry's father John: "I have presumd to send them to you, hoping they will be entertain'd (if not for their own) yet for his sake that formerly ought them, who I am sure was one that did much honour you." In 1659, Browne confirmed "the delight I have formerly had by many serious discourses with my old friend your good father, whose memorie is still fresh with mee, & becomes more delightfull by this great enjoyment I have from his true & worthy sonne."[4] Aside from a residence in Halifax, nothing in Browne's life can explain the friendship that he shared with the Powers, Foxcrofts, Mitchells, and Waterhouses. In addition to the correspondence between Power and Browne, there is also the letter sent to Browne from Halifax apothecary and antiquarian John Brearcliffe on August 24, 1669. In this letter, Brearcliffe presents a catalogue of ancient coins to his fellow antiquary with instructions about how to indicate which ones Browne would like. The document clarifies that the two men have exchanged letters in the past, and both its address and salutation refer to Browne as a friend.[5] Having been baptized in August of 1618, Brearcliffe would have been at just the right age during Browne's stay in Halifax to be impressed (as was young Henry Power) by the intellect and learning of the new physician.[6]

If it is obvious that Browne would seek a place *like* Halifax for his three years of unofficial practice—a town both busy and remote, with patients aplenty but with a minimum of institutional policing—it still remains to venture some sense of why Browne opted for Halifax in particular. According to John Favour (1556/7–1624), who was a Winchester and Oxford graduate like Browne, a relative by marriage of the Powers, and the parish minister in Halifax, the town desperately needed physicians: in addition to his ministry, Favour lamented in 1619, he was obliged to undertake medical services, "in the great penurie and necessitie thereof in the

[4] Keynes, 4.255–70. [5] MS Rawlinson D.391, 77r–78r.

[6] For Brearcliffe, see Walter James Walker, *Chapters on the Early Registers of Halifax Parish Church* (Halifax: Whitley & Booth, 1885), 98; and T. W. Hanson, "John Brearcliffe, the Antiquary," in *Transactions of the Halifax Antiquarian Society* 1908, 321–48. Thoresby spoke of him as "that industrious (and which is infinitely better) religious antiquary" (MS HAS/B/22/27, West Yorkshire Archive, Calderdale Branch, v).

countrey where I liue."[7] The dire need for physicians was driven home by recent bouts of plague in the outskirts, as near as Heptonstall and Ovenden in 1631.[8] Indeed a monument in the church from 1629 evoked the need for medical help, for Brearcliffe's wife, their son Favour, and an infant still in its mother's womb were buried together in one grave. John Favour had tried to ensure medical care for his people after his death, for "in his will he left Edmond Brearcliffe 'Barowe's Phisicke in Englishe.' "[9] But this was hardly a substitute for a trained doctor; Raach's directory of country physicians lists none in Halifax.[10]

It is possible that Browne's key connection to Halifax was Sir Arthur Ingram, a businessman with ties to Browne's London world as well as to West Yorkshire. Commerce between Halifax and London was always strong in this period; indeed, the accounts of the Ishams, key players in the Mercers' Company, clarify just how interactive the two regions were.[11] In the 1630s, Ingram had the greatest influence among the multitude of connections between the Halifax and London areas by virtue of the trade in cloth. In the London of Browne's youth, Arthur Ingram (born before 1571, died 1642) was prominent in the business community as a moneylender, customs officer, and partner of Lionel Cranfield, the powerful merchant and Jacobean officer of the crown against whom Browne's father had run for office in the Mercers' Company back in 1612–13. He may have been Browne's kinsman, for his first wife was Susan, "the daughter of Richard Brown(e) of London."[12] By the time of Thomas Browne's return from the Continent in 1634, Sir Arthur had accrued powerful connections in both Ireland (where Browne's mother and stepfather resided) and the Halifax area.[13] For a brief time, Ingram was the owner of Shibden Hall and had dealings with the Waterhouses and John Power. Later in life, on several occasions, Browne would speak of Sir Arthur's son and heir, also Sir Arthur, with fondness.[14]

Even those scholars inclined to accept that Browne lived in Halifax have been largely skeptical of the claim that he resided at Shibden Hall, and they have gone in search of more remote halls, Upper and Lower Shibden Halls, in Shibden Dale. This search for a house other than the main hall just a mile or so up the hill from Halifax has been motivated by the assumption either that the young doctor would have lived alone or that there was insufficient room for him in the main Hall. But Browne was accustomed to living as a lodger under someone else's roof, and a simple plan of Shibden Hall clarifies that there was ample room for a visiting doctor

[7] Favour, *Antiquitie Triumphing ouer Noueltie* (1619), A5r, address to the reader.

[8] Hugh P. Kendall, "The Plague in Halifax Parish," *Halifax Antiquarian Society* (1931), 3–26.

[9] E. W. Crossley, *The Monumental and Other Inscriptions in Halifax Parish Church* (Leeds: John Whitehead, 1909), 3.

[10] John A. Raach, *A Directory of English Country Physicians, 1603–1643* (London: Dawsons, 1962), 127–8.

[11] Martha J. Ellis François, "A Study in the Manorial History of Halifax Parish in the Sixteenth and Early Seventeenth Centuries," *The Yorkshire Archaelogical Journal* 40 (1961), 250–64; 420–42, here 264–5.

[12] See Simon Healy's entry on Sir Arthur Ingram, *ODNB*.

[13] J. T. Cliffe, *The Yorkshire Gentry: From the Reformation to the Civil War* (London: Athlone Press, 1969), 95.

[14] Keynes, 4.127, 152, 155, 164–5.

and even a study in which he might write. Of the prevailing "H" design of gentry houses in West Yorkshire, it has been noted that, "[j]ust at the time when the diverse elements of the earlier dwellings—hall, chambers, service rooms and so forth—were coalescing into a single block, the constituent parts of the household were drawing apart, each to be provided with more specialist accommodation according to status and function."[15] The tendency in these houses toward the multiplication of parlors serviceable as bedrooms produced ample room and flexibility for a tenant in a house such as Shibden.[16] And the hall was not without fanciful decoration: in the most social rooms of the ground floor, the windows depicted quaint figures such as a bird on a dulcimer, a bird with a wheelbarrow, owls (associated with the Savile family), black pyramids (a Waterhouse image), and a faun, but also a banner with the Waterhouse motto, "Veritas liberabit" ("the truth will set you free").[17] This emphasis on the liberating power of truth was a daily exhortation to an author who would pursue the liberty of philosophizing in his meditations on religion.

Although the hall had changed hands several times in the first years of the century, passing from the Waterhouses to Sir Arthur Ingram in 1608/9, then back again to the Waterhouses, the Hemingway family had purchased the home in 1612/13. By way of a marriage between Thomas Lister and Sybil Hemingway in 1619, the house passed into the Lister family until the nineteenth century. In 1632, upon the death of his father, Samuel Lister, a clothier who was the tenant of Shibden Hall, Thomas (1599–1677) took full possession of the hall. Like John Power, Thomas was employed in the cloth trade; also like Power, he had a son (Samuel, born in 1622/3) who would become a physician. His brother John Lister, who married the sister of Sybil Hemingway, was an apothecary living in Upper Brea. Thomas was a graduate of University College, Oxford so he was no stranger to learning. In short, Browne may not have had many books in Halifax but he had civil and, as it proved, stimulating companionship.

The social context of Halifax played a seminal role in provoking the complex meditations on social virtues, especially charity, in *Religio Medici*. Inextricable from this social dynamic was the cohabitation of potentially conflicting strains in Halifax Protestantism: on the one hand was the local vitality of ancient customs such as maying and rushbearing;[18] on the other were the social engineering and a brand of piety that polemicists would label "Puritan." The marriage between these increasingly hostile tendencies in English religion and social identity served as a crucial foundation for the similar union in *Religio Medici*.

In the 1630s, the Halifax area was still very much under the influence of its most forceful clergyman, John Favour, whose enforcement of strict moral discipline,

[15] *Rural Houses of West Yorkshire, 1400–1830* (London: HMSO, 1986), 7.

[16] John Lister, "History of Shibden Hall," *Halifax Antiquarian Society* (1926), 6.

[17] Lister, "History of Shibden Hall," facing 132.

[18] M. W. Garside, "The Social History of Halifax in the Seventeenth Century," *Transactions of the Halifax Antiquarian Society* 1923, 65–99.

avid commitment to charitable institutions, and encouragement of godly ministers were at once powerful unifiers of his parishioners and an impetus for the area's own strong penchant for independence. Of particular pertinence to the exploration of religious identity in *Religio Medici* was the fact that Halifax parish church of St John the Baptist in town was supplemented by chapelries throughout the outlying areas, in which ministers "enjoyed a great deal of freedom, for they had the right of baptism, marriage, and burial, free from the jurisdiction of the parish vicar."[19] For Browne, the combination of a deeply felt unity of purpose, together with religious tendencies toward individualism, stimulated his meditations on potentially competing Christian priorities—uniformity as against singularity—but also on the social virtues that in Halifax both resulted from and counterbalanced a zealous and scripturally centered piety.

In Halifax proper, the 1630s proved a period in which godly, word-centered ministry and Laudian reform were for the most part synthesized. In the parish church, Henry Ramsden transported Favour's godly legacy from 1629 through 1638. Testimonials to his memory are highly favorable: according to Anthony Wood, Ramsden "had advanced himself much in the theological faculty" at Lincoln prior to his move to London, where he was "much resorted to for his edifying and puritanical sermons."[20] According to his monument, Ramsden was

> a person well known for his learning and probity, the ornament of letters and an exemplar of piety, faithful in the discharge of his function and particularly attentive to the Church's interest for near eight years, exemplary in life and conversation, a zealous defender of the poor, a strenuous assertor of peace, a ready yet impartial dispenser of public Justice, and a principal promoter of the political order and good government of this place.[21]

The fact that he married into the Foxcroft family in June 1630 brings him still closer into the circle of Browne's friends and acquaintances.[22] And from his *A Gleaning in Gods Harvest* (published 1639), comprising four sermons preached in London in the mid-1620s, we find an emphasis on Christian mortification that would have helped to keep Halifax parish relatively free of contention in the 1630s. As the new physician in the parish as well as the author of *Religio Medici*, Browne had much to approve in Ramsden's arresting similes drawn from natural philosophy and the frequent analogies between medicine and mortification.[23] Ramsden's non-partisan tendencies suggest a wider truth about the patterns of religion in Halifax parish during Browne's stay, namely, that a tradition of a fervently godly

[19] Martha J. Ellis François, "The Social and Economic Development of Halifax, 1558–1640," *Proceedings of the Leeds Philosophical and Literary Society* 11 (1966), 217–60; at 217–18. See also William and Sarah Sheils, "Textiles and Reform: Halifax and its Hinterland," in Patrick Collinson and John Craig, eds., *The Reformation in English Towns, 1500–1640* (New York: St Martins, 1998), 130–43.

[20] See Ronald A. Marchant, *The Puritans and the Church Courts in the Diocese of York, 1560–1642* (London: Longmans, 1960), 270; and J. Horsfall Turner, *Biographia Halifaxiensis* (Bingley, 1883), 117.

[21] So says the monument erected by his brother, quoted in *The History of the Town and Parish of Halifax*, 236.

[22] Crossley, *The Monumental and Other Inscriptions in Halifax Parish Church*, 32.

[23] Ramsden, *A Gleaning in Gods Harvest* (1639), 136, 145, 153, 169.

religion need not entail a discord with the rites and decencies of the Church of England, and that this could be the case even in a period when Charles and Laud were alienating the godly with their heightening of ceremony. What is more, records from the 1630s suggest that when it came to reforms such as the physical reparation and ordering of churches, Halifax parish was ready and willing to comply.[24] For Browne, who would project his religious profile as a hybrid of Puritan and Laudian orientations in *Religio Medici*, Halifax's independence from contemporary partisanship afforded a vivid, compelling model.

Any claim that Halifax might make on its status as an extraordinary social and religious unit was heightened by the fact that Browne's contemporaries were apt to stress the remoteness of Halifax, which one early historian characterized as conducive to melancholy.[25] The isolation of the parish was underscored not just by the nearby moors but also by the steepness of the hill that separated the town from parts eastward—several seventeenth-century travelers noted its treachery for navigation; and this sense of isolation was intensified by the area's reputation for the infertility of the land. In a letter to Browne, Henry Power himself remarked on how difficult it was to locate plants within "the barrennesse of our soile" (Keynes, 4.265). Halifax, in short, was no Montpellier. The typical citizen's response to this topography—that industry converts a barren land into fertility—was central to Halifax's contemporary reputation; it corroborated Browne's experiences in Leiden but also contributed to his own conception of intellectual and vocational labor, through which any error or deformity might be transformed into progress, health, and wonder.[26] In its ratio of industry to natural fertility, Halifax struck its observers much as the United Provinces did. For early modern observers, there was something almost miraculous about the prosperity and productivity won *ex nihilo.*

From the beginning, Browne's *Religio* is profoundly concerned with questions of how an affection for ceremony, sacrament, and the beauty of holiness might be reconciled with a word- and sermon-centered spirituality. During his period of residence in Halifax, national trends hardly made this reconciliation an easy achievement. Indeed, as Browne was reaching the conclusion that English godliness would not prosper if it forced people to take sides, the leading citizens in Halifax found themselves contributing to the strangest of disagreements in the 1630s, over that theological virtue, charity, that was supposed to unite all Christians to one another as well as each to God.

2. THE PROBLEM OF CHARITY

What clinched the pertinence of Halifax to *Religio Medici* was the fact that Browne's friends were directly and complexly involved in an extraordinary program of social,

[24] Copies of the Halifax church warden account books, West Yorkshire Archives, Calderdale branch.

[25] William Bentley and Samuel Midgley, *The History of the Town and Parish of Halifax* (1789), 92.

[26] Lister, "History of Shibden Hall" (1923), 107. See also D. Taylor, "Annals of the Parish of Halifax," *Halifax Antiquarian Society* (1972), 109.

putatively charitable, engineering. The local dilemma of defining and instituting charity centered on the chartering in 1635 of the Waterhouse workhouse. Although the workhouse was up and running prior to this year, it was in 1635 that Nathaniel Waterhouse received a royal patent for its institution and control, established its officers, and solidified its modus operandi. The Letters Patent from Charles also reflected the sense of economic crisis to which the workhouse was a response:

> [For] we are given to understand, that the said town of Halifax... is now of late much impoverished, and like to be ruined, by reason of the great multitude of poor people there daily increasing, which hath occasioned many able men within the said town and parish to remove from thence to other places, being oppressed with the heavy burden of the assessments towards the maintenance of the poor within the said parish.[27]

In short, the workhouse was meant to ease the burdens of charity, as well to regulate the morality or orderliness of the town with its immigrant or "stranger" population.

Concerned about what Browne would call with "no breach of Charity" the "great enemy of reason, vertue, and religion, the multitude" (Patrides, 134), Waterhouse aimed his workhouse at ameliorating two problems: poverty and vagrancy.[28] Life in the workhouse was anything but easy. Its work days were long, from five or six in the morning to eight or nine at night with two short breaks for meals, and with the work itself often involving the processing of wool. And the workhouse resembled penal institutions of correction as much as it did almshouses, if not more so, not least since it aimed to quash vagrancy and the vices that putatively accompanied it. To punish transgressions among its laborers, the workhouse used corporal punishment on a regular basis. During Browne's residence, for instance, on December 9, 1635, "It was ordered that Thomas Pearson and Widow Pauldin of Halifax, should be whipped in the Workhouse for begging, and that the wife of Thomas Hold should be whipped for giving Francis Hoylwell a stroke on her ear and felling her to the ground and calling Alice Barraclough names." In July 1636 one Susan Brooksbank was made to toil in the workhouse for desiring that "the Workhouse were on fire and all that is in it, for there were none that belonged to it but bankrupts." One woman was whipped in 1637 for threatening to "hang herself and make such work in the Workhouse on the next Tuesday at night as never was there made"—for the apparent reason that she wanted a fire for warmth against the winter cold.[29]

Halifax records show that the problem of poverty gained a new prominence in the 1630s. Thus the need for institutions of charity was keenly felt, but so too was concern for inventive, equitable, and socially useful solutions to the problem of poverty that, as Browne reminded readers of *Religio Medici*, Jesus had pronounced

[27] Quoted in *The History of the Town and Parish of Halifax*, 163.

[28] T. W. Hanson, "Nathaniel Waterhouse, Great Halifax Benefactor," *Halifax Antiquarian Society* (1919), 73–104; see 104.

[29] T. W. Hanson, "Minutes of Halifax Workhouse," *Halifax Antiquarian Society* (1921), 77–96, see 82–3, 85.

insoluble. This heightened awareness of poverty brought with it a commitment to the establishment of modern institutions for helping the needy, a challenge unleashed by the disestablishment of medieval ecclesiastical vehicles of charity. In this context too, the conception of who was principally responsible for charity fundamentally shifted to the laity in cooperation with the ministry.[30] Here then was the social version of the shift from clerical to lay authority in matters of charity as well as faith that characterized the interpretive work of the *Religio Medici* itself.

The complications and tensions in Browne's treatment of what at first glance would seem an unimpeachable subject, charity, begin to gain in clarity when it is noted that those persons involved in the operation of the workhouse—not least Browne's friend John Power—spearheaded both the critique as well as the establishment of its institutional status and authority. Early on, manorial authorities expressed uncertainty about what to make of the workhouse, for its corporation "was a new authority in the same field and the new governors were not quite certain as to their powers and the relation of their privileges and duties to those of the West Riding Justices."[31] Clarification of authority required a determination of who was, and who was not, a ruffian, for instance in the recognition that given the "power of any Governor to search for ruffians, vagabonds and sturdy beggars," nevertheless the designation of "vagrants and suspicious persons is not to be understood of men of ability, albeit they be for the present, disorderly, but are to be compounded of such as have not whereon to live and are declared vagabonds."[32] In his own way, Browne would also devote sections of *Religio Medici* to sorting out who might qualify as the "rabble" as well as the characteristics and motives of the beggar.

Not every member of Browne's social circle in Halifax was pleased with Waterhouse's new institution and its formulation of charitable obligations. Instead, the workhouse was a controversial institution among the town leaders in Browne's social circle. Its first officers in 1635 were friends of Browne, including John Power, Anthony Foxcroft, and Samuel Mitchell. The master of Shibden Hall, Thomas Lister, also appears on the list of governors. Foxcroft was the man who had married Henry Power's widowed mother and, with her, had lived in Upper Shibden Hall up the valley until official duties took him to Halifax. Foxcroft's involvement in local charitable initiatives was hardly unimpeachable. Having been put in charge of the Brian Crowther Charity established in 1606 on behalf of the poor, he was found around 1631 to have been remiss in his oversight of the fund. But other civic leaders, including John Power, resisted the onerous burdens of governing the workhouse. On September 29, 1637, chosen Master of the Workhouse, Power offered twenty, then thirty pounds to be excused from this office until he finally served for a brief time before his death in 1638.[33] Indeed, as early as December 21, 1635, the

[30] W. K. Jordan, *The Charities of Rural England, 1480–1660* (New York: Russell Sage Foundation, 1962), 236.

[31] T. W. Hanson, "Minutes of Halifax Workhouse," 86.

[32] T. W. Hanson, "Minutes of Halifax Workhouse," 88.

[33] Additional MS 31021, 7r, British Library. John Power was buried in May 1638.

controversy over the new institution was underway.[34] In fact, despite its royal charter in 1635, the workhouse appears enigmatically to have been dissolved or interrupted around 1639 or 1640; and despite the provision for the workhouse in Waterhouse's will (1642), there is a hiatus in its minutes from 1638 to 1682.

Whatever its problems, Waterhouse's approach to charity was built on a bold conviction that would challenge Browne's casuistic wit in *Religio Medici*, namely that "particularly among the powerful and venturesome mercantile aristocracy," the problem of "poverty must be more boldly assailed by raising up institutions for its prevention" (Jordan, 282). In the *Religio*, Browne suggested that such a simplistic preventive ideal might be worse than impossible—that it might in fact subvert the moral utility and spiritual depth of genuine charity. All in all, the Waterhouse workhouse and its social implications provide an immediate framework and an aggressive provocation for the meditation on charity, friendship, the social order, and obligation that we find in the second part of the *Religio*.

Local debates about the workhouse were intensified by the fact that as Halifax church records show, the citizens were far less concerned about the orthodoxy of the chaplains than they were about the unruliness of the congregants, sometimes children (or dogs—one parish office was "dog-whipper"), but often enough civic leaders and church wardens. By all accounts, Halifax parish was unruly even if it was officially conformable. In 1634, John Murgatroyd provoked a "brawl about precedence in his local chapel." In 1635 two church wardens "began an argument during morning service in Halifax Parish Church," with one bidding a "turd in [the] teeth" of the other until "the two men fell out of the pew threshing and brawliong in full view of the congregation," only to be chastised by vicar Ramsden. Fornication, including public acts of it, was commonplace in the Halifax records of the 1630s.[35] As was the case with Browne in *Religio Medici*, local authorities—Browne's friends among them—had to figure out how festivity, moral discipline, and punishment should interact in a Christian society. Clearly Browne had occasion to develop the disregard for the rabble that modifies his enthusiasm for charity in *Religio Medici*. In Caroline Halifax, a reconsideration of the criteria of charity was at once urgent, aggressive, and contentious.

The controversy in Halifax over the promotion of charity drew from national as well as distinctly local causes. Browne's residence in Halifax situated him within a provincial circle at once affected by and autonomous of King Charles's own attempts to redress poverty and to reassert the supreme value of charity. In this context, Browne began his spiritual accounting with the insistence that charity always accompany faith, then once he had turned in the later paragraphs to focus on charity, found that its very conception, let alone its implementation, proved as strangely complex as his profession of faith.

[34] Quoted in *The History of the Town and Parish of Halifax*, 183.

[35] J. Addy, "The Uncontrollable and Ungovernable Parish of Halifax in the Seventeenth Century," *Transactions of the Halifax Antiquarian Society* (1993), 37–40. For the churchwardens' accounts, see J. W. Houseman, "Notes and Comments on Halifax Churchwardens' Accounts, 1620–1714," *Transactions of the Halifax Antiquarian Society* (1925), 137–67.

From the very beginning, the Reformation itself had entailed a major revision of charity. After all, Protestants undercut the redemptive value of works, disestablished the clerical vehicles of charitable actions, and ridiculed the medieval ideal of voluntary poverty and begging, yet they emphasized the obligation of each and every lay person to live with godly discipline and to manifest inner faith in a strong commitment to loving one's neighbors and to improving the Christian commonwealth for the sake of God alone.[36] In the wake of the Elizabethan statutes governing vagrancy and poor relief, English communities in the first quarter of the seventeenth century were charged with applying, interpreting, and adapting those laws to suit local conditions and needs. In this regard, it is worth remembering that Shibden Hall included its own workshop where presumably the able-bodied poor might be employed.

A very practical concern in the reinvention of charity involved the question of which approach to poverty was more efficacious: the creation of institutions such as the workhouse or a centralized collection of poor rates. Browne's Halifax was busily juggling both vehicles of charity. But Halifax was also faced with royal intervention in the implementation of charity so that what might seem a simple Christian virtue steadily grew more complicated, not just on the matters of defining and instituting charity but on conflicts over authority that overlapped with similar questions in regard to faith. At long last, who was divinely charged with making the fallen world more charitable? In January 1631, Charles I had intervened in poor relief by releasing his *Orders and Directions* so that the years of Personal Rule offered a singularly aggressive and comprehensive approach to supplying work for the unemployed and for "looking after the more needy classes when they were suffering from the effects of fire, pestilence and famine."[37] In the 1630s, however, the status of charity in England's Christian commonwealth also figured centrally in polemic—not simply in the longstanding rift between Catholic and Protestant but also in the widening division between partisans within the Church of England itself, especially those accusing one another of "Puritanism" and "Arminianism." It was just such polemic that prompted the strenuous attempts made by writers such as William Chillingworth and Browne himself to salve the wound in the ecclesiastical body. From the "Puritan" vantage, the courtly and Laudian affection for charity as against zealous faith was a dangerous pretense covering the suppression of the very spiritual strength and scriptural focus that could produce a genuinely loving society. From the vantage point of Laudian and Caroline regulation in the 1630s, the "Puritans" were identified as the chief opponents to charity, a theological virtue whose primacy they had traded for an obsession with their own "puffed-up" zeal and knowledge.

[36] For this difficult issue, see Ole Peter Grell and Andrew Cunningham, eds., *Health Care and Poor Relief in Protestant Europe, 1500–1700* (New York: Routledge, 1997), especially the introduction by the two editors and the essay by Grell. The quotation appears in the introduction on p. 3.

[37] E. M. Leonard, *The Early History of English Poor Relief* (Cambridge: Cambridge University Press, 1900), 132.

For both Browne and Chillingworth, the genuineness of charity depended on a flexibility and resourcefulness in English orthodoxy. In the polemical print culture of England in the 1630s, however, Laudian and Puritan visions of social policy simply came apart. For their part, the Laudians repudiated lay agency for the ascendancy of the priesthood; rejected zealous Puritan reform as dangerous apocalyptic restlessness; and stressed ceremony and liturgy on behalf of order at the expense of a driving reformist energy, even going so far as to deny the value of educating the poor, and decrying Puritan reform as the folly of "dreaming of Plato's commonwealth…In the pride of their hearts, [they] imagine themselves to be rather kings reigning with God in heaven, than men living among men on earth."[38] These trends help to account for Browne's own anti-reformist critiques in the *Religio*—for his insistence, for example, that the poor are always with us and that it is impious to nullify the state of poverty—and for his focus on the personal giving of alms as against the top-down thrust of social engineering. "Frequently," Margo Todd writes, "Anglican sermons which initially appear to concern themselves with poverty and benevolence turn out to be spiritualizations of the concept of charity. Donne, for example, defined charity in spiritual terms, and identified the 'best charity' as prayer" (*Christian Humanism*, 251). The same might be said of the thrust of the *Religio*'s final paragraphs, which advertise their subject as charity but have a penchant for spiritualizing, personalizing, and even evading the subject.

To make matters more difficult for Browne, the vocation of learned medicine had its own vexed relationship to charity; the costly medical practitioner was potentially at odds with the general Christian emphasis on merciful care for the sick. As Browne undertook his vocation, however, learned physicians responded to their critics by assailing competition from the putatively charitable. For instance, John Cotta "opposed the argument that a clergyman should cure the sick poor out of a sense of private, individual charity," complaining that "it is manifest that this fluctuation of these men between two callings is offensive to God, scandalous unto religion and good men, and injurious unto commonweales."[39] Whereas he worked out his faith with fear and trembling, Browne had ample reason to work out his charity with indirection and a surprisingly varied set of measures.

3. UTOPIA AND FRIENDSHIP

Crucially for understanding its imaginative power, the social engineering found in Halifax was already the stuff of legends by the time Browne reached the town in the 1630s. From the vantage point of such popular authors as John Taylor the Water Poet, Halifax had a singular fashion of dealing with petty crime on behalf of

[38] The words of Laudian John Carpenter, quoted in Margo Todd, *Christian Humanism and the Puritan Social Order* (Cambridge: Cambridge University Press, 1987), 234.

[39] See Andrew Wear, "Religious Beliefs and Medicine in Early Modern England," in Hilary Marland and Margaret Pelling, eds., *The Task of Healing: Medicine, Religion and Gender in England and the Netherlands, 1450–1800* (Rotterdam: Erasmus Publishing, 1996), 145–69, quotations at 163.

commerce, namely, its infamous "gibbet law," according to which a thief of "any commodity, of the value of thirteen pence halfpenny" would summarily "be taken to the gibbet" on the west side of town "and there have his head cut from his body."[40] Having explained the mechanism of the gibbet, Taylor informed his reader that with the stolen goods brought to the place of execution, the victim of the robbery had a choice of whether to cut the rope: if he chose to do so, then the victim recovered his goods; if not, then the stolen goods would be put to charitable purposes.[41] (See Figure 7.2.) This law and the machine that implemented it were the

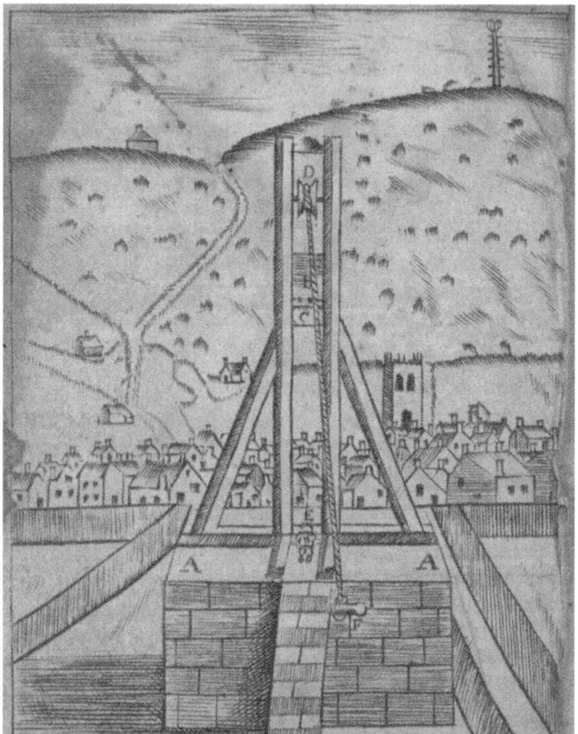

Figure 7.2 Gibbet machine, from William Bentley and Samuel Midgley, *History of the Famous Town of Hallifax in Yorkshire* (1712). Reproduced with the permission of the Harry Ransom Humanities Research Center, University of Texas at Austin.

[40] John Watson, *The History and Antiquities of the Parish of Halifax, in Yorkshire* (London, 1775), 214.

[41] John Taylor, the Water Poet, *Part of this Summers Travels, or News from Hell, Hull, and Hallifax* (1639), 27–8.

stuff of proverbs and helped to turn Halifax in the early modern imagination into something of a Utopia, a distant site in which paradoxical means of social regulation and justice were exercised to the amazement, if not exactly the shame, of "normal" English society. Indeed, in 1648, a pamphlet having nothing to do with Halifax—*Halifax Law Translated to Oxon*—invoked in its title the reputation of the gibbet law as metonymy for an execution of justice without due process in a world turned upside down. The physical, linguistic, and cultural separation of Halifax from the rest of the country lent its unusual means of justice as well as its penchant for strenuous charity a provocative kind of appeal. Commentators might not completely swallow or accept the sagacious nonsense of Utopia, but they were fascinated by and even grudgingly admiring of its bold and paradoxical institutions.[42] During the 1630s, the gibbet law was an endangered custom—its last use would be in 1650. But it still symbolized the remarkably distinctive means by which the people of Halifax sought to control criminal behavior in their midst, and Browne would have had an opportunity to see it in action on May 21, 1636, when one Abraham Clegg was beheaded.[43]

In the simplest sense, Halifax presented Browne with the city-on-the-hill type of "pragmatic utopia."[44] Citing a formulation from 1630, Paul Slack explains that such godly cities were devoted to a " 'a thorough reformation,' and marked by 'their impartial uprightness in executing justice and regarding the cause of the poor.' "[45] From a recognition of Utopia's "nowhereness" arose the suspicion, Browne's included, that comprehensive social engineering and the eradication of poverty neither can nor should take place. Even more than Leiden's, however, the reformist culture of Halifax sobered Browne's meditations with the warning that a Paduan experimentation with ideas and identities might be dangerous (if also pleasing) to the sinful soul. Whereas one of Browne's earliest readers—Abraham van Berckel—praised *Religio* for removing the masks of human vanity in order to "assert the principles of the incorruptible and undefiled truth" (Keynes, 4.336), it is also the case that masks and improvisations pervade the *Religio* in the sometimes ritualized framework of carnival. What makes the *Religio* such an extraordinary work is that fanciful theater interacts with sober reform in complex and dynamic ways.

Young man Browne's complex response to utopian thinking is illustrated by a remark that he makes about Stoicism in *Religio Medici*. The utopian erasure of private property had roots in the Stoic notion that the wise man is a citizen of the world. In *Utopia*, Thomas More's character Raphael locates a noteworthy example of this thinking in Lucan's declaration that "The man who has no grave

[42] James Howell, *A German Diet* (1653), 47; Thomas Fuller, *The History of the Worthies of England* (1662), 189.

[43] T. W. Hanson, "John Brearcliffe," 341.

[44] The phrase "pragmatic utopias" comes from the title of Rosemary Horrox and Sarah Rees Jones, eds., *Pragmatic Utopias: Ideals and Communities, 1200–1630* (Cambridge: Cambridge University Press, 2001).

[45] Paul Slack, *From Reformation to Improvement: Public Welfare in Early Modern England* (Oxford: Clarendon Press, 1999), 29–30, quoting Robert Jenison, *The Cities Safetie* (1630), 25, 20.

is covered by the sky."[46] When Browne quotes the same lines, he partly distances himself from this Stoic whose more radical sentiments are both powerful and threatening to him: "I am not yet so Cynicall, as to approve the Testament of *Diogenes*, nor doe I altogether allow that *Rodomontado* of Lucan; Cœlo tegitur, qui non habet urnam. | He that unburied lies wants not his Herse, | For unto him a tombe's the Universe" (Patrides, 111–12). When, toward the end of the *Religio*, he mixed together the "sovereign amity" of his truly affectionate friendship with the liberation of reason in dreams, Browne compared this quasi-transcendent status to kingship without a crown or wealth without money—the paradoxes of a Stoic wisdom.[47] Both Stoicism and the Pythagorean/Platonic all-things-in-common motif are central to More's construction of his *Utopia* as a paradoxical encomium: praise of nowhere is also, by contemporary standards, a praise of folly. So too Browne's offer to praise the religion of a physician qualifies as a mock encomium in which play and seriousness are inextricably bound together. The method of this paradox shares something with Venetian carnival: it uses inversions—Browne's self-identified tendency—but also improvisations, masked personae, and playful parody. But its ultimate goal is strikingly different: whether properly true or false in itself, paradox seeks to alarm the reader into a new awareness that leads to the reformist transformation of the social order. Returning to England from Padua by way of Leiden, Browne confronted a contrast between carnival and Utopia: the traveler might experience carnival as an occasion for the expansion and liberty of identity and thought within restraining structures that assume the natural valence of seasons or cycles and the Christian-cum-civic warrant of ritual. Yet paradoxical and pragmatic Utopia was committed radically to recasting those structures, subverting those rites, and transforming presuppositions for good, so that human life can be maximally peaceful and fruitful thanks to social disciplining.[48]

Browne's characterization of the setting for the *Religio*, a place without books, resembles Erasmus's claim that the *Praise of Folly* was a *jeu d'esprit* that he tossed off without the aid of a library.[49] But the utopian character of Halifax frames more seriously the high premium that Browne places on friendship in his meditations, in an erotically charged embrace of the ancient adage that friends hold all things in common. While nowhere near to the outright communism of More's fiction, Browne's friendship is deeply embedded in what Kathy Eden has identified as humanism's chief presupposition about the content and method of learning by way of commonplaces and proverbs. Erasmus features the maxim in his *Adages*,

[46] Sir Thomas More, *Utopia*, ed. and trans. Robert M. Adams, 2nd edition (New York: Norton, 1992), 5.

[47] Laurie Shannon, *Sovereign Amity: Figures of Friendship in Shakespearean Contexts* (Chicago: University of Chicago Press: 2002), 225.

[48] Cf. Christopher Kendrick, *Utopia, Carnival, and Commonwealth in Renaissance England* (Toronto: University of Toronto Press, 2004), 86. Browne's library included a copy of the 1629 Amsterdam edition of More's *Utopia*, perhaps suggestive of his engagement with that text in the years of his travels abroad.

[49] Letter to Martin Dorp, printed in *The Praise of Folly*, trans. and ed. Clarence Miller (New Haven, CT: Yale University Press 1979), 144.

and his generation of humanists treasures its ancient legacy in Pythagoras, Plato, and Christ, according to whom community was "rooted in likemindedness."[50] When Browne identifies his attitude toward learning as a treasury to be shared rather than a prize over which he contends and whose riches he seeks to hoard, he frames this view of scholarship in the context of charity and friendship. It is an attitude that Erasmus and More also locate in the most brotherly and pious of the early Christian communities, with its supreme embodiment in the trinity, whose mysterious commonality Browne analogizes to friendship.[51] Whereas idealized friendship of the kind celebrated in the *Religio* might threaten to subvert obligations to parents, spouses, or children, at its noblest it could also be taken as a spiritual marriage that epitomized all the worthy bonds in the godhead, cosmos, and social fabric alike. For staunch defenders of ceremonialism in the Church of England, friendship offered a synecdoche of the ties that bound the visible church as well as the natural world together in a divinely approved peace and harmony. In *Religio*, Browne explicitly compared friendship to the spiritual mysteries of incarnation and the trinity, suggesting that friendship resembles ritual in its capacity to unite heaven and earth, devotion and epistle, universality and singularity, solitude and civility, pensiveness and mirth, spiritual depth and convention. Yet once again Halifax was independent in nurturing a homosocial ethos that endured at least until the early nineteenth century.[52]

Browne's letters to Henry Power suggest that Henry's father John was the friend to whom *Religio Medici* was originally addressed. Information is scarce on John Power.[53] Unlike the elder sons in his family who pursued a vocation in the clergy, younger son John opted for a career in trade. Having married Jane Jennings, he lived with his wife for a period in Annesley, Nottinghamshire.[54] He had some connection with Spanish trade—he was called the "Spanish merchant"—a fact that helps to explain the Spanish books that his son Henry mailed to Browne. A record of his daughter Ellen's birth in 1624 lists him as a gentleman; no record remains of Henry's birth, though Hughes and Adrian Johns believe that it was likely 1626.[55] With his sister married to Favour, John Power came to Halifax, acquired a great deal of property, and leased manorial mills from Sir Arthur Ingram.[56]

Power and Browne's other associates in Halifax were involved in legal controversies in the 1630s. One serious concern was the matter of ulnage, a conflict that

[50] Kathy Eden, *Friends Hold All Things in Common: Tradition, Intellectual Property, and the Adages of Erasmus* (New Haven, CT: Yale University Press, 2001), 4–5, 29, 31–3.

[51] See Eden, *Friends Hold All Things in Common*, 122–7.

[52] For Halifax parish in the history of friendship, see Alan Bray, *The Friend* (Chicago: University of Chicago Press, 2003).

[53] J. Trevor Hughes, "Henry Power (1626–1668) of New Hall, Elland and Experiments on Barometric Pressure," *Transactions of the Halifax Antiquarian Society* 10 (2002), 14–26. See 14.

[54] J. Trevor Hughes, "Dr Henry Power (1626–1668): The Medical Practice of a Halifax Physician," *Transactions of the Halifax Antiquarian Society* 11 (2003), 56–67.

[55] Hughes, "Dr Henry Power (1626–1668): The Medical Practice of a Halifax Physician," 56; and Adrian Johns, "Henry Power," *ODNB*; earlier scholars speculated that Henry had been born around 1623–24.

[56] Hughes, "Dr Henry Power (1626–1668): The Medical Practice of a Halifax Physician," 56; J. W. Clay, "Dr Henry Power, F.R.S., of New Hall," *THAS* (1937), 1–28.

involved Thomas Lister in litigation. Like ship money, which also pitted localities against the crown—Lister and other Halifax families were at odds with the Exchequer over how much ulnage or tax on woolen cloths ought to be paid. Given the recalcitrant barrenness of the Halifax landscape, the woolen industry was vital not just to basic survival but to the sustenance of faith, hope, and charity.[57] As he set out to write *Religio Medici*, Browne interacted with families for whom the woolen trade largely unified the faithful in a time of religious division.[58] In the depositions for the Exchequer, witnesses conflated the woolen industry with "true Religion" as the means to keeping them all "nourished and exercised in godly labour," with "manie poore people and their families honestly mainteyned and vertuously brought up," "a great number of impotent and aged persons relieved," and "many godlie Preachers mainteyned."[59] In 1637, Lister proved a central figure "of sturdy opposition" in the suit of thirty-seven clothiers from four parishes against the Exchequer when ulnagers seized West Yorkshire cloth on its way to London.[60] Among Browne's friends including the Powers, Waterhouses, and Listers, the old controversy over ulnage was especially urgent in the 1630s given their perception that poverty was on the rise. And Browne's friends faced other historically complex legal problems. By the time Browne reached Halifax, the apparatus of manorial rule was experiencing not just its usual jurisdictional conflicts, but considerable resistance from the everyday people who were obliged to it. John Power was in the middle of these conflicts, for he was an agent of Sir Arthur Ingram in the matter of enforcing the manorial rule that all corn be ground in the lord's mills.[61] Power was not only intensely involved in manorial business but he lived in the new Multure Hall, built in 1631 and named for the exaction measured by the "multure dish" to "be taken for the grinding" of a tenant's corn.[62] Having bought the Multure Hall in 1633, John Power worked as an agent of the manor for which he was supposed to mediate conflicts over rights at the mills.[63]

When the new physician Thomas Browne called on John Power, it was then the 1631 Multure Hall that welcomed him, but also a close friend whose own vocational, social, and legal obligations were under pressure. As a lovely in-town estate with a virtually pastoral refuge from the commerce of Halifax, the hall provided an ideal setting for the "many serious discourses" that Browne recalled so many years later. As the eighteenth-century autobiography of Thomas Wright makes clear, the hall "stood not far from the foot of [the] mountain" that rose

[57] John Lister, *Early History of the Woollen Trade in the Parish of Halifax* (1918), unpublished typescript, HAS/B:21/40, West Calderdale Archives. Herbert Heaton, *The Yorkshire Woollen and Worsted Industries from the Earliest Times up to the Industrial Revolution*, 2nd edn (Oxford: Clarendon Press, 1965), 199.

[58] Lister, "History of Shibden Hall" (1923), 106–7.

[59] West Yorkshire Archives, Calderdale, SH:6/WO/11.

[60] Heaton, *The Yorkshire Woollen and Worsted Industries*, 199; Lister, "History of Shibden Hall" (1923), 104.

[61] Ellis, "Manorial History of Halifax Parish," 428.

[62] See the explanation in Watson, *History and Antiquities*, 104.

[63] T. W. Hanson, "The Multure Hall," *Transactions of the Halifax Antiquarian Society* (1935), 1–19; see 10.

abruptly "from the bottom of Halifax" in the direction of Shibden Hall; and its grounds included gardens and orchards.[64] A short walk from the parish church and the workhouse near Hebble Brook on the eastern boundary of the town, it was certainly an impressive hall, with "thick walls, well-formed windows, solid wooden fixtures, with here and there a few carvings, and some glorious plaster work."[65] Appealing in 1637 to the fancy in his visitors, Power added an elaborately decorated plaster ceiling to his residence, a still-surviving and beautiful example of the standard patterns from the 1630s.[66] This ceiling featured, among other designs, the fanciful images of dragons, putti or Cupids with their arrows, mermaids holding mirrors and combs, birds, stags, fish, and flora; the ceiling featured the owner's initials, I.P., in an "eight-pointed star" (Hanson, "The Multure Hall," 5). But the Multure Hall also greeted visitors with sobriety: as Browne entered this estate, he was greeted by a Latin inscription on a still-surviving door lintel from 1631, "Disce Pati": "learn by suffering," "let suffering teach you," or "learn to suffer."

In *Religio Medici*, begun as Browne was poised to turn thirty in autumn 1635, he was accounting for his faith to a friend who had wondered whether there might be some problem in reconciling medicine and religion. This same friend had been directly involved in local attempts to refashion relations among commerce, charity, and true religion. At its best, Browne's friendship might reconcile the personae of the *Religio*: the melancholy yet playful philosopher with the cheerful yet sober and dutiful physician. At its most painful, intense friendship served the critical purpose of reminding the philosopher-physician that neither an intellectual carnival nor sober discipline and reform would by itself suffice for settling accounts with God.

4. THE EARLY *RELIGIO MEDICI*

Of the eight extant manuscripts of the *Religio*, the Pembroke College, Oxford, and the Lansdowne represent the text's earliest phase.[67] Although the Lansdowne is a highly truncated version, it holds the only clue from the two of early provenance. At the top of its first folio, it refers to the author "Mr Browne," then underneath that attribution places in brackets a Greek phrase—"*syn theo*," "with God's assistance"—and a date, 1639. (See Figure 7.3.) The Greek motto is interesting for two reasons: it serves as the only "title" leading into the work, and it appears fairly regularly in the manuscripts of Henry Power. Power, of course, has no monopoly on the motto. Plato uses the phrase in a context that involves bold speech: "to say what one says with the hope that the divine powers both excuse a bold manner of speaking and

[64] Thomas Wright, *The Autobiography*, ed. Thomas Wright, grandson (London: John Russell Smith, 1864), 24–6.

[65] *Halifax Daily Courier & Guardian*, April 29, 1940.

[66] Examples can be seen in Arthur Porritt, *Halifax as It Was* (Nelson, Lancashire: Hendon, 1973), 75; Powers's ceiling is on display at the Bankfield Museum in Halifax.

[67] For the other six, see chapter 8.

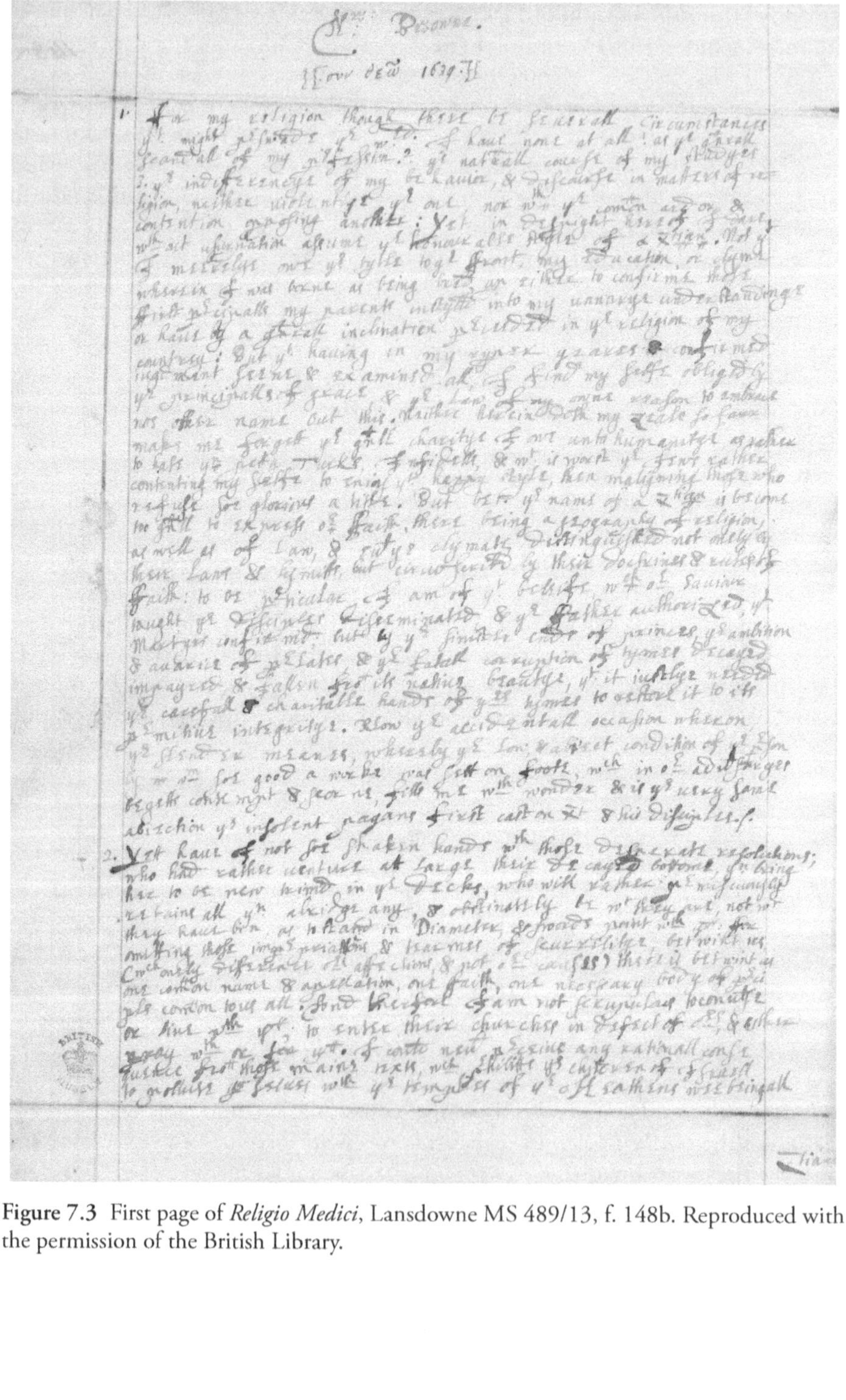

Figure 7.3 First page of *Religio Medici*, Lansdowne MS 489/13, f. 148b. Reproduced with the permission of the British Library.

ratify what is said in its best sense."[68] As a simple motto for Browne's work, however, it serves a double role, first, of articulating the key sentiment expressed graphically in the frontispiece of both the unauthorized and authorized editions of the *Religio*: of an Icarian figure who is being rescued from his precipitous fall by a hand projected from heaven. This is a bold text, and both its author and its reader need divine aid and ratification. Second, it possibly corroborates the view that the *Religio* was first generated in conversations with John Power, the father of young Henry who by 1639 was maturing into teenage and soon expressed his desire to be guided in vocation and intellect by Mr. Browne.

Arguably, the *Religio* moves back and forth between, on the one hand, Paduan concerns about heretical religion and atheism and, on the other, Yorkshire concerns with charity and friendship. This formula is of course far too simple. For one thing, the continental experiences of young man Browne included memories of friendships and presented him with great occasions to consider the sociable and charitable aspects of identity and action. For another, the eventual division of the work between two parts dealing respectively with matters of faith and matters of charity breaks down before we are finished with the very first paragraph. Over the course of the work, the author's social commitments and his spiritual or intellectual contemplations crisscross with as well as balance one another: for instance, friendship is both a vehicle for spiritual meditation and the closest human access to spiritual mysteries such as the incarnation and the trinity; the charity that exists only at the level of social action is for Browne not genuine at all, for charity begins within the devotional self and should retain its focus on the divine.

Even so, the progression from the preoccupations of Pomponazzi to the parish concerns of John Favour and Nathaniel Waterhouse is sufficiently meaningful for Browne to announce it in paragraph 40 of the Pembroke, and the division of the work into two distinctive parts underscores the shift: "Now for that other vertue of charity, without which faith is a meere notion and of noe existence," and then again when, after a discussion of physiognomy, he announces a "returne from philosophy to charity," as though the problems of philosophy amounted at this stage in his text to a digression from the main subject.[69]

Friendship and charity are united at the simplest level by what Browne calls his hereditary instinct to sympathize with all creatures and nationalities. But if the paeans to friendship are usually simple and celebratory, the treatments of charity prove far more intricate and casuistic, in keeping with controversies both local and national in the 1630s. Generally speaking, Browne argues that virtuous action is always complicated by the circumstances of motivation and performance, so much so in fact that we are compelled (he quips) to act virtuously according to moral recipe. But charity proves especially tricky. In the process of declaring his "mercifull

[68] The phrase is "sun theoi eipein"; see R. K. Sprague, ed., *The Older Sophists* (Columbia: University of South Carolina Press, 1972), 72; the Platonic dialogue is the *Theaetetus*, 151B.

[69] I quote the Pembroke manuscript from Jean-Jacques Denonain, *Une Version Primitive de Religio Medici par Sir Thomas Browne* (Publications de la Faculté d'Alger, 36, 1958), 71, 74; cited hereafter in parenthesis. I do not reproduce Denonain's fonts.

disposition and humane inclination which I borrowed from my parents," Browne briefly acknowledges the need "to regulate it to the written and prescribed lawes of Charity" (Denonain, *Une Version Primitive*, 71); but before he can comment on what those might be or whence they might derive, he returns to an anatomy of his charitable nature which recalls passages elaborating his commitment to, yet anxieties about, divine providence from the opening sections of the *Religio*. When Browne insists that he does not blame the winds for his shipwreck, it is his own nature—at once resilient and accommodating—and not divine providence that makes the difference, however. The same holds true for the specter of monstrosity which earlier tests his conviction that providential nature is always beautiful and purposeful. Whether the "Monstrosity" is "the presence of a serpent, scorpion, Lysard, or Salamander"—which does not ruffle Browne's charitable disposition—or "that great enemie of reason, vertue, and religion, the Multitude" (71)—which does, Browne's "generall and indifferent temper" is the guarantor of charity in paragraph 40, even if in paragraph one, the "indifferencie of my behaviour" might strike the multitude as atheistic.

In paragraph 41, however, Browne returns to the requirement that charity should be properly regulated by norms outside the self. Rational or natural charity is but a pale imitation—perhaps even a fraudulent substitute—for the Christian virtue which "must have other ends, motives or impulsives" (72). The workaday giving of alms proves not so simple: one is all too easily motivated by a natural pity in need of contentment or by the hunger of a fellow human being, when it is only the requirement "to fullfill and accomplish the will and command of my God" that should motivate the act. Sympathy and compassion conceal within their "bowells of pitie" the coarsest—even a "sinister and politique"—desire to ease ourselves of discomfort and to exempt ourselves from future misery, in short, to bribe God. This "erroneous course" of charity even manages to pervert Browne's beloved "Signatures" of nature, for beggars or gypsies fixate and prey upon those passersby with mercy in the lines of their physiognomy (72–3).

In paragraph 42, Browne's assessment of charity is both critical and flexible. Having argued that almsgiving alone reflects an impoverished understanding of charity, he does not recommend institutions or policies; rather, he expands the boundaries of the virtue to comprise the countless ways in which human beings "maie bee good" (74). His own preferred branch—to share his copious learning—is celebrated as the act of clothing "the nakednes of... reason." As some of Browne's earliest—and most hostile—readers complained, his meditation on charity is ironically about to lapse into some of the most self-aggrandizing and misogynistic passages in the entire text; even as he chides "such as confine them selves within that narrow principle: Charitie begins at home" (77), Browne's expansive and international disposition persists in returning home to the microcosm, in the inmost rooms of which he dwells alone.

The meditations on charity are persistently torn over the question of whether, or how much, charity should move into the self and upward to God rather than outward to humanity. Far from self-involvement, he tells us, his nature is more likely to weep at the "counterfet griefes" of an actor than at his own real and present miseries (77). In fact Browne assumes such authority in matters of an outward-looking charity that he sets about to rewrite the virtue's disposition as it encounters the competing demands of the world. For one thing, commentators have neglected the uncharitable biases of sexism and national stereotypes so rampant in a satirical age. For another, conventional wisdom has established a hierarchy of obligations—"to love our parents, wives, kinsfolkes, and then our ffriends"—that Browne is keen to invert. He negotiates with the terms of the fifth commandment in professing that "I love my friend before the nearest of my blood, even those to whom I owe the principles of life." Friendship has drawn from him "a true affection" that he has not yet bestowed "on a woman"; its emotional, intellectual, and erotic power solicits from him the language of mystery and providentialism that earlier in the text he reserved for God. Browne goes so far as to assert that true friendship involves a "mysticall" unification on the order of Christ's two natures or the hypostatical oneness of the trinity. Returning to his disregard for the multitude, Browne argues that only noble natures, not "vulgar and common constitutions," are capable of such affection, not least because it penetrates beyond the almsgiving, workhouse emphasis on the body to the soul—to its sorrows, of course, but more importantly, to "that wherein wee all place our last felicity, salvation, which though it bee not in our power to bestow t'is in our charitable and pious invocations to desire, if not to procure and further" (77–8).

This last point—that the form of charity known as true friendship takes salvation as its ultimate aim—proves a turning point for Browne. Having so recently argued that one risk of friendship is that we forget the faces of our absent friends because "they are our selves, and affection makes their lookes our owne," he pursues the goal of salvation in the other direction, toward a public scope that grows from "a catalogue of my friends" to "the fellowship of my neighbour" before widening out to mankind: "I never heare the toll of a passing bell (though in my mirth, and at Taverne) without my praiers, and best wishes for the departing soule." Not just in his cups but also in his vocation, Browne gravitates away from the province of the self into a citizenship of the world (78–9).

Over the next few paragraphs, he chastises his own onetime-restricted moral code and stresses the ongoing need for combat against oneself, for the self is infested by "a swarme of distinct essences," "contrarieties," "private and domestique enemies" and devilishness that prompts Browne to find himself in the thick of his own Battle of Lepanto, not the triumphant one of Venetian ceremony but a complicated and always pending warfare of "passion against reason, reason against faith, faith against the Devill, and my conscience against all." Venetian memories linger in the dilemmas of the soul that Paduan intellectual culture epitomizes, the world of Pomponazzi in which faith and reason stand at loggerheads, and conscience struggles to mediate the dispute only to add to its convoluted treachery. In some of the potentially most embarrassing passages of the text, Browne reels between a suicidal self-hatred that he hopes is "noe breach of charitie" and an ironic arrogance about how his humility has saved him from pride, that "mortall enemie to charitie." He invokes his continental experiences—"I have not only seen severall countries, held the nature of their climes, the geographie of their lands, but understand their severall lawes, customes, and pollities"—yet makes an apology (half-hearted, it is true) for provincialism in the plant-gathering that he did as a child in Cheapside. The restraint of this provincialism is significant, though: the "conceited" pseudo-authorities "that never looke a degree beyond their nests" are at once silly and spirited (79–81).

If Browne is at first prepared to dismiss the fruits of his travels, he suddenly embraces one famous Paduan lesson that strives to make sense of the text's contentious personae and trends, namely, the motto of Cremonini that one should show an orthodox front to the public yet think whatever one wants in the libertine skepticism of the mind. Browne's version of this motto explicitly credits the advanced travels of his life:

> [T]hough our first studies and younge endeavours maie stile us Peripatetickes, Stoicks, or Academickes, yet the solid'st heads prove allmost all at last Sceptiques, and stand like Janus in the fields of knowledge. I confes I have one common authentique philosophy I learn'd ith' schooles whereby I discourse and satisfie the reasons of other men, another more reserv'd and drawne from experience, whereby I content my owne. (81)

This declaration of private independence unites the concerns of both faith and charity, for in both cases the "schools" of respectable, conventional wisdom have tended to get things wrong.

Indeed, in the next paragraph of the Pembroke manuscript, the 48th, Browne conflates the concerns of both faith and charity and resists their enemies together. First comes the specter of monstrosity in nature: Browne's potentially uncharitable distaste for heterosexuality sends him penitently recoiling into celebration of beauty that ranges from the painting of a horse through music—including "vulgar and Taverne Musique," church music, and the music of the spheres—all in a reprisal of his earlier theme, the hieroglyphics of nature, or "an Hieroglyphicall and shadowed lesson of the whole world and the creatures of God" (82–3). No atheist in his prejudice against coition, Browne also insists that he is none with regard to charity, for "I feele not in mee those sordid and unchristian desires of my profession; I doe not secretly implore and wish for plagues, rejoice at famines, revolve Ephemerides and Almanacks in expectation of Malignant aspects, fatall coniunctions and Eclipses" (83). In admitting the failures of medicine along with those of law and divinity, Browne comes close to the type of materialist orientation with which his Galen-obsessed Paduan acquaintance was so vexed, claiming not only that physical diseases can be easier to eradicate than some spiritual ones but even that "I can cure vices by physicke, when they remaine incurable by Divinitie, and they shall obey my pills, when they contemne their precepts" (84). Yet the danger evaporates in Browne's memento mori at the close of the paragraph, according to which our only "catholicke or universall remedie" is death.

This conclusion to the 48th paragraph is one of several that, in the manuscript, is followed by an "&c." The gesture toward finality is misleading, for the unfolding of Browne's intellectual, spiritual, vocational, and social horizons is open-ended, never more so, it turns out, than when it most turns inward in the final paragraphs of the Pembroke manuscript. Starting out in paragraph 49 with the leitmotif of his sun-like disposition to shine warmth on "all men" without respect to their virtues and vices, he warns against self-absorption, for inside he finds infection and the devil, "that unruly spirit that musters up those disordered motions which accompanie our sequestered imaginations" (85). Even the little bit of Spanish into which Browne translates the need for divine protection against oneself suggests his desire to keep outside himself in communication with his most immediate audience, John Power, the Spanish merchant. But the danger of friendship is that it encourages absorption in a sameness with oneself, and in paragraph 50, Browne takes us further than we have been thus far into his inmost corridors, the world of his "happie dreames." On the threshold of the deathlike experience of falling into sleep, Browne offers for the only time in the Pembroke manuscript prayerful verses to his God; upon waking, however, he laments that the liberation is over, that his memory produces only "a confused and broken tale of what hath passed" (86) with his return to the abyss of fallen experience and knowledge.

In the final three paragraphs of the Pembroke, Browne returns to the complexities of charity. In declaring the extravagance of his own liberality, he explains what he calls his "private method" of giving, which requires his greatest financial sacrifice when least he can afford it. On the one hand, this allows him to challenge "severe" Aristotelian notions of liberality and of distributive and commutative justice; on the other, it prompts a distinguishing of "authentique charity"—that New Testament variety depending on "liberall intentions and bountifull good wishes"—from the gaudier charity of those "who have built hospitals, or erected Cathedrals" (89). Browne argues from the biblical dictum that "Hee that giveth to the poore, lendeth to the Lord" comprises "more Rhetoricke in this one sentence then in a librarie of sermons." In this passage at least, the institutions of charity are far less authentic than the intuitions of godliness and common humanity that override the "scenicall and accidentall differences" between the beggar and the giver. Indeed, Halifax civic leaders might well take a lesson from Browne's claim that "Statists that labour to contrive a commonwealth without poverty doe take away the obiect of charity, soe not understanding only the commonwealth of a Christian, but forgeting the prophesie of Christ" (89–90). But the reminder that the poor will always be with us gives way to an "&c." and in the last paragraphs, Browne returns to the private priorities of his affections according to which true friends are conduits to the divine while all other obligations—those to parents, spouse, children—prove "all dumbe showes without reality, truth, or constancy." Having rejected Aristotelian and other worldly theories of happiness, Browne simplifies his desires to "the peace of conscience, command of my affections, the life of my dearest friend, and I shall bee happie enough to pittie Caesar" (90–1). The friendship that has in some measure solicited this stocktaking of a singular, complex conscience also offers the world's only viable means, "syn theo," of salving that conscience this side of dreams and death.

Back in the first paragraph, the solicitation begins, not with action and life—not with charity—but with "religion" and its "severall circumstances," and it signals that Browne is responding to a question posed by the friend who has ventriloquized the objections of the vulgar world to the genuine as well as the orthodox piety of our physician. Nonetheless, charity is present from the very beginning, operating as a counterbalance against a faith-oriented religion with two dangerous penchants: one for presumptuous, disruptive or rebellious zeal; the other for melancholy, potentially impious doubt. Lest our physician insist on his own spiritual authority so far as to border on either sectarianism or atheism, charity is on hand to generalize and externalize either faith or doubt into sympathy for the human condition, amelioration of the reformist harshness, and peaceful tolerance in an age of scurrility. The author's insistence on the value of his own reason not only risks the charge of Paduan godlessness that might accrue with "the generall scandal of my profession, the naturall course of my studies, the indifferencie of my behaviour and discourse in matters of religion" (25); it also skirts the edges of heresy over which sectarian fervor is apt to tumble. Like skepticism, charity is on hand to help ensure that the problems of zeal and doubt remain in the far more innocuous realm of earnest error.

Even though charity can serve as a palliative against the complicated inner circumstances and contestations of faith, the requirement that it be digested into a "method" at a time of controversy proves troublesome for Browne's balancing act between inner meditation and outward civility. Browne betrays this difficulty in the account of his conformity to the English church of the 1630s. At times he sounds resistant to the demands of conformity for its own sake: regarding his "double obligation" to the Church of England, he insists that "Noe man shall wreath my faith to another article, or command my obedience to a cannon more"; and he blames the "the ambition & avarice of Prelates" (28, 25–6). But he can also embrace the irenic charity of a Laudian in insisting that "a good cause needs not to bee patron'd by a passion" (28).

The turning point for charity in its relation to meditation comes, however, when Browne lists the errors of his "greener studies," the first of which—the mortalist idea of the soul dying with the body—smacks of Pomponazzi when Browne declares that "faith, not philosophy can throughly disproove" the soul's mortality. The second error derives from his unwillingness to set limits on God's mercy, a desire that Browne associates with Origen, the church father with whom, according to his daughter Elizabeth, he had been linked in childhood. This error Browne understands as a salve to melancholy fear of a persecutory God. For the third error, Browne credits his own "excesse of charity" with provoking him into unwarrantable prayers for the dead (29–30).

Far from managing an easy reconciliation between the so-called "Arminian" and "Puritan" tendencies of his day, Browne's accounting of himself suddenly confronts the haunting challenge of Paduan epistemology when he offers at least four separate ways of understanding the relationship between faith and reason alone, setting aside for the moment those other contestants in the speaker's inner life such as the senses and the passions. The rich, exploratory, but also uncertain approach that Browne takes to the problem of rationality encapsulates the compelling but sometimes crosshatched experiences and orientations that he has encountered thus far in his thirty years. The first version of rationality offers the stark segregationist policy toward Christianity and natural philosophy that one finds not just in

Pomponazzi but in Galileo's *Letter to the Grand Duchess Christina* and in prominent places in Bacon's Great Instauration. By this account, Browne divides between philosophical discourse, which celebrates the "double-faced" and "paradoxicall," and faith, which amounts to strict obedience to the "great wheele of the church." He is a little careful not to make himself a slave to the church in this passage: his is a "humble" faith but not an "implicit" one, the latter involving an entirely unquestioned assent to doctrine (29).

Having supported his need for humility with the list of his former errors, Browne moves quickly through the three other relations between faith and reason which agree neither amongst themselves nor with the policy of segregation that he has just announced. The first puts "reason" virtually on par with faith as faculties yielding spiritual knowledge in keeping with their heavenly source. But even in articulating this reason's mastery of divine mystery—"the deepest Misteries ours containes have not only been illustrated but maintained by syllogismes and the rule of reason" (31)—he suggests a discontent with the limited or arid scholastic logic into which mystery has been thus translated. Quickly, then, Browne moves to a second notion of reason, according to which it serves as an instrument of faith—one quite subservient to, lower than, and transcended by mystery yet quite supportive of and useful to faith in its stretching exercises. This is the reason that Browne pursues on his way to "an O altitudo," on his way, that is, to the pleasing experience of becoming lost in "those involv'd Enigma's and riddles of the Trinity, Incarnation, and resurrection." Once again quickly, this recreational and serviceable reason is replaced by the evil alter ego of magisterial rationality—in short, by "my rebellious reason," a faculty usurped by Satan on behalf of atheistic doubt and naturalism. To this rebel, faith must respond with contradiction rather than transcendence; this reason must be chastened by Tertullian's paradox that "it is certain because it is impossible," or wise because it is foolish—a declaration made by that church father in his defense of the incarnation against heretics who could make no sense of divinity made human (31). Rebellious reason needs to give up its vain attempts at rigid logic and definition, give in to skepticism, and permit fancy or imagination with its poetics—its "easie and Platonicke description," its "description, periphrasis, or adumbration"—to take over our experience of the divine. The danger, of course, is that fancy itself is ironically keyed to the body's passions and humors: there is a peril in Browne's seemingly innocent claim that "where I cannot satisfie my reason, I am content to humour my fancy" (32).

A more charitable and peaceful world might result from this emphasis on a softer, more accommodated sense of the divine, as well as a world in which singularity is allowed to ride out its errors and explorations, but so too might a less stable and definitive grasp on veracity. In this section of the *Religio*, Browne replays that conflict of Fortunio Liceti between a sublime, evocative hieroglyphics and an Aristotelian solidity and rigor. But unlike Liceti, who writes in different genres even as he carefully mediates between his alternative styles, Browne takes his friend inside the inner struggles of spiritual epistemology. All the while, though, the overriding wit, lyricism, and relaxed, familiar civility purvey a quiet confidence that the physician has a better understanding of what it means to be an orthodox Christian than the scurrilous readers out there in the world of polemic and partisanship.

With a confidence that we should not take the Pauline precept to "Beware of philosophie... in a narrow sense," Browne steadies his religious epistemology with two ballasts: a focus on the attributes of God, and the introduction of the Book of Nature as a potentially unifying supplement to the Book of Scripture which, as he will stress, has a penchant to produce doubts and controversies. Browne turns to nature for vital assistance in linking the inner particularities and singularities of faith to the synthesis and commonality proposed for charity. Right away, though, nature's book is not self-evident. Because the traces of the divine are inscribed "not in capitall letters, yet in stenography, and short character," "wiser reasons" are required if these letters are to prove "Luminaries in the Abysse of knowledge." When the metaphor of light is placed side by side with its partner, the "scales and roundels to mount the pinacles, and highest peeces of Divinity," nature offers "iudicious beliefe" either a clear way through or a direct way out of the morass of book learning which is erroneous, chaotic, and massive (33). Later, indeed, Browne wishes the destruction of the bulk of books extant in the world, especially if he could regain those few lost texts and monuments that promised to summarize the wisdom fractured and occluded after the fall. In the sections that follow his introduction of nature's letters, nature prompts Browne to embrace metaphysical abstractions as a means for contemplating divine wisdom; to celebrate for the first of several times the "humble" experiential basis for natural theology; to situate the very dignity and purpose of man in the contemplation of nature; to revere the final—or purposive—cause amongst Aristotle's four, in stark contrast to Bacon's clarion call for a focus on material and efficient causes at the expense of final; to reassert the "indisputable axiome" that nature never does anything in vain and to single out the microscopic world of the inner workings within "Bees, Ants and spiders" for their special display of providence; to applaud the pagans for their attention to "these common Hyeroglyphicke" and "the flowers of Nature"; and to characterize the divine providence behind nature as artistic, geometrical, and, if roundabout, then "settled and constant" according to "the constituted and foresaid principles of [God's] art," this in opposition to the "Schooles" that define nature according to "the Principles of motion and art" (34–6).

In the Pembroke version, this sequence of the *Religio* has not yet acquired the level of concern that the more elaborate version will convey about the threats to a providentially disposed nature—the threats that involve, for instance, evidence of monstrosity. For the time being, Browne is content simply to modify his emphasis on regulated providence with several reminders that divine dispensation can work in quite a different manner—by miracles and mysteries, by labyrinthine courses unfolded according to divine will and through which maze we have "noe threed or line to guide us." Browne reminds his friendly reader that God has "another way made of meanders and Labyrinths whereof the Divells and spirits have noe exact Ephemerides," a "crypticke and involved method of his wisdome" that can be glimpsed in the lives of the biblical patriarchs as well as in Browne's own history and in the history of nations, including 1588 and 1605 in England (37–8). One key point to emerge from this discussion of nature's stable economy is that human beings have no business carping at nature, no matter how badly we as a species or as individuals deem our treatment.

At the outset of paragraph 16 in the Pembroke, Browne introduces the way in which the study of nature can implicate the student in atheism; indeed, "The bad construction and perverse comment on these paire of second causes, and visible hands of God, hath perverted the devotion of many to Atheisme," though the problem arises not from nature itself but from the epistemological feuding that the student of nature might experience. When Browne explains that he has "allwaies endeavoured to compose those angrie dissentions and fewds of faith, reason, and affection," it is unclear whether "allwaies" pertains to time or means. Nor is it clear whether Browne's metaphor for this attempted composition of enemies—three kings moderated into cooperation and a respect for the boundaries of their several prerogatives—is meant as a paradox bordering on absurdity. The one historical example that he gives—the Roman triumvirate—is enlisted to show how "three competitors...distract the peace of this our commonwealth noe lesse then that other did the state of Rome." Before the paragraph is complete, however, the dangers made possible by the study of nature have given way to general (and intensified) epistemological perils, and then they shift by analogy to those "sturdy doubts and boistrous obiections" in specifically scriptural and Christian divinity. From the outset of this, the most anxious of the sequences in the *Religio*, Browne wants his friend to understand that these doubts have required prayer "on my knees" and strongest resistance to an intimacy with the "unhappies of our knowledge" (40). At this very point, his memories of the Continent begin.

At first Browne offers the conventional defense against atheism that at long last, total godlessness is an impossibility. Yet, it has to be confessed, history testifies to a steady (if small) supply of atheist writings, "all" of which Browne has read, despite the ability of this "Rhetoricke of Satan" to "pervert and loose a preiudicate beleefe" (41). When he turns to his own encounters with continental professionals perverted by this rhetoric, however, the danger, while still isolated in a few "heads," is obviously more familiar, potentially more infectious and more tragic.

In the Pembroke manuscript, naturalism shares any blame for Browne's atheistic tendencies with his brand of scriptural exegesis. Indeed, Browne finds ample reason for doubt—as well as for faith and admiration—in the Bible itself. Browne's Winchester education would have certainly made it thinkable for the young man "bred in the way of study" that he would become a divine. At Oxford, however, the growing controversy over "Arminians" such as Thomas Jackson and the proto-Socinian tendencies of Thomas Lushington clarified for Browne that divinity offered an increasingly vexed and troubled course of life.[70] The Socinian commitment to a biblically based faith was as strong as its insistence that the Bible be read with an unrestricted rationality whose quest for "generally understandable and

[70] For the danger of Socinianism, see Klaus Scholder, *The Birth of Modern Critical Theology: Origins and Problems of Biblical Criticism in the Seventeenth Century*, trans. John Bowden (Philadelphia: Trinity Press International, 1990), 26.

convincing proofs of the credibility of scripture" (Scholder, 34) was no respecter of orthodoxies such as the trinity. Ironically, the Socinian defense of scripture resulted in what was considered, by the 1620s, to be the most damnable of heresies by the major groups of early modern Christendom.[71]

If Socinianism is singled out as the bogey of exegesis in the 1620s and 30s, this choice of a scapegoat manifests a wider anxiety about how to guarantee biblical interpretation at a time when both papal infallibility and a zealous individual appeal to the Holy Spirit offer rival claims of certainty. In the 1630s, Browne joined William Chillingworth in his attempt to compose a specifically English guarantor of the Bible's canonicity and interpretation. At the same time, extraordinary pressure on biblical scholarship resulted from the several fundamental changes in the way in which the world was perceived, and not just from astronomy's upward gaze.[72] Thanks to advances in geography and chronology, historians were exerting pressure on the seamless medieval reconciliation between biblical and world history, according to which the former always regulated the latter. Browne's familiarity with Robert Hues at Oxford helped to inspire his interest in voyages of discovery and in their contribution to the re-measuring and reinterpretation of the world.

The *Religio* testifies to just how intricate and powerful these developments in natural, historical, and biblical studies were to the intellectual coming of age in the first quarter of the seventeenth century. Browne's affection for allegorical significance in scripture and nature alike prevents any simple equation between the *Religio* and the production of a new, utilitarian physico-theology. But for Browne, both allegorical hieroglyphs and providential utility are resources for dealing with his own obsession with doubts as they arise in nature and scripture alike. Having concocted a series of scripturally generated doubts "which a studious atheist could well have made use of," Browne concedes that "there are in Scripture stories that exceede the fables of poets, and to the captious reader sound like Gargantua or Bevis," not least the story of Samson which makes Rabelais read like reportage (41).[73] Offering a theological defense of biblical marvels along the lines of God's inconceivable power, Browne returns to his "Catalogue of doubts, never yet imagin'd, or question'd by anie, which I know, are not resolv'd at first hearing," insisting that these problems are not fantastical trivia. If the point of raising these doubts is once again to criticize a faith that needs historical and rational coherence as its crutch, nonetheless Browne persists in piling on the points of criticism, moving from his own questions to "others more generally questioned and call'd to the barre." In this extended catalogue, the discovery of the new world and research into its natural history play a leading role, as does a panoply of improbabilities produced by accounts of the flood and Noah's ark (41–2). Having defended mod-

[71] For a recent study, see Sarah Mortimer, *Reason and Religion in the English Revolution: The Challenge of Socinianism* (Cambridge: Cambridge University Press, 2010).

[72] William Yarchin, *History of Biblical Interpretation: A Reader* (Peabody, MA: Hendrickson, 2004), xxiii.

[73] Cf. David Norton, *A History of the English Bible as Literature* (New York: Cambridge University Press, 2000), 169.

ern Socinians—"those that now denie our Saviour, though more then Heretiques, are not soe much as Atheists, for though they denie the second person in the Trinity, they hold, as wee doe, there is but one God" (40)—Browne risks complicity with their less-than-atheism when he allows that "There are other points and tenents drawne from Scripture, and generally believed as Scripture, whereto notwithstanding I could never bewray the liberty of my reason" (42). Browne may protest that some doubtful points are inconsequential, but his own experiences with continental and English religious culture have shown him that many others are apt to disagree.

Even Browne's praise for the Bible can prove problematic.[74] Having excused the fabulous tales of the Bible by way of God's will and power, Browne shifts the grounds of assessment from the theological to the literary in order to dismiss the Koran as "an ill composed peece." By contrast, the Bible can be said in literary terms to be a masterpiece of learning, even if its source were human. Theologically, human beings bowdlerize the scriptures with "fallible discourses"; literarily, they can appreciate the Bible as "the most singular and superlative piece that hath beene extant since the worlds creation" (43–4). Between the two, Browne is working out in his own complex way the notion of accommodation—the idea that the Bible is at once divine and fictive.

Extending beyond the scope of biblical history into the history of the church, Browne finds reasons for concern and doubt. Compared to the Jews that Browne has encountered on the Continent, Christians have proved "unstable and malleable," for they "oft transforme [themselves] (not into the severall shapes of Christianity and of the same species but) into more unnaturall, and contrarie formes of Jew and Mahometans" (45). Jewish obstinacy as Browne sees it has been hardened by persecution, the predominance of which in Christian history alone has led to needless suffering, often over very little (for instance, the Antipodes) and probably to ironic ends according to which martyrs move from the flames of their persecution into the fires of hell. Then there is the problem of miracles—have they ceased?—a topic that elicits from Browne both his own dismay at contemporary disenchantment and his own penchant to doubt. Amazed that some skeptics have doubted the Christian explanation of the cessation of the oracles, Browne admits his own bout of that "unhappie curiosity" that insists on measuring "the verity of Scripture by the concordance of human historie." His remedy from this secular antiquarianism involves not reason but laughter—"I laughed my selfe out of it with a peece of Justin"—when the Roman historian's epitome of Pompeius Trogus's digression on the early history of the Jews degenerates into what for Browne seemed farce, the claim that the Jews were exiled from Egypt because of an infectious (and very itchy) scabies. In the same sequence, however, the conclusion to paragraph 21, Browne laughs himself back into doubt with the joke that when it comes to unreliable accounts of the past, "Moses has outgone them all, and left not only the historie of his life, but of his death allsoe" (47–8).

[74] Norton, *A History of the English Bible as Literature*, 169–70.

After this engagement with the problems of reading scripture, theological and natural concerns converge on the question of spirits, angels, witches, and finally, human nature's place in the scale of creation. Faith and doubt fight over reason in this section. Browne professes his strong belief in angels, spirits, witchcraft and the devil, but qualifies this belief in three ways: his epistemological foundation for the belief is often complex (faith, imagination, reason, experience all playing a part); he readily acknowledges limits on spiritual powers (the devil's inability to transform one species into another; the discovery of fraud in the claims "of the maide in Germany"; the extent to which a natural wisdom once owed to the devil in terms of "Magicke and witchcraft" can over time evolve into an innocuous human philosophy); and he allows that theories of angels and spirits, in conjunction with axioms about the scale of creation, can "serve as an Hypothesis to salve manie doubts" (48–9).

Just so, the notion that man is a microcosm with a special position in God's creation is at once elaborately glossed, celebrated, and subverted. On the one hand, man is the ultimate hieroglyph manifesting God's providence in a cosmos that is orderly, beautiful, full, and purposeful. On the other, this notion has struck the Baconian side of Browne's mind as potentially "only a pleasant trope of Rhetorique," the kind of hypothetical salve that makes our melancholy souls feel better in the face of a cosmic disarray, monstrosity, and deformity that extend and evoke our own crooked sinfulness. Throughout the *Religio* Browne often uses the phrasal verb "to make good," but never so problematically as here, where amphibious human nature is responsible for "making good"—for understanding? completing? constituting?—the providential "method of God and nature." The most serious problem with the notion of amphibious man, however, is that far from simply serving as a "great and true" hieroglyph of providence, human nature as composed of the world's "five kinds of existences" is also the world's ultimate monstrosity, hideous to behold and even more miserable to inhabit. At best, man's identity evolves from the lowest, crudest forms to the most sublime; at worst, it accumulates disparate natures, their faculties divided amongst themselves, our best actions implicated in "this riddle and web of sinne" so that "In briefe wee are all monsters." And if this hieroglyph-monstrosity elicits from Browne his greatest optimism and pessimism, it is punctuated by his equivalent concerns about scripture—that it is God's greatest hieroglyph and man's most vexing frustration when even Moses can leave out key information about the universe or leave it for controversy in "a greate deale of obscurity." Even Moses's mysterious paradoxes—divine creation from nothing—can double as resolution and as remedial salve when Browne argues that the Bible has "salved" philosophical controversy (51–2).

More than any other component of God's creation, however, it is the human soul that pressures Browne into reassessing the contents, strength, and circumstances of his faith. On the one hand, the clear affirmation of the soul's immortality and incorruptibility from the more "hieroglyphic," "mystical," or allegorical legacy of Plato outweighs Aristotle's ambiguity. On the other, Browne invokes a contemporary European tendency still to raise doubts about the status and transmission of the soul, whether it be the debate over infusion and traduction "much disputed in the Germane auditories"; the alchemical hubris of Paracelsus with his recipe for producing a "man without coniunction"; or the author's own Liceti-like interest in "those aequivocall and monstrous productions in the copulation of man with beast." This last problem serves to "taunt" him, not least with its elusive epistemological basis: not other authors, he explains, but his own sensory experience, the sensory experience of others, yet also disturbed imagination, "bred amongst the weeds and tares of mine owne braine," that disheveled garden without hieroglyphs of divinity. In his own bout of negative locution, Browne tells his friend that he cannot rule out the soul's dependence on organs in this mortal life of ours, since "for the performance of her ordinarie actions is required not only a symmetry, and proper disposition of organs, but a crasis or temper correspondent to its operation." In one of the most tonally difficult passages in the *Religio*, Browne reports that, like the pagans before him (no doubt Galen of the *De usu partium*), he has found "mysterious" evidence of the divine: the emphasis on "mysterious philosophy" is, however, tricky, since it differs from the natural theology productive and corroborative of a rational understanding of an orderly providence. Browne will return momentarily to the ways in which simple experimentation—with mercury, alchemy, and silkworms—can confirm the mysteries of resurrection and immortality. For the time being, however, he stresses not what he has found in the course of anatomy but what he has not: an "organ or proper instrument for the rationall soule" (53–4).

If this is cause for celebration—the cavities of the brain have nothing to do with the immortal soul—it is also cause for a bemusement bordering on melancholy: "Thus are [wee] men and wee know not how; there is something in us that can bee without us, and willbe after us, though it's strange it hath noe historie what it was before us, nor can tell how it entred in us" (54). With the word "historie," Browne conflates the pressures exerted on his faith by natural philosophy and antiquarianism alike. For if that term evokes the temporality of all human affairs, it also resonates with the recent profiling of "natural history" by Francis Bacon as the material foundation of a pyramid of knowledge that leads laboriously from material causes upward, with formal causes clearly installed in matter itself and final causes left to superstitious theologians who replace a nature contingent on God's mysterious will with a design of their own concoction. In anatomy, Browne has gone looking for the glandular housing of the immortal soul, and he purveys both a relief and a melancholy about the fact that he has not found the residence.

In the wake of this complex failure to resolve the soul's relationship to the body, Browne turns more steadily to experiment. On the spectrum of approaches to alchemy, ranging from the Baconian insistence that it follow a rigorously inductive method to the spiritual alchemists such as Patrick Scot who insist that alchemy is spiritual metaphor,[75] Browne embraces neither extreme. He is committed to the notion that alchemy is both experimental in method and spiritual in value. Two

[75] See Patrick Scot, *The Tillage of Light* (1624).

tendencies of the *Religio* at this point—around paragraphs 28–29 of the Pembroke manuscript—militate against this modest and mysterious alchemy. One is that an almost cynical disregard for human life begins to find a voice so desperate that the more mature Dr Browne removed these passages; the other is that the complaints of atheism against conventional wisdom about nature, morality, and redemption persist in haunting the work. Both arise in paragraph 29, in which once again Browne directly takes stock of his experiences thus far.

At the outset of paragraph 29, Browne confesses his native bashfulness and acknowledges that his "conversation, age, or travailes" have failed to cultivate him out of this retiring tendency. But this calmer, more provincial detachment has its roaring alter ego. "I am not yet soe Cynicall as to approve the opinion of Diogenes" (57): if in a later section, Browne forthrightly rejects the cynical dog's repudiation of worldly honor, in these earlier paragraphs on the characteristics of his faith, he is willing to entertain Cynicism's outrageous asceticism, its disdain for the accoutrements of civilization, its opposition to the conventions of family, marriage, social distinction and political power, its suspicion of intellectual speculation, its primitivism, detachment from life, and its self-sufficiency. In its own right but also repackaged as Stoicism, Cynicism brings with it a sometimes hidden support for Browne's charitable-sociable disposition: it is cosmopolitan in its sense of a homeland (the world is one's home), philanthropic in its acknowledgement that all creatures are integrated in a cosmic whole, and mindful of the common humanity shared by the beggar and the almsgiver. So Browne cannot "alltogether" allow the Cynical-Stoical rejection of "a monument, historie, or Epitaph" for the sake of a more universal shroud under the cope of heaven; and he can allow even less the brand of Stoicism that stresses suicide as an expression of autonomy. Even so, he is drawn to the "singular peeces" of its doctrine, so much so in fact that he can mimic its brazen disregard for life:

> I perceive I doe anticipate the vices of age; the world to mee is but a dreame, or mocke-show, and wee all but Pantaloons and Antickes to my severer contemplations. The course and order of my life would bee a verie death unto others; I use my selfe to all diets, aires, humours, hunger, thirst, heate; cold, I cure not my selfe by heate; when sicke, not by physicke; those that understand how I live may iustly say I regard not life nor stand in feare of death. (58)

This, a more melancholy version of his amenable disposition, negates the value of masquerade; indeed, in the passages that follow, with the poetry of Lucan frequently in his sights, Browne focuses on mortification among other versions of death as the type of response to human masking found in the godly preaching of ministers such as Ramsden. The pretenses of medicine itself are also swept away in this cynical disregard for the earthly means of happiness; even the Cynic's appeal to nature as his guide is negated in an outburst of severity.

In extending his vision beyond death to divine judgment, heaven and hell, and apocalypse, Browne refuses to accept a literal or physical conception of any one of them, as vulgar to him as the memento mori that relies on the presence of a skull. Explaining how the Bible accommodates its mysteries "in a vulgar and illustrative way," however, Browne once again challenges the consistency of the scriptures themselves, which can vaguely characterize the signs of the end times then undercut the reliability of the signs with the notion that Jesus will return like a thief in the night. Once again a Christian's life is one of "unanswerable doubts": and, once again, the doubts pertain to nature as well as scripture (60–1). In paragraphs 32 and 33, the problem of atheism is clearer still: having entertained the question of whether he, or anyone, might live virtuously without the framework of heaven and hell, he decides that the pay-off, resurrection, is essential. Far from arguing the standard line—that natural theology without the mysteries of Christianity refutes atheism at every turn—Browne suggests that Christians are finally locked in a game of chance with the atheists, and the winner takes all. As though to drive the point home, Browne returns to the infamous Paduan distinction between what faith credits and what reason can prove: "How the dead shall rise is noe question of my faith; to beleeve only possibilities, is not faith, but meere philosophy" (62).

In paragraphs 38 and 39, the author's pervasive sense of doubt, not least about his own salvation, takes him also in the direction of a claim that the Church of England is distinguished by its acknowledgement of fallibility and its contentment with a "moral"—less than absolute—certainty in its creed. On the verge of the later paragraphs on charity, Browne stresses the need for doubt to be salved by a Pauline fear and trembling. Having taken his friend on an imaginary journey through a European intellectual landscape, Browne brings him back home again, to the sober godliness of Halifax and its concretization in charity, "without which faith is a meere notion and of noe existence" (71). In a memorable sentence, Browne's often elevated language turns especially mundane as he compares God to a justice, prescribing "a boxe of the eare" for a murderer (67). But the homecoming is fitful, and Browne's revisions of his text show his dissatisfaction with provincialism, even (or perhaps especially) as he settles into his vocational life in Norwich. If, for the sake of bland respectability perhaps, the manuscript's box on the ear is replaced in the printed editions by "Fine," Browne's extraordinary imaginary voyage is far from over. The et ceteras of the Pembroke are to be unfolded with more philosophy, theology, and poetry in the growth of a work that in the decades to come found its vexatious yet powerful way into the hearts and minds of Latin readers throughout Europe.

No matter how freely Browne speculates in *Religio Medici*, Halifax pressured his intellect with a reformist's counterbalance to learned, idle contemplation. The culture of John Favour provoked Browne to reassess the relations of charity to faith and thought, but also to cultivate and criticize paradox in a remote location perhaps absurdly committed to the artificial means of perfecting the social order. Browne's circuitous attempts to value charity aright underscore what was perhaps the most painful legacy of Halifax in the 1630s: that a learned physician seeking to profit from the afflictions of his patients needed always to remember that on questions of charity as surely as on matters of belief, his claims on the godly practice of medicine could never be taken for granted.

However remote it may have been, Halifax boasted famous sons who were celebrated for having achieved the synthesis between brilliant natural philosophy and Christian devotion that Browne pursued in *Religio Medici*. Indeed, the corporation seal of Halifax combined images taken from the town's (dubious) religious and scientific lore: "the maiden hanging from the yew tree and John de Sacro Bosco with a sphere in his hand."[76] Both the tree and the hill on which Sacrobosco was said to have contemplated the stars were commonly shown to tourists in the area; in his diary, Thoresby recalled that the antiquarian Brearcliffe (Browne's correspondent) "showed me...the hill whereupon the celebrated Johannes de Sacro Bosco made his celestial observations."[77] In the seventeenth century, Halifax legend confirmed that Sacrobosco himself had lain on the top of Beacon Hill—up near Shibden Hall—and gazed out at his spherical, geocentric and geostatic cosmos.

If Sacrobosco or "John Halifax" was a distant, perhaps fabulous precursor of the Halifax natural philosopher, much closer to Browne in time and educational context was Henry Briggs, born in 1561 at nearby Daisy Bank, and a high-profile professor in Browne's Oxford.[78] There is, however, an even more immediate way in which life in West Yorkshire appears to have transformed the social and experiential basis of Browne's natural philosophy. In paragraph 22 of the Pembroke manuscript, Browne declares to his friend that "For mine owne part I have ever beleeved and doe now know that thare are witches" (48). As a resident in Halifax in 1634–5, Browne was privy to the intense drama and debate surrounding the notorious trial of witches in neighboring Lancashire. The trial in 1634 concluded against the accused witches, only one of whom had admitted guilt, but the judges were sufficiently concerned to defer to the king's Privy Council, which in June ordered that the bishop of Chester, John Bridgman, question the concerned parties, then in the summer months had the parties brought to London to be examined by medical authorities and midwives working under the guidance of William Harvey. At least two striking details link him to the examining physicians involved in the case: one, that a manuscript of *Religio Medici* is attributed to Alexander Read, and the other, the fact that Browne read Harvey's treatise on generation in manuscript in the 1630s.[79] Even if the findings of the midwives and physicians were wary of concluding that the marks on the women's bodies had anything to do with witchcraft, the accused women were brought back to Lancashire where they were still notorious

[76] T. W. Hanson, "Minutes of Halifax Workhouse," 92.

[77] Taylor, "Annals of the Parish of Halifax," 112.

[78] See chapter 3 in this volume. Another local scientific connection for Browne remains a matter of speculation. Given the Lancashire provenance of one manuscript of the *Religio*, it is perhaps not too much of a stretch to suppose that Browne came into contact with those close friends of the Power family, the Towneleys from the eastern borderland of Lancashire. As one of the most prominent and staunch Catholic families in the area, the Towneleys were also active experimenters in natural studies, though the bulk of the family's natural studies was carried out in the decades after Browne's departure from Halifax by Richard Towneley (1629–1707), the nephew of Christopher and an eventual collaborator with Henry Power. Even so, the Towneley papers include astronomical work from the late 1630s and Christopher was widely and well known for his assiduous antiquarian endeavors, another interest shared with Browne. Not only would an association through the Powers with the Townleys help to make Halifax a stimulating intellectual site for Browne, but his experience of the family's difficulties as recusants would further motivate the sympathy for Catholics in the *Religio*.

[79] See Thomas Smith's letter to Samuel Hartlib in October 1648, discussed in chapter 8.

and languishing in Lancaster Castle in 1636, and some of them remained in autumn of the next year. Letters written by Sir William Pelham during this period reflect just how high the profile of this episode was in the county and its surrounding areas (indeed part of the episode took place at a chapel in Yorkshire, the county of Halifax). Arguably, the whole episode is something of a turning point in the history of witchcraft trials, since the convicted were not put to death and there was no succeeding outburst of witch hunting in the region.[80] If the conflicted responses to the trial anticipate the mixture of skepticism and belief that characterized the 1662 Bury St Edmunds trial in which Browne was directly involved, closer to the event Browne was sufficiently jolted to conclude to his friend that what was once mere belief was now firm certainty. Ironically, an account of the trial in 1677 would both cite and criticize Browne's views on witchcraft.[81]

Even if Browne was unaware of a Northern England and Halifax legacy of natural philosophy and of its synthesis with religion, for Henry Power he came to epitomize and to refashion this legacy. Given family tradition, Henry should have become a clergyman; that he did not was clearly owed to his early influence by Thomas Browne who, from Norwich, guided his young charge in the ways of vocation, thought, and belief.

[80] James Sharpe, *Instruments of Darkness: Witchcraft in England, 1550–1750* (New York: Penguin, 1996), 126–7. The intensity and notoriety of the trial are readily glimpsed in the records of the Lancashire Courts of Quarter Sessions; see Lancashire Record Office QSB/1/170/60; QSB/1/170/64; and QSB/1/170/69. My account of the episode is indebted to Alison Findlay, "Sexual and Spiritual Politics in the Events of 1633–34 and *The Late Lancashire Witches*," in Robert Poole, ed., *Lancashire Witches: Histories and Stories* (Manchester: Manchester University Press, 2003), 146–65.

[81] John Webster, *The Displaying of Supposed Witchcraft* (1677), on some five occasions.

8

Norwich, 1637–1649

The two English cities in which Browne practiced medicine, Halifax and Norwich, shared a penchant for practical civic improvement. Writing some time before his death in 1612, Sir John Harington expressed uncertainty about whether to believe those reports of Norwich as "another Utopia," but he was clear on the civic standards at stake in such a judgment: "The people live all so orderly, the streets kept solemnly; the Trades-men, young and old so industrious; the better sort so provident, and withal so charitable: that it is as rare to meet a begger here, as it is common to see them in Westminster."[1] At least one early modern commentator, Daniel Defoe, saw fit to compare the county of Norfolk to the West Riding of Yorkshire, that is, on the count of a place "so far from London" yet "throng'd with great and spacious market-towns."[2] But Norwich also resembled the city in which Browne had received his medical degree, Leiden, in their mutually neat, earnest, and aggressive commitment to social discipline and reform. Physically, Norwich and Leiden were comparable in their mutually watery environs, for the county of Norfolk possessed not just an extensive coastline, rivers, and fens, but the extraordinary area of shallow lakes known as the Broads. As Thomas Fuller explained in the mid-seventeenth century, there was furthermore a historical reason for comparing Norwich to Leiden: Norwich was filled with Dutch immigrants. In *The History of the Worthies of England*, Fuller knew how much Norwich owed the Dutch for its rare combination of flora and humanity as well as commerce and "pleasurable curiosities": "NORWICH is (as you please) either a *City* in an *Orchard*, or an *Orchard* in a *City*, so equally are *Houses* and *Trees* blendid [*sic*] in it, so that the *pleasure* of the *Country*, and *populousness* of the *City* meet here together."[3] Yet the arboreal splendors of Norwich did nothing to detract from the sophistication of its inhabitants, who "participate, nothing of the *rusticalness* of the [orchard], but altogether of the *urbanity* and *civility* of the [city]." Indeed the county capital served as

[1] Sir John Harington, *Nugæ antiquæ* (London, 1792), 1.147. Cf. Carole Rawcliffe, *Medicine for the Soul: The Life, Death and Resurrection of an English Medieval Hospital St Giles's, Norwich, c. 1249–1550* (Stroud, Gloucestershire: Sutton, 1999), 239.

[2] Quoted in Penelope Corfield, "A Provincial Capital in the Late Seventeenth-Century: The Case of Norwich," in Peter Clark and Paul Slack, eds., *Crisis and Order in English Towns, 1500–1700: Essays in Urban History* (London: Routledge & Kegan Paul), 263–310; see 263.

[3] Thomas Fuller, *The History of the Worthies of England* (London, 1662), part 1, 274. For a description of Norwich and Norfolk in the seventeenth century, see Francis Blomefield, *An Essay Towards a Topographical History of the County of Norfolk* (London, 1806).

"a gathering point and a source of fashionable goods for the county gentry."[4] Its lively civic calendar, often reflected in Browne's family letters, highlighted "a winter season . . . well established, with theatres, shows and assemblies which attracted the surrounding gentry," the summer Assizes, and the inauguration of the mayor. Tourists found many sites of interest: Dutch visitor Willem Shellinks was fairly typical in his diary for 1662 when he singled out for praise the city's walls with their twelve gates, the River Wensum completing the three-mile circumference of the urban area, the beautiful market with its cross and guildhall, the flint churches, cathedral cloisters, hospital behind the cathedral, ducal house (with bowling alley), many Dutch weavers, swampy and sandy environs, and castle views, though he also noted its hilliness, the boat traffic from Yarmouth (bringing coal and fish), the ferry service to Yarmouth for twelve pence daily, and the prisoners crying for alms from the castle jail.[5]

In Norwich, physicians and lawyers often joined the wealthy gentry in living in upscale neighborhoods such as Mancroft and Wymer; but the county gentry also included visits to their physicians (or lawyers) as part of their shopping and socializing expeditions to the city.[6] For this reason, Browne's relations to great county families such as the Le Stranges and Pastons, the Wodehouses, Townshends, and Hobarts, were at once social, professional, and cultural-cum-intellectual.[7] In addition to sharing interests in collecting curiosities, Browne interacted with local gentry in compiling the *Pseudodoxia Epidemica*, receiving verification from Sir William Paston on the question of whether it rains in Egypt, and inspiring Sir Hamon L'Estrange to write a commentary on Browne's work.[8] But Browne also interacted with the lower members of society, seeking information from fishermen, helping the poor with their illnesses, and collaborating with the whole spectrum of medical practitioners.[9]

Adding to the idealization of Norwich was the contemporary observation that its surrounding county, Norfolk, offered a microcosm of what Fuller called "All

[4] John T. Evans, *Seventeenth-Century Norwich: Politics, Religion, and Government, 1620–1690* (Oxford: Clarendon Press, 1979), 4–5, 13.

[5] NRO MC 1628/1 1828X1, an extract (original in the Bodleian). For the combination of features, see *Norwich since 1550*, ed. Carole Rawcliffe and Richard Wilson (New York: Hambledon, 2004), introduction by Richard Wilson (xxi), and essays by Christopher Barringer, 1, and John Pound, 35–6, 45; and John Miller, *Cities Divided: Politics and Religion in English Provincial Towns, 1660–1722* (Oxford: Oxford University Press, 2007), 21. In her introduction to *Medieval Norwich*, ed. Carole Rawcliffe and Richard Wilson (London: Hambledon and London, 2004), Carole Rawcliffe offers contemporary comparisons between the United Provinces and Norwich but also contemporary skepticism about the idealization of the city (xxi–xxii).

[6] See Evans, *Seventeenth-Century Norwich*, 3; Miller, *Cities Divided*, 21.

[7] See R. W. Ketton-Cremer, *Norfolk in the Civil War: A Portrait of a Society in Conflict* (Hamden, CT: Archon Books, 1969), 35–45.

[8] For Paston, see R. W. Ketton-Cremer, *Norfolk Portraits* (London: Faber and Faber, 1944), 23–4.

[9] Frank Meeres, *A History of Norwich* (Chichester: Phillimore, 1998), 79, 80. Margaret Pelling, "Illness among the Poor in an Early Modern English Town," *Continuity and Change* 3 (1988), 282, 286. Also see Anthony Batty Shaw, *Norfolk & Norwich Medicine: A Retrospect* (Norwich: Norwich Medico-Chirurgical Society, 1992). Cf. E. H. Carter, *The Norwich Subscription Books: A Study of Subscription Books of the Diocese of Norwich 1637–1800* (New York: Thomas Nelson & Sons, 1937), 133–47.

England," including "fens and heaths, and light and deep, and sand and clay ground, and meadows and pasture, and arable and woody...so grateful is this shire with the variety thereof."[10] On each side of the city stretched a distinctive landscape or economy.[11] Historically too the county was complex and fascinating. Among the medieval ruins in the area were several abbeys but also the shrine in Walsingham with its fame for "three curative wells, a finger joint of St Peter, milk of the Virgin Mary and, of course, the Holy House."[12] Then there were the antiquarian remains of the Iceni to whom the Romans had granted "the rare privilege of client-kingdom."[13] The county's natural and economic variety but also the archeological layers of its past contributed to Browne's increasing fascination with local and natural history. Even so, its central role in trade gave the region between Norwich and Great Yarmouth a claim on citizenship in the world, a point of considerable significance for Browne since he was eager to learn about and even to experience natural and artistic phenomena from the world at large.

Browne's letters also clarify how busy were his social and professional lives, as well as how bustling proved the human activity around him. With its population rising from 20,000 to 30,000 occupants, Norwich was clearly England's second city, but it was also close by sea or land to the first city, London.[14] Despite these claims on prosperity, the Norwich to which Browne came was hardly placid, bland, or simple. In several respects, Norfolk was a site of serious conflict. As Boyer explains, this "tough, litigious native shire" of Edward Coke was a region "where freeholders pressed lawsuits as tenaciously as their ancestors had pursued private wars."[15] Contemporaries were apt to observe that even the farmers of the shire had mastered the intricacies of law.[16] Religiously and politically, Norwich was not the uniformly "Puritan" haven that historians have sometimes made it out to be. As Matthew Reynolds has recently shown, Browne began his time in Norwich in the company of citizens who had played a contentious and prominent part in the struggle over "the boundaries between conformity and nonconformity, religious orthodoxy and heterodoxy."[17] During the civil wars of the 1640s, Norwich was never placed under siege, but it was far from harmonious, carefree, or peaceful.[18]

In one assessment of the air and health of Norfolk, Browne showed a complex sense of the area in which he would spend the greater part of his life. In *The Natural History of Wiltshire*, John Aubrey commented on the way in which Norfolk's "cleare and fine" air produced both "good clear witts" and a litigious subtlety so

[10] Fuller, *The History of the Worthies*, 402–3.

[11] Allen Boyer, *Sir Edward Coke and the Elizabethan Age* (Stanford, CA: Stanford University Press, 2003), 54–5. Cf. David Dymond, *The Norfolk Landscape* (London: Hodder and Stoughton, 1985).

[12] Dymond, *Norfolk Landscape*, 116–17, 130.

[13] Dymond, *Norfolk Landscape*, 49.

[14] See Evans, *Seventeenth-Century Norwich*, 4–5.

[15] Boyer, *Sir Edward Coke and the Elizabethan Age*, 37.

[16] Boyer, *Sir Edward Coke and the Elizabethan Age*, 55.

[17] Matthew Reynolds, *Godly Reformers and Their Opponents in Early Modern England: Religion in Norwich, c.1560–1643* (Rochester: Boydell, 2005), 255.

[18] See Andrew Hopper, "The Civil Wars," in *Norwich since 1550*, 89.

that even the farmers "carry Littleton's Tenures at the plough taile." In this vein, Aubrey recalled, "Sir Thom. Browne, MD, of Norwich, told me that their eies in that countrey doe quickly decay; which he imputes to the clearness and driness (subtileness) of the aire."[19] As Browne would show most extensively in his master work, *Pseudodoxia Epidemica*, the relations between human advancement and sinful, diseased error were rarely simple in the fallen world. The unprecedented conflicts and turmoil of the decades to follow would only drive that lesson home, and Browne's growing fascination with the amphibious local landscape between Norwich and the sea resonated with his own observation that human life itself was a constant struggle for happiness in "divided and distinguished worlds."

Before Browne could begin his career as a Norwich physician in earnest, he had to incorporate his Leiden degree at one of the English universities and he chose his alma mater, Oxford. Browne was no doubt deemed obviously suitable for incorporation on account of his previous degrees from Oxford but also his prior association with Thomas Clayton.[20] The date on Browne's certificate of incorporation as DM at Oxford—July 10, 1637 during the annual Act—offers the best clue for the time of his transition from Halifax to Norwich.[21] So too does the presence of Justinian Lewin at the 1637 Act, for it was then that Lewin received his law doctorate. According to the *Life of Sir Thomas Browne* included in the *Posthumous Works*, it was around the time of the 1637 Act that Lewin joined "Sir Nicholas Bacon of Gillingham...and Sir Charles Le Gross of Crostwick" in persuading the newly minted Oxford physician to settle in Norwich. As Jeremiah Finch noticed in a 1950 article, this seemingly straightforward claim was not so simple. After all, Wood had already offered a rival account of the persuasion to Norwich surrounding the 1637 Act, namely, that it was Thomas Lushington, Browne's "sometime tutor" who induced the physician to settle in Norwich, and Wood's language about what happened—"where being setled he was much resorted to by patients for his admirable skill in physic, which he practised there with good success for many years"—is replicated in the anonymous life of 1712.[22] Stranger still is the fact that the names of Bacon, Lewin, and Le Gros appear on a cancel or inserted leaf, with a variant copy of the *Posthumous Works* clarifying that the original name, Lushington, had been removed either as a mistake (corroborated by Browne's daughter Elizabeth Lyttleton) or because the tutor's reputation had come to be associated with heresy.[23]

In all likelihood, most if not all of these men played a part in Browne's decision to settle in Norwich, perhaps even at the 1637 Act itself, not least because Norwich's

[19] John Aubrey, *Natural History of Wiltshire*, intro. K. G. Ponting (Newton Abbot: David & Charles Imprints, 1969), 12.

[20] Cf. A. H. T. Robb-Smith, "Cambridge Medicine," in Debus, ed., *Medicine in Seventeenth Century England*, 331.

[21] Oxford University Archives, NEP/supra/Reg Q, 161v. The document includes the certificate from Leiden University with a formulaic report of Browne's success in completing the requirements of his degree. See chapter 6 in this volume.

[22] Wood, *Fasti*, 4.56. Browne, *Posthumous Works*, iii.

[23] Jeremiah S. Finch, "The Norfolk Persuaders of Sir Thomas Browne: A Variant Copy of the 1712 Posthumous Works," *Princeton University Library Chronicle* 11 (1949–50), 199–201.

recent experience with plague reinforced the need for an ample supply of physicians.[24] Baptized in Smithfield, London, Lewin may have been in residence at Pembroke College, Oxford, prior to his matriculation in 1631, since he received his BCL in 1632. On and off an official for the archdeacon of Norwich in the 1630s, he would prove a staunch Royalist during the civil war and interregnum.[25] He had some business relations with the Mileham family into which Browne would soon marry.[26] If Lewin had connections to Lushington at Oxford, so apparently did Nicholas Bacon of Gillingham, for it was he who published the old tutor's treatise on logic in 1651 with testimonials to Lushington's excellence in teaching. Our chief evidence for Browne's view of Bacon, the grandnephew of Sir Francis, derives from the dedication in *The Garden of Cyrus*, in which Bacon is heralded as the handler of massive herbals, as a scholar of such unusual learning that one struggled to find a subject suitably recondite for him, and as a reader apt to appreciate digressive or "collateral" discourses. According to John Evelyn, it was to Sir Nicholas that Browne had addressed as letters the majority of what would become his *Certain Miscellany Tracts*.[27] There is no question that Browne came to know the Le Gros family of Crostwick over the course of his years in Norfolk; Sir Charles was a patient whose son, Thomas, was honored as the dedicatee of *Hydriotaphia*.[28]

The nexus of circumstances inducing Browne to settle in Norwich included not just the ready clientele of the Norfolk area but in all likelihood a prominent family connection, the alderman and prosperous draper-cum-mercer William Browne whose religious and political alliances in the 1630s have also linked him to Lushington. The importance of William Browne for the move to Norwich was first pointed out by Walter Rye, who located the successful draper and respected citizen in the area of Tombland just next to the cathedral.[29] As a member of the "distributive" professions, including drapers, grocers, and mercers, William Browne ranked among the mercantile elite of the city.[30] Among his various moments of local fame, he had been mayor in 1633, and he was a strong supporter of the controversial new Laudian ceremonialism in the 1630s.[31] William Browne died soon after Thomas Browne's arrival in the city, with his burial taking place on April 14,

[24] For the 1636–38 plague, see Pound, "Government to 1660," in *Norwich since 1550*, 55–6.

[25] *ODNB* article on Justinian Lewin by P. O. G. White.

[26] NRO MS 19926, a deed between Lewin and Edward Mileham of Burlingham.

[27] Evelyn's note is found on the first page of his copy of *Certain Miscellany Tracts* in the Colman Collection of the Norfolk Heritage Centre, Millennium Library, Norwich.

[28] According to *Alumni Cantabrigiensis*, ed. John Venn and J. A. Venn, part 1, vol. 3 (Cambridge University Press, 1924), 71, Charles Le Gros entered Caius College, Cambridge, on April 13, 1611; he was son and heir of Sir Thomas of Crostwick, Norfolk, admitted to Gray's Inn in 1614, knighted in 1616, Sheriff of Norfolk in 1627, and an MP for Orford, Suffolk, in 1626, 1628–29, and 1640. He died in 1656. His son Thomas matriculated at Christ's College, Cambridge, in 1631, and was admitted to Gray's Inn in 1632.

[29] Rye, "What Brought Sir Thomas Browne to Norwich?," *Norfolk Antiquarian Miscellany*, 2nd series, 1 (1906), 83–5; 83 for this quotation. See also Walter Rye, *Some Historical Essays Chiefly Relating to Norfolk*, part 6 (Norwich: H. W. Hunt, 1928), chapter 6.

[30] Pound, "Government to 1600," in *Norwich since 1550*, 46.

[31] Major events in his life appear in *The First Parish Register of St. George of Tombland, Norwich (A.D. 1538–1707)*, ed. George Branwhite Jay, revised by William Hudson (Norwich, 1891).

1639.[32] His house, the Samson and Hercules as it came to be called after 1657, had something of a storied past, having supposedly belonged at one time or another to Sir John Falstaff and the Countess of Lincoln.[33] A 1649 document designated his Tombland residence as "a faire howse in the possession of Doctor Browne."[34] With another document locating Browne in North Conisford Ward at the same time that he was in the parish of St George Tombland, it is likely that his residence was positioned either on what is now Upper King Street or on South Tombland.[35] Like his neighbor Arthur Dee, he was a renter not an owner at this time: in collections made during 1644–45 for the forces of Sir Thomas Fairfax, Browne was assessed nothing for real estate and six shillings for his personal belongings.[36] Tombland parish records demonstrate the prominence of the Anguish family, and so it is not surprising that a year later, in 1650, the flourishing physician would purchase for his growing family a large house once owned by Alexander Anguish in the more fashionable parish of St Peter Mancroft. In Tombland, however, the name of which derived from the Danish "tommer" ("vacant") rather than the funereal sense, Browne was at home among merchants and without the ownership of property, much as he had been in Leiden and Halifax. He was also next door to the cathedral and its extensive close whose importance for him would only grow over the course of his life.

1. EARLY MEDICAL PRACTICE

Browne's association with Sir Charles Le Gros of Crostwick Hall offers valuable information regarding the early years of Browne's medical practice in Norfolk. In the spring of 1642, Browne corresponded with Dr Samuel Bave, a Bath physician, about Sir Charles's bad health and, in doing so, epitomized his approach not just to disease or health but to his profession. From the letter's address to Bave, it is clear that Browne had already encountered the German physician if only very casually or "by sight"; this is not surprising, since Bave had received his medical degree from Christ Church, Oxford, in 1628, a year before Browne's graduation from Pembroke across the street. In his Latin correspondence with Bave, Browne

[32] Jay, ed., *First Parish Register*, 108. Another case for Browne's family connections to Norfolk is made in A. Hassell Smith and D. MacCulloch, "The Authorship of the Chorographies of Norfolk and Suffolk," *Norfolk Archaeology* 56 (1974–77), 327–41.

[33] Jay, ed., *First Parish Register*, 220. Cf. William A. Dutt, *Some Literary Associations of East Anglia* (London: Methuen, 1907), 128. See also Basil Cozens-Hardy and Ernest A. Kent, *The Mayors of Norwich 1403 to 1835 being Biographical Notes on the Mayors of the Old Corporation* (Norwich: Jarrold, 1938), 78.

[34] *The Parliamentary Survey of Dean and Chapter Properties in and around Norwich in 1649*, ed. G. A. Metters, in *Norfolk Record Society* 51 (1985), 69. Finch ventures that Browne's residence was "either in Upper King street or on the south side of Tombland" (*Sir Thomas Browne*, 166–7).

[35] F. R. Beecheno, "The First Residence of Sir Thomas Browne in Norwich," *Eastern Daily Press* (Norwich), February 20, 1912, 210. Browne paid 12*d* to a collection for the river and streets in 1649.

[36] NRO NCR Case 71c, May 12, 1645.

reveals key tenets and tendencies of his own medical philosophy, but he also purveys a resourceful and dexterous handling of medical practice as well as an affable and humane attitude toward his colleagues and patients.[37]

Having briefly expressed the honor in which he holds Sir Charles, Browne focuses on the patient's condition as three points emerge immediately. The first is that generous and careful consultation is essential for successful medical practice: indeed Browne and Bave have consulted a third, Dr William Rant, a Norwich native but a London practitioner to whom Browne refers as "our common friend." The second point follows from the first, that is, the recognition that the occasion needs a consultant with expertise on the disease in question or on those afflictions like it (*morbo parem*). In other words, although Browne and Bave both retain a strong and deep commitment to humoral medicine, with its basis in a philosophical system and its reduction of all disease to a single, pervasive etiology, Browne also allows for the possibility that a particular disease can be sufficiently tricky or unusual to warrant specific expertise—and here again one is reminded not just of Browne's concern about new diseases but his recognition that expertise, say, in skin diseases, can prove quite helpful.

The third point is simply that Browne pays close attention to his patient. At one level, such attentiveness is in keeping with the Hippocratic emphasis on assessing the circumstances modifying the case of a disease; this stress has as much to do with climate, setting, or season as it does with the person—and Browne does modify his treatments according to season.[38] Another aspect of his interest in the patient is also standard: Sir Charles's hygiene must be considered, and this requires an honest evaluation of the six non-naturals. Browne is emphatic on this point: no therapy can stand a chance of working if the patient abuses food or drink, lacks exercise and good air or oversleeps, or indulges his anxiety or sorrow (*tristitia*). Bave's letter confirms that on these matters, Sir Charles is a problem: he reads far too much, even all day and night, neglects "exercise of the natural warmth in the open air" that his condition requires, overeats and drinks, and has difficulties with his bowels.

But if it is standard practice for the learned physician to assess the circumstances and habits of his patient—to listen to and learn about as well as to touch or observe the person—Browne also corroborates the view of recent scholarship that early modern patients in general—and those in Norwich in particular—were often actively involved in and opinionated about their own treatment. This proactive stance of patients was obviously something that learned physicians might look on with mixed or even negative feelings, and Browne's initial assurance to Bave about the assiduity with which Sir Charles would doubtless pursue medical care is hard to read for tone: given the honorable patient's apparent unwillingness to alter his habits, Browne might be remarking with a gentle humor about the patient's eagerness to take the baths, to receive the advice of consultants, and to seek out experts

[37] All references from the Bave correspondence are taken from Keynes 4.241–8.

[38] For the general tendency, see Margaret Pelling, *The Common Lot: Sickness, Medical Occupations and the Urban Poor in Early Modern England* (New York: Longmans, 1998), 51.

on his condition. Nonetheless, in Browne's simple remark—that Sir Charles has found greater relief for his condition from baths than from pharmaceuticals—he acknowledges his source to be the testimonial of the patient himself.[39]

Despite the fact that Browne's first point of praise for Rant concerns the latter's understanding of "*morbi speciem et causam*" ("the type and cause of the disease"), it is striking that the bulk of his letter is given over to what he calls "*remedia... tuta, specifica*" ("safe and specific remedies"). So too, despite Bave's praise for Browne's "*mascula...philosophia*" ("manly philosophy") of medicine, it is really their collaboration on a complex, resourceful, and changing therapy that occupies virtually the whole of Browne's attention. Very little time is spent exclusively on pathology, let alone physiology, and for the most part the physical and etiological features of the disease are integrated into a discussion of remedies. Because the disease is so painful to Sir Charles, at times Browne expresses greater concern about immediate relief of the symptoms than hope for a final cure of the affliction. Indeed Browne never quite identifies the disease.[40] It is probable, of course, that Browne and Bave have already discussed the nature of the disease, both together and in consultation with Rant, and also that they take for granted certain assumptions about the basis or causes of the disease. Even so, the condition in question—Browne calls it "μίασμα Scorbuticum" or a scorbutic miasma—bears a certain resemblance to other skin afflictions such as smallpox in which Browne has already shown professional interest, and the way in which it is approached—or even left ambiguous—suggests tensions in medical knowledge that Browne might be glossing over.

Neither the adjective ("scorbutic") nor the noun ("miasma") is helpful in clarifying the nature of the disease. Most broadly, "miasma" means something like "contagion";[41] more specifically it can refer to scabs or corruptions of the skin.[42] Either meaning goes well with the adjective, since scurvy was considered by seventeenth-century commentators both to be contagious and to erupt through the skin into tumors and ulcers. But the adjective, "scorbutic," is at once a typically vague early modern usage and revealing of Browne's humoralism. To take the latter point first: in denying that a disease has its own ontological identity or substance, a humoral theory of medicine always reduces diseases to a minimal slate of qualities or adjectives, especially dry, wet, hot, and cold. Since scurvy was commonly held to arise from poor digestion as it accumulated and then dispersed an excremental melancholy throughout the parts of the body, the "scorbutic" might well serve as shorthand for conventional Galenic wisdom of the kind to be found in Browne's favorite authors such as Rivière and Sennert. Yet these two authors were also famous as mediators between humoral and chemical medicine, and in Sennert's treatment of scurvy, as in Browne's letter to Bave, it is clear that humoral medicine coexists with

[39] Cf. Beier, *Sufferers & Healers*, 116, 121.

[40] Murdoch MacKinnon, "An Unpublished Consultation Letter of Sir Thomas Browne," *Bulletin of the History of Medicine* 27 (1953), 503–11; see 505.

[41] Used thus in Daniel Sennert's *Sixth book of Practical Physick* (1662), 25.

[42] As in Thomas Willis, *Dr. Willis' Practice of Physick* (1684), 161.

the notion that diseases might have their singular—and in this case, potentially slippery—identities and require expertise rather than general physiology and pathology.

Two things are certain in the Le Gros case: Sir Charles's hygiene makes him a prime candidate by seventeenth-century standards for the scurvy; and his miasma grievously mars and afflicts the skin. Browne also stresses that with a chronic as against an acute disease, a long-term plan is crucial, one weighing the pros and cons of each season for treatment. Starting his narrative in the autumn of 1641, when Sir Charles has returned from Bath to his Norfolk home, Browne seems unconcerned about a scurvy patient's potentially contagious and certainly offensive breath; rather, he focuses on the skin's ulcers and spots. With the coming of winter, the dermatological symptoms grow worse (progressing from spots to tumors) but, more problematically, the scurvy begins to dissimulate as it tends to do. It is noteworthy of Browne's problem with the stable, clear understanding of skin diseases that he alters a related passage from the 1646 to the 1650 editions of the *Pseudodoxia*. In the first, he specifies three types of inflammation—"Oedematous, Schirrous, Erisipelatous"—and aligns them with melancholy, phlegmatic, and choleric excess. In 1650, however, he replaces the three adjectives with something far simpler and less committal, "denominable from other humours" (Robbins, ed., *Pseudodoxia Epidemica*, 1.296).

Given a disease whose essential nature is unclear and whose humoral basis involves dissimulation, Browne doubtless found a certain comfort in his focus on the tangible and mostly standard (if sometimes complex) remedies for Sir Charles's affliction. As MacKinnon notes, "the drugs prescribed in this letter are almost all to be found in the *Pharmacopeia Londinensis*, 1618, the exceptions being such plants as leaf of hart's tongue, horse sorrel, and soldanella" ("Unpublished," 505). Making no mention of a course of bleeding for the patient, which after all was often considered the purview of the surgeon, Browne offers his herbal recipe for the autumn. As mainstream herbals such as Gerard's clarify, the herbs in this recipe vary in place of origin, with rhubarb to be found in China, senna in Syria, Egypt, Italy, and southern France, but others (elder, horse radish, and white bryony) pervasive in England. Wherever their origins, these herbs converge as helpful cathartics for diseases of the liver and spleen, and they tend to take on the qualities of hot and dry. For instance, senna is middling in temperature yet dry in the third degree, capable of purging phlegmatic, choleric, and melancholy humors, of opening stoppages in the body, yet slowly and mildly and for all ages and natures. Elder or sambucus purges slimy, gross vapors with greater violence than senna, but it also helps with obesity.

With the coming of winter in late 1641, Browne faces a dilemma. He makes use of local external applications in order to remove the tumors or edemas, but the patient needs to sweat in such a manner that in some measure replicates the benefits of the baths. In ruling out pharmaceuticals at this point, Browne is essentially setting aside plants and turning to the bolder, controversial course of chemical medicine with its focus on mineral, lapidary, or metallic medicaments. Browne has been prepared for this openness to chemical medicine by his medical training, especially in Montpellier, and so it is hardly surprising that he purveys no anxiety over the turn from plants to minerals. Setting aside any mystical or metaphysical pretensions that some of these chemical ingredients are awarded in alchemical discourse, Browne is wholly practical in prescribing "spirits of salt," iron in two forms or modes (pills and tartar or sediment), vitriol, and coral. With the coming of spring, Browne returns from chemistry to botany and reports that his patient is notably relieved ("*egregium levamen*") but not cured. Each in its proper proportions of drams, ounces or maniples, the constituents number almost thirty. In this recipe, Browne is careful to group the ingredients according to the section of the plant from which the medicine is taken, a point of considerable importance in view of the fact that degrees of qualities such as hot and dry vary from part to part. Many of the ingredients have been discussed, though sometimes inadequately, by the ancients; but Browne includes winter's bark, a recent discovery of explorers in the new world.[43] In certain cases such as maidenhair, previous treatments are filled with confusion and instability; Browne sometimes specifies which herb within the nomenclature he means, for instance noting that he wants the polypodium (which grows on old trees and walls) to be gathered from oaks, the best of its kind. Finally, he factors in caraway and coriander seeds with an eye toward helping Sir Charles recover his appetite and digestion after all the purging. The concoction is to be taken in beer.

As his notebooks as well as his work on vulgar errors attest, Browne was dedicated to updating his medical knowledge, both through reading and experience. One sees this not just in his acute awareness of new diseases such as rickets, but also in simpler queries such as "whether hydropicall persons swell most in the increment of the moone," or "whether the urines of healthfull persons have a very good odour, if unsound, not so," with the consumption of asparagus playing a role in the latter problem (Keynes, 3.272). But staying up-to-date and sustaining a busy practice placed a strain on Browne from very early in his Norwich years, a point reinforced for his readers in 1646 when Browne noted that the writing up of his research had been seriously delayed by the demands of his profession:

> Some consideration we hope from the course of our Profession, which though it leadeth us into many truths that passe undiscerned by others, yet doth it disturbe their communications, and much interrupt the office of our pens in their well intended transmissions: and therefore surely in this worke attempts will exceed performances: it being composed by snatches of time, as medicall vacations, and the fruitlesse importunity of Vroscopy would permit me.[44]

In this disregard for "piss-prophets," which he shared with many learned physicians,[45] Browne permits himself to express impatience with the ignorance of his patients, who are apt to violate his "quiet doors and unmolested hours" with urine samples, the analysis of which Browne deems pointless. Even the reference to

[43] See MacKinnon, 511.
[44] Browne, *Posthumous Works*, iii; Robbins, ed., *Pseudodoxia Epidemica*, 1.2.
[45] See Beier, *Sufferers & Healers*, 22–3.

"medicall vacations" serves as something of a slight to his patients, since these hiatuses from medical practice were occasioned by vulgar errors concerning times of the year, such as the dog days, when people generally refused medicine in order to let nature take her course. In *Pseudodoxia*, Browne criticized this basic misapprehension of medicine, deeming the opinion that nature requires breaks from medical intervention "not onely erroneous, but unnaturall" (Robbins, ed., *Pseudodoxia Epidemica*, 1.352–3).

As a manuscript poem testifies, Browne's manner of intervening in the afflictions of his patients was at once vibrantly heroic and finely sensitive. Among the Browne papers in the Bodleian Library is a set of verses entitled "A Cordiall return of thanks unto Dr Brown for the despaired off Cure of Mrs E. S. aged 57 sick of a violent continuall ffever, her body, and spirits almost wasted with a long, continued quartan Ague, still wasting itself with a smart loosness, and possessed by a strong Consumption." The author, N. S., reflects just how closely patients and their loved ones paid attention both to the vicissitudes of a complex disease and to the performances of their physicians.[46] With its opening flourish—"He Came, Saw, Cur'd!"—the poem heralds Dr Browne as a heroic member of the learned medical profession whose Caesarean endeavors have outshone those of Galen, Hippocrates, and London's College of Physicians. The success of the cure depends in some measure on learning—the physician is depicted as delivering a "Lecture o're this Skeliton," the patient emaciated by consumption. But quickly its verses turn to the translation of learning into judgment, and the expression of judgment in gesture or performance. As Browne's "modest eye search[ed] ev'ry part; | Judging, not seeing, how unto the Heart | It [every part] stood affected," his combination of skill and grace also shaped "how his gentle hand | Did prove her pulses (deaths Heraulds) command." Retaining its sense of Browne's heroic intervention, the poem replicates the "exactest care" with which the physician clarified the condition: "That loosness, ffever, and consumption | Each other did oppose, yet all as one | Resolv'd to storm the Ague untaken ffort | Her Heart."

In the climax of the battle for the heart of E. S., N. S.'s version of Browne's understanding of nature is at once pious, imperious, and crafty, turning the diseases against one another: "with Gods help, I'le show | What man can do, And thus, ffever, thy heat | Her Ague & chilness shalt breath out in sweat; | Consumption thou must wast its congeal'd cake; | Thou Loosness must a double office take, | Agues dregs purg; and ffeavers heat abate, | Keeping the body in soluble state." With the hotter and looser constituents of the disease combating the cold, costive ague, the heroic physician saves the heart from a united attack, for success requires his pharmaceutical intervention as well as God's approval: "I'le my best skill employ unto this end | The means apply'd, God may a blessing send." In the author's final exaltation of Dr. Browne, N. S. not only wishes that London's physicians and

[46] The poem is in Rawlinson D.391, f. 33r. The author is probably Nathan Scottow, whose wife Browne recommends to Edward for further medical consultation. Although it is possible that the poem is in fact about Edward, its context—apparently away from London—and its reference to *Religio Medici* suggest father Thomas.

courts had been on hand to witness this cure but summarizes what he has seen as "Religio et Ars Medici."

As early as 1644, prominent Norfolk families were celebrating the skills and authority of Dr Browne; in that year, the correspondence of the Knyvett family included a letter in which a family member is exhorted to "meddle no further with Phissick with out an Apparant necessity and the Advise of Dr Browne."[47] The trust that the Knyvetts placed in Browne was not just medical; in May of the same year, a letter expressed the desire to have his assistance in preventing the seizure of family "goods."[48] The N. S. poem and perhaps another manuscript poem agree that Browne's services were especially welcome for their combination of medical acumen with godliness. In the Browne papers, an anonymous poet urges a renowned physician to "Say on…for none like you | Can Doctor both ye Soul & Body too. | Your equal skill in Both seems so complext, | that you preach drugs, & scarify ye Text." The main point of this is clear enough: the physician has so thoroughly interwoven physic and piety that it is impossible to tell them apart in his performance. Rather less clear is what the poet means by scarifying the Bible. Perhaps the poet simply means to say that the physician's attention to the Bible is wonderfully precise and skillful, yet given the fact that the verb can mean both "to bleed by making slight incisions" and "to subject something to relentless criticism," it is of course noteworthy that *Religio Medici* was already eliciting displeasure in its readers for subjecting the Bible to critique. In any case, the poem goes on to praise the paradox of the physican's "Double Talentte" and "true Galenical Divinity," the inseparability between the physician's patients and proselytes, his concoction of pills so that they "cooperate with Grace," his skill in bodies to rival that of the Council of Trent in spiritual matters, and even his purgation of sin "by way of excrement," a bold encroachment on the territory of divinity that Browne himself dared to make in *Religio*.[49]

As notes in his commonplace books indicate, Browne carefully cultivated the religion of his medical practice. Among his exhortations to a life of constant and ubiquitous prayer, he included the reminder "to pray dayly and particularly for sick patients, & in generall for others, wheresoever, howsoever, under whose care soever, & at the entrance into the howse of the sick to say, the peace and mercy of god bee in this place" (Keynes, 3.325). This list of reminders to pray was predominantly private: "in the night & my dark bed when I could not sleep"; upon waking, whether at the four o'clock bell or at the coming of light (praying from the "collect of our liturgie"); and "in all places where privacy inciteth." Yet it was also public: "in any howse, high way, or streete, & to knowe no street or passage in this citty which may not witnesse that I have not forgot god & my saviour in it, & that no parish or towne where I have been may not say the like"; "upon the sight of any church which I see or passe by as I ride about"; and "after the sermon to take a

[47] Bertram Schofield, ed., *The Knyvett Letters, 1620–1644* (Norwich: Norfolk Record Society, 1949), 136–7.

[48] Schofield, ed., *The Knyvett Letters*, 142.

[49] Bodleian Rawlinson MS D.391, f. 91; cf. Patrides, 151.

thancksgiving & desire a blessing, & to pray for the minister." Browne's encouragements to prayer were not only integral to his consideration of his patients and medical colleagues; they were also responses to the taxing demands of his vocation: "Since the necessities of the sick & unavoidable diversions of my profession keep mee from church, yet to take all possible care that I might never miss sacraments, upon their accustomed dayes." And this program of prayer was also meant to ensure that the medical practice avoided the pitfalls of ambition, worldliness, and an unseemly gain from the misery of others. For Browne, the two caring professions of medicine and ministry overlapped.

As later letters and documents testify, Browne's clients included the poor as well as the rich and middling.[50] And they were scattered throughout the county of Norfolk as well as in the city of Norwich. Browne's purchase of a meadow drives home the significance of the horse that he rode to his patients, and his notebooks and letters are filled with remarks on how his profession removes him from the city into the countryside.[51] Patients were also apt to travel to their physicians, especially if "sufferers were sufficiently desperate or when the practitioner was sufficiently renowned."[52] Browne's charitable disposition toward his poor patients chimed with Norwich's "well-developed social policy with respect to illness and disability among the poor," a legacy that stretched back to Elizabethan times and featured the use of medical contracts.[53] The conditions of these contracts magnified the responsibilities of the physician, who at times "agreed to 'keep' the patient during the cure, and could also accept liability for the patient's future condition—that is, he or she guaranteed to keep the person 'whole' for his or her life, or accept the liability the patient might then represent."[54] Norwich's social policy was sufficiently fine-tuned to specify the need for the care of the elderly as well as of children,[55] with the latter interest dovetailing with Browne's initiation into fatherhood in the 1640s. Norwich also developed a reputation for providing one specialization, lithotomy or the removal of bladder stones, with the Mayor's Court assisting the care of poor children, especially boys, for this affliction.[56] Browne treated some of his distinguished patients, including Sir Hamon L'Estrange and Bishop Joseph Hall, for the bladder

[50] See chapter 11 in this volume. See also Charles Williams, *The Treatment of the Sick in Norwich during the Seventeenth Century* (Norwich: Fletcher and Son, 1903), 4; and Margaret Pelling and Charles Webster, "Medical practitioners," in Charles Webster, ed., *Health, Medicine, and Mortality in the Sixteenth Century* (New York: Cambridge University Press, 1979), 165–235, at 220.

[51] Anthony Batty Shaw, "Sir Thomas Browne's Meadow," *Notes and Queries* 216 (1971), 295–9.

[52] Anne Digby, *Making a Medical Living: Doctors and Patients in the English Market for Medicine, 1720–1911* (Cambridge: Cambridge University Press, 1994), 111.

[53] Margaret Pelling, *Medical Conflicts in Early Modern London: Patronage, Physicians, and Irregular Practitioners, 1550–1640* (Oxford: Clarendon Press, 2003), 246; and on Norwich and the poor, see Pelling, *The Common Lot*, 63–102.

[54] Pelling, *Medical Conflicts in Early Modern London*, 246–54.

[55] See Pelling, *The Common Lot*, 111–75; and Pelling, "Who Most Needs to Marry?: Ageing and Inequality among Women and Men in Early Modern Norwich," in Lynn Botelho and Pat Thane, eds., *Women and Ageing in British Society since 1500* (New York: Longmans, 2001), 31–42. A children's hospital in Norwich was begun in 1621.

[56] See Anthony Batty Shaw, "The Norwich School of Lithotomy," *Medical History* 14 (1970), 221–59, especially 223–8 for the seventeenth century and Browne.

stone by pharmaceutical means. Yet in praising lithotomy as a "great operation," Browne cautioned that actual cutting in these cases should be performed by the physician only if there is no barber surgeon present (Keynes, 4.27).

Browne's commitment to helping his patients sometimes manifested itself as a bemusement both with their peevishness and vulnerability to deception: "Since you are so much unsatisfied with the many rationall medicines which you say you have tried for the gout," he joked in one such moment, "you may imply your curiosity in the triall of many empiricall & odde medicines," the list of which is difficult to read for tone. Since the putatively absurd recipes reveal the unnamed patient's excesses in drink and sex, it is likely that Browne was having a private joke regarding curiosities such as shoes made from lion's skin, owl eggs, a suffocated eel or frog, amulets of "spiders leggs worne in a peece of deeres skinne," waters drunk from the Nile, "gellies of boares & bulls pizzells," and "the Sigill of Paracelsus" (Keynes, 3.269–70). Yet given the fact that learned and chemically minded physicians such as his friend Arthur Dee could easily run afoul of the College of Physicians, Browne must have known that the line between learned and empirical medicine was not always clear. This problem would only intensify over the course of his career as physicians such as Thomas Sydenham touted their own empirical foundation, and researchers such as Browne himself turned increasingly to natural history.[57] Yet Browne does not appear to have let anxieties about disciplinary boundaries overly affect him, even as his own tendency to synthesize medical philosophies and agendas was modified by his emerging campaign against vulgar errors.[58] It is noteworthy that in the preface to the *Pseudodoxia*, Browne is less concerned about the loss of reading time than about the delays in "communications"—in vulgar English, not Latin, at that.

In addition to the medical syllabus that Browne designed for Henry Power,[59] their further correspondence in the 1640s shows the advisor and his pupil striving for a balance between vocational practicality and the philosophical inquisitiveness requisite for a genuinely resourceful medicine. In a letter of thanks written from Halifax in the summer of 1646, Power is keen to impress on his mentor that Cambridge stresses natural philosophy and "Physicall Contemplation" even for its undergraduates. But above all young Henry is enthusiastic about Browne's generous "Communication," going so far as to assure his older correspondent that a trip to Norwich in order to collaborate with Browne on "some practicall knowledge" would be most welcome. Combined in Power's letters with the medical training, narrowly construed, are two intellectual endeavors which merge with yet also rival one another: alchemical Hermeticism and natural history. With his

[57] Pelling, *Medical Conflicts in Early Modern London*, 98n.

[58] See Pelling, *Medical Conflicts in Early Modern London*, 19. See also William Birken, "The Social Problem of the English Physician in the Early Seventeenth Century," *Medical History* 31 (1987), 201–16; Pelling, "Medical Practice in Early Modern England: Trade or Profession?" in Wilfrid Prest, ed., *The Professions in Early Modern England* (New York: Croom Helm, 1987), 90–128; Rosemary O'Day, *The Professions in Early Modern England, 1450–1800: Servants of the Commonweal* (New York: Longmans, 2000), 183–251.

[59] Discussed above in chapter 3 of this volume.

prompt from *Religio Medici*, Power finds himself obsessed with, and disconcerted by, the chemical mysteries by which "an incinerated plant" might be reconstituted or "re-individualled" from the matrix of its form (Keynes, 4.258). In another letter, from September 1648, Power admits that he may be running "into too deepe a beliefe & too strong a conceipt of chymistry (yet not beyond wt some of those Artists affirme) of the reproduction of the same plant by ordinary way of vegetation." But he is asking for more than just for his mentor to make good on ocular demonstrations of the highest, strangest mysteries of the faith, though this would be plenty to ask; the young scholar is also seeking from Browne some guidance about how to approach the future of natural philosophy (Keynes, 4.259–60). In a letter written from Halifax on August 28, 1649, Power recalls the observations in natural history to which he was made privy with Browne on a visit to Norwich: "There were many things wch I tooke notice of in the Vipers head, you pleas'd to shew me when I was last at Norwich, especially concerning the two poisonous Teeth wch moved in the upper jaw upon jemmers, wch shee could lay flat along a little cavity of either side of hir jaw, or erect them as shee pleased." This close attention to the mechanism of the serpent's mouth differs radically from inquiries about the resurrection of a plant from its ashes (Keynes, 4.261–3).

During the 1640s, Browne himself was attempting to stabilize his position on the future of natural studies, a state of affairs made more difficult by three factors. First, there was a growing tension between, on the one hand, those philosophers (such as Browne's friend Arthur Dee) who continued to fight for the legitimacy of Hermetic magic, and on the other those advocates of Francis Bacon's Great Instauration who heralded a radical separation of a true mechanical natural philosophy from the bogus theosophies of Hermes and Neoplatonism. Second, medicine was especially caught in the competition between these tendencies by virtue of its traditional collaboration between theory and practice, with the former still affording ample opportunity for speculation on physical mysteries such as generation which demanded contemplation on how the soul relates to the body. Third, Power and Browne make virtually no mention of the civil wars raging in England in the 1640s, but the traumatic events of the decade exerted an influence on how and why students turned to the study of nature as against law or theology.

Soon Browne's published writings made him into an internationally famous authority with admirers from an exceptionally wide cultural and confessional range of readers. In the interstices between his two personae—local physician and international author—Browne's world of learning expanded even as his sober commitments to family, medical practice, moral discipline, and local flora and fauna anchored him in the watery world of Norfolk. Indeed Browne's patients were eager to unite his two personae as their personal physician and as the famous, exceptionally learned Doctor Browne. Letters such as those exchanged with Sir Hamon L'Estrange epitomize how extremely busy Browne was, how much in demand his opinions were, and how carefully and resourcefully he advised patients throughout the area, those too far away for him readily to visit as well as those neighbors whose humors and habits he knew very well. Back in the early 1640s this state of affairs was only just beginning to emerge: all the more reason, then, for Browne to take control of his *Religio Medici* so that he might shape as carefully as possible his persona of a Christian physician in the public eye.

2. *RELIGIO* REDUX

Despite all the demands of his vocation in the late 1630s and early 1640s, as well as his labors on "vulgar errors," Browne continued to revise the work that would soon become, perhaps had already become, *Religio Medici*. Of the extant manuscripts, six represent a middle stage between the earliest drafts reflected in Pembroke and Lansdowne and the unauthorized editions of 1642 for which one from this middle family of manuscripts, now presumably lost, served as a basis. The provenance of the six is various: an alumnus of St John's College, Cambridge, named Bambridge Dean, who had Norwich connections,[60] a Lancashire family library, and Mimms House, Hertfordshire, for instance. The manuscripts are sometimes bound with others: one with a theological treatise by John Overall, a bishop of Norwich who died there in 1619, but also with a lyric that excoriates Cavaliers who give up on their cause. One of the six ponders the question of its authorship, offering the theory that the Scottish physician Alexander Read might be responsible, yet also criticizing that theory on the basis of the manuscript's elegant English and its devotion to the Church of England.[61] Although they offer no numbers for their paragraphs or sections, they tend to divide the text far more frequently than either the unauthorized or authorized editions, as though Browne were thinking of his book as a set of aphorisms on the order of what would become his *Christian Morals*. And while the manuscripts have their several differences, they concur in their division of the work into two parts (on faith and charity), this change perhaps intended to make the work accessible to a wider audience than just Browne's immediate circle of friends. The attempt in this second stage of revisions to prepare the complex *Religio* for a wider audience is certified by the addition in several manuscripts of marginal glosses. Clarity is also gained from little changes, such as the intermittent insertion of "therefore" into a course of thought, the removal of wordiness, the heightening of parallelism, and the conversion of coordination into subordination.

These revisions, probably made in Norwich from around 1637 through about 1640, offer more than just means of accessibility. Whether Sanna is right in arguing that the addition of passages elevating faith over reason amounts to Browne's reaction against the nearby Cambridge Platonists, she is certainly right that the author's various elaborations of his work suggest the vibrancy of Browne's new life

[60] He became rector of Croswick and Beeston, just north of Norwich.

[61] NRO MS 21268, T134D. Alexander Read (*c*.1570–1641) was a surgeon who in 1616 had published *A Description of the Body of Man*. Incorporated MD at Oxford in 1620, he "was appointed on December 28, 1632 to give an anatomy lecture every Tuesday in the Barber-Surgeons' Hall." His lectures appeared in print in 1635 and 1638. With William Harvey he was on hand for a notorious witch trial in Lancashire in 1634. His findings in the trial were wholly medical (*ODNB*, Shona MacLean Vance).

as a physician in Norwich, no doubt too his maturing thought processes, as well as his concerns about the heightening of political, religious, and military conflict in England and Scotland from 1637 onward.[62] In one passage, Browne traces the history of treacherous sectarianism all the way back to Satan's temptation of Eve (Sanna, 22). In another, he qualifies his disregard for the "multitude" with an observation that "there is a rabble even amongst the Gentry, a sort of Plebeian heads, whose fancy moves with the same wheele" as the vulgar "Mechanickes" (130–1). What follows is Browne's most extended meditation on social rank and nobility, including his argument for the solitary or "forlorne person" over and above the one who craves a following, and his version of the standard maxim that true nobility depends on moral worth rather than genealogy. Other elaborations in the second-stage manuscripts demonstrate Browne's engagement with, and theories of, social dynamics. In one, he elaborates on social relations with a skepticism that reflects the vagaries of reputation in its widening circle of associates: "No man can justly censure or condemne another, because indeed no man truly knowes another. This I perceive in my selfe, for I am in the darke to all the world, and my nearest friends behold mee but in a cloud; those that know mee but superficially, thinke lesse of me than I doe of myselfe; those of my neere acquaintance thinke more" (142). A far cry from the intimate friendship of the Pembroke manuscript, this passage evolves into a reminder of how well God knows Browne's worthlessness, but also into moral generalizations about the ways in which "no man can judge another, because no man knowes himselfe."

As is the case in other passages added at the second stage, Browne traces human behavior back to Adam and Eve—a reflection of his work on vulgar errors—and revels in the paradoxes that such a history can breed ("*Cain* was not therefore the first murtherer, but *Adam*, who brought in death"). But moral philosophy and paradox never completely replace contemporary observation, and the physician offers his analysis of how the humoral complexion of charity, cold and humble, is threatened by "the fires and flames of zeale" (Sanna, 142–3). In smaller ways, too, Browne's revisions register his passionate responses to the changing times: the Reformation has been ruined by "Presbyters" rather than by "Prelates," a sentiment in keeping with the clashes between English prelacy and Scottish Presbyterianism, though Browne reverts to blaming the prelates in the first authorized edition (10). In his irenic distaste for reckless controversy, Browne changes the more sympathetic characterization in Pembroke and Lansdowne—"Many out of zeale unto truth, more conscious of their desires than abilityes"—into the somewhat more hostile diagnosis of "Many from the ignorance of these Maximes, and an inconsiderate zeale unto Truth" (17–18).

Some of the fullest additions elaborate on the constituents of Browne's faith. One passage heralds the mature Browne's subjection of tired, sinful rationality to faith, as well as a list of items from the Bible that only faith, not reason, could ever

[62] See Vittoria Sanna, ed., *Religio Medici: Edizione Critica con Introduzione e Note*, 2 vols. (Cagliari: Annali delle Facoltà di Lettere-Filosofia e Magistero dell'Università di Cagliari, 1958), 1.xxxv–xxxvi. All quotations from her version of the text come from volume 1, either by page or line.

believe (Sanna, 26). Another bout of fideism occurs when he adds the claim that "many things are true in Divinity, which are neither inducible by reason, nor confirmable by sense" (106). Even so, the elaboration proves to possess an epistemological complexity that chimes with Browne's growing concerns about the authorities of knowledge in the *Pseudodoxia*.

One of the most extraordinary additions serves in simplest terms to reaffirm Browne's belief in the art of providence in the face of contrary evidence. Since divine providence is supposed to create a world of beauty, order, and purpose, it bodes ill for the believer if creation includes ugly, aimless, monstrous phenomena. Three times in a row, the added passage asserts the logic of providence over observations or concepts potentially undermining that logic. Thus toads, bears, and elephants preserve a decorum in nature insofar as their putatively ugly outsides perfectly "expresse" their inner natures. The existence of monsters demonstrates that nature is ingenious and playful. As for the primary "Chaos" from which God made the world, there is no question of deformity in a raw material into which the creative God had not yet chosen to inject form. The passage is hardly self-satisfied or complacent with its logic of providence, however. Not only does Browne assiduously invent test cases for his resolution, but his concluding generalization involving art's relationship to nature proves to be one of the work's most exploratory (if brief) passages. Beginning with the mutual service of art and nature on behalf of divine providence, Browne seems momentarily to privilege art in making it the completion ("perfection") of nature, adding that without the creation of the human, "there were yet a Chaos." Having temporarily elevated art, he then segregates it from nature in a kind of peaceful co-existence: "Nature hath made one world, and Art another." With all these possibilities for their relationship in place, Browne concludes with a celebration of nature that makes it virtually interchangeable with art: "In briefe, all things are artificiall, for Nature is the Art of God" (Sanna, 38–9). Under the influence of George Hakewill's defense of providence, but also deeply involved in the Baconian eradication of vulgar error, Browne works hard in this second stage of composition to test and to reaffirm his conviction that natural studies reinforce divinity.

Heightening the more mystical dimensions of his natural studies, Browne interjects a long passage on the possibility of a "common Spirit to the whole world," a paragraph that testifies to his love of Plato and Hermes, to his intensified distaste for sectarian divisions, and to a fervent spirituality, not unlike that of the Cambridge Platonists, that celebrates the presence of divinity in terms of light and heat. This praise for the spirit of God not only features some of Browne's most beautiful prose in the *Religio*, but it concludes with the addition of over twenty verses comparing the radiance of the divine to the powerful heat of the sun. If the additions to *Religio* can delight in poesy, they also relish paradox, for it was at this stage of revision that Browne inserted his witty argument for human cannibalism on the basis of the text, "All flesh is grasse" (Sanna, 83). In counterpoint to this gruesome playfulness, Browne also elaborates on the insights of age and maturity: in one passage, he justifies the desire to outlive Christ yet observes that there is every reason to die young when, after all, "age doth not rectifie, but incurvate our natures, turning bad dispositions into worser habits, and (like diseases) brings on incurable vices" (93). At once, the physician and the moralist face down the most sobering realities of longevity.

If some changes reflect Browne's sense of the growing audience for his manuscript, the process is only partial, for he at times renders the work even more personal than it was before, and he is just as prone to mitigate the stridency of thought with an "I thinke," "me thinkes," "For mine owne part," or "I protest" as he is to depersonalize his notions by removing the pronoun. While many of the changes in syntax and wording illustrate an attentiveness to the details, thought sequences, and rhythms of his prose that Browne would show for the whole of his life, others seem clearly aimed at refashioning his authorial persona. When Browne omits a passage in which he confesses his preference for "hermeticall" and fanciful evocations of death over "those strict definitions of death, by privation of life, extintion of naturall heate, separation, etc. of soule and body," he presents himself as a more mainstream learned physician whose "naturall and experimentall way" is less prone to flights into alchemical metaphors concluding only with an et cetera (Sanna, 89).

In Browne's early Norwich years, *Religio Medici* was making a wider circuit, both spatially and culturally, than previous scholarship has allowed, and Browne appears to have known something about this transmission. Most notably, as Kathryn Murphy has shown, a manuscript of the work was in the possession of John Gauden by 1640; Gauden was the minister who would later become famous as the ghost writer of the prayers attributed to King Charles in *Eikon Basilike*.[63] In 1640, Gauden was sharing news of *Religio Medici* with Samuel Hartlib, who recorded the fact in his diary, and was said to have become acquainted with the work and its author, a "man of excellent parts living at Norwich," by the mediation of Lady Judith Barrington. The manuscript had already acquired a name—*Medici Religio*—as would its author in a second entry in Hartlib's diary. Gauden had not yet developed the staunchly Royalist agenda that he would embrace a little later. The Barrington family was committed to the support of Puritan ministry, while Gauden's attraction to Browne's work appears to have centered on its irenicism. Given Gauden's connections to the publisher Andrew Crooke, Murphy points out that the Cambridgeshire vicar and chaplain to the Earl of Warwick may have served as the means by which *Religio Medici* first came to press. What we can be sure of is that the manuscript audiences for Browne's work cannot be consigned to a rigidly defined profile or demographic. Indeed, Hartlib's was an intellectual network that ranged across a broad spectrum of cultural brokers and intellectuals.

Although Browne retained a number of readings from 1642 for the authorized edition of 1643, he also lamented that the multiplying transcriptions had produced

[63] Kathryn Murphy, "'A man of excellent parts': Browne's *Religio Medici*," *TLS*, July 4, 2008, 14–15. As Murphy notes, we do not yet know exactly how Lady Barrington and Browne encountered one another. "The problem," she notes "is not the lack of possible avenues of acquaintance, but rather the ease with which the prominent families of Norfolk can be used to narrow the degrees of separation between Browne and the Barringtons."

a "successively corrupted" condition (Patrides, 59). Indeed, neither the accuracy of the two 1642 unauthorized editions, nor their relationship to the authorized editions that followed, is a simple matter. Browne retained the publisher and the frontispiece when he regained control of his work. Having achieved the freedom of the Stationers' Company in 1629, Andrew Crooke (*c.*1605–1674) had risen to take the livery of the company by 1638. His shop under the sign of the Green Dragon in St Paul's Churchyard was well known for its publication of plays, as well as for well-loved prose works such as travel narratives or pithy essays like those found in John Earle's *Microcosmographie* and Thomas Overbury's *Characters*—the latter perhaps the genre into which Crooke placed *Religio Medici*. Over the course of the mid-seventeenth century, Crooke would also publish important works in medicine and philosophy, including some works of Hobbes.[64] Crooke also offered for sale certain popular books of piety, including works by the colonial divine Thomas Hooker and the extraordinarily successful *Practice of Piety* by Lewis Bayly.[65] With his knowledge of Latin, Crooke had something of a reputation as a learned bookseller.[66] Whoever conceived the idea for William Marshall's woodcut of a man toppling from a rocky promontory, only to be saved by the hand of providence, it is not surprising that Browne liked it. It resonated with the images of the arrogant tumblers such as Icarus on display in the Leiden anatomy theater; and it embodied effectively the motif of divine assistance that permeates the *Religio* and is suggested by the heading of the Lansdowne manuscript, "*syn theo*." Browne's sympathetic early reader, Henry Bates, found the image evocative in comparing Sir Kenelm Digby's critique of *Religio* to "the fall of Phaeton."[67]

Browne's revisions for the authorized edition manifest some clear but not always consistent trends: sometimes toward neutrality or prudence, at other times toward political engagement with tumultuous times.[68] His expansion of ideas and conceits sometimes leads into or accentuates those perilous grounds on which he stood indicted by his more hostile critics. It is easy to spot the prudence of the newly established professional man and respectable citizen of Norwich. The violence of "cut off my arme" in the rejection of iconoclasm is softened (Sanna, ll. 73–5); ameliorative terms are introduced in order to scale down the size or dogmatism of claims (ll. 76, 457, 459, 1077, 1180, 1865, 2122, 2566, 2669), or to reinforce irenic gestures (l. 78). Brazenness is removed (for instance, "no man shall reach my faith unto another Article, or command my obedience to a Canon more," ll. 120–1), while the extremism of phrases such as "I was inclined by an excesse of charitie" is

[64] Mark Goldie's entry on Andrew Crooke in *ODNB*. See also H. R. Plomer et al., *A Dictionary of the Booksellers and Printers Who Were at Work in England, Scotland, and Ireland from 1641 to 1667* (London: Bibliographical Society, 1907). For the 1642 edition of *Religio*, see also Frank L. Huntley, "The Publication and Immediate Reception of *Religio Medici*," *The Library Quarterly* 25 (1955), 203–18.

[65] See Huntley, "The Publication," 204–5.

[66] Mark Goldie's entry on Andrew Crooke in *ODNB*.

[67] Quoted in Huntley, "The Publication," 218.

[68] NRO MS 4504 55x7 comprises a small fair copy of the passages to be added to 1643, together with the prefatory matter by A. B. and Browne himself.

pruned or rewritten. A certain amount of theological bravado is removed: Browne's challenge to a conventional proof of the trinity from Genesis is excised (ll. 921–7); his hesitation to say that he hates even the devil is redirected towards "any essence but the Devill" (ll. 2389–90); and a metaphysical passage on immortality which begins with a claim about what God will not do is erased (ll. 1935–42). The responsible physician removes his admission to having spent time in taverns (l. 2759).

When Browne comes to adding extensive passages or even entire sections, the 1643 edition can become politically engaged and theologically speculative rather than prudent or platitudinous. The very first major addition, section 8 of part 1, is both engaged and speculative at once. As a mini-history of sectarianism, it decries the fragmentation of the church "almost into Atomes," an image evoking anarchy as well as destruction. And it offers a quasi-medical diagnosis of why heresy is always vexing the church, for there will always be "heads that are disposed unto Schisme and complexionally propense to innovation" (Sanna, 22–3). This lingering on the rending of the church bears directly on what Browne considers the zealous puritanical sickness creating civil war in England. In what seems at first a mitigating concession or afterthought, however, Browne offers one of his boldest paeans to the solitary, speculative mind. Throughout the history of the church, he says, such wits not only have explored theological ideas with "a sober judgement . . . without offence or heresie"; but they have unpacked their "singular opinions and conceits" in such a way as to produce both healthy recreation and extraordinary truth: "for there is yet after all the decrees of counsels and the niceties of the Schooles, many things untouch'd, unimagin'd, wherein the libertie of an honest reason may play and expatiate with security and farre without the circle of an heresie" (Sanna, 23).[69] Whereas Browne's earlier images of orthodoxy involve restrictive circles, including the wheel of the church, here his notion of orthodoxy permits, even encourages, the honest thinker to have fun, to soar, to expand. By seventeenth-century standards, the result may prove extraordinary: religious truth somehow missed over the course of history. Indeed, if some of the additions to the 1643 edition are aimed at prudence, others rank among Browne's most theological and politically daring. Reflecting his work on vulgar errors, for instance, one section challenges the orthodox notion of a physical, locatable hell, venturing to resituate its site in the human heart (ll. 2089–2106).

Browne's location of orthodoxy outside the circle of heresy suggests that heretical thought is always severely limited by the diseased, aggrandizing will of the heretic. By contrast and implication, English orthodoxy licenses well-intentioned philosophers to explore the mysteries of their faith, in full view of the fact that no church can truly claim infallibility. Another implication of this passage is that English orthodoxy is not finally as censorious as the Puritan zealots have made it out to be—Browne is no doubt encouraged in this claim by virtue of the fact that Joseph Hall is the current bishop of Norwich, not the aggressive Matthew Wren,

[69] Sanna's text includes an emendation of "there is" to "there are"; I restore the original 1643 reading.

the bishop upon Browne's arrival in the city. But much later in the work, Browne converts this general observation about singularity into one of the most personal additions to the 1643 when he celebrates the expansiveness of his own thinking: "that masse of flesh that circumscribes me, limits not my mind: that surface that tells the heavens it hath an end, cannot perswade me I have any; I take my circle to be above three hundred and sixty" (Sanna, ll. 3062–4). As Sir Kenelm Digby was among the first to point out, the limitless cosmography claimed for Browne's microcosm might be thought to sit uneasily with his claims to follow doggedly the great wheel of the church. Indeed, the passage dares to boast that "whilst I study to finde how I am a Microcosme or little world, I finde my selfe something more than the great." Then once again it veers toward a radicalism for which he earned the favor of the Quaker Samuel Duncon[70]: "There is surely a peece of Divinity in us, something that was before the Elements, and owes no homage unto the Sun" (ll. 3064–71). In this one passage, all the cross-currents of the 1643 edition flow together: the politically engaged barb cast at those proponents of utter human depravity whose failure to appreciate man's creation in the image of God is a most vulgar error, ignorant of even "the Alphabet of man"; a highly prudent removal of two self-promoting passages in the lines that follow; and a heightened commitment to the playful, paradoxical expatiations of the singular human mind.

Browne's most prominent efforts at controlling the understanding of his work came before the text of the *Religio* itself, in the prefatory material that sought to head off those criticisms and misprisions already beginning to multiply and coarsen. Even on the title page, readers are assured that they now have in their hands "a true and full coppy of that which was most imperfectly and Surreptitiously printed before vnder the name of *Religio Medici*"; the title itself is removed from its prior place next to the engraving, and the spelling of "*coelo*" is changed to "*cælo*." Depending on which of the three states a reader had of the 1643 edition, the work accrued over the course of the year the following apologetic material: Browne's own preface to the reader; a warning from one A. B. to those who have encountered Digby's *Observations on the Religio Medici*; a list of errata; and an exchange of letters between Browne and Digby. As this framework shows, Browne's attempt to regain control over his work was already a game of catch-up that he would quickly lose; he was already becoming his readers, who would remake him in a wide range of starkly contrasting images.

Browne assures his readers that the 1643 edition is "a full and intended copy," that his friends have insisted on the larger moral purpose of taking action against illegitimate printing, that the work itself is not meant to be polished in its learning or dogmatic in its claims, not least because the author himself has undergone—and continues to undergo—personal change; and that the language of the work is not strictly logical, but more loosely rhetorical and metaphorical, the explorations of a young contemplative Christian offered "in a soft and flexible sense, and not to be called unto the rigid test of reason" (Sanna, 7). In the other prefatory

[70] See chapter 9 in this volume.

matter to the 1643 edition, however, it soon becomes clear that the desire for "ingenuous" readers may be too much for which to hope. Digby's own explanation of his observations is one sustained exercise in irony. The inclusion of A. B.'s caution "to such as have, or shall peruse the Observations upon a former corrupt copy of this Booke," tells another story: Digby is a feckless, self-aggrandizing, and even malicious critic who "onely medleth with those points from whence he takes a hint to deliver his prepar'd conceptions" (Sanna, 4). In giving this sober warning, A. B. wants readers to know that Browne has had nothing to do with it: "slighting the refute," A. B. explains, Browne has been forced into publishing an authorized edition that on its own will provide "a sufficient confutation."

Already by 1643, however, the *Religio* was an astonishing publication event: for some readers such as John Aubrey, who recorded how in "1642, *Religio Medici* [was] printed" and "first opened my understanding," it offered a version of Christianity so fresh, evocative, and moving that their horizons of expectations were expanded;[71] for others, the *Religio* became a pawn in the wars of religion both in England and on the Continent, though the players laying claim to the pawn ranged all over the spectrum of contemporary positions, eventually from Catholic to Quaker. For some, it was the best that learned Europe had to offer, so much so that it was instantly honored with translation into Latin and an international, also vibrant, following. For others, both at home and abroad, it was a devilish atheistic poison insidiously proffered by a "Christian physician" in the form of a sweet, seductive rhetoric. Although it would be published eventually as *Medicus Medicatus: Or the Physicians Religion Cured, by a Lenitive or Gentle Potion* (1645), Alexander Ross's well-known assault on *Religio Medici* was first presented in manuscript as by an "Authour in Distresse," obviously a divine whose horrified vindication of the "True Church" exposed the malicious "traps and snares" of *Religio Medici*.[72] Francis Cheynell exhorted the House of Lords itself to "Beware of them that have no more Religion, then is to be found in that unworthy Book, called *Religio Medici, a Book too much applauded by Noble-men*." He had at least one noteworthy reason to worry about the book's threat to the nobility, since Digby's frequently read *Observations* on Browne's work was prompted by the reverence that Edward Sackville, fourth Earl of Dorset, had expressed in late 1642 toward *Religio Medici*, in large part because Dorset found therein the very ecumenical and irenic view of religion that he found to be devastated by the coming of civil war—himself a hybrid of those puritan, papist, and moderate-rational tendencies that the polemics of the civil war tended to manipulate.[73]

[71] John Aubrey, *Brief Lives*, ed. Andrew Clark, 2 vols. (Oxford: Clarendon Press, 1898), 1.37.

[72] *The True Church, Further Vindicated in An Answere to A Book intituled Religio Medici. By An Authour in Distresse*, Bodleian MS Rawl. B.211.

[73] Francis Cheynell, *The Man of Honour, Described in a Sermon, Preached before the Lords of Parliament, In the Abbey Church at Westminster, March 26.1645* (1645), 65. For Dorset, in addition to Digby's *Observations*, see the article by David L. Smith, "Catholic, Anglican or Puritan? Edward Sackville, Fourth Earl of Dorset, and the Ambiguities of Religion in Early Stuart England," *Transactions of the Royal Historical Society* 2 (1992), 105–24; Smith discusses Dorset's hybridity at 106.

As Aubrey's note makes clear, Digby's *Observations* were integrally linked with the *Religio* from the beginning, for Aubrey had taken Browne's work with him "to Eston, with Sir K.D."[74] Over the course of his "occasional" responses, Digby judged either Browne or his work to be "good natur'd" (Digby, 3), "curious" (4), full of "Spirit and smartnes" (4), witty (7), "very gallant, and generous" (51). Browne offered a delightful and "noble... conversation" (4), a "treasury," "strong parts and a vigorous brayne" (24), "a noble & a generous heart" (24), both "æquanimity" and "magnanimity" (29), "worthy motives" (75), and "a *Judicious* piety in making a right use of the blind zeale that Bigots loose themselves in," though it is hard to imagine "blind zeale" as a thing indifferent (6). Yet before ten pages are complete in the *Observations*, Digby has unleashed one of his most humiliating attacks on the *Religio*'s author: as a physician, the author has neither the philosophical depth nor the lofty orientation toward heavenly or spiritual values to do anything other than err ingeniously on questions of the immortal soul, grace, faith, charity, or providence. The upshot of Digby's critique is that Browne's philosophy offers the ridiculous scenario of a manual, if fanciful, laborer pretending to inhabit the social world of an aristocrat as well as the lofty reaches of philosophy: no wonder his views of virtue and charity are so mercantile and debased, so lacking in heroism and overwhelmed by the burden of material existence.

While both Digby and Ross allude only briefly to the "distracted times" (Ross, 79; cf. Digby, 79), both manage to convert Browne's meditations into a living force with an unstable vitality in contemporary England. More privately, readers filled Browne's margins with their complex responses. For instance, Christopher Wren (1589–1658)—the dean of Windsor, brother of former bishop of Norwich, Matthew Wren, as well as the father of the celebrated architect—had both leisure and motive aplenty to explore *Religio Medici* once he had been expelled by parliamentary forces in May 1643.[75] Aside from the extensive underlining and bracketing throughout the volume, Wren's margins betray the reader's enthusiasms, criticisms, confusions, and expatiations of Browne's provocative work. Wren is also fully prepared to delete, alter, and variously tinker with Browne's prose if the results are what Wren thinks are more acceptable and orthodox.[76] As with his annotations of *Pseudodoxia Epidemica*, Wren's responses can be intensely personal as well as learned. If Browne's first work could assist, inspire, and provoke a beleaguered clergyman, it was also having an impact on the bold new thinking of lay philosophers as well; indeed, in a fragmentary manuscript version of *De Corpore*, Thomas Hobbes saw fit to adopt a line from *Religio Medici*.[77] More elaborately

[74] Quotations from Digby come from *Observations vpon Religio Medici* (1643). For Digby's critique of the *Religio*, see Debora Shuger, "The Laudian Idiot," in Barbour and Preston, eds., *Sir Thomas Browne: The World Proposed*, 45–61; and James N. Wise, *Sir Thomas Browne's Religio Medici and Two Seventeenth-Century Critics* (Columbia: University of Missouri Press, 1973).

[75] Reid Barbour, "Dean Wren's *Religio Medici*: Reading in Civil War England," *Huntington Library Quarterly* 73 (2010), 263–72.

[76] Wren's annotation volume is in the Cardiff Public Library, MS 1.160.

[77] See Thomas Hobbes, *Critique du "De Mundo" de Thomas White*, ed. Jean Jacquot and Harold W. Jones (Paris: Vrin, 1973), 449.

one poet George Daniel celebrated Browne's work in rapturous verses while another, John Collop, took it upon himself to defend the beleaguered author from his enemies.[78]

The laudatory mail that Browne received on account of the *Religio* also captured its volatile, unfixed energy. In a letter from Greenwich dated August 28, 1647, Henry Bates professed to speak for all England ("this horizon") in praising Browne's "sublime solid phansie" and the *Religio* as "that incomparable piece of invention and judgment" (Wilkin, 1.353). Private correspondence throughout England testified to the waves made by the *Religio*. In a letter dated April 28, 1645, the year of two new editions of the book,[79] James Howell joked about Browne's desire for procreation without women.[80] In manuscript and print, not only did authors begin to cite or quote *Religio*; they also inaugurated the tradition of imitating it, with Edward Herbert's *Religio Laici* and J. Botrie's *Religio Jurisconsulti* being composed in the 1640s.[81] A few years later, Samuel Pepys would note William Petty's estimation that *Religio Medici* had proved a book "most esteemed and generally cried up for wit in the world."[82]

For all the extraordinary interest in the vernacular *Religio*, however, no single event in Browne's literary life had a greater importance than the work's translation into Latin. In his letter, Bates expressed his desire to undertake the translation, but on a trip to Leiden, he had discovered that a Latin version was already in the shops, the one first published as early as 1644, in Leiden, by John Merryweather. Like Bates, Merryweather intuited that the *Religio* would serve as an excellent English ambassador to the European Continent, though his experiences of marketing the translation impressed upon the translator that, abroad even more than at home, the work would have to make its way through the complicated, often contentious republic of letters.[83] In a letter to Browne, dated October 1, 1649, Merryweather, a Cambridge man, also admitted that he had run into trouble finding a publisher, beginning with a "book-merchant" named Haye, in whose services the great scholar Claude de Saumaise recommended against publication, complaining that while "there were indeed in it many things well said, . . . it contained also many exorbitant conceptions in religion, and would probably find but frowning entertainment, especially amongst the ministers, which deterred him from undertaking the printing." Undeterred, Merryweather presented the translation to two printers,

[78] *The Selected Poems of George Daniel of Beswick, 1616–1657*, ed. Thomas B. Stroup (Lexington: University of Kentucky Press, 1959), 62–3; John Collop, *The Poems of John Collop*, ed. Conrad Hilberry (Madison: University of Wisconsin Press, 1962), 104–5.

[79] See Geoffrey Keynes, *A Bibliography of Sir Thomas Browne Kt. M.D.*, second revised edition (Oxford: Clarendon Press, 1968), 13.

[80] James Howell, cited in Keynes, *Bibliography*, 176.

[81] See Keynes, *Bibliography*, 234.

[82] *The Diary of Samuel Pepys*, ed. Robert Latham and William Mathews, 9 vols. (Berkeley: University of California Press, 2000), 5.27–8.

[83] On the translation, see C. W. Schoneveld, "'The True Anatomy of My Selfe,'" in *Sir Thomas Browne, M.D. and the Anatomy of Man* (Leiden: Brill, 1982), 5–9; and Clarence H. Miller, "Seventeenth-Century Latin Translations of Two English Masterpieces: Hooker's *Polity* and Browne's *Religio Medici*," in *Acta Conventus Neo-Latini Abulensis: Proceedings of the Tenth International Congress of Neo-Latin Studies* (Tempe: Arizona Center for Medieval and Renaissance Studies, 2000), 55–72.

de Vogel and Christian, whose consultants also turned the book down (Wilkin, 1.368). Browne's old Dutch environs were finding the work too abnormal for appropriation into its theological synthesis. Yet Merryweather's conviction of the work's "innate and essential worth," together with his obstinate pursuit of a publisher who would predict its international appeal, led at last to a printer named Franciscus Hackius, "who, upon two days deliberation undertook it" (368).

From 1644 forward, Browne was a celebrity in England and abroad. According to Merryweather, not only were the Low Countries and France rife with false rumors of Browne's death, but in Paris, the Latin translation had been reprinted in 1644 but with "both the epistles left out, and a preface, by some papist, put in their place, in which making use of, and wresting some passages in your book, he endeavour'd to shew, that nothing but custom and education kept you from their church" (Wilkin, 1.367). Famous men such as Guy Patin eagerly sought after and commented on Browne's *Religio* but also on his life and character. As Patin's comments reveal, part of the fascination with Dr Browne resulted from the ways in which the *Religio* eluded convention: "It is a strange and pleasant book, but very delicate and wholly mystical; the author is not lacking in wit and you will see in him quaint and delightful thoughts. There are hardly any books of this sort." Despite his ongoing combat with the novelties of Montpellier medicine, Patin expressed a wish that Browne might lead European intellectual culture toward a new way of thinking and writing: "If scholars were permitted to write freely we would learn many new things; never has there been a newspaper equal to this; in this way the subtlety of the human spirit could be revealed."[84] Yet in another letter, this one from 1645, Patin followed up a comment on the widespread acclaim for the *Religio* with his doubts on the legitimacy of Browne's religion, which (Patin believed) needed a master.

On the Continent in the 1640s, Patin was by no means alone in his attention to Browne's new work.[85] Its most extraordinary early appearance came in a 1646 letter from John Amos Comenius to Samuel Hartlib, in which Browne's views of a "general Synod" figure into a discussion of how education might be wholly reformed according to the scheme of "pansophia."[86] As Browne's own religious identity was being bandied about even in the prefatory material to the various editions of the Latin *Religio*, some of his keenest readers saw through the smokescreen and came to suspect that Browne might hold the key not just to the reformation of learning but also to a seemingly unthinkable European peace. Merryweather's translation served to fascinate its European readers, not least with Browne's defense of "singularity" ("*paradoxi*") or his support for the discovery of unimagined truths ("*integra & intacta*"). The Parisian editor prefacing the pirated version of the 1644 translation was mistaken about Browne's crypto-Catholicism, but he grasped the work's powerful apology for the Christian faith, as well as its defense of the medical

[84] Translation of Patin in Finch, *Sir Thomas Browne*, 114.

[85] For minor references such as those in Jan de Brune's 1644 *Jok en Ernst*, see Keynes, *Bibliography*.

[86] See Kathryn Murphy's discussion of this letter in her essay " 'The best pillar of St Francis': Thomas Browne and Samuel Hartlib," in Murphy and Todd, ed., "*A Man very well studyed*," 273–92.

arts from calumny. Both friends and enemies of the work found ways of shaping the *Religio* to fit their understanding of the European scene: if certain Dutch Protestant readers found the work too "exorbitant" for true religion, so too did the Catholic censors who promptly placed the Latin translation on the Index. Indeed across the frontispiece of one copy of the Paris edition was scrawled the indictment "*hæreticus*."[87]

Given his view of the nature of reading—that a "mans brain is of a ducible pliable nature, easily moulded and conformed to what it is most conversant about"—perhaps Merryweather was especially mindful of shaping the work's reception by means of the choices made in the translation itself.[88] The pliability of young minds in particular was corroborated in a letter sent to Browne from Henry Power's friend Thomas Smith, who informed the now-famous author that he and his mates at Cambridge had been studying Browne's "exact manual" with their Greek professor. That this refers to the *Religio*, and not to *Pseudodoxia Epidemica*, is clinched not simply by Reginald Bokenham's term "enchiridion" in verses added to the Latin translation but by Smith's own digestion of what he has read. Having penned then burned certain observations on the work, Smith is pleased to tell Browne what the manual has meant to him: "Yet must I confesse I never met with the articles of any religion which I could better subscribe to than to yours" (Wilkin, 1.359–69). What is more, Smith is now excited about a career in medicine, having already begun to read the works on the syllabus that Browne has sent to Power. Browne is Smith's standard for all things "rational and solid," a judgment that appears to have begun when his Cambridge professor "copied out" Browne's "exact manual" with instructions for the pupils "to learne *memoriter*."

As Wilkin said long ago, Browne's work was simply too vital, complex, and unusual to be restrained by any one interpreter's control.[89] In the vagaries of translation, the cross fire of religious polemic, the fleeting quips and quibbles of table talk, or the mind-opening enthusiasm of the young, neither Browne nor his *Religio* could be reduced or mastered. Yet even in gossip, readers were keen to get a fix on Dr Browne; for instance, the avid letter writer James Howell passed along a rumor that despite the *Religio's* disregard for sexuality and marriage, its author was reportedly "Wiv'd a little after."[90] Howell was right: whatever his sudden fame, Browne's life in Norwich was newly enriched by a happy marriage and children.

3. MARRIAGE, FAMILY, FRIENDS

It was highly commonplace in early seventeenth-century Norwich for marriages to be formed "between partners very unequal in age," with the elder partner "more

[87] This volume is in the Colman collection, Norfolk Heritage Centre, Millennium Library, Norwich.

[88] John Merryweather, *Directions for the Latine Tongue* (London, 1681), 39.

[89] See Wilkin, *Works*, 1.lxiii.

[90] For Howell, see *Epistolæ Ho-Elianæ* (1645), 91, letter to Thomas Young, dated April 28, 1645 in the 1650 edition.

often a man" yet in a considerable number of cases a woman.[91] Having been born in February 1621 (she would die in February 1685), the woman that Browne married probably in 1641,[92] Dorothy Mileham of Burlingham St Peter, Norfolk, was some sixteen years her husband's junior. The marriage proved a decidedly happy one. Even factoring in rhetorical conventions, John Whitefoot's firsthand testimonial rings true in the light of other evidence, namely, that Dorothy was "a Lady of such a Symetrical Proportion to her Worthy Husband, both in the Graces of her Body and Mind, that they seemed to come together by a kind of Natural Magnetism" (*Posthumous Works*, xxxii). Indeed, the notes that she kept on the sermons that she heard in Norwich reflect that Dorothy was a highly intelligent and intensely spiritual woman.[93] And she would come to support and to participate in her husband's experimental endeavors, not least because cookery, medicine, and natural history were tightly bound together in the Browne household as in so many others in the seventeenth century.

Early in their marriage, the couple sat for a portrait that purveys something of their suitability for one another if also their considerable differences. (See Figure 8.1.) Attributed to Joan Carlile, a woman with a host of connections to Browne's social network in Norfolk,[94] the small portrait distinguishes between

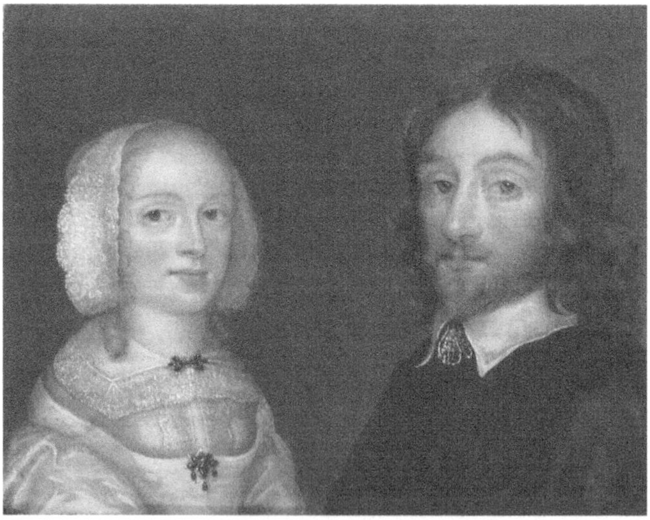

Figure 8.1 Lady Dorothy Browne and Sir Thomas Browne, attributed to Joan Carlile. © National Portrait Gallery, London.

[91] Margaret Pelling, "Who Most Needs to Marry?"; see 34–5.

[92] Browne's monument in St Peter Mancroft suggests this as the likeliest date.

[93] See chapter 9; Rebecca Bullard, "'A bright Coelestiall mind': A New Set of Writings by Lady Dorothy Browne," *Huntington Library Quarterly* 71 (2010), 99–110.

[94] See M. Toynbee and Sir Gyles Isham, "Joan Carlile (1606?–1679): An Identification," *Burlington Magazine* 96 (1954), 275–7; and Toynbee, "Some Friends of Sir Thomas Browne," *Norfolk Archaeology* 31 (1955–57), 377–94. Cf. the article on Joan Carlile in *ODNB* by Arianne Burnette.

the husband, whose faraway stare looks past the viewer's right shoulder, and the wife, who amiably engages the viewer with a welcoming and direct face. One is tempted to see the two as Norwich's version of Milton's social "L'Allegro" and contemplative "Il Penseroso." Yet while the two figures are not interacting and appear on slightly different plains, they are nonetheless painted as equals. Neither person looms above or sits beneath the other. With Dorothy's costume, which includes a headpiece and two brooches, next to Thomas's black outfit with a white collar, the painting depicts the couple as embodying a balance between modest ornament and refined simplicity. Probably because he has not yet published *Religio* and *Pseudodoxia*, Browne is not associated with books or authorship,[95] and there are no symbols or accouterments in the painting. All in all, the pair come across as complementary to one another, strikingly independent yet harmonious in their sense of style. None of their children is portrayed with them, perhaps because the couple was just starting their life together. The provenance of the panel, the L'Estrange family of Hunstanton, affords early evidence of how significant and admired the Brownes would become in their Norfolk world.[96]

Also evocative of Thomas and Dorothy's happiness together is the fact that they had a drawing of Rubens's depiction of Baucis and Philemon in their parlor. Of this work of art Browne made a marginal note next to a poem that he wrote in praise of "a handsome bower of hony suckles over the doore of a cottage of a right good man" who lived "in the countrey a few miles from Norwich." In twelve Latin verses, Browne imagined that the honeysuckle spoke in praise of a simple, healthy country life, then identified its setting as "the blessed [*pia*] threshold of my master and mistress" whose house never entertained sorrow, deception, or violence (Keynes, 3.281). In the Rubens painting, an elderly couple has offered fruit and drink to the gods who are no longer in disguise. The gentle old man discourses with Mercury while the kindly old woman reaches for a goose, presumably with the intention of turning it into supper. Thus the portrait of Baucis and Philemon epitomizes a certain notion of a happy, healthy marriage, in which the household's separate and gendered roles considerably overlap and sustain mutual respect. Crucially, Browne's poem, the painting to which it responds, and the story behind the painting give a humbler, demotic version of a pervasive lesson of *Religio Medici*, that the divine is always closer than you may think, in the scent of honeysuckle or at the hearth of a cottage.[97]

No extant records explain how Browne met Dorothy Mileham, nor does any extant parish record either in Norwich or Burlingham record the event of their

[95] Contrast the Gunton Hall portrait offered as Plate IV in Tildesley, *Sir Thomas Browne: His Skull, Portraits, and Ancestry*.

[96] For information about provenance, see M. L. Tildesley, addendum to *Sir Thomas Browne: His Skull, Portraits, and Ancestry*, 76 bis.

[97] For this notion in *Religio Medici*, see Daniela Havenstein, *Democratizing Sir Thomas Browne: Religio Medici and Its Imitations* (Oxford: Clarendon Press, 1999), 169.

wedding.[98] But Dorothy's home between Norwich and Yarmouth placed her well within the scope of Dr Browne's medical visits and social network. Insofar as Dorothy hailed from a good Norfolk family—a daughter of Edward Mileham and Dorothy Hobart, herself a child of John Hobart of Salle—she certainly did her part to expand and deepen Browne's connections to the leading lights of the county. While the Hobarts of Blickling took a prominent role in the parliamentarian and eventually Whig side of local politics, Dorothy's mother was associated with a Royalist branch of the family, suggesting a conservatism that may well be glimpsed in her sermon notes.[99] Thus the young couple interacted with families ranging across the political spectrum.[100] Given the second marriage of Edward Mileham in 1626, together with the marriage of Dorothy's sister and half-sister into the Tenison family, these connections continued to grow and strengthen.

Whatever the couple's wider affiliations, however, from 1643 or 1644 onward, the birth, death, and rearing of their children occupied a central position in the Browne household. Since the baptisms of their children are not recorded in the parish register of St George Tombland, their birth dates must be pieced together tentatively from a wide range of sometimes unclear testimonies, including Browne's own. Their first child, a son Edward, came into the world in either 1643 or 1644,[101] after which Dorothy would bear probably ten offspring, the last being born in 1662.[102] Only six would live to see adulthood, with four of those surviving their parents. Over the course of the 1640s, the Brownes welcomed the birth (after Edward) of a son Thomas (*c.*1646),[103] then Anne (*c.*1647), Elizabeth (*c.*1648), and Dorothy (buried May 14, 1652).[104] When their sixth child, Frances,

[98] The register for Burlingham St Peter includes only four marriages from the 1640s, including two on the same day in 1648 for Dorothy's twin sisters, Elizabeth and Hobart. No other Burlingham church has a trace of the wedding either. Among the parishes in the Tombland area of Norwich, St George Tombland has a hiatus for marriages between 1642 and 62; St Simon and St Jude's register a gap between 1641 and 1658, for example. St Peter Parmentergate has a 1639 marriage between a George Browne and a Dorothy Chapman, while St Michael at Plea has a 1643 wedding between a William Browne and a Dorothy Cullen or Culler. Many people from all over the county got married in the Cathedral at this time, but there is no separate register and the financial records of the Chapter do not include Browne. Nor is there any record of the wedding in the archdeacon's transcriptions of parish records, or for that matter in the parishes over which Thomas Lushington had charge in Burnham.

[99] For the Milehams, see John Mileham, "Dame Dorothy Browne and the Family of Mileham of Burlingham," *The Norfolk Ancestor* 2 (1982), 104–9.

[100] For further evidence of Browne's county connections, see Toynbee, "Some Friends of Sir Thomas Browne."

[101] His monument in St Botolph's, Norfleet, county Kent, notes that Edward died on August 28, 1708, at the age of 64 ("Aetatis LXIIII," Wilkin, 1.cviii). Had he turned 65 later that year, Edward would have been born in 1643. In a pedigree signed by Browne in 1664, the heir Edward's age was given as 21 (see Wilkin, 1.cxi).

[102] The Williams/Wilkin pedigree judged the total to be twelve, but the assumption of a daughter in 1645 has been disproved; see G. C. R. Morris, "Sir Thomas Browne's Daughters, 'Cosen Barker,' and the Cottrells," *Notes and Queries* 231 (1986), 472–9.

[103] Browne's daughter Elizabeth noted that her brother Thomas had visited France in 1661 at the age of 14 (Bodleian MS Rawlinson D. 391, 81r). So he was born either in 1647 or (in the event that he turned 15 in 1661) in 1646.

[104] Speculation for the birthdates of Anne and Elizabeth is based on the pedigree drawn up by Charles Williams (included as a fold-out in Wilkin). Anne is listed as the elder of the two in the visitation pedigree of 1664. While Anne was married by the end of 1669, Elizabeth did not marry until 1680. Dorothy's burial is recorded in the register of St Peter Mancroft.

was baptized on November 7, 1650, the family was living in the parish of St Peter Mancroft.

In addition to his rapidly growing nuclear family and a network of county relations and associations, Browne developed what might fairly be called intense friendships. Three in particular—with Arthur Dee, Thomas Lushington, and Joseph Hall—convey not only some sense of the wide intellectual range of these friends but also how closely involved with contemporary turmoil Browne's life was. In Arthur Dee, a "great acquaintance" and fellow physician in St George Tombland, Browne met a delightful conversationalist whose life was a sometimes exotic tale and whose intellectual propensities reinvigorated Browne's fascination with the controversial borderland of theology, philosophy, and empirical practice into which natural magic, astrology, Hermeticism, and alchemy could be taken.[105] In a letter to Elias Ashmole, Browne not only spoke of Dee's gift to him of various alchemical tracts, but he recalled their "familiar" friendship: Dee "lived many yeares and dyed in Norwich, from whom I have heard many accounts agreable unto those wch you have sett downe in your annotations, concerning his father"—the great John Dee—"and Kelley," his father's collaborator in magic. For Browne, Arthur Dee offered compelling evidence that he had achieved the most mysterious and elusive goal of natural studies, namely, the philosopher's stone:

> hee was a persevering student in Hermeticall philosophy and had noe small encouragement, having seen projection made; And with the highest asseverations hee confirmed unto his death, that hee had ocularly, undeceavably, and frequently beheld it in Bohemia, and to my knowledge, had not an accident prevented, hee had not many yeares before his death retired beyond sea and fallen upon the solemne processe of the great worke. (Keynes, 4.293)

Browne clearly prized manuscripts from the Dee collection, including medieval studies of the philosopher's stone, as well as works of theory and hieroglyphics which, as Browne explained to Ashmole, bear on the practical work of Hermetic alchemy. Yet often implicit in Browne's memories of Dee is a concern that the dear friend's life has proved delusional, even dangerous, in those obsessions hatched and haunted by his father.

If Dee's flirtations with danger were largely in the past, those of Browne's onetime tutor and associate in Norfolk, Thomas Lushington, grew worse in the 1640s. In a letter to Aubrey from the early 1670s, Browne mentioned in the course of a brief sketch of his tutor's life that Lushington had written "a comment upon the Hebrews" (Keynes, 4.376). The work in question was in fact partly a translation, partly an elaboration and paraphrase of Johann Crell's *Expiation of a Sinner in a Commentary upon the Epistle to the Hebrewes*, published in 1646 by "G. M.," whose

[105] For Arthur Dee see the *ODNB* article by John H. Appleby, which adds to his earlier work published as "Arthur Dee and Johannes Bánfi Hunyades," *Ambix* 24 (1977), 96–109; "Some of Arthur Dee's Associations before Visiting Russia Clarified," *Ambix* 26 (1979), 1–15; and "Dr Arthur Dee: Merchant and Litigant," *Slavonic and East European Review* 57 (1979), 32–55. See also Lyndy Abraham, ed., *Arthur Dee's Fasciculus chemicus*, trans. Elias Ashmole (New York: Garland, 1997); and N. A. Figurovski, "The Alchemist and Physician Arthur Dee," *Ambix* 13 (1965), 35–51.

claim on authorship is both misleading (he says that it was written in English) and ambiguous (he is "moved... to Print and publish this commentary" but never says that he wrote it).[106] Yet in Norwich in the very next year, 1647, a cathedral preacher named Edmund Porter not only criticized the commentary but also identified its author as a scion of Broadgates Hall, punning on the sinful tenor of the hall's name, and attacking the commentator as a viper who "by his personal insinuations" has "perverted many from the saving truth of the gospel, to the evident danger both of theirs and his own soul." Worse still, according to Porter, the Broadgates divine was known to possess such "impious ambition to be the Ring-leader in this blasphemy" that he had accrued across Norfolk "such a Title and Character, as was fastened on *Marcion* the Heretick by *Polycarpus*, when he called him *Primogentium Satanæ*."[107] Although Porter's assault would not be published until 1655, after which the commentary would be released under the authorship of T. L. D. D. (Thomas Lushington, Doctor of Divinity), the date of his preface was March 21, 1647. From that time forward, Lushington would gather such a strong reputation for heresy that by the Restoration he was considered a liability for Royalists and advocates of the Church of England.[108]

Unlike Lushington who, whatever his intentions, generated controversy amongst communities in Oxford and Norwich, Browne's patient and friend Bishop Hall (1574–1656) made peace and reconciliation among Protestants his mantra from the 1620s through the 1640s. (See Figure 8.2.) On the one hand he was solidly Calvinist in theology; on the other, he criticized those "Puritans" who showed "refractory opposition to the ceremonies, rites and customes of the church."[109] This is not to say that he was shielded from controversy, for both the hotter sort of Puritans and the more aggressive sort of anti-Calvinists accused him of defection to the other side. By the time Hall had come to Norwich in 1641, as a successor to Richard Montagu and, before him, to Matthew Wren, Hall was an elderly man who had recently spent time in the Tower. Although he was welcomed at first to the Norwich community, Hall was soon (in 1643) and shockingly subjected to the violence of sequestration and iconoclasm. During the year in which the authorized *Religio* appeared, Hall was undergoing the loss of his clerical incomes but also, by his own account, of the most intimate of personal belongings, even "my children's pictures."[110] Although he was not finally expelled from the bishop's palace until 1647, the years leading up to that final blow were filled with "many insolencies and affronts" (Hall, 1.liv), with what he considered a rabid desecration of the church and a betrayal of careful and moderate reformation. In an often quoted account

[106] For Crell (1590–1633), see H. John McLachlan, *Socinianism in Seventeenth-Century England* (Oxford: Oxford University Press, 1951), 8; on Lushington, 108–17. A decade later, however, Downame insisted that he had in fact objected to certain passages that were not removed or revised according to his requirements; McLachlan, *Socinianism in Seventeenth-Century England*, 112–13.

[107] Edmund Porter, *Θεος Ἀνθρωποφορος: or God Incarnate* (1655), A4r–v.

[108] For the episode in which Dr John Barwick warned Charles II away from Lushington, see McLachlan, 110–11. Lushington continued his retirement until death in Kent, in December 1661.

[109] Quoted in Richard McCabe's entry on Joseph Hall in the *ODNB*.

[110] *Hard Measure*, in *The Works of Joseph Hall, D.D.*, 12 volumes (Oxford: D.A. Talboys, 1837), 1.li.

of the destruction of Norwich Cathedral, Hall recounted how the invading iconoclasts destroyed or mishandled everything from the walls and monuments to the windows, graves, seats, stonework, and organ, with no clear rationale other than an ostentatious humor to commit profanity: "a lewd wretch walking before the train, in his cope trailing in the dirt, with a service-book in his hand, imitating in an impious scorn the tune, and usurping the words of the litany used formerly in the church" (Hall, 1.lv). Even when Hall made his way in 1647 to a house in the nearby village of Heigham, he was assiduous not just in his clerical activities but also in his writing, continuing to publish a range of works from a Latin exhortation to peace, latitude, and charity in 1648 to a study of the inhabitants (angels and immortal souls) in the "invisible world" (1652). The sentiments of these later

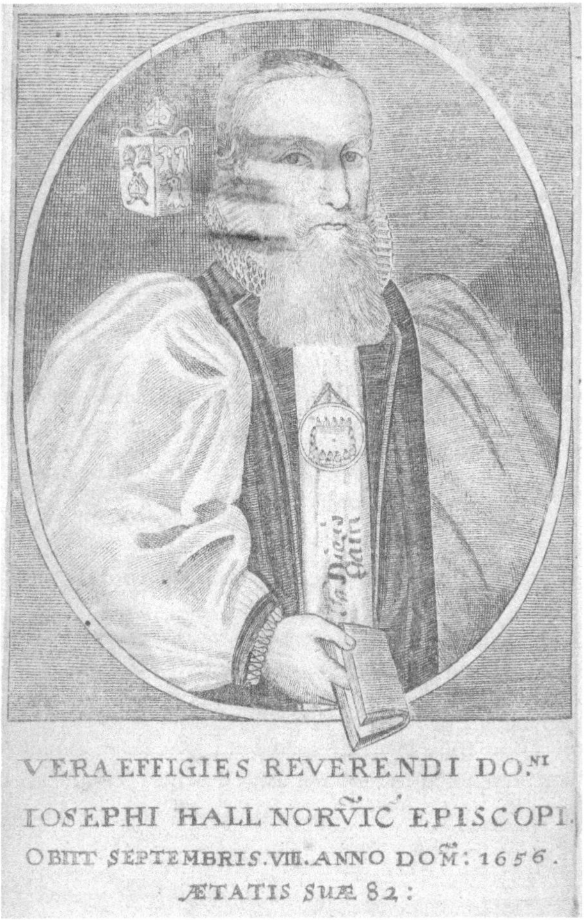

Figure 8.2 Joseph Hall, from John Whitefoote, *Israel agchithanes: Deaths Alarum* (1656). Reproduced with the permission of the Rare Book Division, Department of Rare Books and Special Collections, Princeton University Library.

works intersected with Browne's *Religio*, for instance in the distinction between error and heresy, the clarion call to peace, and the opposition to coercion in religious affairs.[111]

Browne was close at hand to witness the devastating scenes from Hall's later life, and as Hall's physician he was in a better position than most to understand the fragile health of this long-serving divine. In *The Shaking of the Olive Tree, The Remaining Works of that Incomparable Prelate, Joseph Hall* (1660), the editor said of the elderly Hall that,

> after his prevailing infirmities [especially strangury] had wasted all the strengths of nature, and the arts of his learned and excellent physician, D. Browne of Norwich, (to whom, under God, we and the whole church are ingaged for many years preserving his life as a blessing to us,)—after his fatherly reception of many persons of honour, learning, and piety, who came to crave his dying prayers and benedictions,—he roused up hys dying spirits, to a heavenly confession of his faith, which ere he could finish, his speech was taken from him, so that we cannot here insert it.[112]

With his residence in St George Tombland abutting the western side of the cathedral precinct, Browne was a natural choice for the bishop's physician in the early 1640s. Indeed, Browne's familiarity with the medical afflictions of Bishop Montagu makes it likely that he had attended Hall's predecessor too.[113] Browne left a testimonial to Hall in *Repertorium*, that survey of the cathedral that testifies most powerfully to the effect the violent scenes in the early 1640s had on the author of *Religio Medici*:

> My Honord freind Bishop Joseph Hall, Deane of Worcester, and Bishop of Excester, was buryed at Heigham, where hee hath his monument, who in Rebellious times, when the Revenues of the church were alienated, retired unto that suburbian parish, and there ended his dayes: being above fourscore yeares of age.

It is probably too facile to speak of Hall (or Arthur Dee for that matter) as a surrogate father for Browne, but Browne left on record how much Hall's person and works had meant to him in tumultuous times:

> A person of singular humility, patience and pietie: his owne works are the best monument, and character of himself, which was also very lively drawne in his excellent funerall sermon preached by my learned and faythfull old friend Mr John Whitefoot, Rector of Heigham and the very deserving clark of the convocation for Norfolk. (Keynes, 3.134)

Published by the same bookseller, Edward Dod, was responsible for bringing out Lushington's two Socinian commentaries as well as his textbook on logic,[114] Whitefoot's funeral sermon embodies the close fellowship that irenic, reconciliatory

[111] *Pax Terris* (1648), in *Works*, 11.235–7, 255, 261.

[112] Quoted in Wilkin, 1.c–ci.

[113] See the discussion of *Repertorium* in chapter 11 in this volume.

[114] John Whitefoot, *Israel agchithanes* (1656), "A catalogue of some books printed for, and sold by *Edw. Dod* at the *Gun* in *Ivy-lane*," appendix, n.p.

motives kept with the world of deep division, rampant conflict, and neighborly violence that characterized the city of Norwich in the 1640s. As a resident of St George Tombland, as a citizen petitioned for his assistance with wartime causes, and as the physician attending Bishop Hall, Browne could not have avoided involvement with the civil war no matter how hard he had wished for escape. Indeed, his revisions to *Religio Medici* but also his labors over *Pseudodoxia Epidemica* were themselves discursive interventions in a world turned upside down.

4. CIVIL WAR NORWICH

Living just next to the cathedral as he did in the 1640s, Browne resided in close quarters with some of the most volatile scenes of civil war in Norwich. From a Royalist vantage, one Captain Lulman captured how tumultuous the neighborhood became when a company of parliamentary foot soldiers exposed their backsides to the altar "in a deriding manner," or when an old shepherd who loved the cathedral would cry out for God's vengeance for king and church in the streets of Tombland and, having been arrested and brutalized, would continue with his proclamations.[115] In Browne's parish church of St George Tombland, Congregationalists took over the church, destroyed its ornaments, and "scandalously did erect a Gallery with seates over the Communion table, wch is not onely indecent, but alsoe a great hindrance to the light."[116] Nearby, the cathedral was a site of ongoing conflict. In general neither the cathedral itself nor the expansive close around its elongated structure was sealed off from the bustle of Norwich life. The cathedral included sites at which bills might be paid, eventually including one of Browne's own, while its nave "was a bustling thoroughfare and public way into Bishopgate until the early nineteenth century."[117] It was in the close that Browne's boys went to grammar school, and also there, in the green yard, that citizens and city officials gathered to hear sermons as they had at Paul's Cross in the London of Browne's youth. As would be manifested by his later work on *Repertorium*, Browne was profoundly moved by the attacks on the nearby cathedral as well as those on its bishop, and he lamented iconoclasm's erasure of "the distinct places of buryall of many noble and considerable persons" (Keynes, 3.123).[118]

Although Norwich never joined the list of cities under siege during the civil wars of 1642–48, the city was gripped by ongoing fear that it might be. It was, moreover, a volatile alembic of partisan strife. Not only did the city generate a

[115] NRO DCN 107/3, 1r.

[116] Tombland faculty book, quoted by Kevin Killeen in *Biblical Scholarship, Science and Politics in Early Modern England: Thomas Browne and the Thorny Place of Knowledge* (Burlington, VT: Ashgate, 2009), 202.

[117] Roberta Gilchrist, *Norwich Cathedral Close: The Evolution of the English Cathedral Landscape* (Rochester, NY: The Boydell Press, 2005), 202, 221.

[118] For the destruction see Jonathan Finch, "The Monuments," in Ian Atherton et al., eds., *Norwich Cathedral: Church, City and Diocese, 1096–1996*, (London: Hambledon, 1996), 467–93; see 476–7.

steady stream of polemical discourse in the press, reflective of its deepening divisions, but its proximity to sieges in places such as King's Lynn (1643), and an anxiety about the likelihood of an imminent attack, rendered the civil war a painful experience for the city's inhabitants.[119] Anxiety was expressed in newsbooks as well as letters, and ranged from stress over economic depression and mutiny to the fear produced by not knowing how to identify allies or to clarify and express one's own convictions.[120]

As in so many other places in England, Norwich had experienced the upsurge of strife during the second half of the 1630s.[121] The show of support in Norwich for the oft-reviled, hyper-Laudian Wren centered on the very parish in which Browne was living after his arrival in the city.[122] What is more, it appears to have involved in a small role Thomas Lushington and in a prominent one the city leader, William Browne, was probably a kinsman with whom Browne was living. Even in the early 1630s under Corbett, Lushington was useful in helping to oust Puritan lecturers such as William Bridge of St George Tombland; Browne's old tutor had also stirred up controversy in Tombland "by preaching free will, elevating the sacraments above his head in a manner that some present deemed popish."[123] Under Wren, Lushington had been designated among the commissioners "for the advancement of piety" in the archdeaconry of Norfolk.[124] With ceremonialism and anti-Calvinism gaining major support from Wren, William Browne and his neighbors, the Anguish family, were eager to eradicate the hotter sort of Protestant from their onetime stronghold in Tombland.[125] They were rewarded with a minister, Isaac Dobson, who not only supported heightened ceremonialism but also "argued dogmatically that 'wee ought to beleeve as the Church believes, and if the Church said the crow is white, wee must beleeve it.' "[126]

As promising for the new ceremonialism as Wren's bishopric certainly was for Laud and local supporters such as William Browne, its moment of triumph was brief and tenuous, even in Tombland. During Thomas Browne's residence in that neighborhood until 1650, the parish church witnessed the return of Puritan families until "by the late 1640s St George's had become an Independent church and soon afterwards its interior was modified accordingly."[127] As Wren and Richard Montagu quickly gave way to Bishop Hall in 1641, Norwich entered into an explo-

[119] Andrew Hopper, "The Civil Wars," 89.

[120] See Hopper, "The Civil Wars," 97–9.

[121] Kenneth Fincham, "Material Evidence: The Religious Legacy of the Interregnum at St George Tombland, Norwich," in Fincham and Peter Lake, eds., *Religious Politics in Post-Reformation England: Essays in Honour of Nicholas Tyacke* (Rochester, NY: Boydell, 2006), 224–40; see 224.

[122] Matthew Reynolds, *Godly Reformers and their Opponents*, 207–13; and Fincham, "Material Evidence," in *Religious Politics in Post-Reformation England*.

[123] Reynolds, *Godly Reformers and their Opponents*, 207–8. The episode is undated.

[124] Kenneth Fincham, ed., *Visitation Articles and Injunctions of the Early Stuart Church* (Rochester, NY: Boydell, 1998), 2.162–3.

[125] See Fincham, "Material Evidence," 225, and Reynolds, *Godly Reformers and their Opponents*, 207–8; William Browne was an ally of Samuel Harsnet, bishop of Norwich 1619–28, also an anti-Calvinist.

[126] Quoted by Reynolds (212) from Bodleian Tanner MS 220, f. 135.

[127] Fincham, "Material Evidence," 226.

sive decade in which notions of conformity were destabilized[128] and local religious tensions would accumulate until the city, quite literally, experienced an explosion at decade's end. As Browne's ownership of a casuistic work by Hall from 1649 made clear,[129] life in civil war Norwich was not simply a matter of coping with violence both discursive and physical. In a letter to his wife, Browne's associate and patient Thomas Knyvett expressed anxiety about the moral dilemmas that moderates with connections on both sides of the war were bound to face: "I am now in a great strait what to do," for "such is the sad condition of these times, as no man knows how to dispose himself, for now there is so much declared as makes all officers in the kingdom traitors of one side or other; neither are standers-by in any better condition." In these same letters, Knyvett was concerned that his wife consult Dr Browne, not just on medical matters but on help with the sequestration of their property.[130] As a leading physician in the city with patients from both sides of the war, Browne was an excellent choice for informal mediation, but throughout the rest of his life, local reliance on his civility and finesse entailed that Browne would constantly face the moral pressures that Knyvett expressed to his wife.

Early in the course of the civil war, Browne was faced with taking a stand on a strategically important military conflict. The Scots assisting the Parliament in its war with the King had placed the city of Newcastle under siege for months beginning in January 1643, a problem for London and East Anglian economy alike since Newcastle was the key hub for the distribution of coal.[131] In order to break the stalemate, Parliament passed an ordinance to raise money toward the regaining of the besieged city; in Norwich, collectors moved from ward to ward in search of voluntary contributions. In the ward of North Conisford, Dr Browne's name appears amongst those persons declining to contribute to the cause. Little can be inferred about the exact nature of Browne's positions on Newcastle in particular or on the war in general. In fact, a large portion of the citizenry—by no means all supporters of the king's army—decided against contributing. There seems to have been little pressure on them to do so, and their motives for declining "may well have been based on reasons neither political nor religious, such as temporary lack of funds or disapproval of voluntary contributions as a method of taxation."[132] Browne was obviously no supporter of the Puritan-parliamentary cause, but the level of his feelings for the king and the prelacy cannot be determined from the Newcastle affair. On a later occasion in 1645, Browne had no choice but to be assessed for money in aid of Sir Thomas Fairfax, and so he was—six shillings for personal property (as against real estate) in the parish of St George's Tombland.[133]

[128] See Tom Webster, *Godly Clergy in Early Stuart England: The Caroline Puritan Movement, c. 1620–1643* (New York: Cambridge University Press, 1997), 207–14.

[129] For Browne's copy of Hall's *Resolution of Divers Cases of Conscience*, see Finch, *Catalogue of the Libraries*, index.

[130] Schofield, *The Knyvett Letters, 1620–1644*, 105, 118, 142.

[131] See *The Norwich Subscription for the Regaining of Newcastle, 1643*, ed. F. R. Beecheno, in *Norfolk and Norwich Archaeological Society* 18 (1913), 149–60; see 157; cf. Evans, *Seventeenth-Century Norwich*, 132. For Browne's ward, thirteen contributed (including another Thomas Browne), and nine declined.

[132] Evans, *Seventeenth-Century Norwich*, 132.

[133] See Beecheno, "The First Residence of Sir Thomas Browne"; Charles Williams, "Residence of Sir Thomas Browne, M.D. at Norwich," *East Anglican*, n.s., vol. 1, part 3 (January 1886), 194–5. Browne was assessed again in 1649.

In 1650 Browne would move to an area of Norwich, Mancroft, where Royalist sentiment was always high, though the distance from one residence to the other was a matter of a five-minute walk. In the 1640s, he resided in Wymer, an area of the city in which records of taxation "confirm enthusiasm for the parliamentary cause."[134] Even so, Browne's neighbors were clearly not uniformly parliamentarian, while in some cases the documentary evidence is impossible to decipher regarding the loyalties in Tombland. For instance, while 132 took the Solemn League and Covenant in July 1644, the number of those who refused is unknown.[135] Indeed, even the appearance of "Dr Browne" on the document is not entirely clear, since the lack of an *x* by his name probably (but not certainly) means that he did not take the oath.

Toward the middle of the 1640s, the political and religious dilemmas confronting citizens of Norwich positioned somewhere along the large middle of the spectrum were rendered all the more complicated when the Presbyterians and Independents became entrenched in conflict with one another. As the Independents supported the autonomy of congregations as well as ongoing aggression against the king, the Presbyterians were increasingly eligible for a claim as moderate defenders of church reform and of rapprochement with Charles. In Norwich, this permutation in the civil wars found one manifestation in a 1646 pamphlet skirmish between supporters of the now clearly distinguished polities.[136] It is among the names on a Presbyterian document that the appearance of a Thomas Browne has led scholars to wonder whether the author of *Religio Medici* could have supported a national church polity quite different from prelacy.

On the face of it, it seems possible that by 1646, Browne might have seen the Presbyterian option as the one most likely to guarantee peace and moderation. In the 1643 authorized edition of the *Religio*, we have seen, he changed his indictment of presbyters in the second stage manuscripts back to the original charge against prelates. As Evans argues, "the Royalists of Norwich had been living in quiet obscurity for several years, but the coalescing Presbyterian-peace party movement gave them a new lease on political life."[137] The king himself was beginning to see the Presbyterians of his homeland, Scotland, as his own best hope for survival. With Browne's own church soon to become the property of the Independents, it makes some sense to suppose that he might support the Presbyterians against such a devolution into "atoms in Divinity." Yet the name Thomas Browne is far too common in Norwich for us to know whether its inclusion in *Vox Norwici* belonged to him.[138] And while the fifteen "well Affected" laymen in the "voice of Norwich"

[134] Hopper, "The Civil Wars," 100.

[135] NRO NCR 13c/2/2. Arthur Dee's name is ticked with an *x*. It is also possible that Browne was away from home when the visitors came by.

[136] For a quick summary of the skirmish, see Kitty Scoular Datta, "Sir Thomas Browne and *Vox Norwici*," *Notes and Queries* 231, n.s., 33 (1986), 461; for the Independents and Presbyterians in Norwich, see Evans, *Seventeenth-Century Norwich*, chapter 5, especially 154–63.

[137] Evans, *Seventeenth-Century Norwich*, 163.

[138] Datta makes this point with help from Perry Millican's *Register of the Freemen of Norwich*. Moreover, Browne tends to be listed as "Dr Browne" in Norwich city and church documents.

claim to defend orthodoxy in opposition to schism, their pervasive opposition to church ceremony (and not just to Matthew Wren's tyrannical practices) makes it less likely that Dr Browne would have offered his support for the cause.[139] Even if Presbyterianism's heyday in Norwich came and went quickly, at least one Presbyterian author singled out Browne's *Religio Medici* as supportive of his cause. In *England and Scotland Vnited* (1647), one I. H. quoted the authorized edition's criticism of ambitious prelates, blithely unaware that Browne himself had shifted between bishops and presbyters in the course of revising his work.[140]

In keeping with the outbreak of scattered Royalist rebellions in 1648, Norwich finally exploded in the year before the king's execution. Three main groups converged in their anger and frustration: the Presbyterians, the Royalists, and those tradesmen who were perturbed about taxation (Evans, 178). Motivated most immediately by a brouhaha over municipal elections, a crowd began to gather in the marketplace on Sunday, April 23, then by Monday had grown considerably in size. With the emergency arrival of Colonel Fleetwood's troops around 4 p.m., Norwich finally experienced a bloody battle the conclusion of which came when the city's stockpile of ammunition and gunpowder blew up. Whatever their political and religious differences, accounts agreed that "windows were shattered, the whole city shook, and so many bodies were dismembered and scattered that it was impossible to count them" (Evans, 176). The exploding gunpowder was an extraordinarily apt symbol of how profoundly divided the city had become in the second half of the 1640s. In moving to the parish of St Peter Mancroft alongside the marketplace in 1650, Browne may have been taking on a richer neighborhood, but the recent memory of the great explosion in the market could have left him with no illusion that his new home would be any safer than his old in Tombland.

How much Browne knew about the sufferings of his extended family in Ireland in the 1640s is impossible to say.[141] His stepfather had died in 1634, reportedly from the effects of a fight. According to a letter from Strafford to Secretary Coke, Dutton had left his widow and children in financial straits, with Lady Dutton having to sue for two hundred pounds of her husband's pay and to rely on the king's charity for the payment. Although Irish records lack clear evidence from 1635 through 1641, Lady Dutton in all likelihood remained in Ireland for the majority of this period. Then, after the Irish rebellion in 1641, she and her daughter Ellen found themselves in highly dangerous circumstances. The two women were robbed and nearly killed by their neighbors; rescued by Lady Newcomen and Sir James Dillon, Lady Dutton and her household disappeared from the records. In a deposition dated July 14, 1645, one Susan Steele testified that "in April 1642, the Lady

[139] *Vox Norwici* (London, 1646), title page, A2r, 10–11. Cf. Killeen, *Biblical Scholarship*, 193–4.

[140] See *England and Scotland Vnited* (1647), 12. This allusion was discovered by Evan Gurney; see his "A New Allusion to Sir Thomas Browne," *Notes and Queries* 59 (2012), 178.

[141] This paragraph is indebted throughout to Endicott, "Sir Thomas Browne as 'Orphan,'" 199–200. For Lady Dutton's financial problems, see *Calendar of State Papers, Ireland*, vol. 262, p. 81, October 26, 1634; and Strafford, *Letters and Dispatches* (1739), I.257, 309, 348. For Lady Dutton in peril, see Trinity College, Dublin, Longford Depositions, ff. 134, 203–4, 214b; Roscommon Depositions, f. 2.

Ann Dutton, and her daughter, Mrs. Ellinor Browne, and her maid, Mrs. Stubbs, this deponent and the rest of the English, were threatened with death by the said Oliver FitzGarret, Lisagh Farrell, and their confederates." Having secured a warrant, the attackers could not execute it on the Dutton household, including its servants and "other good Protestants" for Dillon removed the whole "to his own house, and from themce sent them all safe to Athlone."[142] In a 1682 letter to Edward, Browne did inquire about his brother-in-law, Thomas Price, archbishop of Cashel, who had married Jane Browne in the early 1630s (Keynes, 4.227). In the 1640s, however, Browne's personal connections to Ireland were recast as evidence for exposing the vulgar errors to which he devoted the bulk of his spare time in the years of civil war. Indeed, the war itself offered Browne the stunning proof that sinful error was rampant.

5. *PSEUDODOXIA EPIDEMICA*, 1646

Published for the first time in 1646, albeit the product of years of research,[143] *Pseudodoxia Epidemica* was Browne's "most considerable work," his "masterpiece," his personal favorite, the modernized encyclopedia in which he set out to answer questions posed in the *Religio*, to assist humanity in eradicating cancerous error, and to stimulate future, collaborative endeavors "to purchase a clear and warrantable body of Truth."[144] It was the work on which he would labor most extensively at revision over the course of his life, and the one that would contribute most to his scholarly and philosophical reputation, even though plans for its translation into Latin never came to fruition. Indeed, as Killeen has argued, Browne intended the work as his most influential and productive contribution to contemporary life, culture, and thought, revising the criteria of biblical exegesis as well as the full range of "intellectual categories" in a time of enormous turbulence and change.[145]

As its very title testified in its diagnosis of "an epidemic of false doctrines," however, *Pseudodoxia* was also Dr Browne's most arduous and audacious work. In an undated manuscript piece, Browne advised a friend undertaking a difficult

[142] Quoted in Mary Agnes Hickson, *Ireland in the Seventeenth Century*, 2 vols. (London: Longmans, Green & Co., 1884), 1.356.

[143] There is no certain evidence for the exact period of composition, though scholars have taken Browne's mention in *Religio* of a catalogue of doubts as evidence that he was already interested in, if not embarked upon, the project in the middle of the 1630s. See Tipton Marshall Westfall, *Sir Thomas Browne's Revisions in Pseudodoxia Epidemica: A Study in the Development of his Mind* (PhD dissertation, Princeton, 1938), 79–80. Given his need for ready access to a large library, however, it is probable that Browne began his work in earnest after he had moved to Norwich.

[144] Keynes, *Bibliography*, 51; Frank Livingstone Huntley, "Browne's Masterpiece, *Vulgar Errors*," in *Essays in Persuasion: On Seventeenth Century English Literature* (Chicago: University of Chicago Press, 1981), 86–96; Ted-Larry Pebworth, "Wandering in the America of Truth: *Pseudodoxia Epidemica* and the Essay Tradition," in C. A. Patrides, ed., *Approaches to Sir Thomas Browne* (Columbia: University of Missouri Press, 1982), 166–77, see 166; Browne, *Pseudodoxia Epidemica* (1646), "To the Reader," A3r; further citations from this edition are parenthetical by page number.

[145] Killeen, *Biblical Scholarship*, 10, 23, and passim.

project to consider his prospect again and again, to train for it as though he were a swimmer confronting a "stormy sea." At the center of this storm was the burden of explicating and clarifying books that were not lifeless and harmless but rather "living things."[146] In Browne's reckoning, the ambitious friend was liable to be attacked by pedants and mockers, by combative critics as well as by narcissistic and envious readers. All manner of wits would assault the work, then one another in a civil war of competing factions and scholarly affiliations. For this reason too, the friend was well advised to toil over revisions and to count himself fortunate if he found the leisure in which to do so. Above all, Browne challenged the friend to devote his energy and time to truth alone, not fame, and he stressed that civility is a critical ingredient in the clearing away of error; scholars are to focus on getting the matter right, not on attacking the persons of the authorities who have humanly erred. Browne advises his friend, too, about confrontations with doubt. With a Baconian understanding that nature daunts us with "twists and turns," with seemingly endless irregularities as well as obscurities, Browne cautions against claiming a total comprehension of things that may begin with a fraudulent certainty but will inevitably leave nothing but doubt. The arduous friend must be prepared to dwell in darkness and doubt, to be patient in the face of nature's labyrinthine intricacies, and not to get ahead of himself in a desire to appear profoundly wise.

As for Browne's two final bits of advice—always consult the learned and find a powerful patron to protect the work—the *Pseudodoxia* saw the light of day in 1646 without the latter but with a keen sense of its need for the former. Although the casual reader would not have connected its publisher, Edward Dod, with the highly controversial work of another author, Thomas Lushington, Browne's preface to the reader announces both "the audacity of the attempt" and the "difficulty" of undertaking the business of advancing learning alone and in one's spare time (1646, A3v–A4r). The subject is both obscure and paradoxical—that is, boldly contrary to received and entrenched opinion, and it is as endless as it is unfamiliar "in the American and untravelled parts of truth" (A5r). Others such as Montpellier's Laurent Joubert or England's James Primerose have disappointed in their pioneering efforts, and Browne captures both the bold heroism as well as the inauspicious odds in casting himself as David, "alone against the strength of opinion . . . to meet the Goliah and Gyant of Authority, with contemptible pebbles, and feeble arguments, drawne from the scrip and slender stocke of our selves" (A5r). This depiction is not quite ingenuous and perhaps not wholly serious, given the fact that Browne intends neither to cast authority as simply an enemy nor to face error without an army of scholars on his side. Nonetheless, the preface to the reader fairly claims that once critical readers are provoked by *Pseudodoxia*, their barbs might come from a variety of directions—from theologians, philosophers, and physicians, for instance—and they will be aimed at him, not at his sources. Rather than combat them as David against the giant, Browne seeks to disarm them by

[146] *Amico Opus Arduum Meditanti*, in Sloane MS 1827; see Keynes, 3.150–55.

inviting them into his civil community of the learned in which they especially might assist the purchase of truth with "experimentall and iudicious knowledge" (A5v–A6r).

As Browne's seven books trace human error through the levels of vegetable and mineral, animal, human, and cosmographical, he is apt to revisit the theme of the work's sheer difficulty. As the first book illustrates, the sources of error in general are many and pervasive—all deriving from sin but ranging from laziness to bad logic, and featuring an addiction to authority. But each sub-topic generates errors as innumerable as the sands (103), for instance, in the attribution of virtues and faculties to plants. In everyday yet sophisticated problems such as the computation of time, not just the instruments by which but the very basis on which to operate can seem hopelessly imperfect, even leading to the admission that there is "no positive or indisputeable ground where to begin our compute" (223). Indeed, throughout the work, the word "ground" tends to refer to the etiology of error.[147] Sometimes, especially with regard to history, difficulty derives from the ruination of original evidence (320). On occasions when natural questions encroach a little too closely on divine prerogative, indeterminacy can prompt Browne to acknowledge that it may well be presumptuous to inquire.[148] Yet as Robin Robbins has said, "religious faith provides both an overall framework and a driving force" for Browne's efforts to move contemporary learning beyond doubt and error.[149] And, much as is the case with Bacon and an early modern culture committed to the essay as a form, indeterminacy itself can motivate not just a desire for truth but also a careful attention to the proper methods and means by which truth might slowly, fitfully be found, and knowledge both carefully limited and wonderfully enlarged.[150] At the end of his digression on blackness, in which there is greater allowance for "contemplation" on a problem that has defeated Browne's best efforts at explanation, he offers the hope that his massive work will be stimulating to others (338). Every individual, especially a busy physician, is bound to be operating on one leg, as Browne puts it, yet each one's searches can produce two forms of collateral by the way, imperfect intimations of truth and the provocation to further, better inquiry.[151]

Browne's "adventures in knowledge" move between what he calls attempts at "decisions" (A3v)—the resolution of puzzles, some of which are posed in *Religio*—and more complex assessments of those conditions and impediments that constitute human knowing. As is the case with all Browne's works, *Pseudodoxia* is filled

[147] See, for instance, 65, 91, 110, 112, and 187 in *Pseudodoxia* (1646).

[148] *Pseudodoxia* (1646), 146, on the beginning of the world.

[149] Robin Robbins, "Browne's Cosmos Imagined: Nature, Man, and God in *Pseudodoxia Epidemica*," in Patrides, ed., *Approaches to Sir Thomas Browne*, 155–65, see 158.

[150] On *Pseudodoxia Epidemica* and the essay, see Pebworth, "Wandering in *the America of Truth*," in Patrides, ed., *Approaches to Sir Thomas Browne*, 166–77. For the assets and liabilities of enlarging human knowledge, see Achsah Guibbory, "Sir Thomas Browne's *Pseudodoxia Epidemica* and the Circle of Knowledge," *Texas Studies in Language & Literature* 18 (1976), 486–99.

[151] For the epistemological assumptions of *Pseudodoxia Epidemica*, see William N. West, "Brownean Motion: Conversation with *Pseudodoxia Epidemica*'s 'Sober Circumference of Knowledge,'" in Browne and Preston, eds., *Sir Thomas Browne: The World Proposed*, 168–87.

with epistemological categories ranging through the evidentiary levels of certainty, probability, and doubt. His recommendations for improving the status of human knowledge can be boldly sweeping—contrary to Plato's dictum that knowledge is remembering, "we must forget and part with much wee know" (A3r). Yet his analyses of human knowing are often remarkably subtle. He is insightful on the question of what twentieth-century critics have dubbed "reader response" but what in Browne's life would have been understood according to ancient literary criticism (for instance, Aristotle on tragedy) as well as Bacon's and other skeptics' scrutiny of the circumstances in which human beings interpret. Not only, then, is Browne aware of how prejudice blinds us to what is "real," but he also explores the ways in which desire, hope, fear, suffering, and shame play a part in the stories we tell, the experiments we pursue, or the explanations we embrace (70, 209, 375–9). Indeed, the very last chapter of the work strangely offers Browne's indulgence in such passions, for he lists fearsome stories so potentially scandalous to human dignity that we would rather not know if they were true (383–6). Far more consistently, Browne is eager to establish a large category of knowledge—moral, emblematic, hieroglyphic, mystical—in which error is legitimately encouraged if carefully used.

Throughout the seven books, Browne repeats certain nodal terms which become a kind of epistemological shorthand. To speak "judiciously," "strictly," "distinctly," or "indifferently" implies an analytical rigor committed to the "real" or to the "things themselves," as the epigraph from Julius Caesar Scaliger announces the standard of judgment. Such precision is set in opposition to imagination which requires either erasure (regarding the thing themselves) or "toleration" as it translates spiritual mysteries or moral precepts into useful myths, metaphors, or hyperboles. "Swallowing" is nearly always bad; speaking "freely" suggests one's openness to scholarly dialogue and respectful criticism. Wonder can be a crucial feature of advanced inquiry or it can be an impediment to the same. "Illations"—inferences—can amount to fraudulent superstructures built on the flimsiest foundations, or to the exhilarating transformation of learning.

In the interplay of terms for the first principles of matter, Browne illustrates the inquirer's inescapable struggle with language, moving between atoms and ideas, seeds and effluvia, in an effort to discover a level of natural reality that he worries will "prove the last leafe to be turned over in the booke of Nature" (58). But he also foregrounds problems of language. In keeping with Bacon's concern that the most recalcitrant of human errors result from the so-called Idol of the Marketplace—involving the ways in which words unmoored in reality or moored unstably distort human knowledge—*Pseudodoxia* is frequently mindful that the vagaries of nomenclature have always figured centrally in fallen humanity's error. Accordingly, Browne identifies how different modes of discourse should pursue distinctive intentions, and he returns to the ways in which proverbs, etymologies, habits of naming, and familiar ways of speaking shape as well as reflect misapprehension. He points out how the smallest constituent of a language, the superlative, can create enormous difficulty in the advancement of learning (315). And he admires the Egyptians for inventing "a language of things," based in the "common notions in Nature," which evaded "the confusion of Babel" (262).

His very choice of English is difficult: on one side of the balance is Browne's concern that English implicates his work in the very vulgarity of the many-headed multitude that he decries. But on the other side, Browne considers that his work can be most immediately productive of change if it can be absorbed in an England never before so fatally wracked by misprision as the country is in the 1640s. It is telling that only one chapter and a scattering of passages focus on the vulgar multitude as a source of error, while the errors of the learned permeate the entire work. Even popular contemporary superstition can prove to have a learned ancient source. Moreover, as Browne moves more decidedly in the direction of natural history, he becomes more attuned to local flora and fauna and, consequently, more open to the observations of all classes of people, even if (as a learned physician) he is often in a position to show them the mistakes of local lore by involving them in experiments, for instance regarding poisonous spiders (177). Iconographic errors are shared by shop signs and masterpieces alike (239). In the first edition, his solution to the problem of the work's linguistic vehicle is to cultivate what he describes as a widespread convergence between English and Latin. Although his prediction—that readers would soon need to know Latin in order to understand English—would run aground as soon as the second edition of 1650, Browne was building on the legacy of the *Religio* in the hopes that a mixture of native and Latinate styles might achieve a candid, flexible, and precise medium for the exposure and eradication of entrenched errors.

For Browne, as for so many of his philosophical contemporaries, questions of language were bound up with questions of knowledge and method. Throughout *Pseudodoxia*, Browne pauses to issue a general statement about the tendencies, prospects, and conditions of human knowledge. At the outset of his discussion of numerology, he notes that understanding and sensation "are differently deceived in their greatest objects," with the former tending to exaggerate, the latter to diminish the dimensions of an object (208). As he begins a consideration of the puzzle of skin pigmentation, he admits that some of the most obvious sensations are especially lost on understanding (322). In an assessment of why dolphins are often depicted with curved bodies, even though they are in fact straight, Browne argues that there are three ways in which to interpret a picture: emphatically (the picture captures the way in which the dolphin appears to the eye); really (the picture shows the dolphin as it is); and emblematically (the picture uses curvature as a symbol of celerity) (235). In some cases, Browne not only generalizes about human knowledge but also instructs the would-be advancer. At times, he cautiously encourages readers to limit error as much as possible, even if that simply entails an attitude of doubt. But defending the rigor of his criticism even in "petty errors and minor lapses," Browne takes a stronger stand, declaring that "as betweene falshood and truth, there is no medium, so should they be maintained in their distances, nor the insinuation of the one, approach the sincerity of the other" (254). Here Browne's absolutism about keeping truth and error apart resonates with the theological framework of his project, one that constructs error as the human labyrinth between divine creation and human judgment. Just as faith should not (and cannot) be manufactured by coercion, Browne concludes, reason and sensation cannot be forced to credit something that they otherwise would not. As the Holy Spirit must genuinely move us to faith in salvation, so reason and the senses must assent freely to claims about the loadstone. At the heart of salvation and advancement alike are "the principles of perswasion" (382–3).

Religion has both a pervasive and a complex presence in *Pseudodoxia*. Offsetting the underlying theme of sin and the devil as sources of error, Browne offers advice for worshipping, representing, and understanding the divine. God is praised as the infallible rule of truth, "for things are really true as they correspond to his conception, and have so much of verity, as they hold of conformity unto that intellect, in whose Idea they had their first determination" (4). As a creator, God is also the source of variety, a quality which according to the imprimatur of John Downame is reflected in *Pseudodoxia* itself. In praises of divine creation, Browne's prose purveys the same love of paradox, the same combinations of Latinate and English vocabulary, and the same affection for carefully wrought patterns in sound and phrasing that it shows in *Religio*: "and so although we say the world was made in sixe dayes, yet was there as it were a world in every one, that is, a distinct creation of distinguisht creatures, a distinction in time of creatures divided in nature, and a severall approbation and survey in every one" (171). But if variety in creation is delightful, it also serves to defy easy understanding, and Browne reminds his readers that physicians are especially skilled at discerning variation among the common ways of the creation (217).

As much as the *Religio*, *Pseudodoxia* stresses that divine creation disposes its variety in carefully planned, always purposeful matrices. With Galen's *De usu partium* as both an explicit and implicit presence throughout, Browne returns time and again to an argument that nature never does anything in vain or superfluously. This refrain is a crucial feature of what Browne means by a "rational" argument; it is used to argue, for instance, that God would not make it fatal to harvest a useful plant (96), that God would not leave an animal without a gall (107), or that nature would not leave an infant bear so badly formed that its mother would be required to lick it into shape (116). Browne is so intent on defending providence that he devotes one of the work's two "digressions" on maintaining the stasis of the earth and mobility of the sun to manifestations of that divine wisdom (290–4). In insisting that the new astronomy of Copernicus would not impugn divine providence, however, Browne introduces a theme—the incomprehensibility of the divine—that modifies his paeans to the rational utility of creative design. Elsewhere in the work, this wonder in confronting the divine takes the form of simple faith: on occasion, readers are urged simply to trust God or his chief spokesperson Moses.[152]

In an effort to manage the conflict between a rational and mysterious God, Browne spends considerable energy on biblical scholarship and hermeneutics. Most obviously, he attacks the sort of hyper-literalism that misses the spiritual depth, moral fables, and figurative accommodations of the scriptures. Thus,

[152] See for instance 274, 278, 282, 343.

Browne complains, the "people" degrade God "into manuall expressions" (9); and philosophers mistake symbols for causes, forgetting for instance that "Hieroglyphically, metaphorically, Illustratively," God makes things in numerical patterns, not by means of them—"not with reference unto action, or causality" (214). In the same vein, Browne devotes a considerable portion of his work to emblematic modes of representation, according to which a good preacher or theologian can imitate Egyptian practices in using an erroneous portrait for the sake of moral and spiritual improvement.[153] Over time, much error has arisen from taking tropes as literal or "strict" versions of the factually real, a fault to be discovered in animal lore as well as saints' lives, and in interpretations of scriptural cruxes or of the iconic legacies presumed to be based on scripture.

Yet Browne's penchant for treating biblical language as a flexible instrument in the hands of moralists and preachers runs into conflict with his even more pronounced insistence on rigor in biblical scholarship. Admiring the critical philology of scholars such as Scaliger and Selden, Browne devotes himself to both firsthand and secondhand understanding of the history of biblical transmission. The professed strictness of such arguments is often directed toward settling simple questions of no doctrinal importance: did Jesus lie down when he ate (243)?; how old was Isaac when his father set out to sacrifice him (245)?; what did John the Baptist wear (254)? As is the case in *Religio*, such queries may be doctrinally safe but they also risk a lapse into idle curiosity, as Browne himself jokes with reference to his discussion of what Eve ate at her fall, a "fruit" after which his "curiosity fruitlessely enquireth" (341). More perilously, the tension between flexible and strict interpretations of the Bible can arise when causation—whether miraculous or natural, spiritual or physical—is in question, whether the topic is fasting, rainbows, or human posture.[154]

As the example of the rainbow suggests, Browne attempts to link interpretive rigor to flexibility in his argument that the more one knows about nature, history, and the Bible, the better one can understand representations of and by the divine. Usually to be found somewhere in this mediation between fact and allegory is Browne's criterion of appropriateness: the more one knows about the rainbow, then the more apt it proves as God's choice for a symbol. As Kevin Killeen has argued, it is on this question of the propriety of representation that Browne's great work intervenes most directly in the contemporary battles of Norwich in the 1640s—in the world in which the polemical war between iconophobes and iconophiles neglects the wide middle spectrum in which most people agree that some form of appropriate representation is useful, pleasing, and godly.[155] On occasion, Browne even goes so far as to offer instructions on religious representation, again with the desire to mediate between the factual and spiritual dimensions of his work. Browne is most emphatic in opposing human representations of God the

[153] See for instance 109, 112, 114, 116, 233, and 247. For the clearest defense of the uses of error, see 361.

[154] See *Pseudodoxia* (1646), 44, 162–3, 179–81, 345–7.

[155] Killeen, *Biblical Scholarship*, 198–9.

Father, not least because such a volatile area of religious culture is partly responsible for the "fecundity of sects" in the 1640s (270). As one way of avoiding the false and dangerous representation of God, Browne reverts to the geometrical metaphors for which he expressed such favor in *Religio*.[156]

The tightest link between religious faith and rigorous criticism in *Pseudodoxia* is methodological. While Browne explains to his readers that error will be judged according to the triple criteria of reason, sense, and authority (114), it is really the first of these—reason—that he connects most carefully to a notion of the divine. At the most basic level, reason apprehends that law of nature which, for Browne, is an expression of divine intellection and purpose. But on one occasion, he also interprets the message of Christ as a matter of "rationall and well grounded precepts"—Christ modeling with his life those "highest rules of reason" that "must flourish in the advancement of learning, and the perfection of parts best able to comprehend it" (10). Throughout the work, reason is attuned to natural purpose to be sure, but it is also that faculty according to which a learned physician comprehends the Aristotelian general principles about animals (104) and faculties of physiology, or the careful observer can discern improprieties in paintings (235–40). All in all, reason ranges in meaning from logic to something like common sense, and includes imaginatively hypothetical as well as moral and theological tendencies.

In Browne's announcements of methodology, sensory experiment is never far from rational precepts, and it is heralded as "the definitive confirmatory and test of things uncertaine" (131). On a steady number of occasions, such "ocular" knowledge is gained from firsthand observation and contrived experimentation. Over the course of the books on minerals, vegetables, and animals, Browne reports his direct involvement with freezing eggs (50), testing magnetism on andirons (60), checking the putative medical benefits of the loadstone (74), and feeding glass to dogs to discover whether it is poisonous (84). He has conducted experiments on pots filled with ashes and water (87); horses and pigeons dissected in a search for their gall (108, 110); kingfishers hung by silk threads (128); gray snails and toads on the question of whether they have stones in their heads (137); the generation of frogs in ditches and pools (138); the generation of vipers, a case in which he has fed them milk, bran, and cheese (144); moles removed from the "belly" of their mother (151); the eating habits of lizards, snails, and leeches, in which Browne has deprived his subjects of food for extensive periods (163); turkeys and poultry cut open but also fed iron or stones in a study of digestion (165). Browne is fully prepared to report when experiments fail to produce clear results. On a very few but noteworthy occasions, he enlists the assistance of statistical measurement in keeping with the work of Santorio and other cutting-edge early modern scientists; such quantification is especially useful when Browne is conducting experiments on animals in order to determine something—say, brain size—about human beings who, he believes, are too "noble" to undergo the experiment themselves (182). Predictably,

[156] For geometry, see *Pseudodoxia* (1646), 270 and 345.

Browne is perfectly willing to drown cats and mice but not human subjects (194–6) in his study of buoyancy.

The greater Browne's commitment to firsthand experience, the more attentive he becomes to Norfolk flora and fauna, and the 1646 *Pseudodoxia* already includes the naturalist's dedication to the local. In a section on the bittern, he refers to observations made by "any that walketh the Fenns" (173); on grasshoppers, he conveys a precise sensitivity to the unfolding of the seasons in the world immediately around him (237). But throughout *Pseudodoxia*, secondhand experience is just as important as direct observation. For one thing, the experience of others stimulates Browne to collaborate in the trial-and-error and the mutual correction that the new science requires. For another, whether the experience derives from his neighbor Sir William Paston, from navigators such as Robert Hues, from ancient authors such as Galen, or from modern experimenters such as Digby and Descartes, experience derived from others permits Browne's encyclopedia to entertain the vastness of God's creation—to comprehend this vastness within a rational and providential framework but also to enlarge human horizons of expectation in directions not yet mapped or understood. Three other corollaries follow from this investment in secondhand experience. One is that Browne tends to enlist experience as an instrument of testing what others have claimed rather than a means of producing new knowledge.[157] The second is that the work is more heavily weighted toward "book-learning" than toward laboratory experience. And the third is that from start to finish, and whatever its focus on a wide array of phenomena, *Pseudodoxia* centers on the human: on human authority, perception, and welfare.[158]

Because extensive reading in scholarship both ancient and modern is the cornerstone of Browne's work in *Pseudodoxia*, his progress depended in large part on the steady accumulation of books over the decade or so during which he composed the first edition.[159] But it also involved certain shortcuts. As Westfall summarizes these tendencies to cut corners, Browne "was likely to draw heavily from a few chapters of his sources," to favor the sections found at "the beginnings and ends of books," to privilege a single source over all others, to offer secondhand "a list of authorities as if they were from his own reading," and even to copy "entire passages from his reading," as Dean Christopher Wren pointed out in his copy of the work.[160] For a work whose range covered crystal and coral, electricity and magnetism, mandrakes and spices, almonds and insects, all manner of animals, a baker's dozen of "popular

[157] See Robbins, ed., *Pseudodoxia Epidemica*, 2.642, 725.

[158] For the value of book-learning, see Robbins, ed., *Pseudodoxia Epidemica*, 1.xxxvii; for *Pseudodoxia*'s human focus within "the vastness of the world it presents," see Robbins, "Browne's Cosmos," in Patrides, ed., *Approaches to Sir Thomas Browne*, 159.

[159] For Browne as reader, especially of Aristotle, see Robert Ralston Cawley and George Yost, *Studies in Sir Thomas Browne* (Eugene: University of Oregon Press, 1965). For the book trade in East Anglia, see David Stoker, " 'To all Booksellers, Country Chapmen, Hawkers and Others': How the Population of East Anglia Obtained Its Printed Materials," in Robin Myers et al., eds., *Fairs, Markets and the Itinerant Book Trade* (London: the British Library, 2007), 107–36.

[160] See Westfall, *Sir Thomas Browne's Revisions*, 85–6.

and received Tenents concerning Man," a wide range of pictorial legacies from antiquity forward, as well as diverse opinions concerning cosmography and history: in such a work, the scholarship was bound to be dazzling. In approving the work for publication, John Downame remarked on its "multiplicity of reading," but Browne's own notebooks have left a trail of how detailed and complex his reading was, especially with crucial authorities such as Aristotle and with favorites such as Athenaeus. As Browne reminds his readers late in *Pseudodoxia*, Aristotle is the most important writer in the history of learning, and no scholar should ever prove ungrateful to him (*Pseudodoxia* (1646), 366). But because of his monumental stature, Aristotle must be read with care—for at least two reasons. For one, as Browne recorded in his notebooks, the canon is both huge and uneven, prompting a principle of selectivity (Keynes, 3.206). For another, Browne characterizes Aristotle as "the wary and evading assertor," a portrait that has more to do with hesitations in particular passages than with contradictions to be found over the whole course of the Aristotelian canon (206). Yet his notebooks corroborate *Pseudodoxia*'s fundamental debt to Aristotle, as well as Browne's use of the works for specifics on a vast array of topics from dice to sleeping, bruising, sounds, shells, tastes, winds, and sneezes (Keynes, 3.205–17).

As the exclusive source of so many ancient writers and customs, Athenaeus is far less conceptually problematic for Browne, if also the cause of an insatiable desire to know more about the past (Keynes, 3.165–81). In his notes on and uses of Athenaeus, moreover, Browne betrays the sheer pleasure and poignancy that he experiences in the vast, varied discursive worlds of ancient encyclopedists. Having retold a story of boys in a Sicilian inn who "are so mad with drink that they think they are sailing in a ship tossed by a wild storm," Browne remarks the amusement of the tale but also its powerful moral that this "ship of Agrigentum is the world, and in it how few are not fools!" (Keynes, 3.173–4). In an indictment of melancholy, Browne decries human madness from the way "we drink in false appearances" to the manner in which we sleepwalk through life. We are all, in short, the vulgar of the stage-play world, the "great rabble" in "the theatre of life." For Browne, Athenaeus epitomizes the very pleasures of reading that entice us into vulgar error, even as careful reading shows us the experimental and rational ways out of error. But Browne cautions that experimenters share with readers the problem of desire (*Pseudodoxia*, 70). Like readers, experimenters bring their passions and presuppositions to the study, and the fact that much experiment is to be found in reading the work of others serves only to accentuate the connection, as does Browne's persistence in referring to nature as a book.

Throughout the first edition of *Pseudodoxia*, Browne's fascination with nature is clearly deepening and expanding. One encounters in its pages Browne's interest in chemistry and anatomy, in botany, zoography, and astronomy as well as medicine. He is impatient with the signatures posited by magicians in the creation, but he never simply repudiates a tradition or legacy of natural studies wholesale. He appears to be behind the curve on plant sexuality and heliocentrism, but clearly open to new knowledge and methods. As scholars have often pointed out, his clearest obsession is with everything having to do with generation. He has been reading William Harvey's book on the subject in manuscript,[161] and he returns to what he calls "the great work" secondary only to divine creation even when he has to draw it in by analogy. As with Harvey, so too with Browne, generation offers extraordinary opportunities to reconcile religious and natural modes of understanding the world, and in this regard *Pseudodoxia* seems self-assured in the mediation between first cause and second in a way in which *Religio* does not.

The roles that Browne plays in the advancement of learning—in recalibrating the relations between religion and natural philosophy and in separating "science" from "magic"—unfold over the final decades of his life, and are often glimpsed in the changes that he continued to make on his master work, the *Vulgar Errors*. As Browne grows and develops in terms of natural philosophy and natural history, however, he also continues to develop a dynamic relationship to the historiographical methods and theories of England and Europe. One sees this development in small ways: in his antiquarian interest in coins and medals, in his indictment of pictures for anachronism, in his praise for the critical philology of John Selden, in his careful attention to ancient customs and to the perplexities of chronology and calendars. As a historian, Browne is attuned to scholarship in cosmography and geography. He takes delight in the witty stories of the past and in the wondrous tales of travel. But he is also apt to question the legitimacy of wit and wonder as the historian inevitably faces the serious doubts raised by evidence—and its lack.[162]

Browne's juxtaposition of natural and historical concerns offered one testimonial, of the several to be heard in mid-seventeenth-century England, that a turn to natural studies was an essential way of coping with, moving beyond, and even capitalizing on civil war and cataclysm. And, indeed, *Pseudodoxia* attracted a widespread, often intensely engaged, and highly various readership. Poets such as John Collop and George Daniel praised it, with the former contrasting the vulgar who "think learning to repeat what's said before" with Browne's exposure of folly and "errors bald pate."[163] At St John's College, Cambridge, a tutor recommended it to his pupils.[164] Readers across England such as Henry Power, Sir Hamon L'Estrange, and Dr Christopher Wren engaged critically with, wrote commentaries on, and added examples to its specific arguments.[165] Correspondents questioned each other about it; and Samuel Hartlib wondered in 1649 whether its second, larger edition would have more to say about Primerose's earlier work on error.[166] By the end of the 1640s, *Pseudodoxia* had exerted such a considerable influence on English intellectual culture that, in 1651, a letter writer named Peter Smith could speak of Browne

[161] Thomas Smith to Samuel Hartlib, October 30, 1648, in Samuel Hartlib, *Hartlib Papers: A Complete Text and Image Database of the Papers of Samuel Hartlib (c. 1600–1662) Held in Sheffield University Library* (Sheffield, Humanities Research Institute, 2002); Smith reports Browne as having read this work, "full of admirable experiments & various learning" some ten years earlier.

[162] For Browne and history, see *Pseudodoxia* (1646), all of Book 6, plus 70, 106, 184–6, 199–205, 208–21, 235, 259, 264–72.

[163] Collop, *The Poems of John Collop*, 105; Daniel, *The Selected Poems of George Daniel*, 61.

[164] See Curtis, *Oxford and Cambridge in Transition*, 133. The tutor was Richard Holdsworth.

[165] For these responses, see chapter 9.

[166] Hartlib, *Hartlib Papers, Ephemerides*, part 3 of 1649.

as "the best pillar of the order of St Francis, which seemes now like the middle region best to fixe the principles of Paracelsus & Aristotle which without this great medium falls in great distempers."[167] As Kathryn Murphy has argued, Smith was reflecting the view shared across the network of correspondents mediated chiefly by Samuel Hartlib—that Dr Browne was a strong force for the ecumenical advancement of learning—and he was interpreting "Browne's eclecticism and syncretism favourably, as a compromise between extremes in the interpretation of nature."[168]

In the second half of the 1640s, Browne worked assiduously at improving and revitalizing his masterpiece for contemporary readers. He read key sources published before, yet missed in the preparation of the 1646 edition—including Scipione Mercurio's study of popular errors—and secured a steady stream of books published from 1646 onward, including works by Athanasius Kircher, Nicolo Cabeo, Pierre Gassendi, John Greaves, Claude Saumaise, and Dr John Bainbridge.[169] Stylistically, Browne was reviewing his decision to keep Latin and English close together in pursuit of philosophical precision, and making considerable efforts to simplify his style according to the growing suspicion of elaborate syntax and floral diction.[170] At the same time, he was intensely interested in physical questions of magnetism, electricity and optics, and in the various theories—atomic and effluvial—that might explicate "a variety of phenomena otherwise inexplicable" involving action over a distance.[171] But he was also poised to move beyond such questions into what would prove a longstanding engagement with the life sciences, with zoology and botany, with physiological questions of generation, digestion, and respiration. Even as Browne removed evidence of personal engagement and cultivated objectivity in his style, he worked hard to give *Pseudodoxia* an aura of immediacy for the readers of the editions that followed from 1650 through 1672.[172] As Browne's later works—*Hydriotaphia* and *The Garden of Cyrus*, *Christian Morals* and *Repertorium*—demonstrate, his pursuit of a more streamlined, less erudite and florid style in the *Pseudodoxia* did not cancel the beauty or vitality of his prose; rather, various styles interacted with one another in a complex dialogue.

Readers such as Peter Smith clearly felt encouraged by Dr Browne to offer advice and criticism, for Smith reports of "that singular piece" that he has asked Browne to correct marginal references and to add an index.[173] But expressions of simple gratitude were also forthcoming; in 1647, Henry Bates "was readie to present an Hecatomb in thankfulnes, and did acknowledge it the greatest entertainmenement the kingdome could afford mee."[174] Bates approached *Pseudodoxia*

[167] *Hartlib Papers*, letter of Peter Smith, April 11, 1650.

[168] Murphy, " 'The best pillar of the Order of St. Francis,' " in Todd and Murphy, eds., *"A man very well studyed,"* 273–92.

[169] See Westfall, *Sir Thomas Browne's Revisions*, 175–80, 184–5, 227–8, 198–200, 206, 210, 233.

[170] Westfall, *Sir Thomas Browne's Revisions*, 120–5, 133–4.

[171] Westfall, *Sir Thomas Browne's Revisions*, 214.

[172] Westfall, *Sir Thomas Browne's Revisions*, 182.

[173] *Hartlib Papers*, Smith to Hartlib, October 30, 1648.

[174] Rawlinson MS D.391, ff. 79–80, in Wilkin, 1.353.

as an active reader, making "bold to Interleafe your Enquiries, and soe insert my blank and empty phansies, vnder the protection of your blanch and cleerer iudgment." As Bates makes clear, the *Pseudodoxia* was a living thing, not just because Browne was promising to revise and enlarge it but also because its clarion call for readers to interject their observations and experiences activated the kind of civil collaboration in the advancement of learning for which Bacon had hoped. Yet if Browne hoped that his encyclopedia would create only harmony among those interested in the "adventures" of learning, he was mistaken. In the very first years after the first edition, writers of all stripes began to cite *Pseudodoxia*, including for the purposes of sectarian polemic in George Masterson's *The Triumph stain'd* (1647).[175]

"Amidst the attacks of his enemies," Wilkin has written, "and commendations of his admirers, the reputation of Browne became so established and extended, that he was applied to on all hands for professional, literary, and scientific advice and assistance."[176] Whether Wilkin was right to conclude that Browne's fulfillment of such obligations deprived him of "much opportunity for further authorship," it is nonetheless fair to say that the singular position of "Dr Browne" in the English world of letters was sealed by the end of the 1640s. On his copy of the 1646 *Pseudodoxia*, Thomas Le Gros inscribed beneath the author's name a reader's sense of Browne's reliability, "*idem prope et procul*," "the same whether near or far." Le Gros included therewith a motto from Ovid, "*Est virtus placitis abstinuisse bonis*," suggestive of Browne's capacity for moral and intellectual restraint in the face of life's temptations.[177]

With the death of King Charles on January 30, 1649, and the decade of political and religious uncertainty and experimentation that followed the regicide, English readers no doubt cherished such an anchor amid the world's epidemic of error and insanity. As Murphy has shown, the image of the rock found on the title page of *Religio Medici* reappeared as a symbol of Stoic constancy amid a turbulent sea of strife on the title page of *Eikon Basilike*, a prayer book attributed to the royal martyr himself who was also depicted on the frontispiece as trading a crown of worldly power for the crown of thorns leading to an exaltation into heavenly glory.[178] But Browne's life was by no means over. In the burgeoning of his family, in the outward growth (all the way to Iceland) of his correspondents, collaborators, and admirers, in the persistent revision of *Pseudodoxia*, in the authorship of some of the best English prose ever written, in the ongoing multiplication of his reading, in the deepening of his commitment to the natural and human history of the local, in his curiosity regarding the events, persons, and phenomena of the entire world, and in the world's curiosity toward and assessments of him: in all these ways, Browne's last

[175] See Nigel Smith, "Sir Thomas Browne and the Levellers," *Notes and Queries*, n.s., 33 (1986), 421–2.

[176] Wilkin, 1.lxix.

[177] Cf. Ovid, *Heroides* (17.98): "it is virtue to abstain from lawful pleasures." K. Garth Huston, "Sir Thomas Browne, Thomas le Gros, and the First Edition of *Pseudodoxia Epidemica*, 1646," *Journal of the History of Medicine* 25 (1970), 347–8.

[178] Murphy, in *TLS*, July 4, 2008, 14–15.

three decades amounted to an extraordinary outgrowth of the forty-five years that had ended up making a London orphan famous. And somehow this worldwide fame depended not just on sophisticated learning or sonorous prose, but on the fact that on March 12, 1649, he was castrating a one-year-old rabbit (Keynes, 3.365) or, a year later, made careful note that "the strawey substances in the stomack of a pigge turned milk well in October 1650, the fresh dung of a goose white did very well, that best wch is whitest probably" (3.452).

9

Norwich, 1649–1660

1. THE REPUBLIC OF LEARNING

In *A Ternary of Paradoxes* (1650) the physician and arbiter of philosophical trends, Walter Charleton, announced the emergence of Thomas Browne into the forefront of English intellectual life as "the now flourishing Dr. Browne." Placed together with Bacon as one of only "two Heroicall Wits" worth mentioning to his patron Viscount Brouncker, Browne was praised for his commitment to proving that English can "be spun as fine and fit a garment, for the most spruce Conceptions of the Minde to appeare in publick in, as out of any other in the World." For Charleton, Browne's "plus ultra" stretched not just outward into the world of natural history but also upward toward those paradoxes that surge beyond rational theology toward mystery.[1] Also in 1650, the Cambridge philosopher Henry More confirmed the best-seller status of *Religio Medici* when he accused the occult writer Thomas Vaughan of inserting poetry into his prose to rival Browne's savory wit.[2] In the 1650s, Browne's fame made itself known in all manner of places and ways, for instance, in Edmund Prestwich's 1656 play *The Hectors*, in which the dupe Le-Gull is instructed to spend a rainy day reading, among other works, the *Pseudodoxia Epidemica*.[3] More flatteringly, Obadiah Walker modeled his own 1659 critique of vulgar errors on Browne's, introducing wisdom from *Religio Medici* and *Hydriotaphia* along the way.[4] The most obvious result of Browne's fame was that a sizable number of his compatriots—learned and unlettered, established and novice—wanted to consult and even to visit him in Norwich. Browne good-humoredly captured this state of affairs in *Amico Clarissimo, de enecante garrulo suo*,[5] in which friendship with an honored but distant addressee is the compensation for being vexed by a bore who has come to visit.

From 1649, when England was suddenly and violently transformed from a monarchy into a republic, Browne's correspondence and impact ramified into the civil, collaborative republic of learning. The citizens of this republic lived in Iceland

[1] Walter Charleton, *A Ternary of Paradoxes* (1650), B2v–B3r.

[2] Henry More, *Observations upon Anthroposophia theomagica, and Anima magica abscondita* (1650), 93.

[3] Edmund Prestwich, *The Hectors, or, The False Challenge: A Comedy* (1656), 50; cited in Killeen, *Biblical Scholarship*, 6.

[4] Obadiah Walker (1616–1699), *Periamma epidemion, or, Vulgar Errours in practice censured* (1659); for *Religio*, see 25; for *Hydriotaphia*, 28.

[5] Latin text in Keynes, 3.181–84.

and Denmark[6] as well as England and France, wrote in Latin as well as English, and discussed the deepest secrets of nature as well as the nitty-gritty details of indigenous plants or fen-draining. Given Browne's vast range of interests, it is not surprising that his correspondents were highly diverse. From the late 1640s onward, Browne's correspondence included letters from admirers: in 1652, for instance, John Heydon (1588–1653), an alchemical theorist and practitioner, wrote the author to praise his two great works, the *Religio* testifying to Browne's sincere, generous, pious and charitable mind, and the *Pseudodoxia* displaying ingenuity, judgment, "reuerence, & zeale to truth & reason." As for the author himself, he was "a person so transcendently qualified, & indowed w:th ye right constitution of a Rationale man: whose true Essence is his Minde."[7] Yet even in the letters in which scholars addressed Browne on more equal terms, they operated under the belief that Browne brought to contemporary times an exceptional wisdom, civility, learning, and judgment. Responses to Browne's work also assumed partisan forms in the Interregnum. However rigidly the Laudian programme had been implemented in Norwich in the 1630s by Wren, it is arguable that Browne was sometimes identified with Laud's doctrinal flexibility as expressed in the archbishop's *Conference with Fisher*, published during the years in which Browne was revising *Religio Medici*.[8] In the 1650s, it was to Browne's *Religio Medici* that the Laudian Peter Heylyn turned in promoting the notion "that, where he found the church had not determined an issue, 'I shall conceive my self to be left at liberty to follow the dictamen of my own genius.'"[9] For supporters of the Church of England such as Heylyn, Browne's sanctification of nature had gained in significance too, now that their church was no longer legally extant.

One of Browne's earliest biographers captured his stature as one of the chief authorities for mid-seventeenth-century intellectuals, virtuosi, and advancers of learning: "He was not only consulted by the Most Eminent Men at Home, but likewise by the Most Learned Foreigners, viz. Gruter; Windet; Theodore Jonsson of Island, & who often writ to him for Solutions of very Critical and Abstruse Points of Literature; and his answers to them always contain'd some very uncommon and curious Remarks." These foreigners not only consulted Browne but also "frequently and personally visited" him.[10] One of Browne's correspondents, Isaac Gruter (1610–80), was eager to extend the English author's influence in the republic

[6] For Iceland see below p. 317. For Copenhagen, see *Breve fra og til Ole Worm*, ed., H. D. Schepelern, 3 vols. (Munksgaard: DSL, 1965–1968), 3.486; and the translation of *Pseudodoxia* into Danish by a royal commissioner for Frederick III, Gabriel Acheleye Knudsen or Knutsen, in the Royal Library, Copenhagen.

[7] Rawlinson MS D.391, 26r–27v. I owe the correct identification of this correspondent to Vera Keller.

[8] See Shuger, "The Laudian Idiot," in Barbour and Preston, eds., *Sir Thomas Browne: The World Proposed*, 45–61.

[9] Peter Heylyn's *Theologia veterum, or, The summe of Christian theologie, positive, polemical and Philological, contained in the Apostles Creed* (1654), 471. Cf. Anthony Milton, *Laudian and Royalist Polemic in Seventeenth-Century England: The Career and Writings of Peter Heylyn* (Manchester: Manchester University Press, 2007), 160.

[10] The anonymous biography, in *Posthumous Works*, xv.

of letters. In a series of letters that came intermittently throughout the Interregnum, the Dutch schoolmaster expressed his desire to translate *Pseudodoxia Epidemica* into Latin so that frustrated readers throughout Europe might be able to read it.[11] In their complaints about delays, difficult conditions, and other scholarly burdens, Gruter's letters make it clear that the project scarcely got off the ground and reveal just how difficult the maintenance and advancement of the republic of letters could be in what Gruter characterizes as an adverse historical period of war and turmoil. During this period too, Browne's most faithful admirer, Henry Power of Halifax and Cambridge University, was parlaying his mentor's assistance into a greater independence of thought with an eye to his own membership in the republic of letters. Sending a letter over "this large distance 'twixt Hallyfax & Norwich" in August 1649, Power refers to his persistent tapping of Browne's wisdom in self-deprecatory terms, yet his queries include his own provisional solutions as well as a confident progress report on his medical studies (Keynes, 4.261–2). By the mediation of Power, another medical man named Reuben Robinson also saw fit to enjoy Browne's "excellent society at Norwich" and then to follow up the visit with enquiries by mail (Wilkin, 1.421).

Browne's correspondence with Elias Ashmole and William Dugdale bears several trademarks of his prominence in the republic of letters in the 1650s. The most obvious is that the republic offered Browne networks of learned "friends" rather than isolated exchanges with individuals. With Ashmole and Dugdale in particular, Browne's dual interests in antiquarian and natural studies converge. This is less the case with Ashmole, whose letters to Browne were principally concerned with Arthur Dee and about borrowing Browne's manuscripts on alchemy and Hermetic philosophy (Keynes, 4.293–4).[12] With Dugdale, however, Browne's interests in antiquarianism and natural history came together in an extended exchange that focused on what for the two men was a world no less new than America: the mutating and mysterious subterranean layers of history, soil, and fossils beneath their very feet. For Browne, too, this exchange helped to consolidate his belief that the local—for instance, the Norfolk broads and fens—could be as rich and strange a subject of study as Egypt.

The impetus of the exchange between Sir William Dugdale and Dr Browne was the former's work on a study of the history of recovering or securing wetlands, a study that would lead to *The History Of Imbanking and Drayning* in 1662.[13] Some of Browne's responses to Dugdale's queries would make their way into Browne's own tract on "artificial hills" in the *Miscellany Tracts*. Both men were established authors, with Dugdale the editor of a first volume of medieval manuscripts recording monastic institutions, *Monasticon Anglicanum* (1655), a project that involved

[11] See Bodl. MS Rawl D.391, 101r–101v; Rawl D.391, 100–6; BL Sloane MS 4062, 138, 141–4, 146, 149, 186.

[12] See also C. H. Josten, ed., *Elias Ashmole (1617–1692): His Autobiographical and Historical Notes, His Correspondence, and Other Contemporary Sources Relating to His Life and Work*, 5 vols. (Oxford: Clarendon Press, 1966), 1.121.

[13] On the date of the letters, see Majl Ewing, "A Note on the Sir Thomas Browne-Sir William Dugdale Letters," *Philological Quarterly* 21 (1942), 425–7.

collaboration with the great polymath John Selden but proved controversial with those Puritans anxious about its tendency toward popery.[14] Dugdale had also contributed to the antiquarian vogue for county histories with *The Antiquities of Warkwickshire Illustrated* (1656). Another work, *The History of St. Pauls Cathedral in London* (1658), anticipated and stimulated Browne's Restoration survey of the monuments in Norwich Cathedral that would become his most straightforwardly antiquarian venture, *Repertorium*.

Although Dugdale and Browne had not met, their correspondence beginning in 1658 readily testifies to their mutual interests and respect. Dugdale's letters offered Browne queries about the wet and subterranean world around Norfolk, sometimes including Dugdale's provisional answers, yet these questions about local history and geology often elicited from Browne a larger view of history and nature.[15] Among Dugdale's questions are these: what did Tacitus mean by the term *emuniendis* in discussing the labors that the ancient Britons performed for the Romans? What sense can we make of hills and mounds which ancient peoples erected without regard to fortification? When the fossil of an apparent marine animal is found where the sea no longer covers the ground, what can we learn about that animal and about the "great mutations" that readjust sea and land? What can the layering of silt and soil teach us about history? What can the gathering of urns, coins, and monuments beneath the earth teach us about nature's mutations? More immediately, might Browne intervene with Selden's literary executors in such a way that Dugdale can gain access to certain manuscripts in London?

In responding to Dugdale's queries, Browne apologizes that for a physician living in a "Restlesse & sickly time," leisure is an "uncertaine" commodity (Keynes, 4.302, 311). Nonetheless, his letters serve as detailed, engaged, and carefully weighed essays in antiquarianism, natural philosophy, and natural history. The most extended piece, an early draft of the tract on mounds, offers a threefold taxonomy of their intentions, as landmarks, sepultures, and protection from flooding, yet Browne accepts and focuses on the first two. Enlisting a criterion—strictness—that he will invoke in the second chapter of *Hydriotaphia*, Browne works through the various people who have resided in Britain from the Romans through the Danes. The neglect of the ancient Britons is significant for two reasons. For one, antiquarianism takes a largely skeptical approach to the old romantic legends that have dominated earlier interest in the worlds of Lear and Arthur. Indeed Browne's skepticism is conveyed in the nuanced vocabulary with which he weighs the various degrees of certainty, probability, and doubt, arriving eventually at the phrase "probable possibilities" as a favorite gauge. Like a good antiquarian, he is eager for material evidence (coins, shards, urns), for manuscript material, and for "ocular exploration," the latter motivating his request that local mounds be cut through, "either directly or crosswise"; and he is keen to receive from Dugdale precise

[14] See William Hamper, ed., *The Life, Diary, and Correspondence of Sir William Dugdale, Knight* (London: Harding, Lepard, and Co., 1827), 475–6.

[15] See Claire Preston, *Thomas Browne and the Writing of Early Modern Science* (Cambridge: Cambridge University Press, 2005), 125.

measurements of a scene in question before he passes judgment on what it means (Keynes, 4.304–5).[16]

The second reason for the neglect of the pre-Roman British is far more subjective: Browne is obviously ashamed of the ancient Britons who, in his view, were barbaric warriors without the prudent intelligence, culture, and industry of the ancient Romans. Browne concedes that this is a problematic stance to take: after all, the Romans were industrious on the backs of the British slaves that they wore out in clearing forests and fens. Moreover, Browne acknowledges the lure of ancient British mystique, one that he connects to the mystery of the fens when he embraces the legend of Queen Boadicea's final escape into the local wetlands, "this being a fast and retiring place in all ages" (Keynes, 4.304). Allowing for the possibility that "the dust of Boadicea the famous Queene of the Iceni may lye about these parts," Browne is also conceding the possibility that the antiquarian may one day find beneath the artificial mounds of Norfolk extraordinary evidence of a pre-Roman civilization. All the same, there is no missing Browne's disregard for the British. No wonder, he says, that Tacitus speaks of the clearing of forests, fens, and other wetlands in ancient Britain, for the Romans were "a carefull & provident people, omitting noe waye to secure or improve their dominions & lands, lost by carelesse ignorance in the disadvantage of sea & waters." Indeed, the Romans used British slave labor to ensure that those lands were "open & lesse fitt for retreat or concealement of the Britans," while their extensive work on clearing and improving the fens served the further purpose of resisting piracy and flooding (Keynes, 4.308).

No doubt one of the reasons why Browne is increasingly drawn to natural history and antiquarian recovery is that these two pursuits allow the civil and learned man to demonstrate his industry and, therefore, to distinguish himself from two nemeses at once. First there are the monkish clerics with whom an antiquarian might be lumped, both for his medieval interests and for his perceived waste of time and intellect. Second, there are the ambitious military Cromwells of the 1640s and 50s who destroy the collaboratively wrought institutions of the past as they exercise their self-serving brutality. In the midst of this intense exchange with Dugdale, Browne signals his realization that the familiar and local can prove as enigmatic and wonderful as worlds distant in time and place, whether America or Egypt. Indeed, in discussing the findings of Herodotus and Aristotle about the artificial improvement of the Nile, Browne briefly remarks that such "fencings, bankings, slucings, & Artificiall streames" make Egypt "a country resembling this," presumably, the wet regions of Norfolk (Keynes 4.314). But the mystery of the local emerges clearly when Dugdale poses the question of whether wetland was once upon a time "firme land," and vice versa. As they work through the question of shifting water and land, they remark on just how mysterious the subterranean truly is (Keynes, 4.323). Indeed, Browne cherishes the letters' orientation downward and locally, to what might be discovered beneath the layers of history and

[16] See also William Clark Library B884L, November 10, 1658 for a letter in Browne's hand. I owe this reference to Claire Preston.

nature "in this place." The mingling of advancement and mystery is clearly powerful to Browne. On the one hand, "manie things prove obscure in subterraneous discoverie"; on the other, "wiser inquirers" now understand the nature of the large fossils more clearly than did those previous observers who attributed them to giants. Indeed, the local and subterranean worlds are mysterious, not just in the past and present, but for so long as the flawed (if industrious) observers will see fit to dig and cut into the earth. And when Dugdale answers Browne's query about whether he plans a local history of Norfolk, the latter rules out the possibility not least because such an undertaking would require far more time, expense, and labor than he has to give (Keynes, 4.309).

Although their priorities might differ, with Dugdale more interested in the preservation of the past, Browne more attentive to hieroglyphic meanings, their exchange epitomizes a civility that, they hope, will mitigate brutal partisanship in war-torn England.[17] Indeed, while antiquarians were not politically united in the 1650s, the very fact that their projects especially flourished in that decade stands as clear evidence that they expressed a backlash against the destructive designs of iconoclasm and civil war: often dismayed by the dismantling of the church, they purveyed the values of friendship, historical scholarship, an appreciation for beauty, and an urgent desire to reassemble fragments. If their methods aspired to critical rigor in the handling of evidence, the antiquarians' projects also conveyed and produced strong feelings of sympathy.[18] In his exchanges with Dugdale and Ashmole, Browne demonstrates the generosity of scholarly communication with his network of "friends."

In no way does Browne's exploration of local history with Dugdale indicate a creeping provincialism in his frame of reference. Rather, Browne appreciates that a history of a place such as Norfolk involves the study of more than one people, even though historians have been apt to homogenize their conception of culture. In a paragraph written in one of his notebooks, on how "the virtuous parts or eccelencies both of men and nations are allowable by aggregation," Browne returned to the Roman use of slave labor, this time noting that perhaps the "Romans" have received more than their fair share of credit.[19] The same truth applied to literature: "So the poets which writ in Latin built up the credit of Latium, and passed for Roman witts. Whereas if Carthage deducted Terence, Aegypt Claudian, if Marseilles should call home Petronius, if the Senecas, Lucan, Martial and Statius should be retored unto Spayne, it would much abridge the glory of pure Italian phancy." From this vantage, the study of a great empire comes to mean very little without the contributions of local history.

Far from depending on provincialism, the flourishing of local histories in seventeenth-century England was made possible by the gentry's access to the kind of humanist education that Browne had received at Winchester and Oxford, and

[17] On civility, Preston, *Thomas Browne and the Writing of Early Modern Science*, 124; cf. 132–33 for the different aims of Browne and Dugdale.

[18] See Graham Parry, *The Trophies of Time: English Antiquarians of the Seventeenth Century* (Oxford: Oxford University Press, 1995), 1–2, 6, 9–14, 17–19.

[19] Norman J. Endicott, ed., *The Prose of Sir Thomas Browne* (Garden City, NY: Anchor, 1967), 468.

it also relied on the network of connections that brought together Browne with the publisher Daniel King in 1656.[20] In his commendatory letter for King's *Vale-Royall of England*, Browne lingers on the difference between local history and provincialism. Addressing King as his "endeared Friend," Browne praises his history of the "County Palatine of Chester" as an "accurate piece of... Geographicall and Historicall Description" and even identifies himself (in respect of his father's people) as "a more unworthy member" of that county (Keynes, 4.394). When he poses a hypothetical question of whether a place owes more to its historian or the historian to his place, Browne urges that King has very good reasons to expend "all your pains and Labour to illustrate beautifie and adorn the place" (Keynes, 4.393). To be sure, Browne argues against provincialism as a credential of the local historian, for travel abroad and comprehensive study are as fertile for the local historian as transplantation into new, rich soil is healthy to a flower.

For Browne, the turn to local history was not provincial because, as Dugdale's evaluation of the difficulty of writing such a history reveals, antiquarians and natural historians operated from the assumption that each and every place in the world was distinctive, complex, and dynamic and that an understanding of one place would profit, if mainly by contrast, from gaining knowledge about the others. In his exchange of letters with the prominent Icelander and Lutheran minister, Þórður Jónsson, Browne had a good opportunity to confirm the wide reach (as well as the depth) of local history. Although only three letters, all from Jónsson, have survived,[21] they convey a clear sense of the kinds of information that the two men cherished from one another. The first, dated July 1651 and sent from Jónsson's home in Hitterdale, details Icelandic trees, flowers, and herbs, the country's climate and diseases, and some of its animal life. In this letter Jónsson is especially keen to set the record straight about Mount Hekla, whose volcanic activity has led to its erroneous association with Hell. As the second letter, from 1656, illustrates, Jónsson is as interested in Browne's world as he is eager to share data about his own. Including a list of questions about Browne's own situation—his marital status and age, his place of residence and profession—Jónsson also solicits information about England, its government, religion, and universities. Above all, he seeks from Browne a narrative of the regicide, which so far Jónsson and his fellow Icelanders have heard about as though it were a dream.[22] Browne worked some of the material from these letters into his writings, including bits on "eagle stone" and burning mountains into *Pseudodoxia*, and notes about migratory birds into his study of fauna in Norfolk.[23] From Iceland, Browne received the sort of information about

[20] See Jan Broadway, *"No historie so meete": Gentry Culture and the Development of Local History in Elizabethan and Early Stuart England* (Manchester: Manchester University Press, 2006). Browne and King are discussed on 106–7. For King, see also 51.

[21] None of Browne's letters is extant in either Iceland or Denmark.

[22] The letters are printed in Wilkin, *Works*, 4.256–70; for a critique of this edition of the letters, as well the misinformation generated by its mistakes, see Shaun F. D. Hughes, "Sir Thomas Browne and Iceland," *English Renaissance Prose* 1 (1987), 25–47.

[23] See Hughes, "Sir Thomas Browne and Iceland," 36–9; Hughes notes that Browne mistakes Jónsson's Latin term for a snipe as a reference to the cuckoo.

Iceland that he would share with the Royal Society in 1663. In that account, Browne covered a wide range of phenomena: driftwood, bears on ice, winter weather, volcanic eruptions, rivers and salmon, and minerals, fish teeth, dog breeds, swimming horses, and coarse wool. Throughout the account, Browne operates on the belief that Iceland has features of its natural history that are "different from any with us," but that this other place, Iceland, is not static across time but subject to changes wrought by nature and human interaction.[24]

In the 1650s, a passion for the study of plants in particular produced learned friendships. As he would recall in a letter to Christopher Merrett in 1668, Browne enjoyed sending the gift of botanical instruction as well seeds and plants as far back as the early 1640s, for it was about then that he sent an account of *Acorus verus* to Dr Goodyear (presumably John Goodyear, d. 1664) (Keynes, 4.344), after which, in the 1650s, he sent specimens to physicians such as William How and Charles Scarburgh, a Royalist ejected from his Cambridge fellowship during the war years and William Harvey's eventual successor to the Lumleian lectureship in 1656. Thus Browne extended his network of friends along the tendrils of his botanical interests and specimens. An Oxonian who had served King Charles in the civil wars, How was by 1655 a London physician and well-known herbalist who was contemplating a second edition of his *Phytologia Britannica*, first published in 1650.[25] In this work, How had assembled a list of indigenous British plants, with English translations of their Latin names, and in many cases with locations identified. To reinforce the legitimacy of the list, How often provided the name of his informant regarding a particular plant. Writing to Browne from London on September 20, 1655, How thanks him for a "rare present," then promises to return the favor "with any faire florall returnes, pacquett of seeds," or by any other means that residence in London can afford (Wilkin, 1.417). In his letter to Merrett, Browne would elaborate on his botanical present to How: "some notes and a box full of the fresh Juli," an "elegant plant" which can be found "by the bankes of the Norwich river, chiefly about Claxton and Surlingham & also between Norwich and Hellsden, so that I have known Heigham Church in the suburbs of Norwich strowed all over with it" (Keynes, 4.344).

There is no sense either in How's published work or in his letter to Browne that the discovery of the indigenous in natural history might have some political meaning or purpose. With Evelyn's far more comprehensive notion of the *Elysium Britannicum or the Royal Garden*, about which Browne was consulted in 1660, the Interregnum politics of gardening comes directly into play.[26] In January 1660, Browne wrote to Evelyn at the prompting of a mutual friend, Robert Paston; having

[24] For Jónsson and Browne, see also Ethel Seaton, *Literary Relations of England and Scandanavia in the Seventeenth Century* (reissued, New York: Blom, 1972), 45, 182–7, 208, 344.

[25] On How, see Charles E. Raven, *English Naturalists from Neckam to Ray: A Study of the Making of the Modern World* (Cambridge: Cambridge University Press, 1947), 304–5; and R. T. Gunther, *Early British Botanists and Their Gardens* (Oxford: Oxford University Press, 1922), 251, though their views of his merits differ.

[26] For the date of these letters, see E. S. De Beer, "The Correspondence between Sir Thomas Browne and John Evelyn," *The Library*, fourth series, 22 (1941–42), 103–6.

been shown an outline of Evelyn's project to comprehend and design a universal paradise, Browne sent what he called "hints & proposalls" for Evelyn judiciously to entertain in the event that the *Elysium* were not already completed (Keynes, 4.273). Evelyn's response, dated January 28, 1660, offers an extraordinary version of what Browne's authority has come to represent for a Royalist virtuoso over the course of the 1650s.

Evelyn begins with an accent on the virtues and qualities that qualify Browne for leadership in the world of letters—his "extraordinary humanity," "communicable nature," and "civility" (Keynes, 4.273–4). A candid note of personal tragedy makes its way into the letter when, having recently lost three children, Evelyn confides in Browne that impediments blocking his progress toward the ideal garden include the sickness of his only son.[27] Having noted some of the motives for his focus in the 1650s on gardening—previously defective treatments, the utility, magnificence, and pleasure of gardens, the excessive artifice "which smell more of paynt then of flowers and verdure"—Evelyn then pulls up the curtain on a grand scheme in which he envisions Browne as a central figure: "our drift is a noble, princely, and universall Elysium, capable of all the amœnities that can naturally be introduced into Gardens of pleasure, and such as may stand in competition with all the august designes and stories of this nature, either of antient or moderne times; yet so as to become usefull and significant to the least pretences and faculties" (Keynes, 4.275). Evelyn's garden holds attractions for the hieroglyphic, mystical Browne of *Religio*, as well as the Baconian Browne of *Pseudodoxia*. And Evelyn makes it clear that Browne is tailor made to become a hero of his garden: "and I would have not onely the elogies and effigie of the antient and famous Garden Heroes, but a society of the Paradisi Cultores, persons of antient simplicity, paradisean and hortulan saints, to be a society of learned and ingenuous men, such as Dr Browne, by whome we might hope to redeeme the tyme that has bin lost, in pursuing vulgar errours, and still propagating them, as so many bold men yet presume to do" (Keynes, 4.275). In a time of military strife, with so "generall a Catalysis of integrity, interruption of peace and propriety," there is reason to worry that "the hortulane pleasures, these innocent, pure, and usefull diversions might enjoy the least encouragement" (Keynes, 4.275). In such fallen, miserable, chaotic times, there is all the more reason for men like Evelyn and Browne to undertake the recovery of paradise. As far as Evelyn is concerned, a princely gardener must rely on exceptional philosophers such as Browne for the way to happiness.[28]

For the learned men in his epistolary network, the authority of "Dr Browne" was not reducible to a staunchly conservative and Anglican Royalism. Indeed, the two sides of his literary output thus far could produce conflicted responses: in *Matæotechnia Medicinæ Praxeos* (1651), Noah Biggs singled out *Pseudodoxia*

[27] For the context, see Gillian Darley, *John Evelyn: Living for Ingenuity* (New Haven, CT: Yale University Press, 2006), 151.

[28] Further evidence of their regard for one another can be seen in the sale of a presentation copy of Evelyn's 1662 *Sculptura* by Sotheby's in 1902, in which Evelyn had inscribed Browne as his "honor'd Friend" (*TLS*, June 5, 1902).

Epidemica for excellence in the exposure of received errors, but he spoke of "*religio medica*" as a begetter of authoritative imposture.[29] Yet as the author of *Religio Medici*, Browne continued to be valuable as a spiritual compass. Nor in the 1650s was such guidance needed only in the internal realm of religious experience. As Gillian Darley has written of Evelyn, the decision about whether to attend church in the 1650s was a difficult one since, "by late 1654 restrictions on mainstream observance were biting hard."[30] In these very years, Browne's parish church, St Peter Mancroft, was embroiled in controversy over a minister with a provocative reputation as a loyalist to the Church of England.[31]

2. MEDICAL PRACTICE AND COMMUNITY IN INTERREGNUM NORFOLK

The case of Sir Hamon L'Estrange serves as a clear reminder that Browne's cultivation of learning in Norfolk was never far removed from his success as a physician. L'Estrange was the author of an extensive manuscript commentary on *Pseudodoxia*; he was also Browne's patient. Browne's letters to this scion of a longstanding Norfolk family, written in 1653, show the signal importance of collaboration and consultation in Browne's medical practice. Having asked his own physician, Dr Samuel Baron, to seek advice from Browne on a case of stone involving Browne's patient Mr. Sayer, L'Estrange learns in March 1653 that Browne is too busy to make the trip to Hunstanton Hall on the far western edge of Norfolk; but Browne has been generous with his advice regarding the "raggs" or "copwebbs" that L'Estrange has witnessed in his urine.[32] On April 17, Baron clarifies for L'Estrange how harmoniously Browne has united humoral and chemical medicine in his understanding of the processes that disrupt or contaminate but also heal and cleanse the body.[33] Despite his busy schedule, Browne took the time to write a series of letters to L'Estrange, and eventually would even make the trip to Hunstanton. In the first letter, dated June 11, 1653, Browne conveys his deep concern for the patient's ongoing afflictions—L'Estrange was in fact in the last year of his life—and warns him about using the widely available and abundant recipes for the stone without clear advice from his physician. As payment for his advice, Browne requests information from L'Estrange about the "spermaceti whale . . . cast upon shoare," a further indication of Browne's growing fixation on natural history (Keynes, 4.285–6).

Browne's turn to natural history and his growing interest in antiquarianism were facilitated in the 1650s not just by the physical world in his county but also by his family's move to a sizable house in the marketplace parish of St Peter Mancroft in 1650. (See Figure 9.1.) By the time Evelyn visited the house in October 1671, he wrote in his diary,

29 Noah Biggs, *Matæotechnia Medicinæ Praxeos* (1651), 227, 4.

30 Gillian Darley, *John Evelyn: Living for Ingenuity*, 139.

31 See below, pp. 325–26.

32 NRO LEST P/20 68r.

33 NRO LEST P/20 71r.

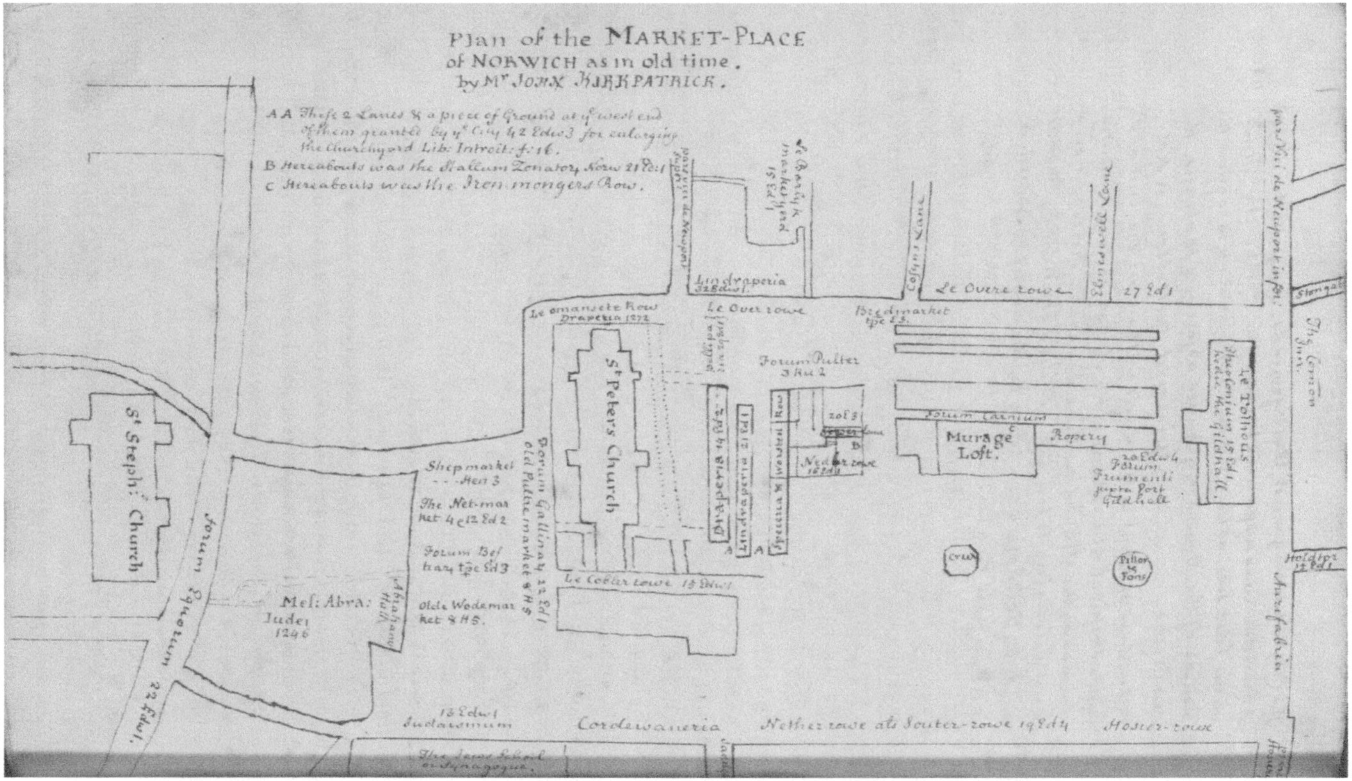

Figure 9.1 John Kirkpatrick, reconstruction of the medieval Norwich Market (*c.*1700), in "Of the Streets & Lanes of the City of Norwich, their antient & modern Names: as also of the Market Place & other Plains, or Void Ground." Reproduced with the permission of the Norfolk Record Office.

> [T]he whole house & Garden [had been converted into] a Paradise & Cabinet of rarities, & that of the best collection, especialy Medails, books, Plants, natural things. [Browne] had amongst other curiosities, a collection of the Eggs of all the foule & birds he could procure, that Country (especialy the promontorys of Norfolck) being (as he said) frequented with severall kinds, which seldome or never, go farther into the Land, as Cranes, Storkes, Eagles &c: & variety of Waterfoule.[34]

Positioned at the southeast corner of the marketplace, on the site of the medieval residence of the high priest for the Jewish synagogue, the house had belonged to onetime mayor Alexander Anguish who made way for the Brownes in the period just before the birth of their daughter Frances on November 7, 1650.[35] According to a document from 1704, the large complex was described as "all that messuage with the appurtenances, and all the edifices, shops, yards, sellars, wayes, passages, stone walls, easements and eavesdroppings . . . all which prmisses were of Sir Thomas Browne, Doctor of Physick."[36] Abutting what was then Rampant Horse Lane and Drapers Row where, by the seventeenth century, the hay carts and wagons gathered, the house was big enough to contain thirteen hearths.[37] Together with the house, Browne's yard came to be filled with plant specimens and a menagerie including "curlews in large cages, sea fowl which he crammed with fish, a pelican ('hanged in my howse'), fish ('hanged in my yard'), the heads of two whales, boxes of flies and of other insects," and many other natural and antiquarian specimens.[38] The complex also comprised the "elaboratory" for Browne's ongoing experiments on a wide range of phenomena in physics and natural history.

Browne's new home was the site of family births and deaths on a regular basis; during the 1650s, he and Dorothy welcomed the arrival and baptism at St Peter's of additional children to his family, but almost just as often lost them to premature death. Baby Dorothy and Frances, born in 1649 and 1650, were buried on May 14, 1652 and September 15, 1651 respectively, with Browne paying ten shillings for the latter's grave.[39] A boy named Charles survived from August 1655 to April 1662. Twin boys Richard and James lived from August 1656 to October 1657 and October 1656 respectively, but their baptism on the very day of their birth suggests that their parents were anxious about their health from the very beginning. For the surviving children, including sons Edward and Thomas, as well as daughters Anne, Elizabeth, and newcomer Mary (born on January 6, 1653), Browne began to oversee what later he conceded was their costly education and rearing. There was the local grammar school for the boys, who studied there under Thomas Lovering; in 1657, Edward was off to Trinity College, Cambridge, matriculating as a

[34] Evelyn, *The Diary*, 3.594.

[35] Francis Blomefield, *An Essay Towards a Topographical History of the County of Norfolk* (London, 1806), 225–6. Charles Williams, *Souvenir of Sir Thomas Browne* (London: Jarrod & Sons, 1905).

[36] Quoted in Charles Williams, "Residence of Sir Thomas Browne, M.D. at Norwich," *East Anglican* n.s. 1 (1886), 194–5.

[37] NRO NCR Case 13a, hearth tax for 1671; only one neighbor in Mancroft, Augustine Briggs, had more hearths at 14.

[38] E. S. Merton, "Sir Thomas Browne as Zoologist," *Osiris* 9 (1950), 413–34, see 413–14.

[39] NRO PD 26/71, f. 429.

pensioner.[40] Browne's family grew and changed in other ways as well, for there is evidence, too, that his sister Mary and her daughters came to live in Norwich after the death of her husband Nevill Craddock in 1651.[41]

Lacking in exterior ornament, Browne's spacious three-story house appears from the surviving images and furniture to have been "sumptuously appointed."[42] Its drawing room included an elaborately carved over-mantel piece, festooned with two bosses of yellow onyx and bearing the arms of King James I, with the motto "*exurgat deus dissipentur inimici*," a line taken from Psalm 68 which beseeches God to arise (as he has in the past) and scatter the enemies of the chosen people.[43] Praised as the father of the fatherless and the helper of the enslaved and oppressed, God is invoked to vanquish those "people that delight in warre." In the abstract, the political edge of the psalm might cut two ways, since it characterizes the enemies of God's people both as kings and rebels. Used on some of the earliest coins in the Jacobean reign, however, the motto had been reinstated on civil-war-era coins depicting Charles holding a sword in readiness for his rebellious subjects. Placed under the Jacobean arms on the over-mantel of Browne's house, its support for a militarized Stuart monarchy on behalf of religious and political unity is impressive. It is unknown when or by whom the Jacobean arms had been installed in Browne's house; but the motto and its biblical source replaced the peaceful emphases of many Jacobean mottoes with the one that stressed the Stuart monarchy's divinely given authority to quash rebellion.

Although the distance might be covered by a brisk walk of five minutes, the move from Tombland near the cathedral to Mancroft on the market brought more than just a shift to a more conservative neighborhood. Browne's new house abutted one of the chief centers of political activism and display in the city, the site of the great explosion of 1648, and the busy concourse at which the provisions of life were for sale. Browne's contemporaries shared a keen sense that the market had witnessed a rich and various history; by the end of the seventeenth century, it had even become the subject of an antiquarian study that noted both continuities with the past (the great Market Cross, for instance) and the extraordinary changes from its medieval beginnings.[44] In 1682, Thomas Baskerville described the market as "a little way from [the] castle on the opposite side of a hill," "the only place where all things are brought to be sold for the food of this great city," and accordingly "vastly full of provisions, especially on Saturdays."[45] As Baskerville observes, Norwich market was essentially different in its unity from London's habit of "allowing markets in several places." And he was not alone in his response to the market; visitors to the

[40] H. W. Saunders, *A History of the Norwich Grammar School* (Norwich: Jarrold and Sons, 1932), 281–5; *ODNB* piece on Edward Browne written by Kees van Strien.

[41] G. C. R. Morris, "Cradock, Amherst and Howell," 11–17.

[42] For the house, see Anthony Batty Shaw, *Sir Thomas Browne of Norwich* (Norwich: Jarrold & Sons, 1982); Batty Shaw identifies the arms as Jacobean, correcting the earlier claims by Charles Williams among others that they belonged to Charles II and that Browne himself had probably requisitioned them when he was knighted.

[43] For a description, see Batty Shaw, *Sir Thomas Browne of Norwich*.

[44] The antiquary John Kirkpatrick carried out this study (NRO Rye MS 9/1). See Figure 9.1.

[45] Quoted in John Pound, *Tudor and Stuart Norwich* (Chichester: Phillimore, 1988), 26–7.

city tended to single out the area "for its size, good order, and for the quantity and quality of goods on sale," with city suppliers competing with butchers and farm families from the country.[46] For Browne, moreover, everyday life was rendered all the more exciting by virtue of the fact that his house was especially close to the gate through which came the traffic from London.

Far more took place in the market than just the sale of highly various provisions on Wednesdays and Saturdays, including civic pageantry, announcements of national significance, and a wide range of entertainment.[47] For the Brownes, the market was also a place of worship, a familiar juxtaposition for a man who had grown up in Cheapside. Built in the fifteenth century, the perpendicular church of St Peter Mancroft was considered Norwich's finest, remarkable for its combination of considerable size and a lightness made possible by its windows. Inside, the unity of the space accentuated one of the most extraordinary features of this church, namely, that its parishioners were autonomous and collaborative in their choice of ministers, fundraising, and governance.[48] For Browne, who in *Religio Medici* had argued for a conformity that permitted the exercise of one's own testing reason, this was a happy state of affairs. Nonetheless, in 1650 the church was suffering from the ravages of war.[49] From 1648 through 1652, churchwarden records were filled with expenses for repair of the church, though, as David King has noted, "[m]oney was clearly a problem, and in 1651 items of church furnishings had to be sold to finance repairs."[50] Such straits in his noble parish church reinforced for Browne how fragile were those ecclesiastical monuments and artworks whose ability to stimulate worship and to preserve cultural memory appeared to him no longer just controversial but in fact imperiled.

On guild days in particular, when the mayor was to be sworn in, Browne would be reliving his urban childhood as families "whitewashed their houses and hung cloths, pictures, garlands, and streamers" in anticipation of the procession that would move from the guildhall to the cathedral, with Snap the dragon entertaining the children, and a panoply of shows, bonfires, and feasting.[51] But the market's neighbors were also compelled to witness humanity in its most shameful guises, with criminals whipped, placed in stocks, or hanged, and with drunken crowds at election time huddled together, according to Browne himself, like sheep. Here too crowds gathered to view a wide variety of human freaks and monstrosities: in the last decades of Browne's life, displays included " 'a monstrous hayrie child'; 'a girl of sixteen with no bones'; 'a child with six fingers on each hand and six toes on each

[46] Penelope Corfield, "A Provincial Capital in the Late-Seventeenth Century," 288–9.

[47] Ursula Priestley, *The Great Market: A Survey of Nine Hundred Years of Norwich Provision Market* (Norwich: University of East Anglia, 1987), 13.

[48] David M. Sharp, *The Church of St Peter Mancroft, Norwich* (Norwich: Jarrold, 1994), 2, 5. NRO PD/26/308 notes that the parishioners had contested Charles I's appointment of a minister in 1638 (43). The churchwardens' accounts give details on Browne's payments throughout the last decades of his life, including Easter and Reparation rates: NRO PD 26/725.

[49] Anthony Batty Shaw, *Sir Thomas Browne of Norwich*.

[50] David King, *The Medieval Stained Glass of St Peter Mancroft, Norwich* (Oxford: Oxford University Press, 2006), lxv.

[51] John Miller, *Cities Divided*, 100.

foot'; 'a little dwarf of 37 years of age'; 'a monstrous man taken from amongst the hills of Corinthia, he feeds on the roots of trees etc.'; 'a monstrous man with 2 bodies brought from the Indies by Sir Thomas Grantham'; and 'a German woman born without arms and hands and does extraordinary things. She doth marvelous things with her feet.'" For the author of *Pseudodoxia Epidemica*, the market also offered opportunities to view unusual beasts from all over the world, as well as a wide range of shows from puppet plays and acrobatics to the hawking of mountebanks. Socially, the market was a contradiction: if the second half of the century bore witness to a certain gentrification of the market area with a promenade and the selection of elite goods, it was also the site of the riot and explosion in the market in 1648, in response to which city officials spent much of the 1650s attempting to preserve a good measure of moderation and stability.[52] When trouble happened, as it did with the trial of Royalist conspirators in 1650, the impact was often felt in the marketplace, where the plotters were hanged.[53] One major threat came early, for a Royalist plot was discovered in October 1650, after which the trial and execution of conspirators unfolded in January 1651.

St Peter Mancroft's role in the tensions of Interregnum Norwich came into prominence when Cromwell sent one of his more aggressive Major Generals, Hezekiah Haynes, to Norwich in 1655 with the agenda of curtailing moderate-conservative gains.[54] Haynes was especially displeased with the role played by a preacher called John Boatman, who was reputed to be whipping up support for the eventual victor Hobart. John Boatman, minister at St Peter Mancroft, had been embroiled in local controversy from 1653, in which year he had emerged as a strident and provocative critic of Presbyterian positions on sacraments, church authority, and Christian community.[55] Indeed, printed access to Boatman's views derives from the polemical works of his opponents, especially the Norwich preacher John Collinges, who in *Provacator Provocatus* (1654) indicted Boatman for his arrogance, failure to attain even an undergraduate degree, and his lack of the proper authority to preach. Yet, for Collinges, this preacher at the greatest parish church in Norwich was no sectary; far from it, he was considered "a great enemy to Sectaries" and even rumored to have a penchant for episcopacy as well as disaffection for Presbyterianism (b3v).

The controversy between Boatman and Collinges placed Browne's old depiction of the Church of England as comprehensive or inclusive in a volatile and immediate context. According to Collinges's reconstruction of a sermon from the notes of others in attendance at St Peter's, Boatman argued for a "promiscuous" Lord's Supper; in other words, Boatman encouraged all persons—that is, all Christians, no matter how sinful—to be communicants in the sacrament. What is more, he reproached those strict Presbyterians, including ministers and elders of a congregation, for their claim to possess the authority to suspend egregious sinners from the service.

[52] Priestley, *Great Market*, 16–17.
[53] Ketton-Cremer, *Forty Norfolk Essays* (Norwich: Jarrold, 1961), 26–7.
[54] Evans, *Seventeenth-Century Norwich*, 213–14.
[55] Evans, *Seventeenth-Century Norwich*, 217; Blomefield, *Essay Towards a Topographical History*, for a list of ministers.

Whereas Boatman argued that a minister could not possibly know which of his parishioners has such sin in his heart, Collinges accused Boatman of refusing to consult his elders for information about the congregation.[56]

In the 1650s, then, the Browne family attended a parish church in which what could have been a peaceful haven in difficult times was continuing to experience discord. During this decade, the church raised money for bell ringing in honor of Oliver Cromwell in 1658, but also for the cakes to be served at the traditional perambulation of the parish boundaries in 1659.[57] While Browne may have connected the controversy over Boatman with the brouhaha in 1620s Oxford over that other brave performer in the pulpit, Thomas Lushington, the only record of his involvement in the Interregnum affair shows his contribution to Boatman's expenses during the latter's suspension in 1656.[58] But Dorothy Browne left behind far more, some seventy pages of notes that she took from the sermons that she heard during the 1650s. As Rebecca Bullard has shown, these notes not only overturn the standard image of Dorothy as simply amiable and virtually illiterate, but also help to account for why hers was heralded in her epitaph as "a bright Cœlestiall Mind."[59] At the simplest level, the notes show how much, like her husband, she prized the sermon as a rhetorical form: she clearly took every opportunity to hear a variety of preachers, only some of whom have been identified, in what may have been a variety of settings—St Peter Mancroft for certain, but perhaps too other churches and possibly even clandestine services in a home. And she is adept at capturing the preachers' distinctive voices, metaphors, arguments, and styles. But the notes show far more than just a literary preference, for Dorothy's responses are often intensely spiritual, insisting as they do on rigorous self-examination, as well as scholarly, since they reflect her mastery of key theological concepts such as the hypostatical union, of Biblical cross-references, as well her readings in authors such as Jeremy Taylor. Dorothy is especially full in her transcription of notes from Boatman's preaching, including his lament that English religion has been diminished by those pretenders who claim to restore its purity.

As a leading physician in the parish of St Peter Mancroft but also more broadly in East Anglia, Browne was called on to help families across the spectrum of opinions in their hours of greatest need. He spent the 1650s caring for the health of families throughout the county, but also helping them cope with illness and death, both in person and by letter. Often sending his prayerful good wishes as well as his medical advice, Browne was a favorite of the Knyvett family of Ashwellthorpe to the southwest of Norwich. Not only did he coach Thomas Knyvett through the administration of clysters, juleps, and syrups—noting their effects but also the means to make them more "convenient" or palatable—but he was frequently

56 John Colllinges, *Provocator Provocatus* (1654), b2v.

57 NRO MC 2577/2/6 984x6, no foliation.

58 NRO PD 26/725, 28r.

59 Rebecca Bullard, "'A bright Cœlestiall Mind': A New Set of Writings by Lady Dorothy Browne (1621–1685)," *Huntington Library Quarterly* 71 (2010), 99–110. Bullard identified the hand of these notes in what is now known as Elizabeth Lyttleton's commonplace book. I am indebted throughout to Professor Bullard for my understanding of these notes.

enlisted to help the family's estate agents and neighbors, for instance, a Mrs. Muriel afflicted with ague or a Matthew Trott whose daughter's death Browne appears to have attended, and Stephen Southall, a business manager, whom Dr Browne set "in a little course of physic."[60]

In 1654, Browne addressed a letter to John Hobart as "your faythfull servant & unworthy Kinsman" in which he professed to have been "at your howse this afternoone to have kissed your hand, & testified my good wishes unto you, wch being in noe waye able to act in proportion to my desires, I am in noe small measure left unto the mercy of your construction." The rest of the letter is given over to medical prescriptions and advice, including pills and syrups for Hobart to have concocted "at any Apothecaries."[61] Without reference to the complications and anxieties of local politics and religion, Browne focuses on his duty to recover Hobart's health or at least to relieve his suffering, remarking of the pills that "you may take them upon occasion when your body is costive, when you find your self stopped, hartburned, hott or find any predominance of choler or salt flegme in your stomack." From the western side of Norfolk, Browne received three pounds from Dame Catherine Calthorpe in 1653, and three times a pound from Lady Alice L'Estrange for his advice on, among other ailments, her husband Sir Hamon's "Numbe Palsye."[62] In 1653–54, he was Framlingham Gawdy's attending physician in the last years of the patient's life; in the early 1650s, he served in the same capacity for father Thomas and son John Windham of Felbrigg Hall, for which, on one occasion, he was paid thirty shillings.[63] With such patients, Browne often shared friendship and a rich array of intellectual preoccupations, a significant matter at a time when he would lose close friends in Arthur Dee (died in 1651) and Joseph Hall (died in 1656). For instance, Browne was not only a consulting physician for William Paston at Oxnead but also his fellow antiquarian, invoking Paston's collection of urns in *Hydriotaphia*.[64] The steady stream of visitors to Oxnead were apt to praise Paston's wide learning, ranging from medicine and math to husbandry and horsemanship, as well as his taste in painting, sculpture, and other arts and crafts. His house also conveyed his "diligent search into the greater curiosities of Nature"; like Browne's own, it was a "*Musaeum* abounding with an infinite variety of the most Choice and admired Rarities."[65]

Browne's medical expertise was regularly sought by consulting physicians via letters in the 1650s: in 1654, by Baldwin Hamey, for instance, and in 1660 by

[60] NRO C3/2/3/5/13, autograph letter from Browne to Thomas Knyvett; Princeton University Taylor Collection RTC01, autograph letter from Browne to Knyvett; NRO Rye 72/284, letter of May 12, 1653 from Trott to Thomas Knyvett; and letter from Stephen Southall to Knyvett from 1656.

[61] Keynes, 4.382–3.

[62] NRO LEST P/12, domestic account books for Dame Catherine Calthorpe, no foliation; LEST P/10, account book for Lady Alice L'Estrange, 80, 111, 141.

[63] Percy Millican, "The Gawdys of Norfolk and Suffolk," *Norfolk and Norwich Archaeological Society* 26, part 2 (1938), 335–90, see 367–8; see *Hist. MSS. Comm. Rep (Gawdy Letters)*, 184. Ketton-Cremer, *Forty Norfolk Essays*, 32.

[64] R. W. Ketton-Cremer, *Norfolk Assembly* (London: Faber and Faber, 1957), 36.

[65] Ketton-Cremer, *Norfolk Assembly*, 37–8. Browne's letter to William Dugdale, Clark Library, B884L, November 10, 1658, also illustrates the ways in which a medical trip (to King's Lynn) could double as an opportunity for intellectual or scholarly exchange.

R. Wolverton.[66] His letters to consulting physicians as well as patients are filled with candor and warmth as well as medical advice. In one undated letter, having testified to the psychological impact of illness on the family, as well as to the nature of the disease, Browne devotes the bulk of his letter to guiding his correspondent through alternative cures, basing his assessment in part on reading and in part on experience (Keynes, 4.389). In a shorter letter, Browne offers a carefully phrased evaluation of the effects of Peruvian quinine, then ends with good wishes "unto al our honoured friends" (4.389). A regular and learned medical correspondent was James Windet who, in addition to consulting Browne about the humoral excesses of a variety of patients, liked to punctuate his requests for assistance with quotations from classic works such as Sophocles's *Ajax*.[67] In one letter written from Great Yarmouth in 1652, Windet corroborated Browne's concern for the mental welfare or attitude of the patient. Practicing medicine in Great Yarmouth before he received his doctorate in medicine, Windet reflected Browne's own view of care—that physicians were treating their patients as whole human beings, not simply as bodies with excessive or impeded humors.

In the 1650s, then, Browne was faced with a mesh of commitments and circumstances—vocational, familial, political, religious, and cultural—through which it was hard to see so clearly as the polemics of a controversialist such as Collinges might insist. Yet the ability to operate effectively and sympathetically within this dense, complex network was essential to Browne's livelihood and sense of Christian duty. The convergence between scholarship, vocation, and friendship is most clearly and extensively expressed in a work that in its posthumous, 1690 first edition came to be titled *A Letter to a Friend*. As Mary Ann Lund has remarked, this was the work in which Browne offered his "fullest picture of the Christian physician in action."[68] This picture, moreover, captured just how complex and demanding the performance of this vocation in context tended to be. *A Letter to a Friend* epitomizes how, for Browne, the truly authoritative physician must move beyond the diagnosis of an obvious consumption and its fatal consequences to a heroic wrestling match with the endlessly varied circumstances in which disease was experienced, interpreted, and applied to future lives. Browne's essential point in *Letter to A Friend* is that even with the most commonplace of diseases and the most certain of prognoses, the true physician faces a swarm of interpretive problems in the service of a wide range of religious, moral, as well as medical roles in a closely knit and intensely felt social context.[69]

The work shares essential qualities with Browne's other major writings. With regard to genre, Browne thought in epistolary terms from the earliest conception of the *Religio* through the various later studies gathered as *Miscellany Tracts*. We have seen that letter-writing served a crucial purpose in his role as public intellectual,

[66] Hamey's letter is BL MS Sloane 1911–13, f. 94. Wolverton's is BL MS Sloane 4062, f. 147.

[67] Windet's letters to Browne are found in BL MS Sloane 4077, ff. 114 and 116; and Bodl. MS Rawlinson D.391, ff. 9–10, and 109.

[68] Lund, "The Christian Physician," in Todd and Murphy, eds., "*A man very well studyed*," 240.

[69] See Barbour, "Sir Thomas Browne's *A Letter to a Friend* and the Semiotics of Disease," 407–19.

much as it would play a vital part in his domestic life as a father. The value of friendship straddled the line between public and domestic; and its centrality in the familiar epistle was arguably made more pertinent because the probable subject of *Letter to a Friend*, Browne's patient Robert Loveday, had published a collection of letters to both family and friends. Yet in *Letter*, the epistle was grafted onto other genres, including medical case reports ranging from the medieval *consilium* to the seventeenth-century "observation," but extending to the moral essay; and it was this essayistic tendency that lent *Letter to a Friend* its key connection to Browne's other works, for instance the *Pseudodoxia*. As N. J. Endicott has put it, the *Letter* proves Browne to be an "inveterate revisionist," one for whom writing was often provisional, always imperfect, and subject to refinement at the levels of word choice, syntax, organization, argumentation, and content.[70]

The text as we have it exists in three forms: a few pieces or paragraphs to be found in manuscript and in Elizabeth Lyttleton's commonplace book;[71] folios 8–25 in MS Sloane 1862; and the 1690 edition overseen by Edward Browne. Although Huntley thought that the elaborateness of 1690 represented an earlier stage from which a more scientifically minded Browne started paring, Endicott argues more cogently that Sloane 1862 "gives us what Browne regarded, probably between 1670 and 1673, as a finished version," but one which he continued to revise, reorganize, and amplify until he had what would prove the 1690 version.[72] Browne's note in Sloane 1862—"this Letter may bee added to the Letters in the folio with red leaues"—suggests that he was organizing his miscellaneous works for publication; 1690's inclusion of explanatory glosses or citations indicates that Browne persisted in getting his epistle ready for a wider audience, even as he continued to expand and revise it. Indeed, the moral "mementoes" elaborated in the latter part of the work became so extensive that, in all likelihood, Browne split them away from *Letter* to include them in the moral observations compiled as *Christian Morals*. As with *Religio* and *Pseudodoxia*, the revision of the earlier version also entailed the excision of passages, in this case three principal ones.[73]

Although Endicott contested the point, Huntley argued compellingly that *Letter* began its life around 1656 as a letter to Sir John Pettus regarding the death of Pettus's close friend, the translator and epistolary author Robert Loveday.[74] Most obviously, Sir John has an important presence in Loveday's letters—not only is he mentioned on several occasions but it is his letter to Anthony Loveday that frames

[70] N. J. Endicott, "Sir Thomas Browne's *Letter to a Friend*," *University of Toronto Quarterly* 36 (1966–7), 68–86; see 79.

[71] Including Sloane 1869, 1885, 1879, and Rawlinson D.109; for the commonplace book, see Geoffrey Keynes, ed., *The Commonplace Book of Elizabeth Lyttelton, Daughter of Sir Thomas Browne* (Cambridge: Cambridge University Press, 1919).

[72] Endicott, "Sir Thomas Browne's *Letter to a Friend*."

[73] For *Letter* in both forms, I use L. C. Martin, *Sir Thomas Browne: "Religio Medici" and Other Works* (Oxford: Clarendon Press, 1964). For these quotations, see 252, 184–5.

[74] On Loveday, the *ODNB* article is by Ross Kennedy, who avers that Huntley's case "has been plausibly but contentiously" made. Huntley made his case most importantly in "The Occasion and Date of Sir Thomas Browne's *A Letter to a Friend*," *Modern Philology* 48 (1950–1), 157–71; reworked in his *Essays in Persuasion: On Seventeenth Century English Literature* (Chicago: University of

the volume—and the Browne family certainly interacted with the Pettus family among their many Norfolk connections. As Huntley noted, Browne speaks about the Pettus family in a 1658 letter to Dugdale, and his reference to Sir John Pettus in a 1681 letter is germane to Loveday's friend.[75] While it cannot be conclusively proven, it is likely that Loveday's exceptionally Latinate letter, addressed only to "Sir," was written to Browne, since it features words ("ventilate") and topics (such as "Plato's year") of relevance to the famous author.[76] Most importantly, Loveday's letters make it clear that sometime before his death, probably in 1656, he consulted a Dr B. in Norwich about the tuberculosis that would kill him. Although Huntley's case worked in part from the characteristics of the patient given in *Letter*—his reputation as "no minor Wit" or "poet"; his facility with French and Italian; his youth and his virtues, for instance—the strongest evidence came from Loveday's *Letters Domestick and Forrein, to Several Persons, Occasionally distributed in Subjects Philosophicall, Historicall & Morall*, first published in 1659.

In those letters, Loveday suffers from a lingering "malady" which by the end of the volume he has begun to associate, albeit anxiously, with consumption. Over the course of the volume, he reports (mainly to his brother Anthony) that early on he has consulted a certain Dr B. whom he knows well and who, as Huntley argues, is *not* the famous Dr Browne.[77] For all the amazing success of this Nottingham physician, however, Loveday's malady is not cured. When his brother Anthony moves to Norwich, Loveday seizes the opportunity to consult by his brother's proxy a Dr B. in that city. At first, the patient simply expresses his desire to know this Norwich Dr B.'s opinion, "from whose advice I fancy most hope of all," and concedes that he would be willing to pay a fee for his cure (Loveday, *Letters Domestick and Forrein*, 106). When next he mentions the Norwich physician, Loveday finds himself under the care of yet another medical practitioner, a confident

Chicago Press, 1981), 114–25. Endicott's answer in *TLS*, September 15, 1966, p. 868, is not convincing, based as it is on its anxiety about the possibility that Browne's imagination dried up after the 1650s, as well as on dubious readings of the "no minor wit" passage and on a mistaken transcription of a church record, one pointed out by the balanced review published in *TLS*, October 20, 1966, 966, by Karl Josef Höltgen, who is still open to Huntley's argument but not yet wholly convinced by it. Endicott's *TLS* piece makes the useful point that the initials "A. F.", printed in one of the notes in 1690, are actually "A. J." in manuscripts, leading to their association with Sir Arthur Jenny and with the date May 26, 1668. For recent doubts about the argument, see Lund, "The Christian Physician," 240.

[75] Huntley, "Occasion and Date," 169. Another piece of evidence for Pettus is that Browne's strange allusion to George Sandys has a pertinence since Sir John's daughter married into the Sandys family. But it is this part of Huntley's argument, the notion that Pettus was the "friend," that some scholars have contested while accepting Loveday as the patient. See R. F. Hall, *Studies in Sir Thomas Browne's Letter to a Friend*, MLitt dissertation, Oxford, 1972, cited by Robin Robbins in his *ODNB* article on Browne. The Sandys allusion was first identified by William Aldis Wright in *Notes and Queries*, 7th series, 4 (1887), 386. Huntley also argues that Pettus's death in 1690 accounts for the date of the first edition of *Letter*: Edward Browne waited until the addressee was no longer alive, perhaps in keeping with a Hippocratic commitment to privacy.

[76] Robert Loveday, *Letters Domestick and Forrein, to Several Persons, Occasionally distributed in Subjects Philosophicall, Historicall & Morall*, first published in 1659, 271–3.

[77] It is probably the "Ma. Brown, Doc. Med." who wrote the poem on Polyander discussed in chapter 6 in this volume, and who published a commendatory poem in the third part of Loveday's *Hymens Præludia* (1655).

"Mr. D., whose Physick I still daily take, (though yet with little apparent success)," yet he chafes to "have a Recipe from Dr. B of some soeveraign lotium," lamenting the fact that his "narrow condition . . . will not suffer me to meet you at Norwich" (186). A few letters later, Loveday has reason to hope that, albeit at a distance, Doctor B. of Norwich has ventured a theory of the disease that bodes well for the patient. Loveday adds his "strong fancy that I shall reap much benefit by those lotions he speaks of, and therefore when you go next to Norwich let me intreat you to take a note of the ingredients from his dictates, for I conceive no time of the year unseasonable to take that kind of Physick." Obviously Dr B. has not yet seen this patient firsthand; even so, Loveday tells his brother that, even though another physician is treating him, he will not "straggle the breadth of a hair from what Doctor B. prescribes" (192–3). Just a little bit later, Loveday is still "resolv'd to consult Dr. B" in Norwich, even as his long experience with this malady, and the suspicion that it may be consumption, have begun to rob him of all hope for longer life in this world (206). Indeed toward the end of the volume, as he prepares himself "to struggle hardest with my malady," he has finally consulted a "rational Physitian in these parts" who has "almost forbidden" him "to hope a perfect Cure" (230). In this letter, Loveday does not say whether he is at home in Suffolk, nor does he identify who this physician is. But at long last he has arrived at the point with which *Letter to a Friend* begins: in observing firsthand the patient in question, Browne knows immediately that consumption will soon kill him, and that the mild experience of the disease has entrenched false hope in the patient and his family. Loveday has also begun to feel the startling emaciation about which Browne speaks, noting to Anthony that "this Cough I find has lately fed upon my flesh, & carried away enough from the poor store I had to make me doubt [i.e. fear] a Consumption" (267).

Comprising only nineteen paragraphs, the manuscript version of *Letter* instantly announces the patient's death with a voice at once candidly personal and learnedly meditative. "I am sorry you understand so litle concerning that worthy gentleman your deare friend," he begins, "that I must also performe that vnwelcome office to tell you Ad portam rigidos calces extendit, hee is dead & buried & by this time no punie in the famous nations of the dead" (Martin, 249). The Latin verse, from Persius's first satire, serves as the transition from the misprision and pain involved in Browne's everyday life to the more mythic, universal sense of death with which the address concludes, a generalizing tendency that Browne stresses in his eventual revisions of the passage.[78] If death allows for hierarchy—the patient is "no punie" among the famous dead in the same way that Loveday was "no minor wit" among the living—its rapid and manifold destruction produces anonymity and obliquity as well. Rejecting the viability of the mystical sorts of intimacy to which he himself laid claim in *Religio*, Browne helps his friend come to terms with the vicissitudes of life, and advises him to "rest content in the vsuall way of knowledge by information." Yet both the recipient of the letter and his immediate community are also

[78] See Claire Preston's essay on *Letter* in Barbour and Preston, eds., *Sir Thomas Browne: The World Proposed*, 220.

confronted with the fact that they have been as naïve as the patient in hoping for recovery. While the physician saw immediately in the face of his patient that the end was near, the healthy friends and family manifested the "strange" tendency to share in the false hope of the patient. Although Browne removes the focus from their error by introducing an analogy to the signs of apocalypse—hard to predict in advance but obvious once they arrive—he presses home the grim distance between what the friends understood and what he did when he notes that in "such languishing emaciations," it is "as dangerous to bee condemned by a physitian as a judge" (Martin, 250). Browne once again introduces classical allusions (to Plautus and Hippocrates), but his main comfort derives not from invoking a larger context but from explaining the good news about "the common fallacy of consumptiue persons"—that they "feele not them selues to dye."

After a paragraph on the elusive history of the disease and its cure—a discussion ranging from the Bible to Paracelsus and the Stoics—Browne yokes his letter back to the painful immediate occasion: "At my first visit of him I was bold to tell his freinds who had not lett fall all hope of his recouery that in my sad opinion hee was not like to behold a grassehopper agayne much lesse to tast another figge" (Martin, 250–1). For the natural historian and author of *Pseudodoxia*, premature death erases ongoing opportunities for both instructive and pleasurable experiences in nature, even as the seasonal images of the grasshopper and the fig summon up the transience of those plants and animals that we would enjoy in nature. Indeed, Browne has already mentioned "that mortall time of the yeare when the figge tree putts forth his leaf like vnto a choughs clawe X" (250), the concluding quincunx of which offers none of the eternal vitality of *The Garden of Cyrus*.

Sad as these losses may be, however, Browne's report on the death becomes graphic and macabre when next he turns to, and lingers on, the emaciation of the consumptive. Although the loss of weight tends to reveal family resemblances (to a grandmother in the manuscript, to an uncle in 1690) that an observer would not see in the healthy man, the skeletal body of the patient has grimmer associations: to the "starved characters" in Dante's portrait of the gluttons in purgatory, a reference that Browne not only gives but annotates in *Hydriotaphia*.[79] Before the end, Browne has moved in and out of various circumstances surrounding the death in keeping with the Hippocratic conventions for reporting a case, but he always preserves a distance from and irony about those conventions. When Browne questions whether astral positions might have affected the patient's end, he recalls how "an old Italian long ago would persuade mee that the greatest part of men dyed" as the "moone was descending from the meridian," and in doing so makes the sources of his medical knowledge both personal and uncertain. In noting the patient's history—that he had suffered from rickets as a child—Browne emphasizes how little is known about relatively new diseases such as rickets and smallpox, this in a paragraph with which he continued to tinker into the 1670s (Martin, 252).

[79] Given in Martin, *"Religio Medici" and Other Works*, 111.

In the final five paragraphs of the manuscript version of *Letter*, Browne returns on occasion to criticizing those friends and families who form beliefs about the patient. He even generalizes their failings in mocking "the heirs & concerned relations" who "gratulate themselves in the sober departure of their friends and though they behold such couetous & mad passages are content to think they dye in good vnderstanding & in their sober senses" (Martin, 254). At the same point, however, Browne begins to allow that there is comfort to be had in human imperfection, a concession that coincides with his turn to the moral dimension of his meditations. His first concession to fallacy concerns the patient himself, whose expression of faith in charitable works was at long last a Christian argument for the validity of intentions: he "was bigge with desires to publick & lasting charities. & surely where good wishes and charitable intentions exceed abilities, Theoricall beneficency may bee more then a dreame." Browne's praise for good intentions moves in the direction of the gnomic wisdom that will fill the end of the 1690 *Letter* and *Christian Morals* as well: "They build not castles in the ayre who would build churches upon earth & though they leaue no such structures heere may lay good foundations in heauen" (Martin, 254–5). Having built this apology for wishes into his claim that the young, noble patient avoided the avarice and meanness of so many who cling to their worldly possessions on the verge of eternity, Browne comes at the end of his letter to the ways in which human flaws and delusions do not prevent happiness and can even enable it. Indeed, at one point Browne makes a case that he also formulates in the final chapter of *Pseudodoxia*—that when it comes to the difficulty of attaining happiness in this world, sometimes delusion goes a long way (Martin, 255). Like the ideal reader of the 1643 *Religio*, but also like consumption itself, happiness by means of error depends on the softness that comes with the misprisions of our lives. What matters for happiness is our sense of belonging to the very community that leads us into error and is always in error about us. The critical rigor of *Pseudodoxia* cannot produce this happiness, not just because it seeks the truth about a world that cannot finally please us, but also because its method serves "strictly to separate" us "from reputed and customarie felicities and to confine [us] vnto the rigour of realities" so that "the consolation of our beings" is narrowed to fit "comfortlesse circumscriptions." While the physician "cannot butt smile" at human error, he might not feel compelled to articulate it to the grief-stricken, raising the possibility that this letter to a friend was never intended for the friend at all. In this regard, Huntley may well be right: that the first edition was published only after the death of Sir John Pettus in 1690.

In the 1650s, and in the context of *Hydriotaphia* and *The Garden of Cyrus*, this apology for human delusion chimes with those works' explorations of our struggles to construct artificial happiness in a world that so often disappoints us. The loss of a major source of artificial happiness—the ceremonies and customs of the Church of England in affiliation with the festivals of "Merry Old England"—adds both point and complexity to Browne's stance, since his critical irony distances him from the very delusions that he also legitimizes. Yet Browne's manuscript letter does not end with these concessions to delusion. In the final paragraph, Browne begins with familiar paradoxes—it is better to be wise and good than old, blind, and vicious; if we reckon only those days that are acceptable to God, "the sonne in this sence may bee elder then the father" (Martin, 256). Then, suddenly, he reasserts a faith in the ability of moral instruction to separate us from our erroneous selves. Not only are we reminded of the desirability of outliving our own "old man," the sinful Adam in us, but Browne raises the moral standard of the work considerably higher than it has been placed. The patient's virtues were not the niggardly ones of "[c]autelous chastitie & cunning sobrietie"; far from it, they were like perfect jewels, "paragon without hayre Ice spot or blemish." It is this paean to perfection that motivates the "good wishes" of moral instruction that will outgrow its original context. As he instructs his reader to "[t]read softly and circumspectly in this... funambulatory tract and... narrowe path of goodnesse," Browne combines the softness of delusion with the rigorous, if flexibly casuistic, demands of moral living. In the manuscript's several signs of revision, however, he practices the virtue of striving for improvement, and then he unleashes his most challenging command: virtues must be pursued for the right reason (service to God) and not for the many false motives with which human beings usually agree to be virtuous (256). As a moralist as well as a physician, Browne knows that he must approach his patient with just the right balance of softness and rigor, of comfort or amelioration and strictures on behalf of a lasting health. What this means is that as Browne reinforces the value of community for human happiness, he also strengthens his conviction that the purpose of a godly life requires individuals to distance themselves from the idols of the community but also, and always, to labor after a transformation of the self.

3. REVISIONS AND RESPONSES

In addition to helping others with their researches, Browne used his correspondence to gather information for his revisions of *Pseudodoxia* and to assist with his ongoing study of antiquities and natural phenomena—as was the case in his 1652 letter to Arthur Bacon regarding his dissection of a whale washed up on a county coast.[80] In the 1650s, Browne's famous works, *Religio Medici* and *Pseudodoxia Epidemica*, were living, thriving entities. In the case of *Religio*, the vitality derived from elaborate reader responses and imitations. With *Pseudodoxia*, the author himself nourished its growth and development.

In a 1652 Strasbourg edition, the Merryweather translation of *Religio* was graced with its own learned commentary from a scholar identifying himself by the initials L. N. M. E. M., that is, Levin Nicolas von Moltke of Mecklenburg-Schwerin. In his preface the annotator testified to the book's avid reception by distinguished men throughout Europe. Having worked for several years at the imperial court, Moltke discovered not only that *Religio* was fervently read but also that its author was commended as a model of sanctity: in triumph over doubts, support for harmony and charity against blind zeal, exposure of the folly of atheism, and

[80] Keynes, 4.381.

testimony to the legitimacy of investigations into the nature of things. This was not to say that Browne is perfect: sometimes he proposed doubts without resolving them, or interjected scruples without removing them. It is on such occasions that Moltke especially saw fit to annotate, confirming his views with evidence from scripture, the church fathers, and other good authors. Moltke's preface also offers a view of Browne's religion as following the tenets of the Church of England as these were established under Elizabeth. In certain matters such as prayer for the dead and pilgrimages, it is true, Browne appears to deviate from the strict path of his church. But Moltke emphasizes that in the prior days of the Church of England—that is, before the horrific civil war that has killed a king and spawned the sectaries—church authorities were careful to ensure that the business of religion was carried out without anger or peevishness. In any case, Browne never promotes his deviations as dogma; such modesty has a way of expiating error. Doubtless the work would have been better had Browne written it in Latin and retained access to a good library.

Early in the annotations, Moltke betrays his Lutheran bias in his argument that Browne, with Luther, stood in a moderate position between Romanists and Anabaptists. The annotations are careful to situate Browne's rejection of iconoclasm in the context of the English civil war, before which (it is argued) reforms were instituted in a moderate fashion. The chief point in Moltke's characterization of Browne's religion in its context is that the *Religio* shows the vanity of angry reform; along the way, Lutherans are praised as the epitomes of peaceful, moderate reform, following the apostolic way of correcting error with mildness. Indeed, Moltke clearly believes that Browne's work offers a commentary not just on the English civil wars but also on the wars of religion in early modern Europe.

Moltke demonstrates both the cultural immediacy and scholarly seriousness with which the *Religio* was interpreted in Europe; indeed, this seriousness was also reflected in critiques of Moltke, including Guy Patin's dismissal in 1657 of the German annotator's delusions of learning.[81] Also critical of Moltke was a rival annotator Thomas Keck, whose English notes were first published with the *Religio* in 1656. Keck claims of Browne's *Religio* that no work "has had better Reception amongst the learned" since "it has been received and fostered by almost all," excepting Ross.[82] Keck is also eager to reclaim the superiority of the English version over the Latin; while he is pleased at the exceptionally warm reception of Browne's work, he complains that the annotator of the Latin has been misled by mistakes in the translation "whereby the Author is much injured." On the whole Keck's annotations reveal two contrasting tendencies on the part of Browne's readership. One is the attempt to concoct a holistic "Dr Browne," a desire that prompts the enlistment of *Pseudodoxia* as a comment on—and completion or resolution of—the *Religio*. On the other hand, Keck is eager to situate Browne in the context of other legacies and to make him less *sui generis*. The most obvious way in which Keck

[81] See Dennis G. Donovan et al., eds., *Sir Thomas Burton and Robert Burton: A Reference Guide* (Boston: G. K. Hall, 1981), 7.

[82] Thomas Keck, letter to the reader, in *Annotations upon Religio Medici*, in *Religio Medici* (1656).

would make Browne less himself is in his ongoing insistence that Browne has derived some of his best sentiments from Montaigne: on the changeability of the self (Keck, 195), grotesques in nature (214), the happiness of political states (217), and on God's ability to do all things without contradiction (245). "Who would not think the Author [Browne] had taken this from Mr. Montaign," Keck muses on the last of these points, coming so close to accusing Browne of plagiarism that Browne himself would later deny knowing very much at all about the French essayist. Yet Browne still allows in this denial that he and Montaigne might share a "coincidence, & concurrence of imagination" in the same way that "Homer should Hebraise & that many sentences in human Authors seeme to have their originall in Scripture" (Keynes, 3.290).

Toward the end of the 1640s and over the bulk of the 1650s, Browne was actively reshaping his *Pseudodoxia* at the same time that readers were busily annotating or otherwise responding to it. Browne's own treatment of his masterwork as a dynamic, changeable intervention in contemporary intellectual culture was also affected by developments in that culture. Efforts were made to produce a 1650 edition that would be typographically more attractive and more accessible to the reader.[83] A steady stream of errors—typos as well as matters of fact—was corrected; thus Seth was restored to his proper father Adam, having been described as Abraham's son in 1646.[84] Browne himself and an appreciative reader calling himself by the frequently used initials N. N. provided marginal annotations or markers.[85] Even with so basic a device, however, the apparatus of the 1650 edition encouraged an active readership. Readers were alerted both to Browne's precision and to the wide range of material that the encyclopedia comprised. What is more, readers of the first edition would notice that both the author's approach and the material approached were undergoing considerable alteration.

In both the 1650 and 1658 editions, Browne cultivated a simpler style in keeping with recent suspicions of rhetorical ornamentation, removing some of the Greek and Latin, pruning away excess or duplicative verbiage and ponderous diction, and reducing the Latinate complications of his syntax.[86] Whereas the first edition had pursued stylistic tendencies tried out in *Religio* for the purposes of philosophical maturity and sophistication, the second reflected Browne's growing sense that post-Baconian critiques of elaborate rhetoric might afford a greater intellectual and experimental precision. This is not to say that Browne's style suddenly reads like a lab report, or that in the works of the 1650s he bid farewell to *Religio*'s Latinisms; rather, Browne developed alternative stylistic practices that might compete—or decorously alternate—with one another.[87]

Equally pronounced was Browne's commitment to keeping the research for *Pseudodoxia* up-to-date. Throughout the second and third editions, Browne

[83] Cf. Wilkin, *Works*, 2.165.

[84] Robbins, ed., *Pseudodoxia Epidemica*, 1.66; see Westfall, *Sir Thomas Browne's Revisions*, 109, for a summary.

[85] The identity of N. N. is uncertain.

[86] Westfall, *Sir Thomas Browne's Revisions*, 121–53.

[87] For decorum, see Westfall, *Sir Thomas Browne's Revisions*, 153.

introduced recent scholarship either missed in the first edition or published from 1646 onwards and, in doing so, testified to the dynamic processes by which learning not only changed but potentially advanced. As he interwove or appended references to the latest work on a wide variety of problems or fields of study, Browne expanded, rewrote, rearranged, and deleted substantial portions of his treatments to keep pace with his revised understanding.

As early as the first chapter of Book 2, on crystal, Browne was adding whole paragraphs to his study of physical phenomena such as congealment.[88] Typically, his additions speak to two aspects of contemporary natural philosophy: theoretical or hypothetical explorations of basic chemical or physical constituents (with words such as "nitrous," "effluvium," "principle," "fixed elements," "volatile and fixed," "spirit," "fundamentall Atomes"); and clarion calls to experimentation both by the learned community at large and by Browne himself. In the 1650 edition Browne is especially keen to extend his explorations of the problems raised by magnetism, introducing research by Kircher, Van Helmont and Liceti, but also his own "iterated experiment" on whether a loadstone will "attract an Iron or Steel red hot."[89] Like Bacon in his natural histories, Browne also recommends future experiments, for instance when he notes that "whether the Magnet attracteth more then common Iron, may be tried in other bodies."[90] In the search for the properties of magnetism, far-flung navigators and merchants as well as the local blacksmith must play a part; but the judicious or rational experimenter will be required to work out the implications of the world's variety for natural philosophy—for "sublimation . . . unto their roots."

Browne's experiments with toadstools and hog dung are detailed as integral means in the search for those natural secrets briefly mentioned in the *Religio*: "The forms of things may lie deeper then we conceive them," Browne adds in a paragraph on the generative properties of manure and seeds, "seminall principles may not be dead in the divided atomes of plants; but wandring in the ocean of nature, when they hit upon proportionable materials, may unite, and return to their visible selves again."[91] In this meditation on the revivification of forms, Browne's language absorbs some of the atomic thought that was being so hotly debated, modified, and Christianized in the 1640s and 50s. Atoms may be alive, not dead as Lucretius and Epicurus claimed, and they might hold the key to nature's sense of mystery and decorum, but they also wander and seemingly "hit" their appropriate materials by chance. In other words, Browne's interventions in and responses to contemporary culture are not always completely controlled or stable; they can embody the tensions or uncertainties in that culture as well as pronounce on them and offer directives for moving beyond them.

These tensions sometimes arise as Browne seeks to follow Bacon's program of recalibrating how theology and natural philosophy pertain to one another. After

[88] For insertions on congealment, see Robbins, ed., *Pseudodoxia Epidemica*, 1.76–83.
[89] Robbins, ed., *Pseudodoxia Epidemica*, 1.96–102.
[90] Robbins, ed., *Pseudodoxia Epidemica*, 1.103–4.
[91] Robbins, ed., *Pseudodoxia Epidemica*, 1.286.

his discussion of Liceti's "excellent Tract" on "those who can live for a long duration without aliment," Browne's 1646 text concludes with a reference to exclusively natural as well as fraudulent instances of this phenomenon. In 1650, however, he ends the chapter with an affirmation of miracles, "for that may be miraculously effected in one, which is naturally causable in another."[92] Working in the opposite direction, 1650 omits a discussion of how the legendary antipathy between man and basilisk might have "expressed first the enmity of Christ and Sathan, and their mutuall destruction thereby."[93] More complexly, Browne deleted from his discussion of the loadstone an extensive concession to the new astronomy of Galileo according to which the earth moved. In 1646, the allowances to heliocentrism had been included in order to argue that it made little difference to theories of magnetism.[94] But in the annotations made by Dr Christopher Wren in his copy of the 1646 edition, the theological motivations for holding onto the old geocentricism are fervently asserted.[95]

In the 1650 edition, Browne's experiments and philosophy converge most forcefully when he speaks as a physician, when what "we have observed" in the "effects" of medicines interacts with what he has read and learned to count as reasonable.[96] In one instance, his call for further experiment even offers an urgent directive regarding public policy; as Browne reviews the evidence for the medicinal value of gold, he adds in 1650 the declaration that "Herein exact and criticall triall should be made by publicke enjoinments; whereby determination might be setled beyond debate: for since thereby, not only the bodies of men, but great Treasures might be preserved, it is not only an error of Physick, but folly of State, to doubt thereof any longer."[97] Over the course of the 1650 edition, however, Browne expands his treatments of a very wide range of phenomena, including the malleability of glass; ballistics; porcelain; carbuncle; Indian stone (with admiring reference to "that eminent Philosopher Licetus"[98]); thorn trees (with reference to one "in Parham Park in Suffolk"[99]); elephants; eyelids; and buoyancy (which entails the drowning of animals, but also confessions that Browne has not experimented with the floatability of "Cripples and mutilated persons").[100] He also expands his discussions of ancient dining decorum; the fancies of Cabala; the legend of St George (with a citation of Peter Heylyn's massive work); the portrait of angels and the cross; Egypt and the Nile (with assistance from Grotius, Greaves, and Alpinus); and he develops a whole chapter on gypsies. Not surprisingly his additions sometimes turn into miscellane-

[92] Robbins, ed., *Pseudodoxia Epidemica*, 1.251.
[93] Robbins, ed., *Pseudodoxia Epidemica*, 1.184n.
[94] Robbins, ed., *Pseudodoxia Epidemica*, 1.87n; and Westfall, *Sir Thomas Browne's Revisions*.
[95] See p. 343 below.
[96] Robbins, ed., *Pseudodoxia Epidemica*, 1.109.
[97] Robbins, ed., *Pseudodoxia Epidemica*, 1.127–8.
[98] Robbins, ed., *Pseudodoxia Epidemica*, 1.138.
[99] Robbins, ed., *Pseudodoxia Epidemica*, 1.150. This tree was still renowned in the twentieth century. In the *Suffolk Chronicle and Mercury*, August 5, 1927, reprinted in *Pocket Histories of Suffolk Parishes* (n.p.: Suffolk Chronicle and Mercury, 1914), 'Yeoman' described a "flowering thorne" that like the one in Glastonbury "not only buds at its usual time, but at Christmas also" (separately paginated, 4).
[100] Robbins, ed., *Pseudodoxia Epidemica*, 1.314.

ous chapters, absorbing material from 1646 while offering a potpourri of vulgar errors or superstitions. All in all, Browne's extensions are as likely to indicate the complexity or elusiveness of a subject as they are to suggest progress toward resolution.[101] In this spirit, perhaps the most noteworthy addition to the 1650 edition is the very last: a closing epigraph from Lactantius which, unlike Scaliger's directive at the opening (to study the things themselves), reminds those readers closing Browne's book that "the first step toward wisdom is an understanding of what is false."[102]

Some of Browne's most significant additions to 1650 anticipate his turn to natural history. For instance, both "good reason" and the "ocular testimony" of others are enlisted in a discussion of ostriches, an animal that Browne had glimpsed as a schoolboy on a trip to Greenwich and about which he would enthusiastically correspond with his son later in life. Clearly the ostrich raised for Browne one of the frustrations of the natural historian, that sometimes pictures, no matter how carefully drawn, would reinforce the limitations of personal experience.[103] Yet additions to 1650 also drove home how testimonials from around the world of nature enriched personal experience, for instance on the subject of "the teeth...of the Hippopotamus, or great animall which frequenteth the river Nilus."[104] Unquestionably, however, Browne's turn to natural history in the 1650s would involve his—and his household's—careful attention to and nitty-gritty handling of the blood and guts of creation. In one addition to 1650, he reports that he has been weighing the brains of sparrows.[105] More typically, he speaks to mysteries of generation—which comes first, the bird or the egg?—with the benefit of some experience with tadpoles and even maggots, whose "daily progresse" Browne has observed in the production of a fly.[106]

In the 1658 edition, Browne persisted in the types of small-scale revisions that he introduced into 1650. Spelling mistakes were caught; verbiage pruned; and word choice refined or clarified. Browne added and extended marginal annotations, some of which were more inclusive of experience, as was the case when the 1658 edition extended the reference to the thorn tree in Parham Park, Suffolk, to take in similar trees to be found "elsewhere."[107] While it is true that from 1658 onward, "the scope of the work was not materially enlarged,"[108] Browne nonetheless continued to add substance to his chapters. Having rewritten his efforts at defining the nature of crystal, Browne added a paragraph in which he considered a whole new horizon—beneath the earth.[109] In the year in which Browne was publishing his study of the historical worlds to be unearthed in urns, his *Pseudodoxia* was challenging readers to consider the complex quasi-life forms beneath their feet.

101 See for instance Robbins, ed., *Pseudodoxia Epidemica*, 1.125.
102 Robbins, ed., *Pseudodoxia Epidemica*, 1.609.
103 Robbins, ed., *Pseudodoxia Epidemica*, 1.255.
104 Robbins, ed., *Pseudodoxia Epidemica*, 1.259.
105 Robbins, ed., *Pseudodoxia Epidemica*, 1.296.
106 Robbins, ed., *Pseudodoxia Epidemica*, 1.379.
107 Robbins, ed., *Pseudodoxia Epidemica*, 1.150n.
108 Westfall, *Sir Thomas Browne's Revisions*, 1.160.
109 Robbins, ed., *Pseudodoxia Epidemica*, 1.83.

In 1658, Browne's turn to natural history comes in all sizes. The addition of an entire chapter on spermaceti whales is the product not just of intensive reading but also of correspondence with local naturalists such as Arthur Bacon who had helped Browne with the whale "cast on our coast of *Norfolk*."[110] At the other end of the animal world is the insect, fascinating to the providential Browne of *Religio* but now also a challenge to the natural historian. For in addition to the praise for the "wisdom of the Pismire" included in the 1646 edition, Browne notes in 1658 that "the prudence of this animal is by Knawing, peircing, or otherwise, to destroy the litle nebbe or principle of germination. Which notwithstanding is not easily discoverable; it being no ready business to meet with such grains in Anthills; and he must dig deep, that will seek them in Winter."[111] As he grew older, Browne was discovering that the arduous physicality of natural history might prove as challenging as the intellectual comprehension of the new conceptual worlds that it promised the determined observer.

In summary, Browne's work on his major contribution to the world of learning was ongoing, detailed, and extensive in the 1650s. His revisions of *Pseudodoxia* reflected longstanding fascinations (with anatomy, geography, biblical scholarship, and Egyptology, for instance) but also his active engagement with emerging physical theories such as the varieties of particulate physics; with newly flourishing fields of study such as optics, chemistry, and electricity; and with shifting stylistic criteria for the advancement of learning.[112] Despite the 1650 edition's intense interest in the physical and chemical basis for natural phenomena, it anticipates Browne's most significant development in the 1650s—into a full-fledged natural historian and a dedicated, careful observer of and experimenter with animals and plants. In this turn to natural history, Browne did not abandon his theological, moral, and theoretical "illations." Rather, he found that the patient, minute study of animals and plants offered a rich means of understanding divinity as well as the inmost mysteries of life itself. No small part of what made the stress on natural history an absorbing development for Browne, however, was the deepening awareness that human ways of thinking or speaking the sacred in relationship to creation were woefully inadequate.

Because the *Pseudodoxia* so fully documents Browne's turn during the Interregnum to what we would call biology and zoology, it has provided historians of science with a treasure trove for the argument that its author was what one scholar has called a "true scientist."[113] Because that turn intermingles in the same work with Browne's interests in iconography, human customs, ancient history, and scriptural scholarship, *Pseudodoxia* has also afforded scholars with an ample supply of evidence that Browne was either a false scientist or no scientist at all, a "humanist." The problem with this debate is that it tends to downplay four crucial factors: the ways in which Browne was perceived by his contemporaries; the interpenetration

110 Robbins, ed., *Pseudodoxia Epidemica*, 1.272.
111 Robbins, ed., *Pseudodoxia Epidemica*, 1.286.
112 See key summaries in Westfall, *Sir Thomas Browne's Revisions*, 155, 184–5.
113 Gordon Keith Chalmers, "Thomas Browne, True Scientist," *Osiris* 2 (1936), 28–79.

between humanism and advanced natural studies, especially with regard to the development of rigorous methods for assessing evidence; Browne's own capacity for change over the course of his career; and the complex, dynamic phenomena that natural studies were in the middle of the seventeenth century, even as followers of Bacon were attempting to clarify and stabilize what counted as true and legitimate research. Indeed Browne's own thinking on key subjects—for instance, the ancient notion of generation from putrefying matter, which he never wholly rejected but, under Harvey's sway, gradually reduced in importance—could be subtle, cautious, and nuanced in its development.[114]

Whether his science was "true," Browne engaged in this period with an astonishingly wide range of what were becoming scientific fields, especially biology (including the commonplace as well as the unusual, and featuring studies of generation and physiological function) but also chemistry, mineralogy, hydrostatics, and physics.[115] A range of specific claims have been made for Browne's savvy as an experimenter: on the color indicator to be found in "the characteristic blackening of iron solutions with an infusion of oak galls," on plant sensitivity in reaction to sunlight, and on chemical embryology, for instance.[116]

Whatever the various defenders of Browne's role in the "scientific revolution" might conclude about the "truth" of his science, they have often usefully reminded readers of Browne's high reputation as an advancer among his contemporaries. Indeed, with the 1658 edition of *Pseudodoxia*, "Dr Browne" became a commodity over which publishers were prepared to compete; and, in the event of such competition, publishers began to compile Browne's various works together so that readers might think about the commodity as a unified source of wisdom and authority.[117] Such competition over Browne was understandable. Even abroad, and despite his opposition to the Latinizing of *Religio Medici*, the great scholar Saumaise was eager

[114] See Westfall, *Sir Thomas Browne's Revisions*, 251–8.

[115] E. S. Merton, *Science and Imagination in Sir Thomas Browne* (New York: King's Crown Press, 1949); Gordon Keith Chalmers, "The Lodestone and the Understanding of Matter in Seventeenth-Century England," *Philosophy of Science* 4 (1937), 75–95; Gordon Keith Chalmers, "Thomas Browne, True Scientist," *Osiris* 2 (1936), 28–79. See also Chalmers, "Three Terms of Corpuscularian Philosophy," *Modern Philology* 33 (1935–36), 243–60; Chalmers, "Effluvia, The History of a Metaphor," *PMLA* 52 (1937), 1031–50; E. S. Merton, "Sir Thomas Browne's Embryological Theory," *Journal of the History of Medicine* 4 (1950), 416–21; Merton, "Microcosm, Epitome, and Seed: Some Seventeenth-Century Analogies," *History of Ideas News Letter* July (1957), 54–7; Merton, "Sir Thomas Browne on Astronomy," *History of Ideas News Letter* 4 (1958), 83–6; Merton, "Old and New Physiology in Sir Thomas Browne: Digestion and Some Other Functions," *Isis* 57 (1966), 249–59; Merton, "The Botany of Sir Thomas Browne," *Isis* 47 (1956), 161–71; Merton, "Sir Thomas Browne's Theories of Respiration and Combustion," *Osiris* 10 (1952), 206–23; Merton, "Sir Thomas Browne as Zoologist," *Osiris* 9 (1950), 413–34. Less keen about Browne's contributions to science are Jane M. Oppenheimer, "John Hunter, Sir Thomas Browne and the Experimental Method," *Bulletin of the History of Medicine* 21 (1947), 17–32; and Walter E. Houghton, Jr., "The English Virtuoso in the Seventeenth Century," *Journal of the History of Ideas* 3 (1942), 51–73, 190–219; see 197. See also Marie Boas Hall, "Thomas Browne Naturalist," in Patrides, ed., *Approaches to Sir Thomas Browne*, 178–87.

[116] Allen G. Debus, "Sir Thomas Browne and the Study of Colour Indicators," *Ambix* 10 (1962), 29–36, see 29; Charles Webster, "The Recognition of Plant Sensitivity by English Botanists in the Seventeenth Century," *Isis* 57 (1966), 5–23; Joseph Needham, *A History of Embryology* (Cambridge: Cambridge University Press, 1934), 110–12.

[117] Westfall, *Sir Thomas Browne's Revisions*, 112.

to find a copy of *Pseudodoxia* in 1648; perhaps he did not connect this work to the *Religio* whose Latin translation he had rejected for publication.[118] In 1651, the physician William Rant wrote to Hartlib that Browne's work was exceptionally helpful, not least because Browne was "very well studyed" and had "made frequent experiments in nature bestowing much time paines & cost to that end."[119] At the other end of the 1650s, in 1661, Robert Boyle praised Browne as a touchstone for the "Sober and Experimental" work of those "wary and considerate Naturalists" capable of "enriching the world with their Observations," declaring himself "unwilling that so faithful and candid a Naturalist should appear fit to be distrusted."[120] A 1657 work called *Nature's Cabinet Unlock'd* attempted to capture a readership for its study of metals, plants and "all Animate Bodies" by appropriating Browne's name and, as an epigraph, his statement in *Religio* that "All things are Artificial, for Nature is the Art of God." Protecting his label, as it were, Browne himself announced the fraud a year later in *Hydriotaphia*.[121]

Like *Religio*, *Pseudodoxia* attracted critiques in print, though the relative modesty with which these were offered to the public suggests Browne's ten-year ascent into high repute. In 1652, *Religio*'s harshest known critic, Alexander Ross, included *Pseudodoxia* in his attack on the neoteric disregard for antiquity that he also associated with Bacon's natural histories in *Sylva Sylvarum* and with Harvey's *De generatione*.[122] Like Ross, John Robinson included his critique of *Pseudodoxia* within a longer work, *Endoxa*, first published in Latin in 1656, then two years later in an English translation by Robinson himself.[123] What Robinson shows more than anything else, however, is that the gently skeptical, strikingly unusual, and brilliantly learned Dr Browne is a celebrity whose association is worth "scribbling" for.

While Ross and Robinson led the charge of those authors attempting to capitalize on Browne's celebrity, *Pseudodoxia* was also engaging Interregnum readers in private. In some cases the results were modest: for instance, one reader set down observations on several of Browne's animals subjects—serpents and scorpions among them—in a manuscript now among the L'Estrange family papers.[124] Richard Shorte sent Browne a set of observations mainly concerned with the etymology of mandrake but dipping into Browne's reference to the army of Xerxes. The frankness with which Browne's readers saw fit to express their criticism of his labors is a testimonial to the candor which they attributed to the author's invitation for

[118] See Keynes, *Bibliography*, 178: Saumaise wrote to Constantijn Huygens for assistance in locating the book, passing on a rumor that Browne resided in The Hague.

[119] Hartlib, *Hartlib Papers*, letter dated September 1, 1651; for Rant, see Browne's consultation letter to Bave discussed in chapter 8 of this volume.

[120] Boyle, *Certain Physiological Essays* (1661), 97–8.

[121] See Keynes, *Bibliography*, 134.

[122] Alexander Ross, *Arcana microcosmi, or, The hid secrets of man's body discovered in an anatomical duel between Aristotle and Galen concerning the parts thereof* (1652), 93.

[123] John Robinson, *Endoxa* (Latin 1656, English 1658).

[124] NRO LEST supp 25ii/1/25A–25L. The manuscript is not in Sir Hamon L'Estrange's hand. I am grateful to Clive Wilkins-Jones for his advice on this document.

assistance.[125] But readers also found considerable hope for the future in Browne's model of scholarship: in a commentary on Lucretius, John Evelyn invoked *Pseudodoxia Epidemica* as a premiere example of how Christian philosophers might rationally resist superstition without lapsing into Epicurean profanity.[126]

Some private responses to *Pseudodoxia* were more elaborate. Although he was reading the first edition, Dr Christopher Wren made his extensive annotations on *Pseudodoxia* over the course of the 1650s, when, as the ejected dean of Windsor, he was living with family members in Oxfordshire.[127] As was the case with his notations in *Religio Medici*,[128] Wren's annotations in the margins and on the flyleaves of *Pseudodoxia* pervade the entire book and are strikingly broad in their learning, personal in their appeals to experience, and candid in their assessments of Browne's achievement.[129] Wren was equally responsive to religious and natural elements in Browne's work.[130] Most poignantly, Wren's personal testimonies turn into memories of England before the civil wars. Despite Browne's own warning about mistaking natural causes for miracles, Wren evokes a time when governors of the church and state shared the floral wonders of England in which plants cooperated with the rites of the church calendar until the civil wars.[131] Perhaps most importantly, Wren appreciates the irenic, encouraging, civil spirit in which *Pseudodoxia* addresses its readers.[132] A far cry from Robinson, for whom *Pseudodoxia* epitomizes the liberty and progress made possible by the rejection of old English institutions, Wren believes that differing perspectives in the learned world can be harmonized in their loyalty to an England where kings and bishops protected and studied God's two books.

In another private commentary on *Pseudodoxia*, dated 1653, Browne's Norfolk neighbor Sir Hamon L'Estrange clarifies why Browne's natural history might matter in a world turned upside down by civil war and regicide.[133] The human relevance of natural history especially emerges when L'Estrange pauses to recreate the surprising wonders and joys of everyday life, as he does in remembering that,

> [A]bout 16 or 20 years since, upon a hot, bright, and cleared aye, (a little before noone,) hapning in the midst of March, as I leaned over my garden wall, and looking steadfastly into my mote . . . I espied sundry small creatures (of a dark or dusky coulour, longwise shaped, and of the forme of beetle or scarabee) to rise out of the mud from the bottom

[125] Shorte's letter is BL MS Sloane 4067, f. 150r–150v. Shorte appears to have lived in Bury St Edmunds, Suffolk, with degrees from Pembroke College, Cambridge in 1621–22 and 1625, and an MD in 1632 (d. 1668). See Venn and Venn, *Alumni Cantabrigiensis*, part 1 (Cambridge: Cambridge University Press, 1927), 68. He also appears to have received a copy of *Hydriotaphia* and *Garden of Cyrus* from Browne; see J. S. Finch, "A Newly Discovered *Urn Burial*," *The Library*, 4th series, 19 (1939), 351n.

[126] Evelyn's manuscript commentary on Lucretius is in the British Library, Evelyn Collection MS 33, 140v–141v.

[127] See Nicholas W. S. Cranfield on Dean Christopher Wren, in *ODNB*.

[128] See chapter 8 in this volume.

[129] Rosalie L. Colie, "Dean Wren's Marginalia and Early Science at Oxford," *The Bodleian Library Record* 6 (1957–1961), 541–51.

[130] Wilkin prints the majority of Wren's notes in his edition, *Works*, in volumes 2 and 3.

[131] Wilkin, *Works*, 2.371.

[132] Wilkin, *Works*, 2.243.

[133] BL MS Sloane 1839.

> of the mote to the topp of the water, and some of them to settle themselves speedily downe againe into the mud, others to rayse themselves above the water five or six inches, others a foote, others more, and some some yards, with a slanting or sloaping mount, and a like descent and falling downe hastened to the bottome.[134]

As he summons his son "to participate and bee a witnesse of this discovery," L'Estrange captures the full appeal of natural history for his intellect, senses, imagination, and emotions, and its place in the life of the family and neighborhood. Both in his exchange with Browne, and in his memory of that day at the moat with his son, L'Estrange reinforces the conviction that a turn to natural history can preserve cohesion in communities imperiled by the paranoia and partisanship of troubled times. That is, the local is not just good for natural history; natural history is also good for the local.

4. URNS AND GARDENS

Published together in 1658, Browne's *Hydriotaphia* and *Garden of Cyrus* shared more than just the covers of the ottavo in which they first appeared. As studies of cremation urns and plant life respectively, the pair shared a basis in early modern notions of *historia* that many early modern authors, especially physicians, had been conceiving for over a century. Browne was one in a long line of learned physicians who worked on antiquarianism and natural history alike, and faced the challenges of methodology and epistemology in these interactive fields. What is more, Browne's two works participated in the early modern rethinking of how history—whether human or natural—should comprise and promote a moral and spiritual dimension, which entailed the exploration of how human artifice was closely related to, but not to be elided with, the natural world.[135]

For Browne as for the line of learned physicians who had moved between antiquarianism and natural history, a chief goal in both cases was the "thorough description" that also characterized the medical case studies and observations published with increasing frequency in the early modern period.[136] As Brian W. Ogilvie has explained, the notion of experience that underlay the value placed on description was a richly layered one, including the historian's "immediate observation," recollections of previous observations, "and the collective experience of the community as expressed in its verbal and pictorial productions."[137] This community of scholars was held together by the affective bonds of friendship as well as citizenship

[134] Wilkin, *Works*, 2.174–5.

[135] For antiquarianism, natural history, and medicine, see Gianna Pomata and Nancy G. Siraisi, eds., *Historia: Empiricism and Erudition in Early Modern Europe* (Cambridge, MA: MIT Press, 2005), editorial intro., 1–2, 6–7. For natural history in England, see F. D. Hoeniger and J. F. M. Hoeniger, *The Growth of Natural History in Stuart England from Gerard to the Royal Society* (Charlottesville: University Press of Virginia, 1969).

[136] Pomata and Siraisi, eds., *Historia*, 2–3.

[137] Brian W. Ogilvie, *The Science of Describing: Natural History in Renaissance Europe* (Chicago: University of Chicago Press, 2006), 141.

in the republic of letters; and they shared a commitment to making careful use of ancient material without either rejecting or swallowing it wholesale. The network of learned friendship was a benefit in extending one's field of experience insofar as the friends shared specimens—for instance, plants and coins—with one another. Like Browne, they understood that the ancients, especially Aristotle, did not present a united front, for instance, on questions of method regarding the study of animals and plants.[138] Mediating personal with communal and ancient observation, the natural historian had to be ready to sojourn into fields and markets as well as into libraries.[139] Those who worked in both fields of study realized the value of cross-fertilization, not just with regard to the methods of accumulating, describing, and making sense of particulars but also insofar as antiquarian evidence could be useful in the natural historian's attempt to weigh contemporary observations against those proffered in the past.[140]

Like Browne, many of the physicians who had contributed to the study of "history" (both natural and antiquarian) had profited from their travels abroad. Travel was deemed important because it allowed a wider field of observation, of course, but travel to medical schools such as Padua also reinforced the methodological commitment to the precise, detailed observation and description of particular phenomena.[141] Yet the value of Browne's Dutch travels ironically reinforced the importance to the antiquarian and natural historian of an enriched description and understanding of the local, for Dutch art, as Svetlana Alpers has shown, concerned itself less with allegorical narratives than with the vivid depiction of a place at a transient moment in time.[142] Both the natural historian and the antiquarian were convinced, though, that their local subjects needed to be described over the course of time—for the natural historian, across the arc of the seasons, for the antiquarian, over the migratory course of various peoples and their customs. Natural historians developed special vehicles, including the garden, the herbarium, and menagerie for facilitating the study of their subjects over time; but they also understood that any such vehicle presented its own problems by removing phenomena from the natural setting in which they grew in association with other specimens. Indeed, one obvious problem in detaching natural history, however incompletely, from the study of the *materia medica* was that the former tended to isolate visual experience from the rest of the senses. For the seventeenth-century natural historian, however, Bacon lent great authority to such removals of specimens from their natural contexts in his insistence that natural history progress from its study of normative nature to the exploration of nature in error or under duress.[143]

[138] This point is made by Pomata and Siraisi in their introduction to *Historia,* 14–15.

[139] Ogilvie, *The Science of Describing,* x, 27–8, 83.

[140] See, for instance, Laurent Pinon, "Conrad Gessner and the Historical Depth of Renaissance Natural History," in Pomata and Siraisi, eds., *Historia,* 241–67.

[141] Peter N. Miller, "Description Terminable and Interminable: Looking at the Past, Nature, and Peoples in Peiresc's Archive," in Pomata and Siraisi, eds., *Historia,* 355.

[142] Svetlana Alpers, *The Art of Describing: Dutch Art in the Seventeenth Century* (Chicago: University of Chicago Press, 1983).

[143] Ogilvie, *The Science of Describing,* 150, 162–3, 165, 182.

For the seventeenth-century antiquarian and natural historian, description was not some dull and lazy substitute for the serious intellectual work of philosophy; the medieval subordination of history to philosophy had given way to the recognition that historical description and collection were challenging, pleasing, and valuable in their own right, in tandem with but also distinct from the need for ancient wisdom and *materia medica* on the part of the physicians who often carried out this work. Surfaces such as skin, a favorite topic with Browne, were observed in such a way as "to astound and expand human perceptions of and assumptions about the ordinary world."[144] Not only did early modern historians acknowledge and celebrate this cultural and intellectual shift; but, with the assistance of technologies of observation, they experienced it with a visceral pleasure.[145] Even so, a concern about the deficiency of language was crucial, since the intense vitality and profusion of new phenomena led in the seventeenth century to three related anxieties: that the human means for communicating natural variety were sorely limited; that previous attempts to convey experience had to be greeted with redoubled skepticism regarding vulgar errors; and that the human mind would need new methods of organizing, clarifying, and classifying the wondrous plentitude and sometimes playful strangeness of nature. Browne and his contemporaries were still indebted to modes of classification found in antiquity, in particular to Theophrastus's division of plants into trees, shrubs, undershrubs, and herbs, as well as to ancient rhetorical and poetic conceptions of description; but they were also busily recognizing the problems with old systems as the specimens and nomenclature proliferated wildly.[146]

While Browne's habits of keeping notebooks owed a great deal to his humanist upbringing with commonplace books, the natural historian and antiquarian insisted on note-taking and the collection of specimens because their sense of being overwhelmed by the diversification of experience called into question the reliability of memory itself in securing the precise yet fleeting facts of time, place, and specimens.[147] Browne was so keen to improve the range and truth value of his historical work that he called on the members of his family to draw specimens or to answer questions from specific sites abroad, and he assiduously collected antiquarian and natural specimens in the cabinet of curiosity into which he converted his house on the marketplace. As his experience of specimens grew more "finely textured," more precise, and more carefully contextualized in place and time, the skeptical pressure to authenticate testimony was heightened together with the need to find new ways of organizing the material.[148] Browne's "Vulgar Errors" was playing a central role in mediating these pressures, but it was also contributing to a rethinking of a problem that *Hydriotaphia* and *Garden of Cyrus* would ponder in complex ways: just how a detailed and accurate account of natural and antiquarian

[144] Cynthia Sundberg Wall, *The Prose of Things: Transformations of Description in the Eighteenth Century* (Chicago: University of Chicago Press, 2006), 71.

[145] Miller, "Description Terminable and Interminable," in Pomata and Siraisi, eds., 360.

[146] For the debts to ancient rhetoric, see Wall, *The Prose of Things*, 15–40.

[147] See Ogilvie, *Science of Describing*, 7–8, 27, 174, 180–1, 209, 215–16, 229.

[148] Ogilvie, *Science of Describing*, 260–1.

evidence might rework the didacticism for which history had always been famous.[149] In mediating between death and life, the antiquities and gardens of the two works are accorded a universal significance, but Browne was still writing in English, with local men as his dedicatees, and with careful attention paid to urns that were dug out of local soil to tell a story about Norfolk history.

There is no question that the pairing of *Hydriotaphia* with *The Garden of Cyrus* had a more than accidental significance for Browne. Even if the side-by-side positioning of the two dedicatory epistles can be chalked up to a publishing ploy, the same cannot be said for equivalent number of chapters—five—in each work, especially since that number accrued such religious, natural, and artistic significance in *The Garden of Cyrus*. Both works share the purpose of consoling the men to whom they are dedicated in the face of deaths in the family.[150] Most expressly, in his dedication of this latter work to Nicholas Bacon, Browne made a case for the unity of his volume:

> That we conjoyn these parts of different Subjects, or that this should succeed the other; Your judgement will admit without impute of incongruity; Since the delightfull World comes after death, and Paradise succeeds the Grave. Since the verdant state of things is the Symbole of the Resurrection, and to flourish in the state of Glory, we must first be sown in corruption. (Martin, 87)[151]

At times in this apology for the unity of the two works, Browne suggests that the garden and the grave were wisely superimposed on one another in this world, much as he had learned in his Paduan medical training to connect the circle of flowers and herbs with the circle of anatomy. In *Hydriotaphia* as well as *Garden*, the geometry of life and death plays a prominent part. In the dedication of *Hydriotaphia* to Thomas Le Gros, Browne stresses the medical interweaving of life and death in explaining that,

> to preserve the living, and make the dead to live, to keep men out of their Urnes, and discourse of humane fragments in them, is not impertinent to our profession; whose study is life and death, who daily behold examples of mortality, and of all men least need artificial *memento's*, or coffins by our bed side, to minde us of our graves. (Martin, 84)[152]

Yet this apology is a little strained in its analogy between the physician's dedication to preserving life and the antiquarian's publication of ancient relics, especially once it is said that the antiquarian in question is ill at ease with his own historical enterprise and has a penchant for jettisoning that enterprise for moral and spiritual ruminations on human vanity and mortality.

[149] See Ogilvie, *Science of Describing*, 149; Ogilvie, "Natural History, Ethics, and Physico-Theology," in Pomata and Siraisi, eds., *Historia*, 75–103.

[150] Robbins makes this argument in his *ODNB* article on Browne.

[151] For the womb/tomb imagery, see Margaret Ash Heideman, "*Hydriotaphia* and *The Garden of Cyrus*: A Paradox and a Cosmic Vision," *University of Toronto Quarterly* 19 (1949–50), 235–46.

[152] For Thomas Le Gros, see John Venn and J. A. Venn, *Alumni Cantabrigienses*, part 1, vol. 3 (Cambridge: Cambridge University Press, 1924), 71; he matriculated at Christ's College, Cambridge in 1631, aged 15; admitted to Gray's Inn in 1632.

This tension in the physician's attitude toward his two subjects can be resolved if we follow Browne in positioning the subject of *Hydriotaphia* at the lower end of a Platonic ladder that stretches toward the vital and sublime universals of *Garden of Cyrus*. This notion is somewhat supported by the probability that *Hydriotaphia* was composed first, in 1656.[153] But as Huntley points out, the movements in the two works are circular as well as upward.[154] As Browne puts them together, he makes no promises that the whole that they form will be an entirely harmonious one. Most complexly, dissonance arises not just between the two works but also, strangely, within each. In announcing the subject of *Hydriotaphia*, Browne admits to Le Gros a certain unwillingness to take on the urns (Martin, 84). After all, Browne is still busily at work on a new edition of his *Pseudodoxia* and, throughout the *Hydriotaphia*, a rift in methods and aims will become increasingly apparent. He is eager for Le Gros to understand, moreover, that the purpose of his antiquarian study is not the typical genealogical one (85). Similarly, in *Garden of Cyrus*, Browne wants Bacon to know from the start that his work should not be taken for a herbal or for a systematic analysis of plant life, as though an association with those utilitarian genres might compromise his work. As its five chapters unfold, *Garden of Cyrus* challenges its readers with two distinctive (if reconcilable) assessments of what nature offers us: a boundless vitality that supersedes the trite categories and "vegetable divisions" into which fallen human minds would cram God's plenty; and a startlingly comprehensive attempt to discover a simple geometrical pattern in all that has been and ever will be.

From start to finish, and even in its marginal notes, *Hydriotaphia* purveys a keen sense of dissonance, irony, and paradox. In the letter to Le Gros, Browne begins with the scene of an ancient funeral where the sorrowing survivor had no way of anticipating the "curiosity of future ages" regarding the ashes of their loved ones, a first of many instances of the ignorance in which human beings live and die. Then the urns in question are demoted to the status of "sad and sepulchral Pitchers, which have no joyful voices"; without the capacity of "Theatrical vessels" to magnify voices in ancient Roman "shows," the urns can only evoke "old mortality, the ruines of forgotten times" (Martin, 83). Before the dedication is over, however, Browne has made a case for the worthiness of antiquarian studies, in part because Le Gros is "no slender master of Antiquities, and can daily command the view of so many Imperiall faces" in his coin collection (83). Indeed, historical study needs a major overhaul in the same way that natural studies do. Yet his other defense of antiquarianism indicts the present times for their dearth of moral exemplars (84). In an age of ambition, perplexity, and duplicity, moderns require a primer for self-fashioning, which they must piece together from the fragments of the past as best they can. In remarking that "A compleat peece of vertue must be made up from the Centos of all ages, as all the beauties of Greece could make but one handsome

[153] Browne refers to a 1653 archaeological dig as having taken place three years previously.

[154] Frank Livingstone Huntley, "Sir Thomas Browne: The Relationship of *Urn Burial* and *The Garden of Cyrus*," *Studies in Philology* 53 (1956), 204–19.

Venus," Browne acknowledges that moral wisdom can only ever be fragmentary in a world devolving into darkness (84).

The tension at the heart of *Hydriotaphia* is that Browne's two defenses of antiquarianism, one factual and the other moral, are difficult to reconcile; and indeed the *vanitas* lessons of the latter tend to subvert the progressive enterprises of the former. This tension arises intermittently in the first four chapters, but it is the very essence of the fifth. In the first chapter, Browne undertakes a brief history of sepulchral practices, focusing mainly on burial and cremation since they are the most sober, least "phantasticall" of human "contrivances" with the dead (Martin, 89–90). Even before this history has commenced, however, Browne confronts his reader with dissonance, irony, and paradox. In what appears to be an exciting announcement of his subject, one that takes us into "the deep discovery of the Subterranean world" (89), he introduces the major theme of nature's relationship to art but quickly declares nature the winner when he relegates the "treasures" of human art, the "Urnes, Coynes, and Monuments," to the most disappointingly shallow region of the earth. It is true that Browne proceeds to conflate art and nature among Time's "endlesse rarities" awaiting human discovery, but by the end of the opening passage, urns serve as a metaphor for the concealment under which "a large part of the earth" continues to hide. Across from this paragraph is a picture of four distinctive urns discovered in the Norfolk field, but the engraving contains a line from Propertius: "*En sum quod digitis quinque levatur onus propert.*" In informing the reader that the urns contain a weight capable of being lifted with five fingers, Browne hints at the vanity of his antiquarian subject and looks ahead to the symbolism of *The Garden of Cyrus* in which nature and its geometry set the standard for human artifice.

In his history of burial practices in biblical and pagan cultures, Browne resorts to a central analytical goal of *Pseudodoxia*: conjectures about the reasons or "grounds" for the development of customs. In *Hydriotaphia*, these grounds can be philosophical, theological, or political; as he sorts them out, Browne occasionally interjects a moral judgment, though in chapter 1 the harshest is reserved for vulgar errors about the natural world, especially those people who "are so thick skinned as still to credit the story of the Phœnix" (Martin, 94). It is in the second chapter of *Hydriotaphia* that Browne is most forthrightly and consistently antiquarian in his approach to the urns. The specimens and their site are carefully described, catalogued, and quantified. The questions of the moment are all matters of fact regarding the historical period and culture responsible for placing these urns beneath a field in "old Walsingham," that is, Great Walsingham near the north coast of Norfolk. Browne's attention is trained on what he calls "strict particulars" of historical evidence. Most pervasively, he keeps the reader apprised of the levels of certainty, probability, and doubt with which assertions can be induced from the physical particulars as they are contextualized by Browne's readings. Like a critical antiquarian, Browne takes it as his responsibility to discredit "Vulgar Chronology" and the unsubstantiated fables of legend, but he is also perfectly prepared to inform his reader when a dearth of evidence provides him with "nothing of more uncertainty" or with "great obscurity." His preference for a Roman origin of the urns may reflect his preference for Roman civility as expressed in the letters to Dugdale, but Browne has a difficult time letting other (British, Saxon, and Danish) hypotheses alone.[155] The careful description of the urns and their accoutrements can be beautiful as well as exact, for instance, in the account of the "blewish" opal which Browne has been sent from one of the urns, or in the description of the "Plates like Boxes, fastened with Iron pins, and handsomely overwrought like the necks or Bridges of Musicall Instruments" (98). But chapter 2 rarely expresses emotion either affectionate or condemnatory, whether the subject be the toiletry items in the urns or the possibility that the ashes belonged to children.

Chapter 3 is a more complicated affair. It proceeds as a descriptive account of various qualities or features of the urns, their size and figure, their color and texture, possible covers and, once again, the objects that they contain. Early in the first paragraph, however, consideration of their "circular figure, in a sphericall and round composure" prompts a brief meditation that can only partly be chalked up to a search for the "grounds" of custom. While any guess about whether the circularity derived "from any mystery, best duration or capacity, were but a conjecture," Browne deciphers the hieroglyph of the shape to his own satisfaction (Martin, 102). A marginal citation of Psalm 63 reinforces the suggestion that the propriety of their shape links the human civility bound up in ritual activity with the wisdom and mystery of divine providence.

Any such lesson from the hieroglyphs of urns passes quickly back in chapter 3 to the sometimes fragmentary assembly of "strict particulars," as well as some speculation based on evidence from the textual record of other discoveries about pieces of the urns that are missing. Over the course of the chapter, Browne's discussion is apt to offer physical and chemical analyses: for instance, about the "piercing Atomes of ayre" rusting the unearthed urns who strangely seem themselves to decay as they "betray their green entrals" (Martin, 104). Browne's study of the chemistry of decay prompts his observation that "in an Hydropicall body ten years buried in a Church-yard, we met with a fat concretion, where the nitre of the Earth, and the salt and lixivious liquor of the body, had coagulated large lumps of fat, into the consistence of the hardest castle-soap; whereof part remaineth with us" (110). Whatever historians have thought of Browne's status as a "scientist," they have agreed that this is one of his most significant episodes as a natural historian, with some crediting Browne as the discoverer of adipocere, "a fatty substance produced in the decomposition of animal substances in moist ground."[156] In chapter 3, however, Browne's chemical and physical observations share the stage with his more morally invested assessment of how and why art represents or ritualizes death.

Browne's sometimes fragmentary, sometimes sonorous prose offers no single or static message about the ways in which ritual, art, and rhetoric mediate the traumas

[155] The urns were Saxon. For a recent summary of archaeological studies of such cremation urns, as well as an exploration of Browne's mistake, see Philip Schwyzer, *Archaeologies of English Renaissance Literature* (Oxford: Oxford University Press, 2007), 175–204.

[156] Henry Watts, *Dictionary of Chemistry* (London: Green and Co., 1918), 1.64, quoted in W. H. Barnes, "Browne's *Hydriotaphia* with a Reference to Adipocere," *Isis* 20 (1933), 337–43, at 340.

of human life in general and of the English 1650s in particular. Whatever their bouts of piety and moral instruction, the first three chapters offer no indication that *Hydriotaphia* is headed toward a mysticism that negates all such physical considerations from the vantage of "true belief." Indeed, this final shift in chapter 5 is so startling that it makes one wonder whether Browne resolved his doubts about human art even while writing the work. Before we come to the final negation in chapter 5, Browne devotes an entire chapter, the fourth, to ritual. The chapter begins with a paragraph that praises Christians for having "handsomely glossed the deformity of death, by careful consideration of the body, and civil rites which take of brutall terminations" (Martin, 111–12). It is true that this handsome care in some measure ignores the belief that such deformity is "reparable by a resurrection," true also that this glossing partakes of the "happy fraud" that Browne will soon attribute to pagan burial practices. But he is quick to point out a Christian ground for the "careful consideration," namely, that Christians "acknowledged their bodies to be the lodging of Christ, and temples of the holy Ghost," for which reason "they devolved not all upon the sufficiency of soul existence" (112). Browne's own support for the "long services and full solemnities" that resulted from Christian care is kept at a distance by his observation that Greek Orthodoxy "seems most pathetically [emotionally] ceremonious." But as he introduces the thrust of the chapter, a survey of pagan rites, he reiterates the Christian ground of funeral ceremonies in asserting that "Christian invention hath chiefly driven at Rites, which speak hopes of another life, and hints of a Resurrection" (112).

As chapter 4 unfolds, Browne continues to scatter observations about the urns from Walsingham in passing. As the physical evidence in question grows increasingly remote, poetic fictions of the afterlife and underworld begin to dominate the discussion. Whether these fictions derive from ancient epic or from Christian "Philosophy" and literature, chapter 4 rides their wave into darkness and doubt. From Machiavelli's claim that Christian virtues render "men cowards" to Dante's struggle to place virtuous pagans such as Epicurus in the *Commedia*, Browne finds error everywhere. The best of the pagans could not help but err, while Christians tend to mistake the significance of behavior in the face of death (Martin, 117). As though weary of the gap between human conceptions of death and its inevitably obscure reality, Browne reverses a bold claim that he has made in *Religio*, the one where he is sorry not to have lived before the time of Christ so as to maximize the potential of his faith in things unseen. Having noted the profound sadness that arises in the case of Dante's Epicurus, Browne concludes that faith profits from having stronger, clearer evidence to go on.

From its opening praise of Christian rites to its closing recourse to "the superiour ingredient and obscured part of our selves," chapter 4 has prepared the way, fitfully and uncertainly, for the extraordinary turn in the finale toward a reality and certainty "above Antiquarism" (Martin, 119). In the final chapter, Browne's urns turn into what we might call negative hieroglyphics, symbols whose métier is their own decay and whose significance is the negation of all the vanity that produced the artifacts in the first place. In addition to his indictment of those who wish for fame in a monument, Browne implicates the methods and aims of the antiquarian who would reconstruct and analyze such vanity as a matter of fact rather than a "memento" of mortality. On the surface chapter 5 makes the gestures toward epistemological critique that chapter 2 does, but the final chapter folds doubt into human vanity while the earlier, antiquarian chapter is keen to reconstruct tentative or probable answers from the pieces. For the most part, Browne concludes his *Hydriotaphia* in the proverbial mode that has begun to rise to prominence in *Letter to a Friend* and that will dominate *Christian Morals*; these adages serve as repetitious (if sonorous) "Emblemes of mortall vanities; Antidotes against pride, vainglory, and madding vices" (118).

Early on, Browne's tendency to use "if-then" formulations to express such vanity might leave open the possibility that readers will reject the logic of life's "sad composition" or the math that makes "our dayes become considerable like petty sums by minute accumulations" (Martin, 119). But it is not long before the adages lose their conditionals. One after another, these truths of human discontent, treachery, ambition, and worldly vanity are lofted at the reader: "'Tis too late to be ambitious"; "The great mutations of the world are acted"; "Our Fathers finde their graves in our short memories"; "Generations passe while some trees stand"; and "Oblivion is not to be hired" (120–1). While the vitality of plants shames our transience, the certainty of geometry encapsulates our finitude, since "Circles and right lines limit and close all bodies, and the mortall right-lined circle"—the theta—"must conclude and shut up all" (120). In a concession to fortuity that links Browne's meditations to Ecclesiastes, he allows that there is no rhyme or reason to the record of history, since worthy lives are as often forgotten as worthless men are remembered (121). In another, looser connection to Ecclesiastes, which argues that pleasure offers solace in the face of pointlessness, Browne allows a respite to be taken in forgetfulness, since hapless humans tend to block out their own past misery in what Browne calls "no unhappy stupidity" (122). But whether the example is a theory (for instance, transmigration) or a practice (mummification), the human "art of perpetuation" comes to the same vulgar error; indeed progress in natural studies, represented by the telescope's revelation of changeability in the heavens, makes the ironic point that not even nature's highest reaches can be relied on to perpetuate our fame.

The concluding two paragraphs are like no other that Browne ever wrote. In the rapturous wonder that they direct toward the divine, these passages resemble the strong bouts of fideism in *Religio*. But there is nothing in that early work to match the utter negation of creatural existence or the dissolution of the self into the numinous evoked in Browne's final return to a conditional in *Hydriotaphia*:

> And if any have been so happy as truly to understand Christian annihilation, extasis, exolution, liquefaction, transformation, the kisse of the Spouse, the gestation of God, and ingression into the divine shadow, they have already had an handsome anticipation of heaven; the glory of the world is surely over, and the earth in ashes unto them. (Martin, 124–5)

Unlike the previous "if-then" sentences, however, the condition is bound to apply to very few of Browne's readers. The phrase "handsome anticipation" hearkens back to the outset of chapter 4, where "Christians have handsomely glossed the deformity of death." Looking back, the reader can perhaps suppose a second meaning to "glossed," that is, to have rendered comprehensible that which staggers human understanding, as well as to have put a sheen on something nasty. Since few of Browne's readers have a gloss of incomprehensible divinity by way of a consuming mystical experience, then they are going to have to rely on a lower form of glossing, one that comforts as a "happy fraud" but also helps us to comprehend the mysteries framing the beginning and ending of life to which we have no experiential or rational access. Ceremony and the "sensible rhetorick" of the dead are as corrupt as they are accommodating; but there is no point in pretending that we can shoulder the "heaviest stone" of our mortality without their assistance (117).

In one sentence from chapter 5, Browne summarizes this complex argument for rites and ceremonies: "But man is a Noble Animal, splendid in ashes, and pompous in the grave, solemnizing Nativities and Deaths with equall luster, nor omitting Ceremonies of bravery, in the infamy of his nature" (Martin, 123). Once again birth and death meet up as human beings strive to compose their ragged lives into a rounded whole. That they work so hard at the art of perpetuity is brave in two senses, both ostentatious and courageous. And the preposition "in"—"in the infamy of his nature"—leaves uncertainty about whether the art in question overcomes natural infamy or participates in it. As Browne has told Le Gros from the beginning, there is more than one kind of nobility, the suspicious kind that finds its worth in family trees, and the genuine kind that looks to virtue. In calling man a "Noble Animal," whose vitality is a "pure" yet "small fire," Browne offers one of his most searching and elusive assessments of why, in making wars and factions over ritual and ceremony, his contemporaries have converted into trauma the imperfect arts by which societies have always managed to survive trauma, if always for just a while.

In two small ways, Browne's 1658 volume practiced the arts of perpetuation for which he made such a complex case in *Hydriotaphia*. For one thing, as Marjorie Swann has pointed out, the marginal notes are filled with the names of Browne's honorable friends, correspondents, and neighbors, as though he were attempting to preserve their names even as he was casting doubt on the possibility of such preservation. That several of these names belong to members of the landed elite reinforces a connection between nature and the social order that *Hydriotaphia* sometimes subverts.[157] In this vein, *Hydriotaphia* is motivated by the same post-civil war urgency to preserve corporate identity that Browne writ large into *Repertorium*.[158] The other way in which Browne works at the art of perpetuity in *Hydriotaphia* has come to light thanks to the careful work of twentieth-century scholars such as John Carter and Finch, who examined a number of presentation copies of the 1658 edition in which Browne or an amanuensis had made a series of

[157] Marjorie Swann, *Curiosities and Texts: The Culture of Collecting in Early Modern England* (Philadelphia: University of Pennsylvania Press, 2001), 121–34.

[158] Swann, *Curiosities and Texts*, 130–1.

careful corrections in the margins.[159] With these corrections, Browne connected two concerns: that the civility of his community might be seconded by the care with which intellectual property is exchanged, and that the author's art might be appreciated all the more for the industry and attentiveness devoted to it.

If Browne's commitment to learned industry and community operates only in the margins and decreasingly in *Hydriotaphia*'s drive toward mystical negation of the world, the reverse is true of *The Garden of Cyrus*, in which assiduous collaboration in the pursuit of truth is increasingly prominent in the work's final chapters. This is hardly surprising, since the *Garden*'s dedicatee, "my worthy and honored friend Nicholas Bacon of Gillingham Esquire," belongs to the family whose name was by 1658 most powerfully associated with the overhaul of natural studies entailing cooperation and labor from its socially differentiated participants. But in the very dedication of the work, Browne puts Bacon (and other readers) on notice that his study of gardens is not to be confused with "phytology," that is, with botanical or herbal inquiries strictly conceived. Rather, his criteria for the study are its newness and the leniency that it affords the "imagination" and a digressive, excursive mind. True, Browne renews the values of *Pseudodoxia*, both in his interest in arriving at "collaterall truths," and in his unwillingness to dogmatize at the expense of exceptions. But the work's stress on delight for its own sake, as well as its obsession with an arcane and geometrical order in nature, art, and religious mystery, tends to compromise the appeal to inductive reason or experience on which, nonetheless, Browne continues on occasion to insist. In the 1650s, Browne's student of patterns in nature faces challenges similar to the physician whose vocation requires that he offer both rigor and comfort to patients and families with their own complex profiles.

As he tells Bacon in the dedication to *The Garden of Cyrus*, Browne is eager to focus on new ways of conceptualizing God's creation, not least because the "temper of these times" as an "ill-judging age" has produced what Browne characterizes as an intellectual nausea over the conventions of thought. Whether the Baconianism popularized by Browne's own work on "vulgar errors" is now implicated in the triteness and imprisonment of thought is a question with which Browne's *Garden of Cyrus* appears to struggle. With an epigraph selected from Quintilian, and a subject whose antiquity is advertised in the work's very title, Browne can be taken at his word when he claims that "of old things we write something new, If truth may receive addition, or envy will have anything new; since the Ancients knew the late Anatomicall discoveries, and Hippocrates the Circulation" (Martin, 86). Yet the first chapter advertises the failure of "Gentile Theology" to account for the third day's creation of plants, that "first ornamentall Scene of nature; the primitive food of animals, and first story of Physick, in Dietetical conservation" (130). And as it unfolds a brief history of prominent ancient gardens from Eden to Babylon,

[159] See for instance Jeremiah S. Finch, "A Newly Discovered Urn Burial," *Library*, 4th series, 19 (1938/9), 347–53, with Carter's response, "Sir Thomas Browne's Autograph Corrections," in the same volume of the journal, 492–3; and John Carter, ed., *Urne-Buriall and The Garden of Cyrus* (London: Cassell & Co., 1932).

Browne explains to his reader that, for one very good reason, the story of Cyrus's garden might be largely untold: the gardener in question was possibly not the famous Cyrus of Xenophon's "memorable work" but a sibling who was "a person of high spirit and honour, naturally a King, though fatally prevented by the harmlesse chance of *post*-geniture." Browne adds that this less famous Cyrus was "Not only a Lord of Gardens, but a manuall planter thereof: disposing his trees like the armies in regular ordination" (131). This is not the last time that Browne will speak of garden "ordination" in analogy with military tactics, though he will also characterize the quincunx as conducive to peace and quiet.

In the first chapter Browne downplays the "mystical" conceptions of the quincunx, offering to skip over the order's appearance in ancient crosses as well as in the Egyptian hieroglyph symbolizing "the processe and motion of the spirit of the world" (Martin, 132). Even so, the epithets with which he often describes the fivefold figure—"fundamentall" and "Originall" for example—suggest its archetypal stature in the mind of God, even as terms such as "handsome" and "elegant" connect its regularity to beauty and pleasure. Browne tells us that he will omit the Hebraic ordination of the High Priest, yet spends a paragraph discussing its significance and later includes Old Testament examples as key instances of the providential geometry. Indeed, in order to assert the deep, Hebraic antiquity of the order, Browne has set aside the tendency in *Hydriotaphia* to proceed carefully where evidence is lacking. For "if it were clear that this [order] was used by Noah after the Floud, I could easily beleeve it was in use before it" (134).

In chapter 1, Browne's most comprehensive statement of the "elegancy of this order" comprises "the severall commodities, mysteries, parallelismes, and resemblances, both in Art and Nature" (Martin, 133), though only the first in this list, the "commodities" or practicalities of the quincunx, is for the most part exempted from Browne's bouts of skepticism. Nature is by far the dominant guarantor of the order's pervasiveness, taking up the longest of the chapters (the third) as well as chapter 4. Since gardens such as Cyrus's combine art with nature, however, it is not inappropriate that Browne begins with those human contrivances of the quincunx. Even before chapter 1 is over, he has made a claim about the "witty Idolatry" and hieroglyphic tendencies of the ancient pagans that will prove a key point of contact between nature and religious mystery: that architecture, including "the constitutions of their temples" as well as walls and pavements, relies on the number five, with five structural parts, types of columns, and "intercolumniations" in buildings such as pyramids, forums, and mausoleums (135–7).

The range of artistic quincunxes is wide: crowns, beds, seats, glasswork, lattices, embroidery, and nets. The number five figures into heraldry, gemology, perspective painting, town planning, military strategy, and sculpture. While evidence for the pattern is both physical (coins, medals) and textual, it bears a complex relationship to nature. Although the Native Americans are said "naturally" to use it, the "untaught finger of nature" found in a spider's web does not: the spider perplexes "the common art of Textuary" and offers Browne's first example of an alternative order by which nature works (Martin, 138). In addition to being "neat" or "noble," the quincunx is also artistically useful, for instance in those medical operations requiring the "contrary ends" of "solution and consolidation" (139). But its uses are also symbolic, for instance in an ancient game board's figuration of "the whole world." Browne also shows an interest in "rurall charms" or "old superstition," including the placement of "chalked Tile at the four corners" and in the middle of fields, by which means farmers have attempted to ward off "*Dodder*, *Tetter*, and strangling weeds" (138; cf. 144). Although Browne is not uncritical of these charms, calling their magical "intention" "ridiculous," he nonetheless appreciates the good sense of "the contrivance" as "a good way to diffuse the magick through all parts of the *Area*" (138). As in *Pseudodoxia*, the vulgar error has a logic or ground; but without the dominant skeptical bent of that earlier work, Browne raises the stature of the charm by placing it among those patterned art works that include not just the "Labyrinth of Crete" but the Hebraic "Ark of the Covenant, the table of the Shew-bread, and the stone wherein the names of the twelve Tribes were engraved" (141).

As he turns from art to nature in the third chapter, Browne raises one question and implies another about the pervasiveness of five in God's creation. The direct question is whether students of nature might sufficiently discern the order among the lights in heaven so as to claim them for the quincunx; suggesting that there is neither way nor need to "look so high as Heaven," Browne nonetheless expresses the desire for such knowledge with such earnestness that he betrays the gratification to be found in patterned, deductive thinking which Francis Bacon made a career of indicting. More implicit is Browne's hesitation about whether the quincunx appears in art by "imitation" of the natural world or "coincidence" with it (Martin, 142). For *Garden of Cyrus*, the difference might matter considerably in deciding whether five is a divinely authorized feature of the creation or a historically transmitted construction that serves a series of partisan human purposes. If the latter, then the quincunx is not unlike the urns in *Hydriotaphia*; if the former, then it transcends antiquarianism.

Whatever can be said for art, however, nature is found to be elegantly quintuple in vegetable and animal phenomena alike. The "subterraneous concretions" that briefly factor into the survey lie far beneath the urns in depth and significance alike. And though Browne makes very little of the methodological criteria that dominate *Pseudodoxia*, it is clear that he spent a great part of the 1650s directly observing the phenomena, especially plants, in search of their "remarkable" geometry (Martin, 143). For instance, he claims to have spent six years observing whether medical plants will lose their properties if submerged in water for extended periods of time (166). In a variety of plants Browne celebrates "how the needle of nature delighteth to work, even in how and doubtful vegetations" (144). In tracing their designs, he writes with an inventive, often Latinate, vocabulary that ranges over "uncous" and "calicular," "abstersion," "favaginous," and "spicated." The density of these words is matched by the largesse that he finds in putatively lowly, miniaturized worlds: Browne peels back petals and finds a palace: "The Arbustetum or Thicket on the head of the Teasel may be observed in this order: And he that considereth that fabrick so regularly palisadoed, and stemm'd with flowers of the royall colour; in the house of the solitary maggot, may finde the Seraglio of Solomon" (144). On occasion he makes personal references to his aging or poor eyesight, which prompts the reminder that the observer will profit from having a magnifying glass or microscope at hand. But unlike his friend Henry Power, who was at work on a microscopic study of tiny phenomena, Browne shows less interest in *Garden of Cyrus* than he will in later editions of *Pseudodoxia* in the assistance of such devices. Rather, his mode of perception moves across a sliding scale of contemplation, judgment, and observation. That he is prepared to include "doubtful" things in the geometry of artful nature underscores his desire to think of nature as overcoming adversity even when nature's productions appear to be monstrous, an essential lesson of Fortunio Liceti.

The Garden of Cyrus often claims to omit examples that it nonetheless manages to include in the act of jettisoning. The work is also mindful of digressions, which Browne marks as "by the way." These diversions from the repetition of quintuplets sometimes point out an experiment that Browne has undertaken, for instance, with the "abstemious" maggot. He makes it clear that he has spent no small portion of the previous decade gazing into glasses of water in order to observe some natural event or specimen. But the most sizable digression, the one that dominates chapter 3, forthrightly recognizes that the wondrousness of nature is neither static nor always fivefold. This digression on generation features two main points: amazingly little is required to do much in the "originall production" of plants, and nature uses a "strict rule" but not the quincunx in unfolding the "plastick principle" that resides in the seminal "nebbe" or single, most prominent point. The vegetation under discussion is commonplace fare—beans, acorns, walnuts, and grains—but Browne's example shows just how acutely and patiently observant we must be to apprehend and appreciate the beauty, order, and wonder of the everyday. By gazing on the seminal casements of duckweed in water, the observer can glimpse the "first and rudimental stroaks" of generation and, in doing so, come as close to witnessing the divine creation as mortals are ever going to come. Browne also marvels at the way in which the sun is able to find out "seminall powers" no matter in what dark, remote, or barren location they are situated, whether the fern polypody in stone walls or the stinging nettle in sandy highways (147).

Returning to "the higher Geometry of nature" (Martin, 151), Browne interrelates circles with his quincunxes, and proceeds to survey those animals in which "nature Geometrizeth, and observeth order in all things" (153). The focus on honeycombs elicits a passing political resonance in the appreciation for "the edificial Palaces of Bees and Monarchical spirits." Yet in the same discussion, Browne expresses a certain skepticism about the inclination of "a pliant fancy to credulity of similitude" (152). In its reminder that the varied experience of particulars often subverts our desire for patterns, this passage ranks among the work's most Baconian, and it implies a warning about bending nature to the fantasies of anthropomorphism. When Browne turns to human examples of quincuncial design, he places no special stress on its role in the list of reticulate designs also found in the elegance of flies, butterfly eggs, snake skin, beaver tails, and fish scales. Even so, the analogical network of correspondences so crucial to *Religio Medici* is not simply a "pleasant piece of Rhetoric" in *Garden of Cyrus*. Browne advertises how "Studious

Observators may discover more analogies in the orderly book of nature, and cannot escape the Elegancy of her hand in other correspondencies" (156).

With the opening of chapter 4, Browne includes religious "mysteries" together with "delights, commodities," and "other concernments of this order." Utility dominates the opening discussion, which covers considerations of plant nutrition and shade, as well as problems arising from entangled roots, inadequate wind to assist vegetable perspiration, and insufficient exposure to the sun and moon. As he works though a wide variety of examples, Browne sometimes introduces details of his own experiments: for instance, he recalls how "in tender plants from mustard-seed, sown in the winter, and in a pot of earth placed inwardly in a chamber against a South-window, the tender stalks of two leaves arose not erect, but bending towards the window, nor looking much higher then the Meridian Sun" (Martin, 160). But suddenly Browne is imagining a garden far distant in time and place, Solomon's own in Jerusalem, with the city wall on the garden's west side. Even though so many of his examples seem homely and local, Browne pauses in chapter 4 to caution against confining one's apprehensions to the narrowly local: regarding ivy, for example, Cyrus's Babylon could not grow it, and ancient writers such as Galen and Virgil are interested in kinds other than the one found in the north. As chapter 4 unfolds, it becomes increasingly clear that Browne is somewhat torn between an emphasis on the vital, abundant variety and dynamism of the natural world—qualities not wholly imitable or controllable by art—and the noble elegance of geometry. Within the quintuple itself, he begins to parse variations in the rhomboidal arrangement, which after all is by definition always varied in its obtuse and acute angles. One way in which Browne combines vitality and regularity is by remarking that while nature is geometrical, it never works in strictly defined right angles, or that its geometrical work unfolds in motion over time and against creatural adversity (163, 165).

In the course of his celebration of the delightfulness of quintuple order, Browne returns to its appearance in architecture, only this time with an eye toward the kinship between groves and the pillars in "famous buildings." In reference to the porticoes of ancient structures, Browne briefly imagines the spaces in which "men discoursed, walked and exercised" (Martin, 165). It is at this point in his work, with cloistered passageways linked to the healthy arrangement of trees, that Browne suddenly offers the most sustained defense of divine providence in the 1658 volume, one that manages to find new, uplifting significance in the darkness of *Hydriotaphia*.

The immediate subject of Browne's apology for providence is optical: an arrangement of trees or columns as a quincunx facilitates vision with its combination of "long parallels" with intervening shadings. Thus sight is neither "diffused" by too much light and openness in a vista nor impeded by too much shadow or by too many intervening objects. From this point about commodity, Browne argues that "therefore providence hath arched and paved the great house of the world, with colours of mediocrity, that is blew and green, above and below the sight, moderately terminating the *acies* of the eye" (Martin, 165). So providence observes moderation in its careful attention to our needs but also those of vegetation too, since just the right balance of sun and shade is critical for the prosperity of seeds as well as mature trees. It is this point that prompts Browne to reclaim darkness from both the mortal vanity and the negative mysticism with which it was burdened in *Hydriotaphia*, for darkness as well as light contributes powerfully to life: "Darknesse and light hold interchangeable dominions, and alternately rule the seminal state of things." From vegetation, Browne moves outward into the cosmos at large, including those stars that before were relegated to the unknown, then even further into religious mystery before returning to optics—in each case reclaiming darkness for the realm of the living. If we cannot posit a quincunx in the patterning of the heavens, then the quincunx allows us to see the stars, since "it is no wonder that this Quincunciall order was first and still affected as gratefull unto the Eye: For all things are seen Quincuncially," a notion whose optical geometry Browne proceeds to explain (167).

The example of light and shade in religious mystery instills a confidence about biblical typology that Browne has so far lacked in *The Garden of Cyrus*: "The greatest mystery of Religion is expressed by adumbration, and in the noblest part of Jewish Types, we finde the Cherubims shadowing the Mercy-seat" (Martin, 167). Disinclined to pursue the typological significance of Hebraic ordination in chapter 1, Browne adverts in chapter 4 to that Christian theory of history that conceived of Old Testament events and rites as shadowy anticipations of Christian events and truths, with the latter fulfilling and completing the former. What is more, he chooses as the "noblest" of these types that lid or cover of the Ark of the Covenant that God required to be framed by golden cherubim. In this holiest of places, only Aaron the High Priest and his descendents were supposed to communicate with God, and especially to offer sacrifices of atonement for the sins of the people. In Christian thought, in keeping with the words in Hebrews 9:3–5, Christ was understood as the true High Priest whose incarnation, new covenant of grace, and sacrifice on the cross would spiritually atone for the sins of humankind.

As Browne invokes this passage, its focus on the "cherubim of God's glory, overshadowing the place of expiation" serves to reclaim the value of two things that *Hydriotaphia* abandons in its final chapter. One is the spiritual (if imperfect) value of artifice and ritual; the Ark replaces the urns, and atonement supplants funerals as the centerpieces of Browne's imagination. The other is the patterned coherence of history. If in *Hydriotaphia*, history is at best irrelevant to the mysticism with which the work concludes, in the *Garden of Cyrus* it shares in the providential order that Browne has been tracing in art and nature. And history gains in significance as it unfolds rather than as it dwindles into triviality and vanity.

As chapter 4 comes to an end, Browne prepares the way for the transition from nature and art to mysticism that takes place in the final chapter. He devotes a paragraph to "ascending and descending Pyramids" by means of which "geniall spirits" were "mystically" represented as moving back and forth between heaven and earth, and serving as the media of reciprocal influence and correspondence that played a crucial role in the philosophy of Renaissance magic. More elaborately, Browne explicates Plato's chiasmic vision of the world soul, including a circle as the symbol of "the motion of the indivisible soul, simple, according to the divinity of its nature";

the crossing lines of the chi as "respecting the motion pertaining unto sense, and vegetation"; and the point at which they cross, "the central decussation," as "the wondrous connexion of the severall faculties conjointly in one substance." From this "Systasis or harmony" of the body and soul, Browne moves to Justin Martyr's claim that this chi "had the honour to characterize and notifie our blessed Saviour, as he [Justin] delivered in that borrowed expression from Plato." Once again, Browne offers his view that pagan and Christian—here Plato and Justin—themselves criss-cross at the "mystical expressions…of Ægypt" (Martin, 169).[160]

As he affirms the mystical stature of the quincunx, Browne introduces his revision of an analogy that William Harvey boldly offers in his treatise on generation. While Harvey directly analogizes procreative conception to mental conception, Browne ends up arguing that generation and intellection operate differently. Generation, we have seen, is the extraordinary mystery of nature, the one with the best adumbration of divine creation, but it does not share in nature's love of fives. By contrast, mental conception operates quincuncially, with "things entring upon the intellect by a Pyramid from without, and thence into the memory by another from within." In this way, mental conception connects us not just to the world soul but to Christ who comes to save the world that God has made but that we have wrecked. What is more, the pyramidal geometry of thought opens up the possibility that one day we might be able to understand (and to correct?) those "irregular apprehensions of things, perverted notions, conceptions, and incurable hallucinations" (168) that continue to make Browne's an "ill-judging age."

In the fifth chapter, Browne begins his treatment of "the mysteries and secrets accomadable unto this number" with a resolution against the excesses of an "inexcusable Pythagorisme" (Martin, 169). In keeping with this caution, he offers his examples of moral and spiritual symbolism as the ones that he "cannot omit." Indeed, nature and art continue to claim his attention as though to pull the discussion back down to earth, with even the wonders of generation proving to have connections to the number five. If Browne has not wanted his discourse to be associated with a standard herbal, he also tends to distance it from what he considers an embarrassingly excessive natural theology.

With its unwillingness to overindulge the mystical flights of numerology, chapter 5 never quite gets off the ground. Rather, it devolves into a long list of further inquiries from nature, art, and religion that Browne's readers might pursue. These topics range widely across the fields of medicine, astrology, Cabala, music, magnetism, magic, theater, chiromancy, and botany. But whatever the inquiry, Browne makes it increasingly clear that he is concerned to enrich the lives of his readers. He would prevent them from having to spend their "hours in vulgar speculations," or "to fall on trite or triviall disquisitions" (Martin, 173). For "acuter enquirers," Browne diagnoses a tendency in the late 1650s toward "nauseating crambe verities and questions over-queried" (173–4). Reversing his desire in *Religio* to be read in

[160] For the Platonic heritage behind Browne's quincunx, see Kathryn Murphy, "'A Likely Story': Plato's *Timaeus* in the *Garden of Cyrus*," in Barbour and Preston, eds., *Sir Thomas Browne: The World Proposed*, 242–57.

a "soft and flexible sense," Browne relegates flexibility to boredom and triteness: "Flat and flexible truths are beat out by every hammer; But *Vulcan* and his whole forge sweat to work out *Achilles* his armour." In this image, Browne mythologizes both the labor and artistry required to fashion a truth worth having. Earlier in *Garden*, Browne associates Vulcan with making the net in which to trap Venus and Mars, a myth which he says might yield "no vulgar speculation" regarding its allegorical significance. But the context of Vulcan (Hephaestus) and the armor, Homer's *Iliad*, book 18, is especially ripe with import for Browne's readers in 1658. With "whole forge" Browne is referring to Homer's point that Vulcan deployed all twenty bellows in the contrivance of the armor to replace that lost by Patroclus in battle. The request for the armor comes from the goddess Thetis to the sweaty god whose lameness makes him an appropriate surrogate for Browne's sense of the human artist, elegant in what he can produce but also decidedly flawed in who he is. While the description in the *Iliad* reminds readers that Vulcan has crafted an extensive line of extraordinary metalwork, from jewelry to the furniture of his home, Homer focuses book 18 on the contrivance of Achilles's shield, with its five layers an obvious prompt for its inclusion in *The Garden of Cyrus*.

Although its occasion is the grievous strife of war, the shield includes scenes of tragic conflict within the larger context of a cosmos that manages to bring artistic concord out of discord. On the shield the limping but nimble craftsman hammers out the earth and the sea, the heavens and the stars. He depicts human life in a variety of scenes: a city in the midst of celebrations and marriages but also settling a conflict in assembly; another city torn by war; a rural picture of plowmen at work, this one featuring the kind of shadowing that Browne has earlier praised in sculpture; another image of farmhands working for a king, this scene giving way to feasting and ritual sacrifices; a vineyard with musical performances, a pasture, and a joyous dance, with all this cosmic whole surrounded by the River Oceanus. If Browne's acute inquirers are to imitate Vulcan, then, they are responsible for using all their skill and might to fashion a quintuplet cosmos in which strife is but a phase or season in the whole.

So it goes in *Garden of Cyrus*. Contrary to his resistance to the wars of truth in *Religio*, Browne directs his "acuter enquirers" to don the armor that they have made and fight for truth. In keeping with appeals to experience in *Pseudodoxia*, Browne argues that "sense and ocular Observation" should figure prominently in the arsenal (Martin, 174). It is not enough to be handsome in battle; like Vulcan, one must be prepared to get sweaty and dirty. Introducing another myth, Browne also reminds his team of blacksmiths—the Cyclopes assisting Vulcan?—that they also must be ready to get lost as they "erect generalities, disclose unobserved proprieties, not only in the vegetable shop, but the whole volume of nature." The truths that they find can offer pleasure, he promises, but attentive observation will also offer a level of certainty, "the surest path, to trace the Labyrinth of Truth" (174). All in all, Browne's summons to move beyond the nausea of "flat and flexible truths" offers a rebuke to the fifth chapter of *Hydriotaphia*, in which Vulcan's artistry might be reducible to trinkets, and the heroic effort for the sake of truth deemed just so much human vanity. As Graham Parry has noted, antiquarian discovery was often given a heroic cast in early modern England; yet in the late 1650s, Browne rediscovers the urgency and sublimity of learning in glasses of water containing duckweed rather than in urns containing bracelets.[161] With Vulcan, the emphasis is clearly on the artistic fashioning of the cosmos within the orderly contrivance of set-pieces in the service of partisanship in war. With observation and the labyrinth, truth is something we find, not make; its pattern is something we fitfully, cautiously discover, not feverishly impose with a hammer or chisel in the forge of our imaginations. Even so, in his insistence on revising both works in the 1658 volume, he emulated Vulcan in his own way, prizing his own artistry even as he recognized the feebleness of the human artist with his vanity and bleary, aging eyes.[162]

In the final paragraphs, however, Browne finds a way to unite the two heroics, and to revisit the apocalyptic finish of *Hydriotaphia* at the same time. Noting that the hour is approaching midnight in his corner of the world, he insists on ceasing his work on the quincunx lest he dream of the pattern afterwards. In *Religio Medici*, the dream offers the most liberating and transformative opportunity for human thought, but also the most inaccessible for the waking. At the conclusion of *The Garden of Cyrus*, Browne objects to the way in which "phantasmes of sleep" create "Cables of Cobwebbes and Wildernesses of handsome Groves" (Martin, 174). On the one hand, this image demotes the geometrizing of the work to a delicate but lightweight fiction that sleep will wrongly coarsen but also actuate. On the other, dreams are accused of disordering the lovely, patterned designs of the quincunx into an unreliable version of the truth-seeker's labyrinth. Given his claim that "All things began in order, so shall they end, and so shall they begin again; according to the ordainer of order and mystical Mathematicks of the City of Heaven," it is clear that Browne laments the loss of truth as well as beauty in our abandonment to sleep.

Browne is eager for his readers to stay awake, to resist the lure of dreaming that one finds in the Interregnum poetry of Henry Vaughan. Such a dream of the apocalypse haunts the end of *Hydriotaphia*, with its mystical kiss amounting to the annihilation of human identity, agency, and artistry. But in *Garden of Cyrus*, the apocalypse offers us the greatest reason to stay awake against the temptation of cultural retreat and slumber (Martin, 175). In sleep, Browne explains, we are never going to experience the pleasures or vivid sensations that we can gain in our waking hours; dreams deaden, rather than liberate and accentuate, our experiences. As Browne prepares for sleep, he remembers the strange fact that in Homer, sleep served to wake up Agamemnon. But he also remembers that even as he sleeps, somewhere in the world, in the new world of America in fact, the hunters are ready to begin their searches.

On May 13, 1658, Samuel Hartlib wrote to Robert Boyle that Browne's 1658 volume "seems to be no ordinary book."[163] Although the two works in that volume

[161] See Parry, *The Trophies of Time*, 1.

[162] Keynes published notebook passages relevant to the two works in *Works*, 3.246–48. See also Jeremiah S. Finch, "Early Drafts of the *Garden of Cyrus*," *PMLA* 55 (1940), 742–9.

[163] In the *Hartlib Papers* database.

came nowhere close to the instant fame of *Pseudodoxia* or *Religio*, their power was certainly felt by contemporaries; one year after Browne's death, a member of the Norfolk gentry named William Windham "recorded the planting of forty-nine trees in a formal pattern described as 'the Quincunciall, Lozenge, or Net-work Plantations,'" clearly an attempt to carry on the geometrical legacy that Browne had revived.[164] Writing to Browne about the newly published volume in 1658 and 1659, Henry Power was obviously stimulated—"extimulate" is his word—to further thought by *The Garden of Cyrus*. In a response written in June 1659, Browne appears less eager than his younger self to relegate their inquiries to the realm of fancy, noting that much of what they are discussing can be had "by playne & rurall observation" or "by an easie way of experiment" (Keynes, 4.268). In other words, Browne's letter associates *The Garden of Cyrus* with the criteria of the *Pseudodoxia* far more than with those of the *Religio*. He insists that he has spent hours gazing at duckweed "kept in thinne glasses" filled with water, all in an effort to "perceave any alteration or Atome as bigge as a needles poynt" as it is followed "within 3 or 4 howers" by the appearance of the entire plant (Keynes, 4.269). There is no place for slumber among those inquirers who would "narrowlie" observe the generation of new life.

Browne's letter to Power of June 1659 honors dynamic process in two distinctive ways. For one thing, even if the conception of life is all at once whole, that whole is "discoverable successively" as human investigators make their way through the labyrinth of truth. If the time required for discovery hardly counts as a ringing endorsement of history, the second way in which Browne and Power support the virtues of process serves as a perhaps unintended retort to *Hydriotaphia*. In the fifth chapter of the work on urns, as in the *Religio* before it, Browne demotes the value of family—of generation understood genealogically rather than botanically—by arguing that children readily forget their parents. In the *Religio*, the doubt cast on family memory was part of Browne's celebration of the intimacy of friendship that he now recalls sharing with Power's father. Having received some Spanish books in the mail from Henry, Browne not only remembers his friend but celebrates John Power's continuing vitality in his son (Keynes, 4.270). As Browne shares with his protégé the wonders of generation in plant life, he expresses a faith in the vitality that memory can lend not just the names but the spirit of the past. With children, it seems, memory and heritage could prove as vital—or "fresh"—as seeds and plants. As the word "spirit" appears prominently in the letter, Browne finds in his most longstanding and devoted correspondent a way to connect natural history to history so that the past contributes to the hope of the future. In the last twenty years of his life, Browne abandoned his old grievance with family and discovered in his sons, daughters, and grandchildren the point at which nature and history intersected and fertilized one another.

[164] Dymond, *Norfolk Landscape*, 192. Cf. Elizabeth Griffiths, ed., *William Windham's Green Book, 1673–1688*, in *Norfolk Record Society* 66 (2002), 11–12.

10

Norwich, 1660–1671

The final two decades of Browne's life were his most intellectually diverse as well as the most richly documented. With *Christian Morals*, these years also produced Browne's most mature spiritual and moral ruminations, his last advice for a world that he had influenced so complexly. In offering his 1683 edition of *Certain Miscellany Tracts*, Thomas Tenison connected the miscellaneous, piecemeal tendencies of Browne's late writings to the intensity with which Browne pursued his life and vocation in the final decades. Tenison did his best to impose order and method on the highly various, "beginning first with Plants, going on to Animals, proceeding farther to things relating to Men," yet even this scale of creation, like that found in *Pseudodoxia*, finally gave way to "matters of a various nature."[1] As the trove of letters from Browne and his wife Dorothy to their children underscores, Browne's life of learning was inextricable from his domestic concerns in Norwich: although he continued to collaborate on projects within the republic of letters, to revise *Pseudodoxia* so that it might engage the latest in the advancement of learning, and mentally to explore the human and natural history of the entire world, the older Browne's seemingly inexhaustible curiosity about, and command of, the macrocosm began and ended at home.

1. RESTORATION AND WITCHCRAFT

At the outset of 1660, as General Monck made his way to London without having made his intentions fully clear, the gentry of Norfolk and Norwich presented him with what Evans has called the "boldest and the most defiant" of the several petitions he received.[2] Beginning with the gentry's dismay at "our sad Distractions and Divisions, both in Church and State," the Address decries "the Miseries of an unnaturall Civil War, The too frequent interruptions of Government, the Impositions of severall heavey Taxes, And the loud out-cryes of multitudes of undone and almost famished people, occasioned by a generall decay of Trade, which hath spread itself throughout the whole Nation, and these Counties in particular."[3] Amid the

[1] Thomas Browne, *Certain Miscellany Tracts* (London, 1683), A2v.

[2] Evans, *Seventeenth-Century Norwich*, 223.

[3] *An Address from the Gentry of Norfolk and Norwich to General Monck in 1660: Facsimile of a Manuscript in the Norwich Public Library*, intro. Hamon Le Strange, notes by Walter Rye (Norwich: Jarrold & Sons, 1913), 12–13.

often cramped columns appear the names of many families with whom the Brownes interacted, including Hobart, Townshend, Bacon, Le Strange, Pettus, Bendish, Woodhouse, and Le Gros—and three times the name Thomas Browne. Although none of the signatures can confidently be assigned to the famous author,[4] this document potently captures the climate in which virtually all the leading persons of Browne's county and city stood together for Monck, the Long Parliament, and ultimately for restoration as the best means for the recovery of the nation's health. When that restoration finally came, Browne was attentive to, and often vocal on its complex ramifications.

With the Restoration, Norwich expressions of monarchism included a parade as well as the jettisoning of any Interregnum arms of state; less officially and decorously, citizens burnt fires and celebrated raucously. At Browne's parish church, St Peter Mancroft, the church wardens recorded payments for the painting of the king's arms, along with bell ringers for the event at which the painting would be erected and for the proclamation of the king.[5] Browne would, of course, be assessed for these items, as surely as, during the 1660s, he would be assessed for support of the militia,[6] the poor,[7] maimed soldiers, reparations, the relief of mariners, and subsidies for the king and his army.[8] Living on the marketplace as he did, where civic processions, disorderly gatherings, and some public punishments (in the pillory) were often centered, Browne had an optimal vantage from which to view the extraordinary changes. In letters to his son Thomas, who was traveling at the time in France, he was full of the news both good and ill. "Some riseings there have been in London of the Anabaptists, fift Monarchie men and others," he noted, "but soon suppresd and 13 Executed" (Keynes, 4.5). Amid advice on how to travel in France, news about brother Edward's progress at Trinity College, Cambridge, and records of additions to his collections (especially coins), there is a steady stream of current events: the supplanting of aldermen who gained offices "in the usurpers time"; the "humiliation and fast" to prevent divine punishment "for the Abominable murther of King Charles the first"; the reparations of and return to worship in the cathedral, not least on coronation day in April 1661, when the Restoration "will be observed with great solemnity Especially at London; a new Parliament on the 8 of May and there is very good Choice almost in all places" (4.5–19). Yet while Browne was pleased with the victory of two Royalists in the city elections to the Parliament, he also recognized a profound division in local society that would remain largely underground until the last years of his life. Even in 1661, the two Royalists were selected for Parliament "against all opposition that could possibly bee made."

In letters to his son Thomas from April 1661, Browne captured the diverse effects of Restoration. The return to Lent was good for the fishing industry; control

[4] *An Address*, 19. For a recent assessment of this document, see Killeen, *Biblical Scholarship*, 193–4.

[5] NRO MC 2577/2/6 984x6, no foliation.

[6] In June 1665, his house and grounds were assessed at 2*s*.10*d*; his personal property at 2*s*. 0*d*.

[7] NRO NCR Case 20c.

[8] NRO PD 26/725.

over the militia was "in good hands through all England"; clergy returned to "the Liturgie or Common Prayer," and began to hold communions. With the impression (at least in Browne's circles) that "by degrees most will come to Conformitie," Browne painted a picture of the jubilation and charity, with some retribution thrown in for good measure, with "Cromwell hangd and burnt every where, whose head is now upon Westminster hall, together with Ireton and Bradshows" (Keynes, 4.19). Perhaps the two most important bits of news from Norwich were indicators of the future. On June 24, 1661, Browne reported to Thomas that "in Norwich the Court of Aldermen and Common Councell have made a law to resort to the Cathedrall every Sunday, and to be not only at Sermon but at Prayers wch they observe" (4.10). In this kernel lay the future conflict between drastic measures for forcing conformity (with the relatively conservative Presbyterians conflated with other nonconformists into the category of Dissent), as well as counter-measures from both sides of the religious spectrum on behalf of toleration and inclusiveness. Then, in August 1661, Browne reported that "affairs goe quietly on with us both in Religious and Civill Concernments." In Norwich at least, such peace and calm would persevere into the 1670s, then come undone for the rest of Browne's life.

As though already aware of the precarious and fleeting nature of human events and news, Browne dismissed such matters as "these small things" and redirected Thomas's attention to his Latin studies and to moral and spiritual concerns. Even so, news is everywhere in the letters addressed to this future member of the British Navy, for instance, the diseases afflicting people in France and Norfolk; the fetching of the queen from Portugal; the recall of Commonwealth money; the high price of corn; and the regular presence and preaching of "my loveing friend" Bishop Edward Reynolds in the cathedral where "he sitteth in his seat against the pulpit, handsomly built up and in his Episcopall vestments, and pronounceth the Blessing or the Peace of God etc at the end, where there is commonly a very numerous Congregation and an Excellent sermon by some Preacher of the Combination" (Keynes, 4.14). In a sermon delivered at St Peter Mancroft on September 22, 1661, Reynolds epitomized the spirit of reconciliation when, in celebrating the rites of ordination, he rejected the extremes of self-aggrandizing, tyrannical clergy and wild sectarian preachers alike, and praised those forms of worship that aspire to both external decency and scriptural simplicity.[9]

In 1662, Browne himself made news when his testimony in a witchcraft trial confronted him with the severe implications of his learning. Prior to the trial of Amy Denny and Rose Cullender in Bury St Edmunds in 1662, Browne had tended to insist on certainty regarding the existence of witches while conceding that each case presented ontological as well as judicial dilemmas.[10] Although Browne never wavered in his belief in witchcraft, and asserted that belief against Denny and Cullender at the trial, he sometimes purveyed a keen awareness, even at the trial, that

[9] Edward Reynolds, *Twenty-Five Sermons Preached upon Several Occasions* (1663), separately paginated, 19–20, 32.

[10] The most important account of this trial is Gilbert Geis and Ivan Bunn, *A Trial of Witches: A Seventeenth-Century Witchcraft Prosecution* (New York: Routledge, 1997).

any honest explanation of witchcraft was bound to be complex and potentially confusing. Insofar as parents of afflicted children often summoned medical advice, it was frequently left up to the physician to decide when medicine needed to give way to spiritual and judicial remedies—when what was thought to be disease was held to be enchantment.

Five things made the interpretation of witchcraft problematic for learned Englishmen such as Browne. One was that medical learning specifically, but also natural studies more generally, were implicated in magic and so liable to some of the suspicions of devilish work that were affixed to witches. A second was that English Protestantism was divided over what might be done to counter witchcraft—over the extent to which acceptable spiritual means such as prayer might still require forms of counter-magic against the devil's devices.[11] Although, in *Pseudodoxia*, Browne credited the tendency of witches to speak with dogs and cats (Robbins, ed., *Pseudodoxia Epidemica*, 164), and cautioned about the devil's self-interest in dissuading us from a belief in witches ("whose concession infers his coexistency," 65), he also treated the breaking of eggshells "to prevent witchcraft" as a childish superstition (425). A third was that each case presented those involved with social pressures: charges of witchcraft were commonly made in relatively small or tightly knit communities. As in the case of the Bury trial, the charges were often made by well-to-do citizens, habitually against poor, elderly, and isolated women with a reputation for witchery. To participate in a trial was to face the intensity of these neighborly relations, not least because the sessions of the Assizes where witches were often tried were major social events that drew huge crowds. English accounts of witchery were far more apt to stress the altercation between neighbors than they were to focus on a pact with the devil or strange doings at a black Sabbath. And they were apt to invoke gossipy conveyances of reputation as hard evidence against the indicted.[12] Making the social dynamic all the more charged was the fact that the afflicted were often children ill-equipped or unable to speak for themselves—indeed in the Bury case, much of the crucial testimony came from parents on behalf of their children. Browne's concerns about witchcraft would have been heightened by virtue of the fact that pediatric medicine and childcare were central to most cases.[13]

Fourth, the effects of witchcraft needed to be distinguished from those of possession, and on this dilemma Browne seemed especially worried. In his notebooks, he argued that

> We are no way doubtfull that there are wiches, butt have not been alwayes satisfied in the application of their wichcrafts or whether the parties accused or suffering have been guiltie of that abomination, or persons under such affliction suffered from such hands. In ancient time, wee reade of many possessed & probably there are many still, butt the common crye & generall opinion of wiches hath confounded that of possession,

[11] James Sharpe, *Instruments of Darkness: Witchcraft in England, 1550–1750* (New York: Penguin, 1996), 88.

[12] On gossip see Sharpe, *Instruments of Darkness*, 163.

[13] On childcare and witchcraft, see Sharpe, *Instruments of Darkness*, 175.

> men salving such strange effects from veneficiall agents & out of the partie suffering. Many strange things have been done beyond the salvo of human reason wch might proceed as well from possession as veneficatio. (Keynes, 3.294)

The question of just how possession interacted with but also differed from witchcraft was a highly vexing one in seventeenth-century England, not least because possession might be thought to require some special priestly (and papist) exorcism.[14] Related to the problem of possession was the fifth difficulty, that Francis Bacon had called upon new philosophers applying his inductive method to examine cases of nature at its borders with the preternatural—cases that included witchcraft.

For Browne, then, there were intellectual, professional, social, spiritual, and moral challenges to be faced if a case of witchcraft were to be judged aright. Recent local history resonated in 1662 as well: in the first decade of Browne's life in East Anglia, the 1640s, the pursuit of witches carried out by Matthew Hopkins had shown just how destructive the cry against and opinion of witches could prove in a community, and it is quite possible that this legacy hung over the proceedings at Bury in 1662.[15] To make matters stranger, there was in the Restoration a national decline in witchcraft prosecutions, yet leading spokesmen for advanced learning such as Joseph Glanvill and Henry More had come out unequivocally in support of a belief in witches as a major defense against the encroachment of atheism.[16]

According to one observer, the Bury trial was a long one, lasting for seven or eight days, with each day of the proceedings lasting well into the evening.[17] We learn from the same source that Sir Matthew Hale had enlisted the advice of "divers Physitians, and other learned Men."[18] In his testimony against Denny and Cullender, Browne expressed his belief that while witchcraft was very real, it was far from simple. As reported in *A Tryal of Witches at the Assizes Held at Bury St. Edmonds* (London, 1682), Browne's involvement happened like this:

> There was also Dr. *Brown* of *Norwich*, a Person of great knowledge; who after this Evidence given, and upon view of the three persons in Court, was desired to give his Opinion, what he did conceive of them: and he was clearly of Opinion, that the persons were Bewitched; and said, That in *Denmark* there had been lately a great Discovery of Witches, who used the very same way of Afflicting Persons, by conveying Pins

[14] Sharpe, *Instruments of Darkness*, 209.

[15] For another local trial at the time, see James M. Rosenheim, ed., *The Notebook of Robert Doughty 1662–1665* (*Norfolk Record Society*, 54, 1989), 89–90.

[16] See Sharpe, *Instruments of Darkness*, 244–6; Geis and Bunn, *A Trial of Witches*, 6.

[17] In the extant records of the Suffolk Assize (National Archives, ASSI 16 4/1), the indictments are found on small rectangular slips. The Latin texts use words such as "fascinatrix," "incantrix," "diabolica," "males et diabolicas," "fascinac[i]ones," then offer English translations of the key terms such as witchcraft, charms, enchantments, incantations. There is an indictment for each charge so that both Rose Cullender and Amy Denny have several each; the year is given as 14th of Charles II, that is 1662. In the Suffolk Record Office (Lowestoft, MS AR 992/1) an eighteenth-century compilation of materials concerning the trial includes some anecdotes passed down through the decades but nothing pertinent to Browne's involvement.

[18] Preface to *A Collection of Modern Relations of Matter of Fact Concerning Witches & Witchcraft upon the Persons of People* (1693), A4r.

> into them, and crooked as these Pins were, with Needles and Nails. And his Opinion was, That the Devil in such cases did work upon the Bodies of Men and Women, upon a Natural Foundation, (that is) to stir up, and excite such humours super-abounding in their Bodies to a great excess, whereby he did in an extraordinary Manner Afflict them with such Distempers as their Bodies were most subject to, as particularly appeared in these Children; for he conceived, that these swooning Fits were Natural, and nothing else but what they call the Mother, but only heightned to a great excess by the subtilty of the Devil, co-operating with the Malice of these which we term Witches, at whose Instance he doth these Villanies.[19]

One obviously important, yet tricky feature of this testimony is that it is depicted as an intervention ad hoc: Browne is "desired to give his Evidence" at a certain point in the proceedings "after this Evidence" and "upon view of the three Persons in Court." The phrasing of this passage leaves open the possibility that Browne's testimony was not considered an inevitable or a necessary part of the trial but a timely show of "great knowledge" as a rhetorically effective instrument of prosecution (Geis and Bunn, 82). This reading is reinforced by Geis and Bunn's recovery of what was meant by "the three Persons in Court." For if they are right, the prosecution was running aground because three leading men were skeptical that the women on trial were actually guilty. On the other hand, Browne was about sixty miles from his home in Norwich: did he just happen to be nearby on his medical peregrinations? Or was he in fact summoned by Sir Matthew Hale, with whom he had coincided for a few years at Oxford, or by someone else involved in the trial, for instance, Sir Edmund Bacon or a friend that Browne shared with Samuel Pacy, Sir John Pettus?[20]

It has always been known that at least one man—Sir John Keeling—was critical of the prosecution. Prior to Browne's testimony, the case had unfolded as follows. In February 1662, Samuel Pacy, a merchant and nonconformist from the Suffolk coastal town of Lowestoft, had secured an indictment against Amy Denny and Rose Cullender from county Justice of the Peace, Sir Edmund Bacon, in the inland parish of Redgrave. Bacon's involvement might help to explain how Browne became involved; after all, Browne had dedicated *Garden of Cyrus* to his uncle and had praised the JP himself as "my true and noble friend" (Geis and Bunn, 21–2). Pacy was not alone in his complaints against the women; the indictment included fourteen counts concerning several families, with the most dramatic charges stemming from Dorothy Durrant's claim that back in the 1650s, Amy Denny had suckled and sickened her infant William (the only male victim) and caused the death of stepdaughter Elizabeth.

After the Durrant business, Samuel Pacy testified that his two daughters (Elizabeth, 11, and Deborah, 9) had been bewitched by the two women. The father did all the talking for the girls, with the older so overwhelmed as to be unable to testify, while the younger was deemed too feeble even to come to court.

[19] Geis and Bunn, *A Trial of Witches*, 223.
[20] For these possibilities, see Geis and Bunn, *A Trial of Witches*, 21–2 and 82.

Yet it was precisely the drama of their performances of bewitchment—including the report of Elizabeth's counter-magical scratching of Denny's face—that prompted Sergeant Keeling at the very least to have his doubts (Geis and Bunn, 55). Pacy, however, provided this portion of the trial with a gravitas that impressed the reporter: he was a wealthy merchant with substantial ties to the fishing industry and to real estate ventures who also happened to carry himself with unimpeachable sobriety and Christian faith. He himself would run afoul of the Restoration authorities on account of his nonconformity, but in 1662 he was still considered a pillar of the community.

Pacy's daughters were characterized as overcome by apparitions and fits, the variety of which was as noteworthy as the most extraordinary effects—the vomiting of pins and needles (Geis and Bunn, 67–70). After the Pacys, there were other witnesses to the witchcraft yet the two Pacy daughters proved crucial, and other witnesses helped shore up the evidence for their wild afflictions, including the testimony "that Amy Denny had predicted (and therefore presumably caused) Elizabeth Pacy to have her mouth opened with a tap in order to feed her" (Geis and Bunn, 77). Above all, it was the claim that the Pacy girls would be sent into fits by the touch of the accused that led to expressions of skepticism, a trap laid by the skeptics, and the crucial question of how Browne's testimony factored into the trial.

Because Sergeant Keeling had a reputation of being adversarial to Hale in particular and mean-spirited in general, his isolation in the 1682 report as the one skeptic at the trial made a certain sense. Yet this singling out of Keeling left it unclear why the report at first listed three "known persons," including Sergeants Erasmus Earl and Robert Bernard together with Keeling. A manuscript discovered among Richard Baxter's papers maintains that all three of these men were unhappy with the evidence "and thought it not sufficient to convict the prisoners" (quoted in Geis and Bunn, 79). It was all three by this account who tricked the Pacy girl into swooning (while blindfolded) at the touch of a neutral party, and therefore a group of distinguished men rather than a solitary hothead whose skepticism Browne's learning was meant to impress.

We cannot be sure of course that Browne's testimony occurred at precisely the point in the trial where the 1682 report places it, and questions about its placement have fortified scholars in their attempts either to accentuate or to minimize its pivotal import.[21] Also unclear is what Browne had in mind in summoning corroborating evidence from Denmark. One possibility is that Browne is referring to a notorious case of a boy bewitched in Bergen, Norway, though a major account of the trial, Thomas Bartholin's, would appear only a year later in 1663 (Geis and Bunn, 85).

[21] For Browne's supporters, see Dorothy Tyler, "A Review of the Interpretation of Sir Thomas Browne's Part in the Witch Trial of 1664," *Anglia* 54 (1930), 178–95; and Malcolm Letts, "Sir Thomas Browne and Witchcraft," *Notes and Queries*, 11th series, 5 (1912), 221–3, which points out that we cannot be certain when Browne was actually in court other than for his testimony (222). Edmund Gosse figures among the long line of condemners.

Three things, however, *are* clear about Browne's testimony. First, the prosecution hoped that his learning and reputation would overwhelm any doubts to the contrary: if the chief diagnostician of vulgar errors supported conviction, how could a jury have doubts? Second, Browne provided the basis for a guilty verdict without ever once declaring that Denny and Cullender were guilty. Third, even if the defendants were judged to have been guided by lethal malice rather than menstruation, Browne set a standard for the complex analysis of causation that argued for the devil's natural modus operandi: the devil created heightened effects from the materials of our excessive humors, in this case those associated with young female's menstruation and hysteria, and he did so at the malicious solicitation of older women whom "we term witches." This naturalizing of Satanic evil is not surprising from the author who in *Religio Medici* derived some legacies of natural philosophy from a devilish origin. What is less clear about Browne's recourse to a mixed etiology is what role he would find for a physician in its remedy.

Hale's summation to the jury shared in Browne's combination of a "deep and unquestioning religious faith" and learned caution (Geis and Bunn, 99). In the case of Denny and Cullender he refused to synopsize the evidence lest he distort it. In a half an hour, the guilty verdict was rendered, the accused having never said very much in their defense and without any legal representation whatsoever. They were hanged on March 17, 1662. One thing about his recorded testimony underscores the difficulty that Browne experienced in mediating among the claims of faith, medicine, charity, and duty: even if he corroborated the bewitchment of the victims, he never claimed to know whether Denny and Cullender were responsible.

As his library shows, Browne continued to study the problem of witchcraft: witness his ownership of *The Opinion of Witchcraft Vindicated* (1670).[22] As Browne's testimony made clear, thinking about witchcraft was for him an extension from other areas of thought, in part metaphysical and epistemological but also more specifically medical, since Browne's training in Montpellier had inaugurated his fascination with questions of menstruation, generation, and motherhood. Yet, inasmuch as Browne's medical practice involved him in the care of local families, his authority on witchcraft was also implicated in the complex ties that bound East Anglian society together.[23] By the 1660s, moreover, Browne's connections to leading families in the county were legal as well as vocational, social, and personal.[24] Closer to home, the subtle evils in the world were of enormous concern to Browne now that he was a dedicated father as well as a caring physician whose overriding source of anxiety was the moral, spiritual, economic, physical, social, and educational welfare of his children and patients.

[22] Finch, *Catalogue of the Libraries*, 52.

[23] See Keynes, 4.122, 192, 222; and NRO MC 107/1, f. 12, discussed below. The Dr Browne involved in a controversy over a contested clerical living in the Doughty family is probably Dr Thomas Browne, DD, canon of Windsor (NRO BL/Y/1/21 37r).

[24] See for instance Derbyshire Record Office D231 M/E 507 and D231 M/T 407, title deeds relating to the Norfolk and Suffolk estates of the Okeover family of Okeover, Derbyshire, which includes a transaction between, among other parties, Browne and Sir Thomas Pettus.

2. HEALING AND PARENTING

As a physician in the Restoration period, Browne treated leading families from across the political spectrum in Norwich and Norfolk, an act of implicit mediation that would only become more challenging when in the mid-1670s local politics became bitterly divisive. Although little remains of Browne's own political activities from the first half of the 1660s—in 1662, he donated £10 for a voluntary gift of funds to King Charles II[25]—he served as a thread of continuity among local families who, for the most part in the 1660s, managed to maintain what John Evans has called an "uncommonly tranquil" co-existence until bitter rivalry broke out in the last years of Browne's life.[26]

Among Browne's prominent patients was Sir Robert Paston, whose chronic bad health insured that Browne had much ado to assist him against pain. But physician and patient shared much more than the medical challenges posed by the latter's girth. Already in the 1650s, Paston had been instrumental in introducing Browne to John Evelyn. As a 1662 letter from Paston makes clear, the two men also shared a wide range of intellectual interests, from the collection of medals and manuscripts to chemical experimentation. Paston's massive collection of paintings, sculpture, jewels, books, and curiosities at his estate, Oxnead Hall, offered a larger version of Browne's own residence, so much so that Sir Robert was constantly struggling with debt.[27] A letter from Paston to Browne conveys something of the exuberance which prompted this state of affairs. The letter also makes it clear that the two men have discussed alchemical experiments at length.[28]

Browne continued to serve as a physician for Sir John Hobart, writing to him in August 1666 with preventatives and remedies for the plague, as well as with an expression of solicitude toward and comfort for the family in a time of great anxiety. In the later 1670s and early 1680s, Hobart's Whig leanings would make him a prominent rival to Paston in local politics, with insult added to rivalry by virtue of the fact that Hobart's Blickling Hall would profit from Sir Robert's financial straits in the form of statues and fountains that were secured from Oxnead.[29] Yet in the 1660s, Hobart was too busy trying to overcome his affiliations with Cromwell to pose much of a contrast to Paston, and both their homes figured prominently in the king's visit in 1671. Browne also served as a physician for, among other leading families, the Knyvetts and the Townshends, whose estate at Raynham Browne praised as the "noblest pyle among us." Both families entered the Restoration with clear and obvious Royalist credentials, yet Sir Horatio Townshend would be subsumed by what James M. Rosenheim has called "the precociously fevered character of Norfolk political life" in the 1670s and fall

[25] See Phyllis Mary Williams, *Norwich Subscriptions to the Voluntary Gift of 1662*, *Norfolk Record Society* 1 (1931), 69–86, at 85.

[26] Evans, *Seventeenth-Century Norwich*, 245.

[27] See Robert Wenley, "Robert Paston and the Yarmouth Collection," *Norfolk Archaeology* 41 (1991), 113–44.

[28] Paston's letter, from Rawlinson 391, is printed in Wilkin, *Works*, 1.409.

[29] For the letter, see Keynes, 4.383–4; for the rivalry, Ketton-Cremer, *Norfolk Assembly*, 216–17.

short of his desires for royal favor.[30] Among other families, the Cokes figured among Browne's patients; despite a grinding schedule of consultations "daylie out of the towne & not returning before night," Browne was eager around Christmas time to attend the ailing Madame Coke (Keynes, 4.390).

In East Anglia Browne's medical services were much in demand. Writing to his brother from Yarmouth in March 1661, one George Harper expressed the family's desire that all possible means be enlisted to secure Browne's services for their mother; in the event that Browne cannot make it that week, Harper cautions, Dr. Robinson should be substituted but "Lett not Doktor Robbenson know that we haue sent to Doktor Browne."[31] Browne was called on for mundane tasks such as filling out certificates of sickness.[32] But families also looked to him for an understanding of, and hope in the face of, disease. Thus Elizabeth Rous wrote in a letter to her father Thomas Knyvett that, given the latter's increasing pain, "I hope docter browne will find both ye cause, and remedie."[33] Browne's Christian and medical duties were most cohesively united in Norwich's public policies for the care of the indigent, for St Peter Mancroft was often assessed for funds that would pay for the services of medical experts such as Browne in attending to the various ailments of the poor.[34]

Browne's skill at navigating the social context of his medical profession can be seen in his interaction with Lord and Lady Maidstone. On the one hand, in 1670, Browne was treating Elizabeth, Lady Maidstone for the fluor albus or "white flux," a condition that required the physician's greatest delicacy and care, not least because the patient had a "weake & tender body," might in fact be pregnant, but lacked any experience with the changes that her body would undergo during parturition, including miscarriage.[35] On the other hand, Browne's son Edward and daughter Anne were enlisted in 1670 to support the testimony of their friend Lady Maidstone in a scandal involving another prominent patient of their father's, Lady Maidstone's brother, William Windham of Felbrigg Hall. Having already taken their fair share of her brother's resources, Elizabeth and her husband claimed in 1670 that Windham had promised them £5,000. But from Windham's business manager, Robert Pepper, we learn that more than money was involved, since Anne Browne, now Fairfax, had "asserted that Windham had injured her reputation." Pepper was blunt in informing Windham that "Mrs Fairfax is openly your Enemy

[30] James M. Rosenheim, *The Townshends of Raynham: Nobility in Transition in Restoration and Early Hanoverian England* (Middletown, CT: Wesleyan University Press, 1989), 7. For Browne's attendance on Thomas Knyvett of Ashwellthorpe, Norfolk, there is a letter in the Princeton University Library with Browne's medical message involving "things convenient for clyster & Julep & Syrupes" as well as advice concerning diet. The letter is in the Robert Taylor Collection, RTC01.

[31] NRO MS Y/L 13/17.

[32] NRO CON 21, 1663–66, a holograph: "These are to certifie that Mr Iohn Cromwell hath been dangerously sick and still remaineth under such weakenesse that hee cannot expose himself unto the Ayre, or go out of his chamber or house without great danger."

[33] NRO KNY 750–84 372x5, no date.

[34] The workings of this policy are laid out in the Mayor's Court Books, NRO MF RO 81/4, 1654–66, and NCR Case 16b. For Browne's specific services, see chapter 11 in this volume.

[35] Browne's letter on this case is in Sloane MS 1833, f. 119.

and pretends you have mightily wrong'd her..., and she will have satisfaction too."[36] Despite Browne's obvious dilemma, he alienated neither Windham (who would model a garden on Browne's *Garden of Cyrus*) or the Maidstones, about whom Dorothy Browne cheerfully spoke to Edward as late as 1679 (Keynes, 4.116).

Over the course of the 1660s Browne's medical travels around the county were regular and demanding; indeed, in 1669, he would secure the lease of a meadow for the horse that he rode on medical travels.[37] Nor was Browne's medical sphere of influence confined to the local area. In the 1660s, for instance, Browne's recipes were appearing among the notes of other physicians.[38] In August 1668, he was consulting with Dr John Maplet on the case "of a little boy who cannot speak" and whose body was wracked by weakness (Keynes, 4.250). A letter of recommendation for a chirurgeon lent Browne an opportunity to write the famous astrologer William Lilly in February 1670, though therein Browne pled some ignorance regarding both the skills of the man in question and the circumstances in which medicine was practiced in London, where a surgeon would be "much confined and restrayned unto companies" (Keynes, 4.295). In addition, Edward's travels abroad would soon extend Browne's consulting to an international scope: on February 22, 1669, he wrote to Mr. Jenkinson of Hamburg on two medical problems, a friend's "Gonorrhœa non virulenta" and Jenkinson's own "colica labora" (Keynes, 4.386).

At home in Norwich, considerations of parental love and duty prevailed in Browne's life, as well as his continuing leadership in the city's medical vocation. With the baptism taking place on September 5, 1662, the family welcomed their final child, daughter Frances (the second child so-named), to join siblings Edward, Thomas, Anne, Elizabeth, and Mary.[39] In the 1660s, however, family was also a source of grief, for a son named Charles was buried on April 13 of the same year. In the 1660s, Browne's extended family would suffer losses—including Dorothy's father in 1661. By decade's end, his immediate family would also experience a marriage, Anne's, with the result of Browne's first grandchildren. Browne carefully listed all six surviving children in their proper birth order in a pedigree that he filled out in 1664.[40] He was less knowing or careful in inscribing his ancestors. During the visitation made by Sir Edward Bysshe, the Clarenceux King of Arms, Browne laid claim to the entitlement to bear arms, described as "argent, two bendlets sable, between as many pellets."[41] The crest was given as a lion sejant. While the

[36] See R. W. Ketton-Cremer, *Felbrigg: The Story of a House* (London: Rupert Hart-Davis, 1962), 52. Cf. Griffiths, ed., *William Windham's Green Book*, 26.

[37] DCN 24/3, the chapter book of Norwich Cathedral for 1669, f. 90r, where Browne is granted the "little meadow...now in his occupation during his naturall life" at the cost of ten shillings per annum; in 1670, chapter records note that he will have the meadow for twenty-one years "from this day" (100v). Less clear are the reasons why in March 1660, he purchased marshland from his kinsman Edward Mileham.

[38] See for instance the recipes for one Mrs. Clement, April 1663, in Sloane MS 175, f. 3r.

[39] Recorded in the parish register for St Peter Mancroft.

[40] I am grateful to Robert Noel, Lancaster Herald in the College of Arms, for confirming the details of the original document of the visitation.

[41] See Walter Rye, *Some Historical Essays Chiefly Relating to Norfolk*, part 6 (Norwich: H. W. Hunt, 1928), 454; and A. W. Hughes Clarke and Arthur Campling, eds., *The Visitation of Norfolk Anno Domini 1664* (Norfolk Record Society, 1934), vol. 1.

differences between these arms and those of his father's Cheshire family were relatively slight,[42] the pedigree offered to Bysshe on this occasion erroneously derived his paternal line from a Richard Browne.[43]

While Browne's life in his house on the marketplace involved him in the most mundane of domestic concerns,[44] his children were already proving sources of fascination but also anxiety for the aging physician. Browne's one letter to son Edward from 1665 indicates that the horrible plague of that year is still upon them, "the sicknesse being great still" (Keynes, 4.27). In a postscript to the letter, Browne purveys the fatherly and professional dilemma that he faces in deciding whether to abandon Norwich for healthier climes. Given the affection that Edward, like brother Thomas, expresses for his sisters Anne (Nancy), Elizabeth (Betty), Mary (Mol), and Frances (Frank), it is not surprising that Browne wants to assure his son of their safety: "The sickness wch God so long withheld from us is now in Norwich. I intend to send your sisters to Claxton, & if it encreaseth to remove 3 or 4 miles of, where I may bee serviceable upon occasion to my freinds in other diseases" (Keynes, 4.28). Although the question of whether physicians, among other leading members of society, should abandon their plagued cities had long been a complex matter for casuists and commentators, Browne seems quite clear that there is little if anything that he can do about the plague, and that his primary obligations are to family and county friends, whose other ailments he might be able to remedy.

Of his two sons, Edward and Thomas, Browne took more delight in the one, Thomas, that epitomized the vitality of his father's spirit rather than (in the case of Edward) the trajectory of his vocation. When young Thomas travelled on holiday through France, Browne offered him ongoing advice about the keys to happiness, health, social success, a rounded education, and a sound Protestant faith. Browne was in Yarmouth in December 1660, ensuring that Thomas's travel expenses would be covered, but he was also penning his strategies for the traveler to avoid melancholy, minimize expense, thrive with the civilized French, worship both privately and publicly in an acceptable way, and observe as well as record and draw the particular or "remarkable" sights of Bordeaux in a maximally informed and attentive manner. Browne's letters are brimming with moral exhortations, social guidelines, intellectual or educational directives (especially about learning Latin and French)—and obvious, deeply felt admiration and love. Readers of these letters hardly need Dorothy's words to her son that "yr father was well pleased with yr account of yr Voiage and it will Please very much if you Continue informing of him still what you observe there" (Keynes, 4.6). But Dorothy also conveys a sense

[42] In the *Chester Courant*, November 15, 1899, William Ferguson Irvine noted that while Browne's arms comprised argent, two bends sable, in sinister chief and dexter base a pellet, the Cheshire Brownes had two bendlets between as many mullets.

[43] See Wilkin, *Works*, 1.ciii.

[44] In August 1663, the Norwich Assembly Book recorded Browne's request that the six posts he had erected to support his house not be removed by the city, which approved his request but required his heirs or assignees to pay a fee for the posts annually at Michaelmas (Assembly Book, 1642–68, 247r, in NRO).

of the tightly knit family unit, not just in her news of Thomas's siblings but also in her remark that "All the servants present their Loves to you and are mighty joyd to hear of you and will observe yr Commands" (4.6). Unlike later letters to Edward, with whom Browne's interactions were more complex, these missives offer no sign that Browne is guiding his son toward a career in medicine. Rather, Browne seems far more interested in a well-rounded education in civility, whether this involves knowledge of antiquity or numismatics, an appreciation for "Coynac wines," the practical study of salt works, wines, and viniculture, proper punctuation, ongoing interaction with "Civill Company" (4.7) or behavior which is "Patient Civil and debonair unto all" (4.9). The letters from home are attended by packages for the darling boy who sends his father "pritty stones and insects" for his collection (4.15). No doubt Thomas's journal recording these travels in France was pleasing to his father, who urged his son to notice the world with the careful particularity that can be found, for instance, in Thomas's catalogue of the curiosities in the treasury of Chartres Cathedral (Wilkin, 1.22). Yet in this list, something more than antiquarian empiricism comes through: Thomas manages all at once to suggest a suspicion of vulgar errors side by side with a romantic evocation of wonder. This combination of critical acumen and intensity of experience was more fully on display in an account of the tour Thomas and Edward took of the English counties between Norwich and Chester in September 1662.[45] Although the account may well have been a collaboration of the two brothers, Thomas's dynamism and engaging sense of adventure are palpable in the often first person singular narrative.

Thomas's service in the Navy, beginning in 1664, did a great deal to reinforce Browne's idealization of his character. Yet Thomas's military exploits also worried Browne who, with Dorothy, expressed anxiety as well as pride regarding Thomas's resolve to join the Navy against the Dutch. On November 25, 1664, Browne attempted to moderate and direct his younger son's zeal for military heroism:

> I presume you are in London where you may satisfie yourself in the buisinesse. Do nothing rashly butt as you find just grounds for your advantage, wch will hardly bee at the best deservings without good & faythfull friends; No sudden advantage for rawe though dangerous services. There is another & more safe way whereby Capt. Brookes & others come in credit, by going about 2 yeares before they were capable of places, where I am not well acquainted. God & our good freinds advise you. (Keynes, 4.17)

It was rarely that Browne found himself completely out of his depth, but in the protocols of military advancement, let alone the rigors and extremities of sea battle, Browne's indirect social acquaintances—he knew Captain Brooks's brother Sir Robert—and extensive reading in ancient naval conflicts were clearly inadequate

[45] Thanks to Antonia Moon for her advice on this manuscript. The written account of the journey is not definitely Thomas's; the handwriting of the manuscript resembles Edward's more than his brother's, though it may well be a copy of an original, made with an eye toward presentation to their father. One piece of evidence for its being a copy is that the scribe left several pages blank for the insertion of verse couplets on the Devil's Arse caves in Derbyshire. Wilkin claimed to have found internal evidence supporting Thomas's authorship, but did not say what it was (1.lxxv).

if movingly well intentioned. Even so, Browne persisted in his heartfelt advice to his younger son and namesake: against wearing periwigs, on learning Latin, and (of more immediate importance) regarding the mastery of "practicall mathematicks & use of Instrume[nt]s."

In his letter to Edward of September 1665, Browne was eager to correct any mistaken reports that Edward may have received about the progress of the Dutch war:

> Whatever your gazett sayth that the Indian fleet is come in without seeing any of our shipps, wee are sure wee have 2 of their best in England beside other shipps making up in all the number of thirtie, & what shipps ether of warre or marchands came home unto them were such as wee could not meet or not reach, having got the start of us: it holds still that the prisoners amount to about 3 thousand. (Keynes, 4.27–8)

It is a revealing moment in Browne's correspondence. Unlike the First Dutch War under Cromwell in the 1650s, the Second was going to prove a disaster and disgrace for the English Navy in whose service young Thomas Browne had staked his life and honor. It was, moreover, a controversial war falteringly pursued. Browne was keen to give Edward the optimistic English take on the action, lest his elder son be misled by European journalism into doubting the success and esteem of his brother's enterprise. Yet neither learning nor wishful thinking would save Thomas from a premature, if honorable death.

In March 1665, a letter from the Dutch translator of *Religio*, Abraham van Berckel, clarified why Browne was bound to have been conflicted about his son's involvement in the Second Dutch War. Writing from Leiden, Berckel underscores the deleterious effects of the war on scholarly communication between the two nations. By contrast, Browne's disposition is twice compared to the sun's capacity to warm and invigorate all sorts of men. As a universally acclaimed and magnetic force in the commonwealth of letters, Browne offers the very antithesis to a war that touts "grave differences and dangerous contentions between the King of England and the States of Holland." For Berckel, Browne represents learning and virtue, friendship, the unity of "pious and learned minds," and a Stoic honesty that rejects disguise in order to "assert the principles of incorruptible and undefiled truth, and penetrate with not uncertain step to its sacred threshold."[46]

Browne's son Thomas showed no such opposition to the Dutch war and appears to have embraced his naval service with fervor. In the last letters which survive from Browne's correspondence with his son, and despite the fact that Thomas may never have matriculated at Cambridge,[47] the father fashioned his son into a paragon yet with lingering fears for a suicidal rashness that Browne himself had expressed in early versions of *Religio*. "I am glad to you like Lucan so well; I wish more military men could read him," Browne wrote in February 1667,

[46] Translation of this letter is in Keynes, 4.335–9.

[47] He was admitted pensioner at Trinity College on May 22, 1663, but there is no record of his matriculation.

> Butt I hope you are more taken with the verses then the subject, and rather embrace the expression then the example. And this I the rather hint unto you, because the like, though in another waye, is sometimes practised in the Kings shipps; when in desperate cases they blowe up the same. For though I know you are sober & considerative, yet knowing you also to bee of great resolution; & having also heard from ocular testimonies with what undaunted & persevering courage you have demeaned yourself in great difficulties, & knowing your Captaine to bee a stout & resolute man, & withall the cordiall friendshippe that is betweene you, I cannot omitt my earnest prayers unto god to deliver you from such a temptation. (Keynes, 4.21)

Having argued against a Stoic's suicidal resolution in the face of despair, Browne details the "various accidents" that a soldier may well have to face, above all imprisonment, and he is eager to have his son understand that "after a due resistance," captivity "is no disparagement." Urging Thomas to find examples of honorable captivity in his memory of Plutarch, Browne reminds his son of his best characteristics: "God hath given you a stout, butt a generous and mercifull heart withall, & in all your life you could never behold any person in miserie butt with compassion & releif; wch hath been notable in you from a child." Although this means that Thomas is in good favor with God, Browne repeats that he must trust God to protect him in the event of a "disaster" and on a divine schedule to remove Thomas from the life through which God has guided him. Browne had ample reason by this time to worry about the disastrous. In stark contrast to the English triumph over the Dutch navy in the 1650s, and despite some initial high spirits on the part of the English hawks, the tables had been decidedly turned in the second war.[48] Disillusionment with the war was not eased by the just perception that, although the ideological relations between the two countries were considerably complex, there was no getting away from the fact that the war was grounded in a longstanding commercial rivalry.

Thomas's letters reflect the severe challenges of the war, not least the thunderously violent and gory experience of naval battle itself, but they also encapsulate his resolution to confront the disastrous with heroic intensity. Eager to keep his father informed of the goings-on, "especially being now so neare the grand action, from which I would by no meanes bee absent," Thomas testified on July 16, 1666, from on board the *Marie Rose* that "I extremely long for that thundering day; wherein I hope you shall heare wee have behaved ourselves like men, and to the honour of our country." What follows is a frank and vivid re-creation of human experience under duress (Wilkin, 1.129). If Edward's reports from his travels tend toward straightforward observation and record, Thomas offers a soldier's version of religio medici, complete with an "o altitudo" as well as the more workaday features of human experience. Thomas's letters show his desire to be a scholar according to his father's wishes and to entertain his father with stories and observations, but scholarship proves difficult to pursue on the high seas of battle. A letter from September 1666 is dire in its reports of hostile weather, the casualties suffered in battle, and

[48] For the Second Dutch War, see J. R. Jones, *The Anglo-Dutch Wars of the Seventeenth Century* (New York: Longman, 1996), 145–78.

above all soldierly discontent at the lack of pay, which prompts from Thomas a paean to personal charity on the order of his father's *Religio* (Wilkin, 1.133). Although this letter ends with a testimonial to Thomas's studies, as well as to the profound learning of an "honest Moore," it is clear that the Second Dutch War has made it especially difficult for the sincerest of men to retain their sense of honor and purpose.

In the last surviving letter from Browne to Thomas, the father attempts to help his son cope with bitter disappointment. Having exhorted Thomas always to thank God "for your great deliverances in so many fights, and dangers of the sea, whereto you have been exposed upon severall seas and in all seasons of the yeare," Browne sets out to frame Thomas's naval career and moral philosophy in ancient terms. First he recalls their readings in the history of naval battles, notes about which are extant in the Browne family papers. This Latin study of the ancient sea-fight begins and ends with scholarly imperatives and moral observations. As "memory slips away, age, time, events pass mostly into oblivion," it is crucial for scholars to keep those events alive, not by setting them down in some alternative order in a commonplace book, "but from a fresh reading of books to set down an abstract in free style, to include all that is difficult and worthy of note; whatever the author himself, the memory of like things, or natural genius supplies" (Keynes, 3.158–9). Here is Browne's typical desire for scholarly transmission to give new life and a fresh, productive context to old knowledge, a context fertilized by the note-taker's own associations, experiences, and projects in collaboration with the other ingenious scholars of his age.[49] In addition to notes on the rites, ship types, and battle accounts that he includes, Browne concludes his engagement with the writings of "Bayfius, Revius, and Scheffer" with the generalization that

> [t]he cause of this war was that of all wars, excess of prosperity. As wealth spreads, spirits rise, and lust and greed of power appear; thence men lose their sense of moderation, look with distaste on the prosperity of others, revolve disquiet in their mind, and throw over all settlement, for fear lest their enemies' wealth be firmly established, they put their own at risk; and finally (as happens in human affairs) fall into slavery when they seek to impose it, and earnestly courting good fortune, experience disaster. (Keynes, 3.162)

Whether Browne intended this final observation as a comment on the Dutch war, it is impossible to say. In a set of English notes on naval battles, Browne sought to answer the questions of an unnamed inquirer as well as to propose questions for further consideration, now with regard to more modern as well as ancient battles of the kind found in those histories of various peoples—of the Turks, or the Venetians, for instance—that Browne so enjoyed in his later years. In these notes, Browne generalizes that "in most navall fights some notable advantage, error, or unexpected occurrence hath determined the victory"—this, without saying anything about how providence might be involved (Keynes, 3.253).

[49] Cf. Antonia Moon, "'A Fresh Reading of Books': Some Note-Taking Practices of Thomas Browne," in Murphy and Todd, eds., "*A man very well studyed,*" 67–86.

Having reminded his son of such readings in naval history, Browne quotes an Aristotelian definition of fortitude that he gave Thomas as a rule when first he took on military service, and which now Browne repeats in order to praise his son for achieving the standard. Taken from a spurious work in the Aristotelian canon, the definition maintains that bravery resists the fear of death, shows constancy in the face of danger, and chooses an honest death over base servitude, a concession to the attractions of the Stoic's honorable pride. The definition adds that the brave man seeks to be the source of victory, and commits himself to labor and endurance. This latter emphasis, on toil and the endurance of difficulty, is one which the definition repeats in its conclusion, for in addition to daring, spiritedness, and confidence, the brave man must embrace "diligent activity" ("*industria*") and tolerance for difficulty ("*tolerantia*"). This capacity and eagerness for difficulty is instrumental in helping Browne to harmonize soldiering with scholarship.[50]

A major portion of Browne's celebration of his son Thomas derives from the wide range of witnesses with whom Browne has conversed; from them father has learned that his son is a valiant, resolute soldier but also a keen observer, a scholar, and a man of sympathy (Keynes, 4.22). As Browne records them, the range of witnesses to this ideal in his son is impressively wide: a chaplain, high ranking officers such as Sir Jeremy Smith and Sir Thomas Allen, a captain characterized as "a meere rough seaman," and "Mr. W. B. of Lynne, a stout volunteer in the Dreadnought" who "sayd in my hearing that you were a deserving person and of as good a reputation as any yong man in the fleet." A captain but also the Lord of Sandwich himself testify to Thomas's perfect valor (Keynes, 4.23–4). But the final framing of Thomas's character is Browne's own: "beside these I must not fayle to tell you how well I like it, that you are not only *Marti* butt *Mercurio,* and very much pleased to find how good a student you have been at sea, and particularly with what successe you have read divers bookes there, especially Homer and Juvenal, with Lubines notes." Browne is extremely proud of his son the courageous soldier, but he is clearly eager for militarism to be overcome by scholarship, and even for the virtues of the military man finally to funnel down into an industry that transfers to learning. "You are mightily improved in your violin," Browne observes, having sent his son the instrument back in 1666. The sweet music of strings is allowable while, Browne warns, the trumpet is not, "for many reasons." As for fencing on board, it "may bee" of use "against the scurvie, butt that knowledge is of little advantage in actions of the sea" (Wilkin, 1.152).[51]

The avid letters that they exchanged make it patently clear that Thomas Sr. and Thomas Jr. shared a profound sympathy that manifested itself in their mutual attempts to help the other see the world more vividly. Whether it was father describing with exactitude a comet in the sky (Keynes, 4.19) or son recounting his adventures between northern Africa and Spain (Wilkin, 1.120–8), the two men

[50] Browne gives the definition in Latin with one Greek term; see Keynes, 4.22; for a translation, see J. Solomon, trans., "On Virtues and Vices," in *The Complete Works of Aristotle*, ed. Barnes, 2.1983.

[51] For Thomas Jr. in the navy, see J. J. Keevil, *Medicine and the Navy, 1200–1900*, 3 vols. (London: E. & S. Livingstone, 1958), 2.91, 126, 159, 165.

inspired one another to be more careful in their observations, honorable in their values, and intensely alive in every moment of their existence on earth.

When at the outset of 1664, Edward began to record the events of his life at home and abroad, he would paint the picture of an elder son whose closeness to his father in space and career trajectory produced a far more complex dynamic than the simpler affection that Browne conveyed for the younger son. (See Figure 10.1.) Edward's journal begins with a starry-eyed account of Christmas revelry with Henry Howard, the Duke of Norfolk's brother, "at the duke's palace in Norwich, so magnificently as the like hath scarce been seen" (Wilkin, 1.44). The palace was located just a short walk to the north toward the river from the Browne home in the marketplace. Terminating the glorious nights of dancing, drinking from gold, and beautiful ladies with a *Sic transit Gloria mundi* on January 4, Edward already has his father's combination of curiosity and sobriety. Alongside such revelry with "our greatest beautys" are the anatomies that Edward carries out with his father: "I cut up a bull's heart and took out the bone"; "I opened a dog"; "Mr. Osborne sent my father a calf, whereof I observed the knee joynt, and the neat articulation of the put bone which was here very perfect"; "Cutting up a turkey's heart"; a dog

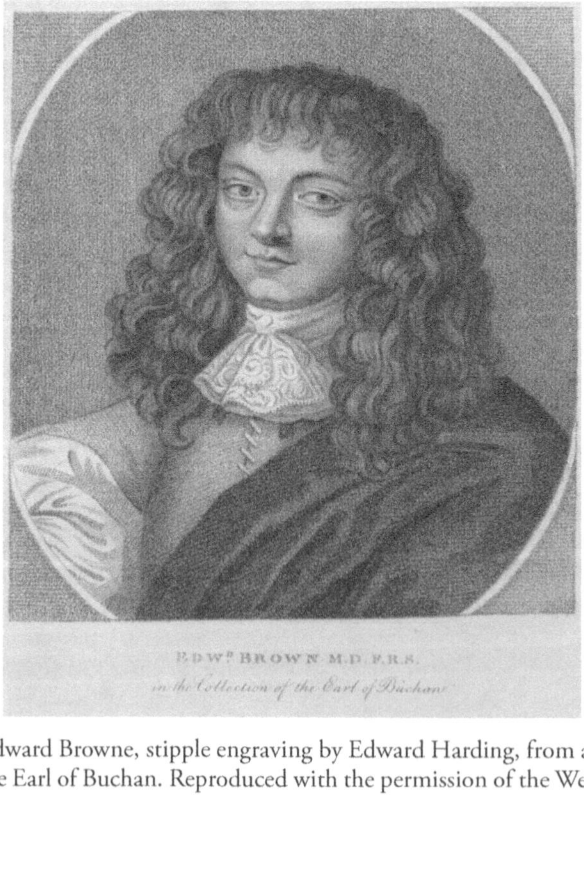

Figure 10.1 Edward Browne, stipple engraving by Edward Harding, from a portrait in the collection of the Earl of Buchan. Reproduced with the permission of the Wellcome Library, London.

and monkey; a sheep and oxen at the butcher's; a hare and pike on the same day; a hedgehog and a badger.

It is clear from his journal that Edward was attempting to experience life as intensely and attentively as his father. On January 3, he "took notice that the sun rose in an elliptical or oval figure, not round, the diameter was parallel to the horizon" (Wilkin, 1.45). The days included serious dinner conversations ("there was some discourse of Drabitius' prophecy"); readings about faraway places such as Egypt and China; interesting animal specimens both for dinner (the "weed fish, very like to an haddock") and for collecting; letters from Iceland; interesting visitors (including Dr de Veau, who brought news from France and Italy, played the guitar, and "shewed a powder against agues"); a steady stream of sermons; ideas for experiments such as "a magical cure for the jaundise"; the correction of vulgar errors (for instance on a map provided for Caesar's *Commentaries*); plant specimens found in gardens but also at the sea; medical operations ("I saw a polypus taken out of Mr. Townsend's nose" by Mr. Croppe); medical visits (including Edward's "first fee" on February 16); and miscellaneous wonders: for instance, "I went to see a serpente that a woman living in St. Gregories church yard in Norwich vomited up, but shee had burnt it before I came" (1.49). With his MB degree from Cambridge in July, 1663, Edward spent time in London before resuming life with his father in pursuit of dissections, plant observations, churchgoing, chemical experiments, medical visits, connoisseurship with Mr Howard, and conversation with a chirurgeon called Flatman about life and customs in other countries of the world. On March 28, he once again set out for London whence, on the evening of April 2, he departed for the first of three visits to the Continent and, eventually, for fame as a travel writer. On this first journey he would see Paris, then Italian cities including Genoa, Rome, Naples, Bologna, Padua and Venice, then French cities from Arles, Montpellier, and Toulouse up through Rochelle and then back to Paris.

Edward's skill and eventual recognition as a travel writer were clearly a tribute to his father, for it was Browne who had taught his son what in the world to observe and how to observe it, and it was for Browne that Edward originally recorded his travels.[52] As his Parisian journal makes clear, this accountability was a source of anxiety for Edward as a well as an inspiration. Even so, the steady supply of letters to and fro makes it perfectly clear that the family, siblings and parents alike, are tightly knit for better and worse.[53] At one point in the journal Edward's characterization of his plans as fanciful dreams, Platonic forms, or recalcitrant passions does not disguise the fact that he finds his father an impediment to his happiness. Yet Browne proves a somewhat negotiable burden, since Edward continues his journeys into Italy, at first "ordered" by his father "to goe as soon as I could to Montpelier" (Wilkin, 1.26). Being the son of the famous Dr Browne had its benefits as

[52] For an example of Browne's financial support of the travels, see Bodleian MS Lister 3, f. 19, Thomas Briggs to Martin Lister, which mentions Browne's assistance with his son's travels in August 1665.

[53] "Journal of a Visit to Paris in the Year 1664," ed. Geoffrey Keynes, *Saint Bartholomew's Hospital Reports* 56 (1923), 1–34; at 20.

well, as Edward discovered on July 30 when a chance encounter with Guy Patin in a Parisian shop yielded Edward a welcome attention: "Bouillet [the shopkeeper] told [Patin] whose son I was; hee saluted mee very kindly, asked mee many things concerning my father, whom he knew onely as Author of *Religio Medici*, discoursed with mee very lovingly, and told mee hee would write to my father" (1.31). Later, in Padua, Edward was given access to advanced anatomical training thanks to Sir Henry Finch's admiration for his famous father (1.92). From Paris at the end of September, Edward reported that a mathematician named Peti "hath got your *Vulgar Errours* translated, but tis halfe into English and halfe into Latin, so that it cannot be printed so; hee doth not understand English, but hath got this done for his owne satisfaction." Edward added that "I beleeve he will present you with one of his books de Cometis, which he hath lately written, upon an hypothesis of his owne, different from Des Cartes" (1.113).

Browne's letters are filled with travel advice about what to see while abroad, in no small measure based in travel writings as well as personal experience, and Edward's with elaborate details about the past and present of what he has seen, from antiquities, churches, and gardens, to cabinets of curiosity and Mount Vesuvius and the plants round about it. He also tells his father about people he has met (the courteous Athanasius Kircher, for instance, or the "low and fat" Queen of Sweden), with an emphasis on traveling companions who are "all persons of good quality" (Wilkin, 1.89)—such as Christopher Wren, John Ray, and Philip Skippon—and cultural experiences he has had, such as his attendance at Jewish circumcisions in Rome and Padua (1.86, 94) or the "madness" of "carnauall time" (1.89). Specific strategies for making the most out of travel—for instance, for living with an apothecary in Montpellier—are owed to father Browne who also speaks in the sobering voice of professional responsibility, family obligations, and financial exigency. Through his father's mediation, however, Edward finds a further way to justify his travels: by converting experiences abroad into the advancement of learning at the Royal Society.

In Browne's correspondence with his elder son, one gathers occasional details about life at home in Norwich, for instance, from Edward's reference to the picture of Icarus that hangs in their home. But only one of Browne's letters to Edward from this period has survived. In September 1665, father wrote son that it was a good thing that Edward had witnessed operations for the stone, and that he should see other surgical as well as chemical and anatomical operations. Browne was especially relieved that Edward had recovered from smallpox, "wch may now so embolden you, as to take of, at least abate, the solicitude and feares wch others have." Browne encouraged his son's interactions with Guy Patin, and he offered both encouragement and advice for Mr. Briot's proposed translation of *Pseudodoxia Epidemica*, to which there would be some additions or changes, he pointed out, but from which "there is litle to be expunged or totally left out" (Keynes, 4.27).

While Browne was trying to find comfort in Thomas's "hard service" against the Dutch, he was overseeing Edward's progress as a physician and observant student of the world. Before he had settled into a steady practice in the capital, Edward embarked on a second journey abroad which, having begun as a short trip to the Netherlands, gradually expanded into a year and a half (August 1668 to Christmas 1669) in which he journeyed through "Germany, Austria, Hungary, Serbia, Bulgaria, and northern Greece, where at Larissa he saw the court of the 'Grand Seigneur.'"[54] Browne's messages to his son are also fairly mixed if nonetheless repetitious. On the one hand, there is the "solicitous" father, the one ready to do anything to help his child yet anxious for and insistent on the son's return to England and the medical profession. On the other, there is the ambitious scholar inciting his son on how best to convert his journey into credit with the Royal Society and eventually into a published account. Somewhere between the father who would severely restrict "wide excursions" and the one who thrives on the advancement of learning is the affectionate parent who entrusts his son to God's providence and offers him cautious advice about how to rest while in motion and to preserve his health while in foreign climes.

Not surprisingly, father and son range across a wide spectrum of subjects for observation as the travel letters unfold. Browne is eager for Edward to supplement his firsthand observations with secondhand conversation and germane reading; indeed, one of the ways in which Browne combines caution with encouragement is to advise Edward on when to rely on the secondhand. Edward is encouraged to attend to plants but also politics. The letters have a special regard for mines, minerals, and mineral waters, but also for "fish and fowle in markets"; "defences agaynst sea inundations"; "various Animals"; "speciall medicines & preparations"; "evidence of alchemical transformations and projections"; "granates & other stones"; museums of "rarities & what is remarkable in any private custodie"; "the manner of the executions in all places"; "what proportion Lutherans, calvinists, catholicks, Jewes are in Germany"; and methods of dyeing. Edward's letters report on "the varietie of habits in [Vienna]...as of Hungarians, Transyluanians, Grecians, Croatians, Austrians, etc." (Wilkin, 1.159). Edward takes note of the Holy Roman emperor's "Austrian lipp," of musical performances and instruments, and of the "magicall glasse" perhaps associated with John Dee at the emperor Rudolph's court. Edward sometimes helps his father follow his travels on the map by providing an outline of the route. But more often, he gives his father snapshots of people, customs, technologies, and natural phenomena: the dress of Hungarian women, for instance, or a plant book assembled in Padua.[55] No doubt strategically, Edward is apt to point out the wide regard for his father as expressed by a nun in Brussels or by the emperor himself and his librarian in Vienna.

One delightful feature of the letters from Norwich is that they often prove collaborative family compositions carried out by Dorothy Browne as well as her hus-

[54] Kees van Strien, "Edward Browne," in *ODNB*.

[55] For a plant book put together by both Edward and his father, see the manuscript Hortus Siccus, 108 in the Sloane Herbarium (the Natural History Museum in London), described in *The Sloane Herbarium*, ed. J. E. Dandy (London: British Museum, 1958), 99. Father and son threaded into this book a number of specimens from England, the Continent, and the New World alike, sometimes providing English versions of the Latin names but mostly offering Latin nomenclature for flowers whose habitations were as far-flung as Virginia, Iceland, and Crete.

band, and most notably by three of Edward's four sisters, Elizabeth, Mary, and Frances. Anne is the vehicle for the transmission of some of Edward's letters from her residence with the Barkers in Clerkenwell, London. Sometimes the news is worrisome—on December 2, 1668, Frances is "lively and cheerily, butt leane, and another sharpe fever might soon take her away" (Keynes, 4.32). But the trinity of daughters provides an especially vital and intelligent presence in the letters. The three concoct arguments attempting to bring their brother home, all of which amount to expressions of love. Elizabeth or Betty is often commended for her skills in various arts and crafts—in "limning" but also in "washing in black and colours," for instance (4.33). In one letter from summer 1669, Edward addresses his three sisters separately. For Mary, he expresses his desire that she should have accompanied him to Holland. The message to Frances is more flirtatious. But the longer characterization of Elizabeth clarifies why, for father as for son, she was exceptional: "Though I make many journeys, yet I am confident that your pen and pencill are greater travellers. How many fine plaines do they passe over, and how many hills, woods, seas doe they designe? You have a fine way of not onley seeing but making a world; and whilst you set still, how many miles doth your hand travel!" (Wilkin, 1.190). In these lines, Edward seems to say more than just that Betty is a gifted or precise graphic artist. The fineness with which she makes worlds as well as sees them anticipates her role as Browne's preferred reading companion in the last years of his life, especially featuring books of travel in their impressive list.

With Edward having been inducted into the Royal Society on January 2, 1668, it is hardly surprising that a desire to supply the Society with information appears early and often in the letters. On December 2 of that year, Browne advised his son that "it were well you could observe anything in order to the Royall Societie" (Keynes, 4.33), and the father repeated this advice a few weeks later, specifying medical knowledge but cautioning against the overtaxing of Edward's "spirits" (4.37). Having urged Edward to establish "an ingenious & inquisitive" correspondent in Vienna, Browne reported on April 28, 1669, that he had "sent the figure of the soles parelli to the Societie wch was very well taken. Dr Merret presented it for you" (Keynes, 4.45).[56] This material on mock suns or parhelia, the bright spots formed by refraction on both sides of the sun, was published in the *Philosophical Transactions* in May 1669.[57] On June 25, Browne's report of sending "your observations of damps in the mines of Hung[ary] to the R.S." acknowledged that he had added material from other letters to fill out the submission, and that he had heard from Secretary Oldenburg (Wilkin, 1.172).[58] On July 21, Edward had also heard from Oldenburg who was expressing the excellent reception of the Browne material with a warm invitation for further submissions from abroad.

[56] Thomas Birch, *The History of the Royal Society*, 4. vols. (London, 1756–57), 2.357, gives the date of the presentation as April 1, 1669.

[57] May 10, 4.953.

[58] See Birch, *The History of the Royal Society*, 2.337, for the December 1668 meeting at which Oldenburg read the letter in which Edward volunteered his services. Other communications from Edward or from Browne are in the same volume, 353, 357, 376–7, 399, 418, 422, 427.

A letter from Oldenburg to Robert Boyle on March 3, 1668 indicates that Browne had also taken it upon himself to send the Society "severall curiosities, to be lodged in our repository, as a great Bone petrifyed, a whole Egg in an Egge, a Stone-botle, wch 7. years agoe was filld full wth Malaga-sack, and well stopped, but is now empty, though said never to have been opened, and ye outside of it is all cover'd over wth a thick mucous Coat, having stood in a corner of a Wine-sellar all that time."[59] Assigning the date of February 27, 1668 to this donation, an account found in *Philosophical Experiments and Observations of... Dr. Robert Hooke* explained that the bone had been discovered in the year 1666 "on the Sea-Shore, not far from *Winterton* in *Norfolk*," uncovered there after a landslide provoked by flooding. As for the double egg, it was owed to a goose and comprised "nothing but the White" in its outer layer.[60] In addition to this donation, Browne sought to assure the Society that his family was prepared to serve the advancement of learning in whatever way possible. In his own letters to Oldenburg, Browne prefaced the informative papers with news of Edward's travels, including characterizations of the considerable dangers and difficulties his son had faced for the sake of gathering information (Keynes, 4.365–9).

Having returned to England around Christmas 1669, Edward continued to consult with his father on travel-based submissions to the *Philosophical Transactions* (Keynes, 4.49). Especially impressive was the letter sent from Edward to the Society in January 1670, in which he enclosed correspondence from the emperor's librarian Peter Lambecius, "presenting his service to the society, and sending a catalogue of divers chemical manuscripts in the Imperial library, and offering them the liberty of transcribing any of them, and even his readiness to send the books themselves upon caution given."[61] As of March, 1670, the minerals gathered in Edward's travels—from Carinthia and Schemnitz in particular—had arrived in boxes to the Royal Society.[62] Browne also began to advise his son about how best to prepare the "historicall and narrative observations concerning your last travayles" for publication (4.49), with directions concerning what should be included (4.54–5).

In 1670–71, Browne was helping his son settle into medical practice in London; accordingly, their letters often revert to consultations about patients, including an electuary, pills, and regimen for Mr Burwell; an assessment of "Plethoricall young persons or scorbuticall or such as discompose their blood by strong liquours or irregular diet" (Keynes, 4.52); prescriptions for Ms Crosse's bloodily phlegmatic cough (4.52); and an asthmatic condition experienced by Mr Bernard, in which case Browne cites his old favorites, Sennert and Rivière. Browne is living an exceptionally busy life; in one letter, in the course of narrating the death of Dean Crofts, Browne tells his son that "I have half an howers time wch opportunity I would not lett passe, this being the post day" (4.49). In this letter Browne momentarily seems

[59] Oldenburg, *Correspondence of Henry Oldenburg*, 4.224.

[60] W. Derham, ed., *Philosophical Experiments and Observations of the Late Eminent Dr. Robert Hooke... And Other Eminent Virtuoso's in his Time* (London, 1726), 31–2.

[61] See Birch, *The History of the Royal Society*, 2.418.

[62] Birch, *The History of the Royal Society*, 2.427–8. On May 20, 1670, Edward provided a letter with a further gift of minerals.

nostalgic for a better, more pious time. Consoled by the fact that his afflicted dean "found much good in drincking the clarified juices of urtica & plantago in milk for his bleeding," Browne also mentions that his friend has bequeathed him "his chariot and harnesse" (4.50). A gift of a chariot might well be pleasing to an aging physician no longer wholly prepared to make long journeys on horseback. Indeed, in these letters, Browne informs his son that he is growing old: "Though my foot bee very paynfull & disableth mee from going, yet my hand is free & I thanck god I am not sick... though as yeares growe upon me I cannot butt expect more frequent returnes of these or worse infirmities" (4.51). In her postscript, Dorothy elaborates that "your Fathar haveing layd out the last night have gatt some Could and it is fallne into his foutt and is very painefull to him. Hee has complained of his back a good while and I sopos it is now fallne into his foutt." To make matters worse, the pervasive sickliness of the city and county has meant that Browne "has not much rest," and the letter expresses a mother's desire for her son's assistance, even as she is just now helping her husband to bed "and can say no more" (Keynes, 4.51). In 1668, Browne's protégé Henry Power had already died; Browne had survived far longer than his youthful *Religio* seemed to predict or even to desire, yet irreversible decline was now quite viscerally real in Browne's life.

On one matter—an affection for the second son and younger brother Thomas—Browne and Edward were in full agreement. Among other things, the brothers shared their father's delight in poetry: for instance, Thomas Jr.'s verses from "aboard his Maiesties shippe the Marie Rose" expressed a wanderlust—"The Ocean we must Cut through every place"—that moved both sons, even as these verses stress their difference in vocation: Edward would be fighting against disease but travelling for pleasure, while his brother would be pursuing the military "enemie."[63]

While Edward was abroad, Browne also kept his son abreast of noteworthy recent, often medical, publications, for instance, John Mayow's book on respiration and rickets (Keynes, 4.37). Browne's reports on the latest books include Christopher Merrett's *Neri de arte vitraria*—a translation and elaboration of a work on glassmaking—as well as anticipation of the revised edition of his *Pinax rerum britannicarum*, supposed to be a catalogue of the plants and animals in Britain. In natural history as in antiquarian studies, Browne did not need to travel in order to heighten his widespread authority. As translations of *Religio* and the great reputation of *Pseudodoxia* continued to accrue acclaim far and wide for their author, Browne's profound grasp of local flora and fauna also served to magnify his stature as a public-spirited and ingenious savant.

3. THE REPUBLIC OF LETTERS

As one of the inaugural honorary members of the Royal College of Physicians—the rubric was created in 1664—Browne was inducted within a controversial context

[63] See BL MS Sloane 1833, f. 235, for the naval poem.

and figured into the College's attempts to strengthen their reputation—and their finances.[64] The College was facing new competition from the Royal Society, whose body was rapidly growing. In December seventy-three honorees were inducted, supplying money for the banquet and their admission.[65] At a remove from London, Browne was shielded somewhat from the intensity with which a rivalry between the Royal Society and the Royal College had heated up by the late 1660s, and more generally from the conflicting claims of experimentalists on the one hand and the learned physicians of the College on the other.[66] Clearly, in 1664–65, the latter the year in which Browne actually was offered his diploma, the acclaimed author and physician from Norwich was selected from the provinces for the prestige that he offered the College.[67]

As early as January 1663, Browne was contributing information to the Royal Society in an effort to connect with that world of modern learning into which Power was officially inducted in June 1663. On the basis of letters received from Þórður Jónsson, Browne compiled "An Account of Island, alias Ice-land," in which he included data about driftwood, animal life, winter weather, volcanic activity, mineral springs, rivers, agriculture, plants, rocks and shells. Among other things, Browne noted how local shepherds are eager for a fox-headed dog brought from Iceland but also how an Icelandic horse, "kept in the pastures by Yarmouth in the summer, would often take the sea, swimme a great way a mile or two, & returne." Having concluded his report, Browne signed off with the promise that "I shall bee very ambitious to serve the noble societie whose most honouring servant I am."[68]

On at least one occasion, Browne's medical practice was brought to Oldenburg's attention when, on April 25, 1667, Nathaniel Fairfax wrote to the Secretary about the case of Margaret Girling of Rumborough, Suffolk, a young woman of twenty-four whose medical history for the past decade included green sickness, disconsolation, and a chronic sickliness over the death of her parents and the "misbehaviour" of a brother, then a chest so "clogged" that Margaret had found the least exercise, especially in windy weather, to be onerous. Together with other Norwich physicians, Browne had offered her a number of remedies, to no avail. Although Fairfax did what he could to relieve Margaret, she eventually died of her strange clogging ailment; with her permission secured in advance, Fairfax performed an autopsy in search of the cause, his very first. Whereas the rest of the letter offers a detailed account of this procedure, it also makes clear that Browne continued to consult with Fairfax during the autopsy, remarking that he had "mett with ye like in an

[64] See Sir George Clark, *A History of the Royal College of Physicians of London* (Oxford: Clarendon Press, 1964), 1.312–15; and Harold J. Cook, *The Decline of the Old Medical Regime in Stuart London* (Ithaca, NY: Cornell University Press, 1986), 76, 144–5. As Cook points out, there was "some precedent" for the designation (144).

[65] For the conditions, see Cook, *Decline*, 145.

[66] Cook, *Decline*, 179–82.

[67] Clark, *History of the Royal College*, 1.315. For accounts of the other honorary members, see William Munk, *The Roll of the Royal College of Physicians of London* (London: the Royal College, 1878), 1.315–51.

[68] Keynes, 3.345–6; the original is MS Sloane 1911–13, f. 90. Cf. Wilkin, *Works*, 4.254; the letter is also found in the Royal Society's archives.

Italian author" and offering advice about how best to proceed.[69] Fairfax helped account for the importance of consultation in the autopsy by admitting that he was rendered nervous by virtue of his medical inexperience, his inexperience with women, his promise to the parents and patient not to mangle the body, the strangeness of the disease, but also his "remembrance of yt playfellowship" with the deceased "wch neighbourhood & equality of years had occasioned in ye days of Childhood."[70] Later supplementing the "Worthy" physician's account of local trees, Fairfax looked to Browne not just as a highly skilled doctor but also as a trustworthy, sympathetic mentor.

Fairfax's letter to Oldenburg also suggests that although Browne never became a fellow of the Royal Society, his extensive network of associates locally as well as in London prevented his sphere of activity from becoming provincial or remote. In the first years of the Restoration, Browne continued to correspond with, and to receive notices from, various contributors to the republic of letters. Some were new presences in his life. In March 1661, Browne received a letter from Samuel Sainthill regarding their mutual interest "in the Cantabrian Language," in the poet-priest Don Rafael de Micoleta,[71] and in the phenomenon according to which a relatively minor language such as Basque is "interwoven" with a major language such as Spanish. As "one of those that has walked under the Livery of [Browne's] reason a long time," Sainthill shows considerable sympathy with Browne's fascination by the complex mixtures of, as well as divisions between, the world's many peoples, cultures, and tongues.[72] In 1664, Thomas Lawrence published a letter that he had sent to Browne as *Mercurius Centralis: or, A Discourse of Subterraneal Cockle, Muscle, and Oyster-shels, found in the digging of a Well at Sir William Doylie's in Norfolk, many foot under ground, and at considerable distance from the Sea*. Between Lawrence and William Dugdale, with whom Browne continued to correspond, Browne was considered an expert on the realm of the subterranean.[73] In answering questions about subterranean shells apparently prompted by a conversation with Browne, Lawrence also heralded Norwich's great savant as a pious promoter of creation's putatively insignificant phenomena.[74] Also in 1664, Browne's protégé Henry Power credited his mentor with leadership in the appreciation of and attention to the miniature or microscopic in nature. In *Experimental Philosophy in Three Books, Containing New Experiments Microscopical, Mercurial, Magnetical*, Power chastised "those sons of Sense" who "were not able to see how curiously the minutest things of the world are wrought, and with what eminent signatures of Divine Providence they were inrich'd and embellish'd, without our Dioptrical assistance."[75] Connecting his focus

[69] Oldenburg, *Correspondence of Henry Oldenburg*, 3.401–3.

[70] Oldenburg, *Correspondence of Henry Oldenburg*, 3.402.

[71] Already in the seventeenth century, Micoleta's name was sometimes mistaken as Nicoleta. His Basque grammar, *Modo breve* (1653), was possessed in manuscript by Browne (now in BL).

[72] The letter is found in MS Sloane 1911–13, 154r–v.

[73] Pembroke College, Oxford, has a letter of September 11, 1661 from Browne to Dugdale, with thanks for the latter's gift of the second volume of *Monasticon Anglicanum*.

[74] Thomas Lawrence, *Mercurius centralis* (1664), A4r–v.

[75] Henry Power, *Experimental Philosophy*, reprint of 1664 edition, intro. Marie Boas Hall (New York: Johnson Reprint Corporation, 1966), a3v–a4r.

on the tiny both to new optical technologies and to theories of corpuscles and atoms, Power quotes Browne's *Religio* on the preference for "Regiomontanus his Fly beyond his Eagle," with the suggestion that Browne had early recognized the "miracle" of the narrow and miniscule whilst "ruder heads stand amazed at those prodigious and Colossean pieces of Nature, as Whales, Elephants, and Dromedaries" (b3r). Power is willing to correct mistakes in his "ever honoured friend['s]" *Pseudodoxia*, but he is keener to enlist that work in the service of an enthusiastic defense of modern advancements in learning.[76] To this end, Power diverts a passage in *Religio* from its theological focus: having adjusted Browne's assault on "this numerous piece of Monstrosity (the Multitude onely)" so that it centers on impediments to modern learning, Power praises the heroism of the naturalist by insisting that "There are not difficulties enough, in Philosophy, for a vigorous and active Reason" (*Experimental Philosophy*, 184, 190–1). Browne, of course, had assigned this vigor to faith.

Over the course of the decade, Browne's influence continued to spread and his authority to figure widely, variously, and prominently. Among the manuscript responses, Power himself heralded Browne's work on coagulation in a manuscript entitled *Historia Physica Anatomica*, putting his mentor in the company of Descartes and J. B. Van Helmont.[77] In his commonplace book, Thomas Hughes of Trinity College, Oxford, wrote out his notes on *Religio Medici* while Sir John Cotton, second Baronet of Landwade, attempted to solve a theoretical argument with Browne's "ingenious and learned" view of the multitude in the same work.[78] In his diary, one Thomas Gooch recorded a conversation with his friend Mr. Money in which the latter had praised Thomas Fuller's *Holy War* at the decided expense of Thomas Browne.[79] In print, Robert Bayfield dedicated a section of his treatise on tumors to "*famosissimo philosopho Thomæ Brown*"[80] while Thomas Blount featured Brownean language as a key source for his *Glossographia: or a Dictionary Interpreting All Such Hard Words.... as are now used in our refined English Tongue* (1661).[81] In 1663, Edmund Gayton published his own version of *The Religion of a Physician*[82] while, in 1670, Browne's kinsman Thomas Tenison enlisted his learning on world population in *The Creed of Mr. Hobbes Examined*.[83] Browne's mediations between natural philosophy and religion were useful to Restoration attempts to rethink their proper relationship. For this reason, the Hermetical-alchemical Thomas Vaughan joined Browne's enterprise of refuting vulgar errors, and Thomas Fuller noted in *The Worthies of England* (1662) that *Pseudodoxia* was helping to

76 See Power, *Experimental Philosophy* (1664), 8, 37, 42, 58.

77 Sloane MS 496, f. 29. The date on the manuscript is 1666.

78 Bodleian MS Eng d 3615, ff. 171–2; Folger Shakespeare MS V.a. 344, f. 88.

79 Sloane MS 161, f. 16; the date is March 15, 1671.

80 Bayfield, *De Tumoribus* (1662).

81 Most of the words were taken from *Pseudodoxia Epidemica*; I am grateful to Nathan Stogdill for this reference. This Blount (1618–79) is not to be confused with the Thomas Blount who included Browne in his natural history.

82 See Lund, "The Christian Physician," in Todd and Murphy, eds., "*A man very well studyed*," 233–5.

83 See Tenison, *Creed of Mr. Hobbes*, 215.

vanquish errors about the devil's powers.[84] At the outset of the Restoration, Robert Sharrock invoked *The Garden of Cyrus* as a famous model for the new natural history of vegetation.[85]

Whereas *Pseudodoxia* may have qualified Browne for affiliation with the Royal Society, *Religio* was more problematic. Restoration pundits might consider it a seminal work of irenic religious discourse, yet often with regard to a previous, naïve generation of wits. Thus, whereas Sir William Petty could tell Pepys in 1664 that the *Religio* was one of the "most esteemed and generally cried up for wit in the world," Petty concluded that "the wit lie in confirming some pretty sayings, which are generally like paradoxes, by some argument smartly and pleasant urged—which takes with people who do not trouble themselves to examine the force of an argument which pleases them in the delivery, upon a subject which they like." Others found humor in its quaintness: in 1661 Alexander Brome quipped that "Physick and preaching ill agree | There is but one Religio Medici," and Oldenburg remarked to Boyle on November 5, 1664 that Browne's fine work now needed updating: "After yt Religio Medici is growne stale, we have lately printed Religio Stoici, wch hath some strains of wit, and some very honest and healing maxims for broken Christianity."[86] In Robert Wild's poems of 1668, *Religio Medici* once again figured among the jests of Restoration wit; some of Browne's contemporaries appreciated his performance of, indeed his insistence on, the comedy of human life.[87] Even *Pseudodoxia* found its way into satire: in *Hudibras*, Samuel Butler offered not just topics from Browne's encyclopedia but a sample of his most ponderous diction.[88] One vivid indication of a certain cognitive dissonance between Browne and the Restoration mentality was that when Sir Samuel Tuke visited him on behalf of the Royal Society in the autumn of 1663, Tuke found him "good-natured" but unintelligible.[89] But in this letter Tuke was perpetuating a running joke with Evelyn, whom he grouped with the abstruse philosophers that lay men of affairs could barely comprehend. Tuke expressed his intention to solicit from Browne a more straightforward version of his forthcoming contribution to the Royal Society and otherwise expressed his affection for both Browne and Evelyn between whom he acted as a messenger, carrying information about

[84] Thomas Vaughan, *A Brief Natural History... with Refutations of such Vulgar Errours as our Modern Authors have omitted* (1669), 94. For Fuller, see Keynes, *Bibliography*, 190.

[85] Robert Sharrock, *History of Vegetables* (1660), see 142–3 (misnumbered 140–1).

[86] *Correspondence of Henry Oldenburg*, 1.211 (letter of March 1659); Pepys, *Diary*, 5.27; Keynes, *Bibliography*, 187–91; *Correspondence of Henry Oldenburg*, 2.291–2. On the prospect of translations of *Pseudodoxia*, see also *Correspondence of Henry Oldenburg*, 1.396.

[87] Cf. Robert Wild, *Iter Boreale* (1668), 68.

[88] Samuel Butler, *Hudibras*, ed. John Wilders (Oxford: Clarendon Press, 1967), 6–7 for Adam's navel; and 30 (Canto 2, line 47) for Browne's term "Tollutation" (cf. note on this line, p. 342). For Browne's response to Butler, see chapter 11 in this volume. It is possible that Browne's son Edward wrote verses indebted to Butler; see OSB Shelves B1115 in the Beinecke Library at Yale University. I am grateful to Claire Preston for this reference.

[89] For this episode, see Darley, *John Evelyn: Living for Ingenuity*, 183. For his part, Browne seemed not to notice the effect he had on Tuke (see Keynes, 4.280), who joked with Evelyn that "we lay men cannot tell how to melt [i.e. understand] you Schollars."

timber from Browne to Evelyn and "Cases of birds wth their feathers" from Evelyn to Browne.[90]

In the early 1660s, *Religio* factored, sometimes dramatically, into continental religious debates, as can be seen in Theophilus Spizelius's *Scrutinium Atheismi* (1663). In section 25, Spizelius turned to Browne while discussing the fifth source of contemporary atheism, a concentration on second causes rather than on God, which included the attribution of all human actions to the temperament of the body.[91] In the 1660s, *Religio*'s potential for European influence was heightened by its translation into the vernaculars of Dutch and French. With the 1668 French version a rendering of Abraham van Berckel's 1665 Dutch, both volumes framed the work as especially committed to defending the Church of England and anticipated that the translation would be controversial and, according to some parties, condemnable.[92] While van Berckel had credited *Religio Medici* with elevating his piety and virtue, he also knew that its reputation for heresy was already pronounced, that is, that "it does not sit too well with many, and its name is not too good." Also adding to the spread of Browne's fame was a Dutch translation of *Pseudodoxia Epidemica* in 1668; it too was subject to the ire of Browne's harshest critics such as Jacobus Koelman.[93]

If Browne's influence was not entirely in his control, sometimes that influence was so unsettling to him that he did what he could to recover some slender thread of that control. The most striking case involves the Quakers. Of the countless letters of comfort, prophecy, instruction, and invitation sent out by Quakers in the 1650s and 60s, one was addressed to Browne. Written to Browne by a well-known Norwich Quaker named Samuel Duncon in the period during or just after 1659, the brief manuscript document reads in its entirety as follows:

> ESTEEMED FRIEND, Haveinge perused a booke of thyne called Religio Medici (and findeinge these sound assertions followinge—'To aske whare heauen is, is to demand whare the presence of God is'—'Moyses committed a gross absurditye when with these eyes of fflesh he desired to see God.' Wee are much contested agst by some, because we can't comply to their tenett in that particular, viz. that with their ffleshly eyes they shall see God. 'There is a piece of divinitye in us, some thinge that was before the elements'—'That God loves us for that part which is, as it were himselfe, and the traduction of his holy spirit.') Judgeinge thee juditious, I therewith send thee

[90] See BL Additional 78306: Sir Samuel Tuke to Evelyn, 28 September 1663 (on timber, 110v): Oct 7, 1663 (on trees, 111r–v) October 14 (113v; Tuke to Evelyn: "I pray procurre mee the receipt for the p[re]serving of the Cases of birds wth their feathers for my freind Dr Browne & I will pay you wth something as good"); and Nov 30 1663 (116r; "I have made yor Complement to Dr Brown who takes it in good part", offering to give the Royal Society some contribution "if at least i can make him fasil, hee is a good naturd man, but wee lay men cannot tell how to melt you schollers").

[91] Theophilus Spizelius, *Theophili Spizelii Scrutinium Atheismi Historico Aetologicum* (1663), 11–13.

[92] As the title page of *La Religion du Medecin* (1668) put it, the work comprised a "Description necessaire par Thomas Brown, Medecin renommé à Norwich; touchant son Opinion accordante le pur service Divin d'Angleterre." In Dutch, the latter phrase was "gesuyverde Gods-dienst van Engelandt." For the Dutch reception, see Rosalie L. Colie, "Sir Thomas Browne's 'Entertainement' in XVIIth Century Holland," *Neophilologus* 36 (1952), 162–71.

[93] For the translation of van Berckel and the controversy with Koelman, who especially objected to the notes added to *Religio Medici*, see Colie, "Sir Thomas Browne's 'Entertainement,'" 168–9.

a booke to peruse; and if thou desire any personall conferrance with me, or any of my friends concernynge the principalls of our religion, (which we believe is the immortal religion, though generally accounted herisie) I shall indeauer it, in the same loue I present this booke to thy vieue, who am a lover of mankind in generall, and thyselfe in particuler.[94]

Despite Browne's prominent (if complex) pronouncements of his commitment to the Church of England, and despite *Religio Medici*'s scorn for "insolent zeal," Duncon looks past what he would consider the carnality and formality of Browne's work and finds three seeds of spiritual wisdom that have convinced Duncon that Browne is ready to be a friend to the Friends.[95]

In his invitation to Browne, Duncon appeals to an essential impartiality purveyed by the persona of *Religio Medici*: the claim that its author tests all positions on his own, that he is therefore unbiased and not to be misled by contemporary constructions of heresy, indeed that he himself has frequently considered unorthodox ideas, and that even if he has moved beyond some of those as error, he is prepared to credit men of singular visions whose wisdom captures truths either long forgotten in the church or never before properly grasped. In Duncon's letter, Browne is at once the most unbiased and welcoming of readers, as well as the most spiritually rigorous and inwardly exploratory.

1659 was a wildly successful year for the Quakers, not just generally but specifically in Browne's Norwich, which prior to that year had proved difficult ground for the Friends to cultivate. But it was also the year in which the pervasive and intense fear of Quakerism—as witchcraft, mania, and anarchy—reached its peak.[96] Tension over the Quakers often impinged quite closely on Browne's neighborhood in Norwich. Earlier in the 1650s, one prominent confrontation took place at Browne's own church in the market, St Peter Mancroft, between leading Quaker George Whitehead and the parish minister John Boatman, whilst the market itself, the site of Browne's home, was a frequent location of Quaker evangelizing.[97] Yet with the Restoration, soon after which the Quakers were singled out for oppressive legislation, the Friends were so maltreated that their emphases and tone drastically changed, becoming more passive and pacifistic, more accommodating and apologetic, less apocalyptic and more inwardly divided about mundane questions such

[94] The letter is found in Rawlinson MS D. 391, f. 52; printed in Wilkin, 1.352, from which I quote here. In the manuscript a small portion of the letter is inserted in the left margin.

[95] For more on this letter, see Reid Barbour, "Thomas Browne, the Quakers, and a Letter from a Judicious Friend," in Anne Dunan-Page and Clotilde Prunier, eds., *Debating the Faith: Religion and Letter Writing in Great Britain, 1550–1800* (Dordrecht: Springer, 2013), 37–48.

[96] For 1659, see Barry Reay, *The Quakers and the English Revolution* (London: Temple Smith, 1985), 81–100.

[97] For the Quakers in Norwich 1659, see Arthur J. Eddington, *The First Fifty Years of Quakerism in Norwich* (London: Friends' Historical Society, 1932), 26–7; cf. George Fox, *The Journal of George Fox*, ed. Nigel Smith (New York: Penguin, 1998), 270–1. For preaching and prophesying in the market, see Richard Hubberthorn, *The Testimony of the Everlasting Gospel Witnessed through Suffering* (1654), 4; and George Whitehead, *The Christian Progress of that ancient servant and minister of Jesus Christ* (1725), 34. For Whitehead and Boatman, see Whitehead, *The Christian Progress*, 34.

as organization.[98] Duncon's letter to Browne is still heady in its hope that the famous citizen of Norwich will join sides with the Friends, but it is also fully aware that the often anti-intellectual and egalitarian Friends need learned and prominent support, and that the bulk of contemporary East Anglian society is very much against them.

There is no record of Browne's direct response to Duncon, no extant letter and no mention by Browne of Duncon to anyone else in the extensive correspondence that Browne left. But arguably we do have one indirect response. Another piece of evidence supporting 1659 as the *terminus a quo* of Duncon's letter is the fact that *Religio Medici* was published twice in that year, once together with the *Hydriotaphia* and *Garden of Cyrus*, but also in its own fifth and annotated edition. Crucially, no further edition of *Religio* would appear until 1669, in which edition one of the passages singled out by Duncon has been seriously altered. Up through 1659, one reads the sentence essentially as it is quoted by Duncon "that God loves us for that part which is, as it were himself, and the traduction of his holy spirit." In 1669, this has been changed so that God "can love nothing but himself, and the traduction of his holy spirit." Yet at the same time, Browne retains the three other citations that Duncon has culled out: Moses is still absurd; heaven is not really a specific place; and "there is a piece of divinity within us, some thinge that was before the elements." Has the quotation about divine love been altered by mistake? Or was there something a little too bold about claiming that God loves himself in us, or that our souls are traduced from the Holy Spirit as against from our parents and ultimately from Adam and Eve, the hereditary basis of our fallen state which Browne cannot forget in one of the several discussions of monstrosity in *Religio Medici*? Whatever the case, the publication history of *Religio Medici* confirms that Browne's work had a way not just of appealing to readers of widely ranging religious persuasions, but also of testing, even pressuring the boundaries of orthodoxy itself.[99]

In other avenues, Browne's most vital contributions to the republic of letters took the form of correspondence. John Evelyn continued to serve as a favorite correspondent for Browne in the republic of letters. Having sent Evelyn a tract on "garlands, and coronary or garland-plants" in 1660, Browne followed up with a letter and a "catalogue of plants" in response to which "experiments might bee attempted by insition & wayes of propagation." Advising Evelyn on nomenclature for his garden of "great fishes," he was clearly serious about his position as a cultural and intellectual arbiter, and as Antonia Moon has noted, Browne was eager to transform his learning into fertile material for growth in the heads and laboratories of correspondents.[100] In an October 1663 letter, Browne shared with Evelyn his

[98] For this shift, see H. Larry Ingle, *First Among Friends: George Fox and the Creation of Quakerism* (New York: Oxford University Press, 1994), 190.

[99] For further evidence of Quaker interest in Browne, see John Perrott, *Battering Rams against Rome* (1661), 11–12; and Nigel Smith, *Literature and Revolution in England, 1640–1660* (New Haven, CT: Yale University Press, 1994), 226.

[100] Letter to Evelyn is in Keynes, 4.279. Evelyn's copy of Browne's 1683 *Miscellany Tracts* is in the Norfolk Heritage Centre, Norwich. For Moon's work, see " 'A Fresh Reading of Books'," in Todd and Murphy, eds., "*A man very well studyed*," 87–103.

observations of the large trees in Norfolk, including oaks (mainly disappointing), a huge lime tree ten miles outside Norwich at Deopham, and a poplar, recently blown down, "at Harling by Thetford at Sr William Gawdie's gate." Browne's specification of precisely where each tree resided shows how carefully he experienced God's creation in the form of the local. As the demise of the poplar conveyed, the local could be highly dramatic, and indeed one of Browne's most extended notes from the period was a description of a storm on June 28, 1665.[101] The fury of this storm was extraordinary, and the damage to his property detailed in the note offered a clear sign of how hapless human artifice could prove in the face of nature's power (Keynes, 3.240). The storm was so noteworthy that it, and Browne's account of it, were recycled in the July 20 installment of *The Newes*.[102]

In a letter from March 1664, in gratitude for a present of Evelyn's *Sylva*, Browne divulged why "ingenious" men such as Evelyn were so valuable to him in a profit-driven, "lower minded world." For Evelyn's work would stimulate even those baser wits to attempt "the handsome wayes of Improvement . . . wch may bee commodious unto them selves, & usefull in consequence unto succeeding generations." For Browne, it was Evelyn's combination of "Ingenuity Learning & publick spirit" that made his relentless pursuit of "noble works" so crucial for the future into which Browne's familial and intellectual heirs would be making their way. Such leading lights of England's republic of letters would simply have to face the fact that they would be ending their days without much rest "as occasions shall arise" for improvement and advancement (Keynes, 4.281). It was as a central personage in this restless endeavor on behalf of learning that Evelyn as well as William Dugdale conceived of Browne, a reputation motivating far-flung ingenious, public spirited men, to seek him out.[103] For instance, as a clear expression of Browne's importance as a naturalist, John Ray paid a visit to him in Norwich, in all likelihood in August 1660.[104] In 1667, Warden Woodward of New College, Oxford, dropped in on Browne during an itinerary that included Norwich's cathedral and castle.[105]

Having informed the reader of *Sylva* of the helpful letter from the "learn'd, and obliging person" of Dr Browne, in 1671 Evelyn would have, and record, the complete Browne experience.[106] "Next morning I went to see Sir Tho. Browne," he wrote in his diary for October, "whose whole house & Garden being a Paradise & Cabinet of rarities, & that of the best collection, especialy Medails, books, Plants,

[101] Keynes, 3.238.

[102] See Keynes, *Bibliography*, 192; and P. J. Dobell, *Books of the Time of the Restoration* (London: P. J. and A. E. Dobell, 1920), 36.

[103] Cf. Dugdale's invitation, "Sir, if your occasions should bring you to London, I should thinke myself happy to wayt on you." Letter of April 5, 1662, in Keynes, 4.326–7.

[104] Noted in Finch, ed., *Catalogue of the Libraries*, 210, but based on Charles Raven, *John Ray, Naturalist: His Life and Works* (Cambridge: Cambridge University Press, 1950). Ray speaks of having been shown "shrub-stonecrop" by Browne; see Ray's *Catalogus Plantarum* (1670), 313.

[105] *The Progress Notes of Warden Woodward 1659–1675 and Other 17th Century Documents Relating to the Norfolk Property of New College, Oxford*, ed. Michael Woodward and R. L. Rickard (*Norfolk Record Society*, vol. 22, 1951), 97.

[106] John Evelyn, *Sylva* (1664), 152, with reference to the lime tree.

natural things, did exceedingly refresh me after last nights confusion."[107] Reinvigorated and clarified in paradise, Evelyn singled out Browne's egg collection for special commendation, citing his host's view that the promontories of Norfolk abounded in those left by "Cranes, Storkes, Eagles &c. & variety of Water-foule." Then the two men ventured out, with Browne the guide, into the streets of Norwich, almost as though into an extension of Browne's museum: "He likewise led me to see all the remarkeable places of this antient Citty, being one of the largest, & certainly (after London) one of the noblest of England, for its venerable Cathedrall, number of Stately Churches, Cleanesse of the streetes; & buildings of flint, so exquisitely headed & Squared, as I was much astonish'd at." As they toured, Browne expressed a sense of loss: "Sir Tho: told me they had lost the art, of squaring the flint, which once they [were] so excellent in: & of which the Churches, best houses, & Walls are built." Yet on the whole, Evelyn came away from the guided tour with a sense of renewal far stronger than melancholy: "The suburbs are large," he concluded, "the prospect sweete, & other amenities, not omitting the flower-gardens, which all the Inhabitans excell in of this Citty, the fabric of stuffs, which it affords the Merchants, & brings a vast trade to this populous Towne"—this, in the year after town recorder Thomas Corie had exclaimed that "the small pox rageth still amongst us, and poverty dayly invades us like an armed man, soe that want of health and wealth makes us in noe condition to entertain such guests" as the strolling players.[108]

4. NATURAL HISTORY AND ANTIQUARIANISM

As a member of the Royal College of Physicians, the curator of William Harvey's library-cum-museum, and an original fellow of the Royal Society, Oxonian Christopher Merrett (1614–95) had just published the first edition of his *Pinax* (1666–67) and was entering into a period of litigious turbulence which would last for the remainder of his life.[109] Although the blemishes and gaps in the original edition of the *Pinax* were so severe as to provoke criticism from leading naturalists such as Ray, Browne took an entirely different tone when, in one of his most gently aggressive letters, he introduced himself to Merrett on July 13, 1668, and offered his services in the revision of the catalogue. Wasting little time with niceties, Browne establishes his credentials regarding nature in Norfolk by pointing out not only that "I have observed and taken notice of many animals in these parts" but also that for three years, he has been compiling an account of these matters for a now-deceased friend (Keynes, 4.343). Then he dives right in, beginning with local bird, fish, insect, and testaceous life omitted from the *Pinax*. One of the most extensive corrections in the first letter involves the location of sweet-flag or *Acorus verus* near

[107] *The Diary*, ed. De Beer, 3.594.

[108] *Correspondence of Thomas Corie, Town Clerk of Norwich, 1664–1687*, ed. Robert H. Hill (Norwich Record Society, 1956), 30.

[109] See D. E. Allen's entry on Christopher Merrett in *ODNB*.

Lynn, an amendment of special import to Browne since its discovery there is attributed to him. Briefly remarking that no one is likely to have found this plant near Lynn, Browne offers a full paragraph in which he remembers his own history with the plant, details precisely where it can be found outside Norwich, makes note of success at its transplantation, and sketches something of its elegance and bounty, with special attention to the production of its *julus*.[110] A precise and evocative sense of place pervades these letters, as does the precision of Browne's memory for where, when, or how many times he has encountered an item. Sometimes he offers a sense of smell, noting that a certain beetle, contrary to authority, "to me... smelt like roses, santalum, & Ambergris" (Keynes, 4.343). Perhaps the most pervasive concern of the letters to Merrett is with nomenclature, in both the learned (Latin) and common (vernacular) uses. Although Browne often transfers the authority to name specimens over to Merrett, he also carefully models the practice of naming according to the principle of obvious and immediate marks of difference.

Browne's care in nomenclature is not lost on Merrett. In one of his two surviving letters to Browne, he praises how "fully" his correspondent has "expressed... the cours to bee taken in the imposition of names, viz. the most obvious & most peculiar difference to the ey or any other sens" (Keynes, 4.360). But Browne is also aware that sensation varies from viewer to viewer, and that some specimens are especially hard to name. In the naming of a fungus, for instance, he concedes that "unto some it seemed to resemble some noble or princely ornament of the head, & so might be called *fungus regius*; unto others a turret, top of a cupola, or lanterne of a building, & so might bee named *fungus pterygoides, pinnacularis,* or *lanterniformis*. You may name it as you please" (4.345). Concerns about naming according to the descriptive "differencing" (4.348) of specimens entail that Browne juxtapose what he has seen, felt, smelled, and dissected firsthand with what has been claimed and depicted in authorities such as Clusius, Jonstonus, and Aldrovandus. But he also converses with seamen whose assistance he values albeit, as with the learned sources, not uncritically.[111] One benefit of problems with nomenclature in the face of a rare or unknown bird is that Browne's descriptions become especially detailed, as is the case with "a very rare bird... sent mee kild about Crostwick" in May 1664, with three claws in front and one behind, and "the head neck & throat of a violet colour the back upper parts of the wing of a russet yellowe the fore & part of the wing azure succeeded downward by a greenish blewe." Of what Browne guesses is "some kind of Jay," he continues that "on the flying feathers bright blewe the lower parts of the wing outwardly of a browne inwardly of a merry blewe the belly a light faint blewe the back toward the tayle of a purple blewe the tayle eleuen fethers of a greenish coulour the extremities of the outward fethers thereof white with an eye of greene" (*Notes and Letters on the Natural History*, 30). With such color gradation

[110] Responding to *Pinax*, p. 2, Browne's account is in Keynes, 4.344. In *Catalogus Plantarum* (1670), John Ray adjusted the account of Browne's encounter with sweet-flag (7).

[111] *Notes and Letters on the Natural History of Norfolk... from the Mss. Of Sir Thomas Browne, M.D.*, ed. with notes by Thomas Southwell (London: Jarrold & Sons, 1902), 14.

a crucial part of coming to know this bird, it is no wonder that Browne is critical of graphic representations in books but also in the pictures produced in his own household.

While Browne is eager to describe the various parts, shapes, sizes, and colors of his specimens, he also characterizes their habits and behaviors. He is especially interested in migration, with a sense of nature's dynamism that pervades his extensive notes on Norfolk natural history as well as his correspondence with men like Yarmouth's John Wakeman.[112] Not only are some birds "of a migrant nature & exchange their seats according to the season," but their movement takes place in a mixture of several flocks together.[113] Among the distant sites of migration, the Faro Islands figure prominently in their position to the north of the British Isles; in fact, a letter from Wakeman confirms that Browne has been inquiring about the names given to birds there.[114] As for other aviary behavior, Browne has observed out in the Broads that coots will face down an enemy fowl by gathering

> in strange numbers when if the Kite stoopes neare them they will fling up [and] spred such a flash of water up with there wings that they will endanger the Kite. & so keepe him of agayne & agayne in open opposition. & an handsome prouision they make about their nest agaynst the same bird of praye by bending & twining the rushes & reeds so about them that they cannot stoope at their yong ones or the damme while she setteth. (*Notes and Letters on the Natural History*, 15)

Sometimes birds are distinctive for their notes, as is the case with the specimen "calld a stone curlewe" or the so-called yarwhelp (a black-tailed godwit) (25).

Browne usually notes if, in what context, and for what duration he has kept a specimen, alive or dead and dried, in his domestic collection. There are, for example, the eagle which he "kept 2 yeares, feeding it with whelpes cattes ratts & the like" yet not providing the bird with any water;[115] the "fenne" eagle "so tame that it went about the yard feeding on fish redherrings flesh & any offells without the least trouble";[116] the pelican "wch stuffed and cleansed I yet retaine";[117] and the bittern which "I kept in a garden 2 yeares feeding it with fish mice & frogges." Curious eggs, for instance the one from a bird referred to by Browne as a dorhawk, are a happy consequence for the collector of birds. As the case of the endlessly feeding knot suggests, the birds are of value not just for their presence but also for the experiments that can be conducted on them (19).

As Browne's corrections, additions, and donations of specimens and drawings accumulate, Merrett waxes bold to enlist Browne's help in supplying the losses caused by the great fire. For one melancholy moment, Browne gives the reasons why this might be difficult for him, for "many of my old assistants are dead & sometimes they fell upon animals, scarce to bee met with agayne." Indeed, the let-

[112] Cf. Southwell, ed., *Notes and Letters on the Natural History*, xvi.
[113] Southwell, ed., *Notes and Letters on the Natural History*, 2–3.
[114] See Sloane 1911–13, 112r.
[115] *Notes and Letters on the Natural History*, 3.
[116] *Notes and Letters on the Natural History*, 4.
[117] *Notes and Letters on the Natural History*, 17.

ters are attentive to the possibility of extinction. And there have been disasters in Norwich too, with the plague leading "the person intrusted in my howse" to incinerate or jettison some forty specimens "hanging up in my howse" (Keynes, 4.362). Yet even though the letters are filled with the shooting, stuffing, and drying of living things, they are wonderfully alive with the richness of nature in the small space between Norwich, its suburbs, and the sea. Indeed, part of the savor of this material comes from Browne's strong interest in cookery and cuisine. He recalls the crane served "in a bill of fare when the maior entertaind the duke of Norfolk" (*Notes and Letters on the Natural History*, 6); the herne "much desired by some palates" (17); and the godwit ("accounted the dayntiest dish in England & I think for the bignesse, of the biggest price," 19). And Merrett is quite frankly surprised by the newness with which Browne allows him to see the natural world, whether that novelty consists of whole species or variations, of the sense of rarity or commonality, or of some corrected mistake about a putatively well-known breed.

Browne's watery world of fens, broads, estuaries, marshes, as well as ocean, is often inextricably part of his experience of the bird and its behavior, as is the case with kingfishers: "The number of riuulets becks & streames whose banks are beset with willowes & Alders wch giue occasion of easier fishing & slooping to the water makes that handsome coulered bird abound" (*Notes and Letters on the Natural History*, 22). With starlings, the season and time of day factor into the scene:

> I haue obserued about the Autumne when they roost at night in the marshes in safe places upon reeds & alders. wch to obserue I went to the marshes about sunne set. where standing by their vsuall place of resort I obserued very many flocks flying from all quarters. wch in lesse than an howers space call all in & settled in innumerable numbers in a small compass. (28)

Not that the scenes are always soft and pleasing: in a letter to Merrett, Browne sends a sampling of flies whose abundance in the marshes of Norfolk is especially marked in "unhealthfull years about the first part of September" (Keynes, 4.351). Yet there is an expression of hope in Browne's gathering of the flies in a box, labeled for the sake of memory, with the insects converted into the shared material for learning.

With the study of fish, Browne acknowledges, water is rather an impediment than a vital and revealing context. "It may well seeme no easie matter," he notes, "to giue any considerable account of fishes and animals of the sea wherein tis sayd that there are things creeping innumerable both small and great beasts because they liue in an element wherein they are not so easely discouerable" (*Notes and Letters on the Natural History*, 31). This modest caution notwithstanding, Browne asserts that across the world, including America and other "barbarous nations," humankind has always been so "addicted to fishing" that "after this long nauigation search of the ocean bayes creeks Estuaries and riuers . . . there is scarce any fish butt hath been seen by some man." This assertion that the obscure might be better known than the obvious has little of the ring of paradox that Browne offers in works such as *Religio* or *Hydriotaphia*. The point here is simply that all humanity has collaborated in overcoming a pervasive obstacle to the advancement of learning. Throughout these notes on marine life, Browne once again records his own dissections, with close attention to the eyes in particular. He rates the specimen for the purposes of cuisine; juxtaposes observed specimens with those found in authoritative books; records the specimens collected at his house, as well as the experiments conducted there; and notes local names. Sometimes, a specific memory matters more than classification or naming: "Concha anatifera or Ansifera whereof about 4 yeares past were found upon the shoare no small number by yarmouth hanging by slender strings of a kind of Alga vnto seuerall splinters or cleauings of firre boards vnto wch they were seuerally fastned & hanged like ropes of onyons." As Browne proceeds with his careful description, he even notes what the "spectators fancy" to be the case (*Notes and Letters on the Natural History*, 48–9). In moments such as these, the study of nature involves a happy communion of Norfolk society, with water making each of nature's parishes continuous with all the others nearby. But the observation of nature is, for Browne, an often solitary and contemplative experience.

When Browne includes Camden's report "that in former time there haue been Beuers in the Riuer of Cardigan in wales," then goes on to assert the presence of otters as a "great destroyer of fish" in local rivers and broads (*Notes and Letters on the Natural History*, 56), he briefly connects natural history to antiquarianism. In making this link, he suggests a certain affinity with Izaak Walton, the author of the *Compleat Angler* and of the lives of Anglican divines, whose cultivation of an irenic, contemplative, yet empirical study of fish and angling is one side of an ethos whose other side is an idealization of the former Church of England before the civil war. So it is that Browne laments the passing of Dean Crofts as a churchman in the old style, presumably of Joseph Hall. In the books that he has ordered from bookseller William Oliver in 1671, we find Robert Sanderson's sermons (Sanderson, one of Walton's subjects); Heylyn's life of Laud; and "an endeavr to rectify some prevaylinge opinions contrary to the Doctrine of the Church of England" (Keynes, 4.386–7). Indeed, Browne's library contained a 1676 edition of *The Universal Angler*, a collaboration of Charles Cotton and Robert Venables with good old Walton.[118] As a clue to the likelihood that Browne's ideal church remains relatively inclusive in a Restoration world in which Presbyterians have been lumped in with other nonconformists, we also find Richard Baxter's work on the holiness of the Sabbath. In the same vein is Browne's admiration for Bishop Edward Reynolds (1599–1676). From 1638 onward, Reynolds had accentuated the need for comprehension, peace, and unity in the church. Having participated in the Westminster Assembly, he took up the cause of reconciliation between Presbyterians and Anglicans for the sake of a reformed and reduced episcopacy.[119] In Reynolds, that is, something of old Bishop Hall persisted in a living, preaching hero, a point which Browne made explicitly in *Repertorium*:

[118] Finch, ed., *Catalogue of the Libraries*, 52, item 155.

[119] Quotations and account of Edward Reynolds from Ian Atherton's essay in *ODNB*.

"My Honord freind also, Bishop Edward Reynolds, was not buryed in the church butt in the Bishops chappell, which was built by himself.... A person much of the temper of his prædecessor, of singular affability, meekenesse and humility, of great learning" (Keynes, 3.134).

Browne's continuing antiquarian interests can be seen in little ways, in the letters that he shared with other coin collectors such as John Brearcliffe of Halifax in the late 1660s or with a Mr. Talbot in an undated letter.[120] But Browne also composed a much reduced follow-up to *Hydriotaphia*, the so-called *Brampton Urns*, in which his focus is exclusively on the facts about the antiquities. This 1667 work shows that the aging Browne is increasingly concerned simply with preserving a past which the Restoration cannot and will not reconstitute. Despite a certain dismissive attitude at the outset—"I thought I had taken leave of urnes" until an associate requested his description—he eagerly calculates that millions of urns still buried in English turf "may still satisfie the curiosity of succeeding times and arise unto all age" (Keynes, 1.233, 237).[121]

In carefully setting the scene of discovery—near Paston's Oxnead park "in a large arable feild lying between Buxton and Brampton"—as well as the occasion (work on enclosing land with ditches), Browne immediately registers the fragility of the specimens, not just from the carelessness of the diggers but also in the hands of careful antiquarians such as Browne (Keynes, 1.233). Registering sounds (hollowness) as well as sights, textures, and smells, he interweaves cautious, detailed description with inference and conjecture. Thus the shallowness of the burial implies "that in all this time the earth hath litle varied its surface, though this ground hath been plowed to the utmost memorie of man." The numerousness of the urns suggests that the area was not wooded in antiquity, since groves were reserved for the burial of special persons. Not surprisingly, the presence of coins prompts consideration of dating burial practices; the inclusion of a nail in one urn leads to the hypothesis that one can learn about the vocation of the body from the accouterments in or "figures" on its burial vessel (1.236). Although the inscriptions at the Brampton site are neither many nor clear, Browne notes that they "commonly signified the name of the person interred, the names of servants officiall to such provisions or the name of the Artificer or manufactor of such vessels," calling on Liceti's guidance regarding how to tell the difference (1.235).

Lingering over the variety in "their magnitude, figure, colour, posture, &c.," Browne draws cross-references with other antiquarian findings, invoking authorities from Casaubon to "the learned Licetus" (Keynes, 1.233–5). But as he seeks to situate the specimens before him in a larger historical context, Browne purveys with these remains the same sense of unusualness that he brings to the evidence of certain birds in local waters. For two substantial paragraphs, he describes what

[120] MS Rawlinson D.391, 77r; Keynes, 4.387–8.

[121] First published in *Posthumous Works* (1712), *Brampton Urns* exists in several manuscript versions, and Keynes has made principal use of MS Sloane 1862, with insertions from MS Rawlinson D. 391.

at first is called "an observable peece of work" but which proves to be an elaborate structure of something resembling brickwork which comprises a series of holes on its sides with pots in some of the holes, "mouths downeward" (1.237). As Browne numbers the holes and measures their size, he also captures the experience of exploring this unknown structure: the workers feel through the holes into the hollowness, then clear away impeding earth and begin to break open the structure from the top moving downward through a series of floors composed "of a slatty not bricky substance" (1.237). Employed by Browne's friend W. Marsham, the workmen must employ "hard blowes for the breaking of the floares"—no delicate procedure, this discovery of the past—and Browne is on hand to describe what they uncover: "and in the last partition butt one a large pott was found of a very narrowe mouth, short eares, of the capacity of 14 pints which lay in an inclining posture close by, and somewhat under a kind of arch in the solid wall" (1.237). When the pot is removed intact, it is found to be "almost full of water, cleene, & without smell & insipid, which being poured out there still remaines in the pot a great lump of an heavie crusted substance" (1.238). As *Brampton Urns* moves toward its conclusion, we are left with a mystery consigned by Browne to "better conjecture," with cross-references to the republic of letters (his correspondent Gruter) yet with the clear sense that the fragmentary state of human knowledge, like the truncated, uneven shape of Browne's own notes and essays, might after all be a good thing for the future. In Browne's notes, shards are converted into seeds then plowed by the constant revision to which he subjects his notebooks, yet ready to be transplanted into the soils of fresher minds.[122] With the constant activities of migratory birds, of shifting earth, of workmen digging, and of landowners enclosing, the future looks bright for those curious children such as Edward Browne who can be trained to observe and inquire into the palimpsest of natural and human history.

The variety of Browne's fascinations in the Restoration period can lead to an astonishing combination of items on any one manuscript page: notes on coition run cheek by jowl with fragmentary musings on prelacy, twins, the inhabitants of the moon, charity, and figs.[123] But in this miscellaneousness, Browne focuses intensely on all that lives, not just in the larger sweep of history but in the smallest sites of nature, for instance, the "2 yellow stupid caterpillars taken from the eare of rie" that produced "great store of rough & woollen substance ouall like egges." For Browne, attending to life entails learning from death as well: "they both dyed butt out of these came in fewe days great numbers of small flies[—] strange it is there should bee 2 seurall productions from them."[124] In turn, Browne's contemporaries—both famous and obscure—honored him for his unsurpassed capacity to discern the ways in which God's creation was wonderful.

[122] This notion of Browne's notes as generative has been formulated by Antonia Moon in her essay, " 'A Fresh Reading of Books': Some Note-Taking Practices of Thomas Browne," in Murphy and Todd, eds., "*A man very well studyed,*" 67–86.

[123] BL Sloane 1843, 42r, 44r.

[124] From Sloane MS 1875.

5. KNIGHTHOOD, 1671

On Thursday, September 18, 1671, King Charles II, together with the Queen and the Dukes of York, Monmouth, and Buckingham, and a large retinue of courtiers and servants, paid a highly anticipated visit to Norwich.[125] Having departed from Newmarket on the 26th and visited Yarmouth on the 27th, the king arrived late on a rainy day for his tour of one of England's greatest provincial cities. The visit began awry, with the separate entrances of king and queen provoking city officials to scramble so that both parties might be met and then united. Once together, they were entertained at the Duke of Norfolk's palace by Sir Henry Herbert. On the 19th, the king attended service in the cathedral, then, after time spent in the bishop's palace, ended up at the Guildhall in the marketplace on which Browne lived. Appearing before the people and observing the troops, his majesty continued on his merry way to entertainments offered by the city at New Hall, by the Hobarts at Blickling (where he knighted Sir John's oldest son, Henry), and finally, for the evening, by Sir Robert Paston at Oxnead. On the 20th, Charles visited the Townshends at Raynham, though the queen returned to Sir Henry Howard in Norwich. According to Thomas Corie, the king took the time to touch citizens for the king's evil, an opportunity for which physicians such as Browne were required to provide certificates, and the queen condescended to let all manner of people kiss her hand.

In the midst of all this fanfare for the royal family, at the city feast in New or Blackfriars Hall, the king made a knight of Dr Thomas Browne.[126] (See Figure 10.2.) Transformed after the Reformation from the nave of a Dominican church into a place of civic assembly (the old chancel still serving as a place of worship), New Hall was a short walk toward Tombland and the cathedral from the marketplace where Browne lived. According to one account, Browne was conferred this honor "at the same time" that the mayor, Thomas Thacker, declined it.[127] But both *The London Gazette* and Matthew Stevenson's poem on the occasion stressed that the knighthood was self-evidently deserved: the king "was pleased to confer the same honor on the famous Dr Browne," and "There the *King* Knighted the so famous *Brown*, | Whose worth & learning to the world are known."[128]

For all the boisterous acclaim and city-wide shows of loyalty that greeted the king that September, Charles II's standing had never been more controversial, the king having agreed on the sly to convert to Catholicism for the sake of French support, and including a brand new mistress in the traveling retinue. When, on

[125] Planning began in April 1670 and the actual visit was postponed in April 1671. The three main sources for the visit are a letter by Thomas Corie, a poem by Matthew Stevenson, and a report in *The London Gazette*.

[126] See Trevor Hughes, "Sir Thomas Browne's Knighthood," *Norfolk Archaeology* 43 (1998–99), 326–7, which corrects the misunderstanding fueled by Blomefield's famous account that Browne was selected only after the mayor declined.

[127] Francis Blomefield, *An Essay Towards a Topographical History of the County of Norfolk*, 11 volumes (London: 1805–10), 3.413–14.

[128] *The London Gazette*, 1671, 613, September 24–October 2nd, 2; Matthew Stevenson, *Norfolk Drollery* (1673), 30.

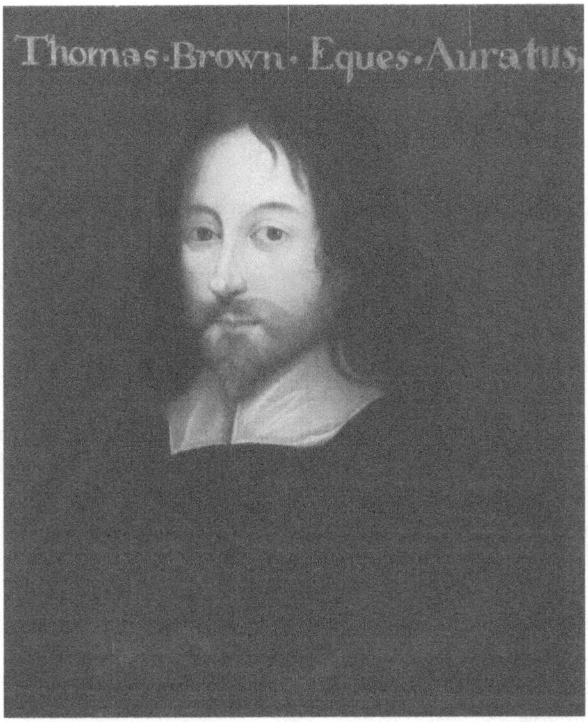

Figure 10.2 Sir Thomas Browne. © Royal College of Physicians.

March 4, 1672, Warden Woodward reported on another visit to Browne that his knighthood was bestowed "to Dr Brownes prejudice," it is impossible to know whether that judgment was meant to suggest extraordinary favor or unfounded scorn.[129] Even though few physicians had ever been knighted,[130] the citizens of Norwich no doubt believed that their famous doctor deserved the honor. The question further raised by the mayor's declining this honor was whether King Charles deserved an association with Browne.

What Browne thought about receiving an honor from this particular (and infamously lecherous) monarch—as against the Tudor Elizabeth, the last ruler to make a visit to Norwich—is hard to say. A year after he was knighted, Browne did make sure that young William Wotton "read a Stanza in Spencer very distinctly, and pronounce it properly" (Keynes, 4.399), and Elizabeth was of course the Muse of *The Fairie Queene*.[131] By 1679, still writing out certificates so that scrofula patients

[129] *Progress Notes*, ed. Woodward and Rickard, 99.

[130] See Hughes, "Sir Thomas Browne's Knighthood," 327, for Charles's reputation, and 330, for physicians and knighthood.

[131] Wotton's education, but also Browne's part in it, were the subjects of Henry Wotton, *An Essay on the Education of Children in the First Rudiments of Learning* (1753); for Browne, "not only famous for his Practice, but illustrious as well in Philology, as Philosophy," see 58–9.

might receive the king's touch, Browne was reporting a widespread pleasure that the king was leaving Newmarket prematurely—not just because "the country is still sickly" or "the wether uncertaine" but also, though Browne steers clear of actually passing judgment, because the place itself, with its focus on cockfighting, plays, and racing, epitomized the fecklessness of the Restoration court. Yet whether he liked it or not, Browne's responsibility for mediating between scrofula victims and the king required that he play a part in the contemporary myth-making of monarchy.

In briefly narrating the events of his life to John Aubrey, Browne jumped from his travels on the Continent to his induction into the Royal College followed by his knighthood (Keynes, 4.376). Clearly it was a major milestone in his life. In recalling the event of his knighting to Edward, however, Browne set it in the context of natural history and domestic life in Norwich. On June 14, 1676, he reminded his son of the dolphin which they dissected during the king's visit to Norwich. "Dr Clark was at my house," Browne recalls, "when you tooke a draught of severall parts very well, wch Dr Clark had sent unto him." The most vivid memory of the moment comes next, when Browne notes to his son that "your mother hath an art to dresse & cooke the flesh so as to make an excellent savory dish of it, & the King being at Newmarket I sent collars thereof to his table, which were well liked of" (Keynes, 4.60–1). Perhaps it was his modesty that led Browne to subordinate honor to dissection and cuisine. But as the 1660s gave way to the 1670s, it is a safe bet that he cherished the guts of a dolphin or the ancient art of cooking, like the art of stone masonry, more than he did the denuded rituals of a world now sadly lost.

Cooking and cuisine, like dissection and anatomy, were themselves bound up in ritual according to Browne's training and reading. Among the manuscript notes that he left behind, Browne recorded details from the history of cooking, an extension of his deep engagement with Athenaeus's *Deipnosophists.* As Karen Edwards has argued, this work offered Browne "a model of fluent urbanity that forever defers a confrontation with a diminished political and social context.... The point is to keep the conversation going in such a way that it will not have to confront what has been lost."[132] Browne's reading notes on Athenaeus explicitly lament the loss of a whole world of learning, wit, and humor that the many citations in the *Deipnosophists* evoke. In catching glimpses of so many almost obliterated writers, he can only wish that time were somehow less corrosive. Browne's is never a pure or simple nostalgia; in the same notes, he urges the courage to shape language anew. With his notes focused on cookery, however, it is readily apparent that eating and drinking are, for him, so subject to horrible abuse and immoderation that such abuse serves as a synecdoche for the human tendency to sleepwalk through life. But the experience of dinner, like the experience of rites, of reading, or empirical observation and dissection can be as wonderfully meaningful as their perversion is foolish, diseased, and sinful. Not one to criticize his king at any length, Browne concedes in a letter to Edward that "the King or gentlemen will bee litle taken with

[132] See Karen L. Edwards, "Engaging with Pygmies: Thomas Browne and John Milton," in Barbour and Preston, eds., *Sir Thomas Browne: The World Proposed*, 112–13.

the Anatomie" of an animal, "butt are like to take more notice of some other things wch may bee sayd upon the animal & which they understand" (Keynes, 4.206). Browne was sagely preparing his public figure of a son for a reduced political culture.

Explaining to Aubrey that "an understanding singing-man of 91 yeares" was assisting him with the record of cathedral monuments, many filched "in the late times" and all vulnerable to "oblivion," Browne dismissed Restoration religious culture with his remark that today's "churchmen [were] litle minding such things" (Keynes, 4.374). In *Repertorium*, he remarked on Elizabethan monuments violated "in the late times" (Keynes, 3.124) or on the high quality of those Elizabethan bishops who "lived as Bishops should do, and were not warriars like B. Spencer their predecessor" (3.132). More than once in the last years of his life, he reverted to the famous weeklong visit to Norwich paid by the virgin queen in 1578—once, in *Repertorium* where he commemorates the attractive noble arms beautifying the cathedral, created just after that visit, and damaged during "the late times" yet preserved in "a draught of them all I have by me" (3.137–8). In a letter written to Edward in October 1680, Browne uses the visit to anchor his contrast between contemporary extravagance and the simplicity of older times. Unlike the coach-obsessed moderns, Queen Elizabeth had paid her week-long visit to Norwich on horseback with only "a coach or two in her trayne." "When I was a youth," Browne continues, "many great persons travelled with 3 horses, butt now there is a new face of things" (Keynes, 4.166). In November, Browne was at it again, sorry for the death of "the old man beyond Scoale Inn, who wayted on the Earl of Leicester when Queen Eliz. came to Norwich, and who told me many things thereof" (4.169). Reporting to Edward on local events, Browne was apt to make note of the king's presence at Newmarket, especially since he had to attend to certificates for the touch. But he was also increasingly dismissive of the tasteless expensive ways there, at the amounts of money that people were willing to pay for bad accommodation or "very bad claret" (4.218).

Yet Browne was never ready to give himself over wholly to nostalgia, which simply did not suit the author of *Pseudodoxia*, the natural historian of an ever new and mysterious watery world, or the hopeful grandfather and father. And so in his notes on Athenaeus, Platina, and Apicius, in juxtaposing ancient with modern cuisines and tastes, Browne defended the moderns. "I wish we knew more clearly the aids of the ancients," he said of their "sauces, relishes, flavours, digestives," and so forth, then concluded that "I do not know whether they would have surpassed salted sturgeons' eggs, anchovy sauce, or our royal pickles." Both the elaborate delicacies promoted by Apicius and the austerity of the Stoics are dissatisfying to the modern palate. Yet Browne is not simply rejecting the ancients either. Most obviously, he is proposing the changeability of taste, its unpredictability or even its lunacy. If Browne's appetite is far more squeamish than he claimed it to be in *Religio*—he "would have had [his] stomach turned by the sausages, tripe, morsels and coarse greens of Apicius" (Keynes, 3.179)—this is simply because human preferences are unstable, even absurd factors in historical change.

But change is not the only keynote of these jottings on culinary reading. At times Browne proposes an ethical principle or calculus according to which we ought "to soothe appetite and satisfy nature" ("*orexim leniat et naturæ satisfaciat*" [Keynes, 3.176, 179]). And he offers guidelines in delineating extremes. We would be foolish to expect the "Trojan pig," which he glosses as "a hogge Roasted with great varietie of other flesh in the belly; so called from the Trojan horse, which concealed so many men in its cavitie" (3.176). But this does not mean that we should heed the taste of ascetics whose severity would have us return to what they suppose was a sauce-less world "before the flood" or to the paltry diet of "cabbage and cheese" (the Epicurean diet) or of legumes now reserved for cattle (3.175, 178–9). If Browne is not ready for such a reduced fare, however, his is not a heavenly palate in need of ambrosia or asphodel. He is neither one of Penelope's extravagant suitors nor the Pythagorean Empedocles whose vegetarian ways led him to celebrate an Olympic triumph with "beef made of myrrh, incense and aromatics" (3.179). "I am sure," Browne jokes, "that at the race-feast few of those who enjoy feeding their stomachs rather than their noses, stretched a hand to this."

The Olympic context of that last jest is important for Browne's setting of dinner as part of a triumphant social context. At issue is not just the criterion of taste but the value of appropriate ritual. Like cooking, Browne suggests, ritual should be neither ridiculously elaborate nor wholly denuded by iconoclasm—whether the context is domestic and social or ecclesiastic and divine. By looking to Athenaeus in particular for guidance, Browne seems to recognize that the middle ground is harder to come by in contemporary times. Yet in their home, Browne and his wife Dorothy worked side-by-side to create such a social context, a collaboration that one sees most clearly in the modest form of a household book preserved by the Harbord family who, from 1676, resided at Gunton Park where Browne continued to attend them. As the Harbord family papers show, Browne had been their physician since at least the period of his knighthood: in a letter dated January 14, 1673, Sir Charles Harbord, who in 1648 had purchased Stanning Hall in Norfolk, confided in his son John that he was perplexed about why John should be troubled by the scurvy since he has been so active in his recreations. Then Sir Charles exhorted, "Pray neglect not to observe Sr Tho: Brownes advise." In another letter during the same month the father is still worried about recurrence "of the stuffing in [John's] breast"; recommending a remedy, Sir Charles urges that "if that give you not ease try Dr Brownes remedyes."[133]

[133] Norfolk Record Office, GTN 5/4/3/32 and GTN 5/4/3/37. In his *Compte Tout mes despens Com[m]encent en May 1670* (GTN 5/4/4), John recorded a number of payments to Dr Browne: January 16, 1673 two pounds "at several tymes" (no foliation); March 1675, a pound; twice on the 20th and 30th, a pound; 14 May 1675, 0.10.6 to Sir TB for physic; August 30, 1675, 1.1.6; November 21, 1676 0.10.0; October 16, 1677, again 10 shillings. One payment for shoes and other household goods given to "Dr Browne" in March 1677 may refer to Dorothy, since she often sent shopping orders off to London for her neighbors, and John Harbord tends to refer to Thomas Browne as "Sir" by this date.

In this manuscript, the family recorded seven medical prescriptions dictated by Sir Thomas, each with its carefully delineated steps of preparation and ingestion. As is so often the case in the seventeenth century, medicine and aliment belonged together in the reference manuscripts of the household, with pharmaceutical ingredients including roses, caraway seeds, marsh mallow, sea holly roots, fennel seed, honey, raisons, currents, china root, anise seeds, barley water, chamomile, quinces, betony, harts horn, and so forth.

Given Browne's concern for children's diseases, it is noteworthy that one of the Gunton recipes is designed for "a child of 6 years old" and urges the attendant to be careful with quantities "according to the age & strength of the Person" (Keynes, 3.463–5). Yet this prescription for ague demonstrates how even the most familiar remedies can have complex features. In its inclusion of a "Confection of Alkermes," the child's recipe purveys its highly commonplace nature as well as Browne's own training in southern France, for it was in Languedoc that one often encountered the type of oak on which grew an excrescence thought at the time to be an insect-producing berry. But the mystique of its Arabian origins, as well as the uncertainty of its basic species and the intricacies of its preparation, meant that a level of uncertainty was often admitted when it came to the use of this famous drug.[134] So too with Browne's prescription of "9 grains of Gascoigne Powder or Lady Kent's." As the Countess of Kent's version of "Gascons own Powder" made clear, the ingredients for the medicine were not simply herbal: "Take a pouder of Pearl, of red Corral, of Crabs eyes, of Harts horn, and white Amber, of each one ounce, beat them into fine pouder, and searce [sift] them, then take so much of the back toes of the Crabs clawes as of all the rest of the pouders, for that is the cheif worker." The recipe distinguished between necessary ingredients and those "added by some for curiosity."[135]

An additional Gunton entry has Lady Browne's advice for the broiling of a tench:

> Take a large Tench, scoure him & wash him clean in warm water, then slit him down the belly all the way, then take a pretty deal of winter savory & parsly, wash & shred them fine with an onyon, then mix it with a good peice of butter & some salt & turn the Tench the inside outside & sew it up with the butter & herbs in it, & broyle it upon a gridiron till it be brown enough on all sides, then take a good peice of butter & melt it with an anchovy, then take the herbs out of the belly & put into the butter, dish it & poure the sauce over it. (3.465)

Diners from antiquity, or those in future days to come, might not recognize or appreciate every aspect of this preparation; but in his notes on cooking, as in his praise for Joseph Hall and Edward Reynolds, Browne made his case for the grounds on which all sane human beings might find genuine (if limited) meaning, loving community, and rich experience in their short lives on earth. Whether

[134] See John Gerard, *The Herbal or General History of Plants* (facsimile of 1633 enlarged edition, New York: Dover, 1975) 1342–3.

[135] Elizabeth Grey, Countess of Kent, *A choice manual of rare and select secrets in physick and chirurgery* (1653), 172–3.

medical, culinary, or devotional, the rites of living not only needed to be moderate or temperate, a virtue that Browne would accentuate in the letters of his last decade; they also profited from being flexible, bending to meet the circumstances in which a complex life unfolded, and open to the new discoveries that the inquisitive were and would be making. Thus Browne worked out the ways in which he might reconcile worship with the demands of vocation, or adapted his medical advice according to the profile of the patient. And thus too Lady Browne understood that good cooking was attentive to circumstances and occasions; in a letter written to Edward later in the 1670s, she apologized for not considering her daughter-in-law's pregnancy when she seasoned a plate of venison (Keynes, 4.88).

By the early 1670s, Lady Dorothy and Sir Thomas Browne were indeed looking to the future through the birth of their grandchildren. But as was the way with the dangers of seventeenth-century childbirth, the hope of the future was often so simply erased. Having married Henry Fairfax of Hurst in Berkshire toward the latter end of 1669—he was the son and heir of Henry Fairfax, second son of Thomas Viscount Fairfax—Anne had her first child baptized in her parents' parish church on August 30, 1670, then gave birth to a son called Barker in 1671 in the parish of St James' Clerkenwell, London,[136] but the next decade would bring a good deal of grief in the death of her offspring. Anne had met her husband while living with the Barker family in London.[137] For his part, Edward married Henrietta Susanna Terne, his anatomy mentor's daughter, in the spring of 1672.[138] For the rest of his life, Browne would take great delight in Edward's son Thomas, but he knew more than ever that children were fragile: "God blesse my daughter Fairfax my daughter Browne & the litle ones," he wrote to Edward one winter's morning in the 1670s (Keynes, 4.58).

But in the early 1670s, Browne was looking to the future of Norwich in particular with regard to another type of offspring, a copy of his 1672 *Works* that he corrected for donation to the Norwich City Library. Having donated to the same library a multivolume *Opera Omnia* of the scholar and philosopher Justus Lipsius in 1666, Browne wanted to ensure that local readers, above all the clergy who made greatest use of the Norwich City Library, would be reading *Religio Medici* and *Pseudodoxia Epidemica* as at long last Browne wanted them to endure. Most of the changes were miniscule: words occluded by the printing press written in; mistakes corrected; punctuation altered; and syntax smoothed. In one instance, in a translation of Latin verses in *Religio Medici*, the term "cunningly" was altered to "purposely" for a characterization of divine providence, perhaps simply because the dominant meaning of the

[136] Baptism registered in *A True Register of all the Christeninges... in the Parishe of St. James Clarkenwell*, ed. Robert Hovenden, Harleian Society Publications (London, 1884), 9.251.

[137] For Anne or Nancy and her marriage to Henry Fairfax, see Morris, "Sir Thomas Browne's Daughters, 'Cosen Barker,' and the Cottrells," *Notes and Queries* 231 (1986), 472–9. See also Charles Williams, "The Pedigree of Sir Thomas Browne," *Norfolk Archaeology* 15 (1904), 109–13.

[138] Their license was dated April 29.

word "cunning" had degenerated from learnedly skillful to covert and sly.[139] Browne may well have been drawn to the city library as a repository for his works because its members tended to override religious divisions, with the now ejected Presbyterian John Collinges joining forces with the St Peter Mancroft loyalists to the Church of England, George Cock and John Whitefoot. The future archbishop Thomas Tenison would join up in 1674.[140] It was a modest way to affect the future, but it suited Browne's increasingly rich and powerful understanding that the advancement of learning began in one's city, county, and very home.

And indeed Browne's notebooks and letters from the last decades of his life were filled to brimming with people and places of his homeland. There were kind neighbors such as Augustine Briggs; colleagues such as Drs Brady, Blincolme, Witherly, and Croone; apothecaries such as Dey; surgeons such as Crop and Dade; George Rose the bookseller; Mr Beecroft the carrier; and Mrs Green the sugar baker. So many Norfolk places filled Browne's memories and imagination: the cliffs at Winterton; the fens, marshes, broads, rivers (the Yare, Bure, Wavenly, and Wensum or "Norwich"), and shores; the rabbit burrows in Norrold; herring fisheries in Yarmouth; chalk pits and meadows but also the bridges and parish churches; and so many towns, from Lynn and Hunstanton on the west side of the county to Cromer at the northeast corner, and down to Thetford, many associated with specific flora and fauna. Of Norwich itself, Browne wrote of the dunghills and churchyards with a special fascination; of neighborhoods such as Timber Hill, churches such as St Stephens and St Leonards, gates including Bishops and Pockthorpe; and of course the cathedral and the marketplace—he could always see the spire of the former from his home in the latter. As Browne approached death and his Norwich became ever more divisive, he grew in the intensity with which he found a world of wonder in a little meadow and a profound experience in the place where he had settled. Although Browne's knighthood offered him a boost of self-esteem, the portrait made of him in the wake of the occasion (Figure 10.2) struck its earliest viewers as anything but a show of hubris. One observer noted that for all his widespread fame as an author, his celebrity as a successful physician, and his universal learning, Browne purveyed in this portrait a "most amiable sweetness of aspect, grave without Dulness, thoughtfull without sourness; and with a most engaging Blush of Modesty suffused over his Countenance"; in

[139] See Patrides, 114, for "cunningly." The corrected copy of 1672 is in the Norfolk Heritage Centre, Norwich, see p. 34. The correction to "purposely" is also found in Elizabeth Lyttleton's commonplace book. The history of the Norwich City Library, and the known facts of Browne's donations, are given in Clive Wilkins-Jones, ed., *Norwich City Library, 1608–1737*, in *Norfolk Record Society* (2008), 73. The minister at St Peter Mancroft, George Cock, was in attendance with Browne's friend John Whitefoot at the donation of the Lipsius on May 14, 1666 (73). The copy of Browne's *Works* was received from Whitefoot on January 12, 1674 (83).

[140] There is some disagreement over the identity of the Thomas Browne who assisted Collinges, Cocke, Whitefoot, and Robert Harmer in reviewing the merits of a proposal for a second grammar school by one Mark Lewis; see H. W. Saunders, *A History of the Norwich Grammar School* (Norwich: Jarrold and Sons, 1932), 211.

short, his was "a remarkable tenderness of Disposition."[141] While the wording of this passage owes something to Whitefoot's remarks in the prefatory material to *Posthumous Works*, it is noteworthy that even with Browne's elevated social status, his admirers read in the characters of his face the same foundation of honor in virtue that the by-now famous physician had once praised as an obscure man in *Religio Medici*.

[141] BL Additional MS 4221, 191v.

11

Norwich, 1672–1682

In February 1672, Sir Thomas Browne received a fortnight's visit from a Suffolk gentleman named William Acton. While it is unclear whether the visit was mainly professional or personal, the two men conversed about honor. Browne had recently been awarded a knighthood from the king, and Acton was in consultation with the heraldic authorities over his family coat and crest. Unlike Browne, Acton was (he wrote in a letter) "a single man" and "younger brother" enquiring on behalf of a nephew. But like Browne, Acton had a growing sense that it was too late for him to concern himself very much with worldly honors since he was "goeing out of ye world." Making this remark on February 23 after his visit to Norwich, perhaps Acton had received less than rousing news from the famous physician.[1]

By the end of 1673, the value of honor had never been so dubious in the Browne household. For in all likelihood it was from wounds or sickness received in the disastrous Battle of the Texel, August 11, 1673, at the climax of the Third Dutch War that Browne's dear son Thomas died.[2] With the war itself in part motivated by an exchange of insults, and with Prince Rupert in denial about the dire

[1] News of the visit is found in a letter from Robert Clarke to Sir Edward Bysshe, the Clarenceux Herald who had overseen the visitation of the eastern counties in 1664. See J. J. Muskett, "From a Herald's Letter Book," *The East Anglian* 13 (1909), 88. The letters are drawn from a manuscript in the British Library, Sir Edward Bysshe's Correspondence 1653–76.

[2] Evidence for Thomas's condition after the battle derives from National Archives ADM 7/778, a list of wounded and sick men transported from various ships to a vessel called *The Gloucester*. While Thomas's name was a common one, the list noted the more important of the men involved, and Thomas of course was a lieutenant. The fact that these men were brought to hospitals in London in late August helps to explain the one thing that we have known about Thomas's death for years now, namely, that he died "unmarried" and was buried in the London parish church of St James Clerkenwell (this from an early eighteenth-century pedigree drawn up by the antiquary Peter Le Neve (printed in Wilkin, vol. 1, as pedigree 2)). Because the old St James's Clerkenwell was torn down and replaced in the eighteenth century, no monument remains, if ever there was one. Thomas's sister Anne had lived with the Barkers in Clerkenwell in the 1660s and worshiped at St. James'. It should be noted as evidence against the 1673 death that the parish register of the old church lists for June 9, 1667, the burial of "Master Browne, a gentleman, bur[d] in the Chancell" (*A True Register of all the Christeninges, Mariages, and Burialles in the Parishe of St. James Clarkenwell, from the Yeare of our Lorde God 1551*, ed. Hovenden, vol. 5, 5). But the Le Neve pedigree includes the date September 1 for the burial, which works well with the Battle of Texel on August 11, 1673. Registers of sea officers held in the National Maritime Museum, Greenwich and in the Pepys Library, Magdalene College, Cambridge (PL 2941) tell us only that Thomas was commissioned as a lieutenant by Prince Rupert and the Duke of Albemarle in 1666 for the *Marie Rose*, but these lists are incomplete regarding commissions and the deaths of those so commissioned. See also J. R. Tanner, *A Descriptive Catalogue of the Naval Manuscripts in the Pepysian Library at Magdalene College, Cambridge* (London: Naval Records Society, 1903), 1.330. I am grateful to Mike Bevan (Royal Museums Greenwich) and to Phillipa Grimstone (Magdalene College) for help with these registers.

consequences of fighting for the sake of reputation, it is not surprising that contemporaries expressed dismay at, as one put it, so "many valiant men sent into th'other world, without any cerimony besides peales of Thundering Ordnance." To make matters worse for the Browne family, some reports had it that the ship known as the *Saint George*—the one on which Thomas in all likelihood saw action—was shameful for the men's lack of experience and for their failure to "stand by their Guns" under heavy attack.[3]

Despite tragedy and his own encroaching frailty, Browne remarkably never eased up on his intellectual vigor, professional commitment, and fascination with the world around him. In one letter from this period in his life, written to Madame Susan Hare about her sick daughter, Browne vividly expressed just how eager he was to help his far-flung patients: "I am sorry to understand your daughter is fallen ill & hath a cough for above a fortnight & now lately raysed a little blood.... I am glad Dr Edwards doth sometimes visit her and I shall bee ready in my utmost assistance." It is true that the horses that must carry him the thirty miles from Norwich to Broomsthorpe are not yet sufficiently "in case" (in the right physical condition) to make the trip, and that Browne's own business requires his presence in Norwich "at four or five aclock." Nonetheless, Mrs Hare has his assurances that Browne will be with her and the patient on the morrow and that, in the meanwhile, he has sent the girl a "thinne syrupe" as well as a "plaster to be applyed to the mould of her head, the hayre being shourn or clipped very close on that part."[4] In the last decade of his life, Browne's vocational intensity was matched by the richness of his intellectual, social, and experiential engagement.

During the 1670s, Browne sensed that English society was changing in irreversible, drastic ways, and he was not alone. Sir Edward Dering agreed with a considerable number of observers that 1672 represented a turning-point in English politics.[5] Even those not sharing Dering's viewpoint tended to agree that 1672 was a watershed year for the nation. As John Miller argues, 1672 prompted many observers to conclude that "the rest of the reign was to be unsettled by fears that the king and his advisors wished to establish 'Popery and arbitrary government'."[6] Far from floating free of this contentious partisanship, Norfolk ranked among the most divided localities of all. In religious matters alone, the period from around 1674 onward was highly contentious. With Bishop Sparrow declaring Norwich as "the worst corporation I thought that I had met with" in 1678, the more aggressive supporters of the Church of England renewed their resolve to suppress dissent, all of which helped produce the rift between Whigs

[3] CSPD, August 12, 1673, Rupert to Lord Arlington; SP 29/336/2 f. 155; and *Journals and Narratives of the Third Dutch War*, ed. R. C. Anderson (London: Naval Records Society, 1946), especially 339–94. For further evidence of Thomas on the *St George*, see National Archives ADM 33/97.

[4] This letter, written between 1668 and 1682, is in the NRO, Norfolk and Norwich Archaeological Society Collection, C3/7; it is transcribed by Paul Rutledge in "Doctor Thomas Browne," *Norfolk Archaeology* 44 (2005), 712–13.

[5] *Diaries and Papers of Sir Edward Dering, Second Baronet*, ed. M. F. Bond, HMSO (1976), 125–6; quoted in John Miller, *The Restoration and the England of Charles II*, 2nd edn. (New York: Longman, 1997), 108–9.

[6] Miller, *The Restoration*, 68.

and Tories in the 1680s.[7] The clash between sides came to a head in the last year of Browne's life, 1682.

Browne was no distant observer of these developments in local affairs; the major players on both sides and in the middle belonged to families—the Pastons, Hobarts, Townshends—who were his friends, patients, and kinsmen. It was Browne who twice afforded Bishop Sparrow with letters excusing him from making official trips to London (Keynes, 4.399–400). In the Paston letters, one finds Dr Browne amid the ongoing accounts of partisan politics, "caballing," and social networking. In September 1677, there is Dr Browne confiding in Henry Beddingfield that the heirs of two Paston estates are unlikely to survive to maturity, a piece of news greeted with self-interested glee by the benefactor of this morbidity, William Paston.[8] On April 14, 1678, Lord Yarmouth wrote of Lord Townshend that the latter "has had a suddene fit of ye gow^t^ & stone both together or rather ye strangerie, butt as I heare was left somewhat better on friday By Sr Thos Browne who was sent for to him."[9] Paston's letters also betray the weariness and paranoia that Norfolk partisanship was producing in Browne's patients in a culture where friendship, loyalty, and the civility underwritten by scholarship as well as tradition could no longer be taken for granted.[10] To the end of his own life Browne brought comfort to Yarmouth who on September 25, 1682, told his wife that "this day heere came in Sr Thomas Browne and stayd with me till now."[11] On the other side of all the contentiousness was the Hobart family, to whom the Browne family was related, to whose illnesses Browne continued to dedicate his "mite" (Keynes, 4.383), and whose letters are as filled with contemporary strife as the Pastons'.[12] Whereas Browne was placing a high value on neighborliness in his own letters, Lord Yarmouth referred ironically to the Hobarts of Blickling as "neighbours" from whom he was glad to be hearing "neither newes nor noyse."[13]

Even when Browne was not riding out to heal the families of Norfolk, their conflicts were barging into his life, as they did on February 18, 1678, when the marketplace at Browne's doorstep was once again the site of what one biased observer called "fanatic impudence" and villainy in the wake of a hotly contested election.[14] Thus St Peter Mancroft's domination by conformists—according to a 1676 census—did not shield Browne from the voices of dissent, nor did it conceal the fact that the defenders of conformity could show more violent zeal than those sympathetic to dissent.[15] When Browne expressed "content" at the results of the election in February 1681, it is hard to tell whether that registered his response to a conservative victory or to the astonishing fact that the event had "passed quietly

[7] Quoted in Evans, *Seventeenth-Century Norwich*, 268. [8] NRO B/Y/2/27, September 2, 1677.

[9] NRO BL/Y/2/68. [10] See for instance NRO BL/Y/2/48 and BL/Y/2/57.

[11] BL Additional MS Section B 27,448, f. 134. [12] NRO WKC 7/6/1-77 404x1.

[13] NRO BL/Y/2/68.

[14] Reverend John Gough, letter to Lady Yarmouth, in NRO BL/Y/2/60.

[15] According to the census, St Peter Mancroft comprised 800 conformists, 4 papists, and 40 nonconformists (see *The Compton Census of 1676: A Critical Edition*, ed. Anne Whiteman, assisted by Mary Clapinson (London: Oxford University Press, 1986), British Academy Records of Social and Economic History, XI, 218.

without opposition" (Keynes, 4.183). As a newsletter from 1681 illustrates, Browne himself could be appropriated in the partisanship: in *Strange and Wonderful News from Norwich*, one T. W. quipped that the good citizens of Norwich have sent "an Address against Popery" to newly elected MPs—despite the fact that "we like *Religio Medici* very well."[16] But Browne also attracted intense loyalty as the very embodiment of a kindness, trustworthiness, and civility that were endangered virtues. Browne's fellow physician Richard Clarke, a friend with whom Browne had collaborated in anatomical exercises on a dolphin, had it inscribed on his monument in Marlingford parish church that Clarke was "as one might expect the faithful servant and companion to that great Aescalapius of Norwich Sir Thomas Browne."[17] At Gunton House one could see a portrait of Browne posing with his hand on a copy of *Religio Medici*.[18] Among the loose papers of the Woodhouse family was Sir Thomas Wodehouse's anagram that Browne was *Ter bonus, cordatus homo*, with the remark that this witticism would serve as an apt eulogy.[19] But the most commonplace testimony to Browne's favor in the eyes of his neighbors was the credit that his medical success tended to receive, for instance in a May 1677 letter from William Heveningham to his mother, in which William expressed his gratitude to "docter Browne" for recovering his strength after a bleeding and medical "advice" had "carried away my feauour."[20] For Browne's part, healing patients such as William Heveningham was part and parcel of concern for all the circumstances of their lives, and so it is not surprising to find him writing Edward in July 1676 about the marriages and other happenings in the Heveningham family (Keynes, 4.66). In Norwich, too, physicians such as George Colebrook eagerly consulted Sir Thomas on a wide range of their neighbors' diseases and afflictions, from a malignant fever and diabetes to ulcers and a nose scab.[21]

As he took notes on Samuel Butler's satirical *Hudibras*, Browne attempted to locate contemporary polemic within the ancient tradition of burlesque, arguing that the "ludicrous way of transferring Verses of famous Poets into a Jocose Sense and Argument" represented "no new inventions, but old Fancies reviv'd" (Keynes, 3.245). It was an interpretation of that poem which was deemed sufficiently noteworthy by Browne's executors to be included in the *Posthumous Works* of 1712. As his many letters to his son Edward reveal, Browne was disturbed by the normalization of vicious partisanship in the political intercourse between Norfolk and London, and amongst neighbors in Norwich itself. At times he registered his concern as bemusement, a state of uncertainty maximized by its principal source of

[16] T. W., *Strange and wonderful news from Norwich* (1681), n.p.

[17] In Latin "utpote magne illius apud Norwicenses Aesculapy Thomae Browne Equitis Aurati fidus minister et Comes" (quoted in Batty Shaw, *Sir Thomas Browne of Norwich*). On a deed from June 14, 1676, Browne served as a trustee for a property on behalf of Clarke (NRO MC2577/6/9/1–3 984x7).

[18] This portrait is now in the possession of St Peter Mancroft.

[19] NRO MS KIM 9/3.

[20] NRO MC 107/1 f. 12. Although the NRO catalogue speculates that this Browne might be Edward, this seems unlikely since Heveningham is writing from Ketteringham, four miles from Norwich.

[21] Royal College of Physicians, MS-COLEG/208/1, the *Consilia medica* of George Colebrook.

information in newspapers and gossip. Browne was constantly trying to peer through the haze left by the various newspapers that he read, including the ones generated from coffee-houses as well as the one he considered as standard, generic, or "common."[22] When rebellion threatened in Scotland over anxieties that Protestantism was imperiled by popery, Browne complained that "the coffie & common newes letters tell us something of the rebellion in Scotland, but I thinck very imperfectly. A litle more time will better informe us of that businesse" (Keynes, 4.119). At times the word "news" seems to slide into "noise," for instance in a letter of November 1679, when Browne remarked that "all the noyse heere is of the new plot sett up to make nothing or litle of the former, which I perceave no contrivance can effect" (4.137). Yet unlike conventional notions of opinion, fame, and gossip, which tended to suppose a constant truth untouched by infectious misprision or "vulgar error," Browne's fascination with news had a way of colluding with a political culture in which perception shapes reality, even as he harped on the moral and devotional means by which his offspring might preserve their integrity in a world of trouble, discomposure, and confusion. It was a dilemma that he had been confronting ever since his Oxford tutor had commenced a sermon with a provocative request for news, only to fill his teachings with sophisticated estimations of the languages of faith. In Browne's life, news had a way of exaggerating the imperfect means by which human beings strove to arrive at truth.

1. LETTERS FROM HOME

In lieu of certainty about events, Browne periodically offers his own analysis in letters, as he does in the case of the Scottish unrest (Keynes, 4.119). In January 1681, he surmises that "the calling of the parliament at Oxford will make citizens & tradesmen the less earnest to bee Burgesses in corporations" (4.181). Browne is frequently concerned about the volatility and temperature of the English Parliament itself and especially attentive to the progress and prospects of elections, in reference to which he begins to use the term "party," for instance in describing the "rude and boysterous" seamen who "take in with the country party, as they call it" (4.93). In April 1679, he explains to Edward the "late differences" among his own friends in Norfolk politics and elections, including Sir John Hobart's charges of "illegall proceedings" by Lord Yarmouth, so that when the letter goes on to mention the same "parties" standing again, it is not quite clear whether the word is confined to the meaning of "persons" (4.101). Contentiousness comes to be taken for granted, the question remaining only as to degree. Of election results, he often expresses regrets rather than satisfaction,[23] even analyzing the partisan perceptions that sway elections: of one candidate he points out that "hee lost it the last time because though the Gentry were much for him, yet the people feared hee would prove a meere courtier" (4.93). Increasingly he comes to expect what he calls a

[22] For this distinction, see Keynes, 4.99. [23] See for instance Keynes, 4.97.

"hard canvas" during election times (4.181–2). And he worries, in this context as in others, that the affairs of the world are beginning to prey on the composition of brains or minds as much as on the social temperature generated between the rivals (4.101).

Browne's letters convey something of the excitement that attends waiting on the latest news from London for a gauge of the nation's political health. A world governed by news is one of heightened expectation (Keynes, 4.101). Yet he is also clear that such a visceral rush is no substitute for social harmony, neighborliness, friendship, and a shared estimation of life's means and ends. In April 1679, noting of another election that "there is like to bee a great endeavoring for the places," Browne worries that such intensity "will still keepe open divisions wch were to wide before, & make it a countrey of Guelphs & Ghibellines" (4.102). By "countrey" here, he means Norfolk, not England. Elections, he knows, are highly contingent affairs, depending for example on the weather (4.182). So too is office: intermittently concerned about the strength of the navy and the integrity of its officers, Browne laments the botching of the recent Dutch wars, then prays that "God send faythfull, valiant & sober commanders, well experienced and carefull; above all, if places bee sould or given by favor only, such virtues will concurre butt contingently" (4.141). The corruption of the navy, not surprisingly given his son Thomas's death, is strongly felt, as Browne lambastes the English command "who thought it sufficient to fight upon any termes, & carry to many gentlemen & great persons to bee killed upon the deck, & so encreaseth the number of the slayne & blott their victories" (4.141). The recurring memories of his late son over the course of the letters suggest that the politicization of contemporary society has threatened to darken the glow of Browne's sociable and charitable disposition.

Nonetheless, like the Guild Day, Assizes, or Fairs, elections retain in Browne's mind something of their character as a civic rite attended by exuberant holiday, each sector of society with its own proper role to play yet all united by a common vision of English welfare. In May 1679, Browne is pleased to report of the election that "I never observed so great a number of people who came to give there voices, butt all was civilly caryed at the hill, and I do not heare of any rude or unhandsome caryadge." The marketplace at Browne's doorstep is the scene in which the winners, including Sir John Hobart, are paraded "in chayres about the markett place after elven o clock, with trumpets and torches, candles being lighted at windows, and the markett place full of people." "There was a strange consumption of beere and bread and cakes," Browne remarks after giving the final numbers of the voting, and "abundance of people slept in the markett place and laye like flocks of sheep in and about the crosse" (Keynes, 4.104–5). If the tone with which he characterizes these sheep is hard to pin down, Browne obviously prefers such communal festivity to the routine ways in which common humanity is being fractured into rigid, irrational political constructs. He takes delight in telling Edward that grandson Tomey surprised a gentleman by declaring to support "all four" candidates. The gentleman's reply is cynical, for all its humor: "answerd like a physitians sonne," implying presumably that the lad has already learned to trim his sails in the hopes of securing the maximum number of clients (4.106).

Browne's anxiety about the conspiratorial and partisan corruption of political culture in the late 1670s and early 1680s is rarely absent from the letters written in the last decade of his life. Despite his obvious hunger for news, Browne is dismayed by the leak of a bold parliamentary speech into the public domain (Keynes, 4.177). This sentiment—that freedom of discourse has its proper place—harks back to Browne's dismay over the publication of *Religio* in the context of the early 1640s in which political discourse has degenerated in national affairs. In the letters of the 1670s and 80s, however, the publication of disrespect is no longer shocking; it has become routine, an integral part of human affairs. At the end of one letter, after giving the tallies of a vote, Browne generalizes about the future: "Tis probable there will bee alwayes some opposition, though without successe: the people delight in it and saye it will bee the better for the towne, as causing more concourse of persons & more mony to bee spent in the towne" (4.184). Political partisanship has replaced communal (if raucous) festival as a boon to the local economy.

In an extended comment on conflicts over money between Parliament and king in February 1681, Browne converts the folly of this dissension into a fable: "Two earthen bottles floating upon the sea with this motto, si collidimur, frangimur, is applyeable unto any 2 concernes whose interest is united & is to conserve on[e] another, which makes mee sorry for this dissention between the King & the people, that is, the major part of them, as the elections declare" (Keynes, 4.185). Despite his prayers that God will "send a happy conclusion & bee reconciled unto us & give us grace to forsake our sinnes, the *boutefeus* & Incendiaries of all" (4.185), such a call for national repentance is rare in the letters; rather, his tendency in these letters is to teach Edward a moral program aimed at minimizing the damage in Edward's professional, familial, scholarly, and inner life. After all, those bottles washing around in the sea have no control over their collision; agency is now resigned to larger, perhaps haphazard forces. When his son Thomas was expressing exuberance about the "hurly burly" and adrenalin rushes to be experienced in the navy, Browne had urged, with only moderate success, that Thomas learn more precisely the laws governing the motion of sea and land, or the proportions that make up a perfectly designed ship (Keynes, 4.19; Wilkin, 1.130). But in his letters to Edward in the 1670s, he stresses that such bewildering times require a maximum of personal control. In one letter, Browne puts a positive reading on what it means to be a physician in such a contentious age: "God send us to number our dayes and fitt our selves for a better world, times looke troublesomely, butt you have an honest & peacable profession which may employ you: & discretion to guide your words & actions" (4.144). This last bit of advice—to follow discretion or prudence—is no small matter for the son who attends Lord Rochester in his final days and who practices his profession near the center of power. Here is the political version of a larger moral issue that crops up in the letters: how to break bad news to psychologically complex or volatile patients.

Indeed, a major theme of Browne's letters comprises his moral and spiritual advice to his son. His son's understandable interest in the Epicurean poet Lucretius prompts from Browne a warning parallel to the cautions about Lucan's Stoicism that he once offered Thomas: whereas the father feared his naval son's extension of valor into reckless self-destruction, he worries that Edward will be infected with the materialism and anti-providentialism widely appropriated by Restoration rakes such as Rochester. The cleric Thomas Tenison, Browne adds, has produced "a good poem" against the "Lucretiuses of our times," "illustrating Gods wisdome & providence from Anatome" and, moreover, dedicating the poem "to mee & Dr Lawson" (4.57). As a remedy, Browne directs his son to the unimpeachable treatise on duties by Cicero, even reminding Edward that the book, a compendium of "good matter" in a charmingly small printed format, was either Edward's own or his brother Thomas's. When young Robert Bendish has a mental breakdown in a London coffeehouse, "breaking windowes and doing outrageous things, so that they were fayne to laye hold of him," Browne not only sympathizes with a father's sacrifices ("charges") and pain, but he also shapes this episode into an example of mental "distraction" that occurs as "the sad ends of many dissolute & governelesse persons, who, if they bee of a sheepish temper, runne into melancholy or fatuity, and if proud, haughtie & obstinate, into maniacall madnesse" (4.103). In the last year of his life, Browne is still concerned about the cultivation of temperance against "the common excesse of the times" (4.217). Far more frequently, Browne cautions Edward to be frugal and temperate in every aspect of his life: in his intake of drink, "bewiching" tobacco, or sauces (4.139), in his managing of money, indeed in all his personal habits including the non-naturals such as rest.

One of Browne's most extended offers of spiritual and moral guidance to Edward is prompted by the death of latter's infant in December 1678. Beseeching God to lend them all sufficient patience, the father veers into the advisability of prudence with money. "Least repentance come to late upon you," he presses on with warnings about the "accidentall charges" to which an uncertain world makes us prey, and with cautions against foolishly putting off until "impotent age" the practice of saving. Suddenly the lessons to be learned are the ones that Browne neglected:

> The christening & buryalls of my children have cost mee above 2 hundred pounds & their education more; beside your owne which hath been more chargeable then all the rest putt together, and therefore consider well that you are not likely to playe in this world or in old age, & bee wise while you are able to get & save somewhat agaynst a bad winter & uncertaintie of times. (Keynes, 4.88)

In some letters, Browne appears to be highly anxious about his own responsibility for his extended family's welfare, writing in French (to keep members of his household from reading it?) that the sustenance of his family is a matter of considerable vexation in his old age (4.141). A similar moment of confession—and quasi-recrimination—arises in August 1680 when Edward reports that he has had a good year financially. Cautioning his son that next year might not be so lucrative, since the stature of one's patients can change from year to year, the father gives his son a litany of advices about frugality, temperance, and the laborious demands that earning a thousand pounds a year places on the physician's "body and mind," so much so that his life is "not much lesse paynfull & laborious then that wch the meaner sort of people go thorough" (4.156). Complaining that excess in consumption has weakened the virtue of charity, Browne nonetheless admits that he himself should have been more savvy in his investments. "I thought myself rich enough," he remembers, "till my children grewe up" (4.156).

This is not to say that Browne wants his son's life to be defined by confinement and negation. For one thing, the father is constantly seeking to stimulate Edward's mind via proposals for reading and experimenting (Keynes, 4.69). For another, Browne is eager for his son to pursue his career ambitiously. When Edward takes on the office of censor for the Royal College, Browne advises him on how to carry himself or converse with "some gravity" (4.92). He urges Edward not only to gain access to a certain febrifuge, but advises him to have it "privately made" so as to maximize his proprietorship of the same (4.60). On the word of an acquaintance, Browne expresses a concern that Edward "were not over modest in this world where that virtue is litle esteemed," adding that "I am afraid that unreasonable qualitie makes you decline the freindshippe of my Lord B. of London, which others would thinck themselves happy in" (4.101). As the same letter's disregard for political shenanigans lets on, modern partisanship is one thing, but patronage among civil and talented gentlemen is quite another. It is one thing for Edward to know how to discuss geography with Vossius, or to let his good parts and education, well expressed in civil conversation, make appropriate inroads for the young physician among the "knowing." It is quite another, however, to imitate those hungry for prestige and power who make their way by money, self-aggrandizement, and empty yet constant bustle. To clarify the difference, his letters revert to the recipe for success: "Tis good to take notice wherin men excell & to rayse examples of imitation from the same, as farre as every mans genius & proper Minerva will enable." Such good old humanist emulation, modified according to an individual's proclivities, is the key to self-fashioning: "Hee that buildeth himself up by the modell of the best parts of men is like to become no ordinary man" (4.112). Yet Browne also worries that Edward's successes—his offices in the Royal College and his anatomy lectureship—tend to produce what Browne seems to consider is one of the greatest dangers of the age: mental perturbation, obsession, and "trouble."[24] Indeed, there is something about holding an important office that consumes "allmost all your thought," entailing that a talented young man renege on the comprehensive learning and unsaddled investigation so important to Browne's view of a proper life (4.187). Whether or not his father had advised it, Edward took one ambitious step in marrying Henrietta Terne in 1672. Often a subject and addressee in letters from Browne and Dorothy, especially regarding their grandchildren or when Dorothy was seeking an item of merchandise in London, Henrietta was the daughter of Christopher Terne, whose lectures on anatomy to the Barber-Surgeons' Company Edward had taken in during the 1660s.

The most pervasive—and invasive—way in which Browne encouraged Edward's ambitions was in collaborating on—or even assuming the reigns of—the writing of his public lectures and the revision of his travel book. To the very end of his life, the father was correcting, not to say commandeering his son's contribution to a

[24] See the reference to "troublesome office" in Keynes, 4.133; 4.135.

new translation of Plutarch. Browne's work on Edward's anatomy lectures for Surgeons' Hall begins in the very first month—June 1675—of his son's office, when Browne writes that he has "returned the first of your lectures" (Keynes, 4.56). In addition to revising the lectures, Browne gives advice on how to go about revision, constantly recommends books, and even composes segments for inclusion, offering guidance about when and how to introduce the material, about performance and delivery, including pointers about what specific groups in the audience will need from him.[25] Notes for these lectures tend to adopt the first person when Browne is showing his son how to introduce first-hand experience from his travels, as he does, for instance, in a section on observing circumcisions in Amsterdam, Rome, and Vienna. He is concerned that his son's lectures be entertaining, suggesting materials for jokes such as the one about the utility of multiple penises for generation, to which Johannes Benedictus Sinibaldus retorted that one was far too many (4.61).

One special and relatively unusual focus taken by Browne is on the skin, a longstanding interest that has already ranged from marring diseases such as smallpox to ordinary natural phenomena such as pigmentation.[26] Browne's fascination with dermatology conveys his openness to emerging fields of medical knowledge as well as with advances in old fields. In every case, the study of human anatomy is worked out in analogy with the animals—from dolphins to wolverines—whose dissection Browne is constantly discussing; the letters are filled with directives such as "take notice of the penis of a catt" (Keynes, 4.118). Yet Browne incites close, even quantitative attention to human anatomy as well, challenging what many anatomists often take for granted (in the case of skin) but also inviting Edward to "waygh the head of a man, braynes, scull, and other parts, & the scull & brayne distinctly, that you may knowe what proportion it hath to the body, at least with some latitude, although you do not waygh the trunck" (4.63–4).[27] What is more, he instructs his son on method by encouraging him to keep consistent notes over time so that, with the help of this diary, he can expand his expertise by way of observation (involving the circumstances of a peculiar case) and analogy (4.76, 4.175). And Browne demonstrates the value of analogy in difficult or unfamiliar illnesses by calling on the case of the Suffolk woman whose "julking and fluctuation in her chest," audible to bystanders, was reported in the 1667 *Philosophical Transactions*. Browne now finds that this daunting case is useful in examining a Suffolk man with similar symptoms, and consults with Edward on finding a chirurgeon who might be willing to tackle a tricky operation (4.146–7). Stressing the value of direct experience by way of anatomies, Browne urges his son to pay careful attention to afflictions such as deafness that are not yet fully understood (4.98). Over the course of the 1670s, the Browne family papers include accounts of, or references to, the performance of autopsies: of a 19-year-old boy in Norwich; of Sir

[25] For instance, the barbers will need theory to add to their practical knowledge (Keynes, 4.62). For enunciation, see 4.102.

[26] See Keynes, 4.66, 69–74, 113, 3.338–40.

[27] This reflects the influence of Sanctorius; see, e.g., 3.339.

Thomas Pettus of Rackheath in 1675; and of a woman with child at Ratcliff down the Thames from Edward's London in July 1674.[28]

Browne is also intensely involved in the revised editions of Edward's travel book as well as in his collaboration on a translation of Plutarch. As for the former, the father gives his son material for inclusion, for instance, on medical history in Thessaly which will be appealing "especially unto physitians and schollars" (Keynes, 4.117; cf. 3.306–7), and on explorations of the location of the famous Pharsalian fields (3.262–4) and of other geographical problems. Browne adds descriptions and identifications to Edward's drawings of "Citties and considerable places which I haue seene,"[29] fills in book learning on Hamburg and Prague, yet exhorts Edward to learn firsthand as much as he can about Vienna, since it will outpace the other points of the journey in a widespread interest among readers (3.266–7). In letters and notes, Browne once again ventriloquizes Edward's voice, writing passages on Hungary that speak from the vantage of his son's experiences yet filled out with material from books (4.129).[30]

Browne does far more than just assist revision when it comes to Edward's opportunity to deliver the annual Harveiean lecture for the Royal College; in this case, the father does his son's homework for him, writing out the entire oration. In the letters, one finds Browne studying previous examples in an effort to size up how much substance and how much encomiastic fluff they contain (Keynes, 4.169). Clearly the latter dominates, as Browne's composition shows.[31] Yet amid the honors bestowed on College benefactors, previous orators, and Harvey himself, Browne's speech—one which Edward never delivered—includes some incisive formulations of how Browne views his profession at its best. For one thing, oratory is significant as a means of commemorating the heroic physician, of protecting this ideal against obsolescence by fixing it in mental and institutional place with "the beam bolt of ordinance and custom."[32] The heroic physician is characterized as possessing that "upright and godlike" mind that holds "nothing dearer than to look on others with widespread benevolence and moreover with open hand" (3.197). Harvey is especially precious to the profession because he carries on the ancient ideal of philosophy as the foundation of medicine, a born philosopher whose curiosity about nature spurs him to "search out realities not images with wise scrutiny and perspicacious industry, bring many things to light and place them in the open, discover much or add to what has been discovered, judging best not from traditional dogmas or the words of others, but from repeated observation and tried

[28] All in Sloane MS 1833. [29] BL Additional MS 5233, 12r.

[30] Edward published *A brief account of some travels in Hungaria, Servia, Bulgaria, Macedonia, Thessaly, Austria, Styria, Carinthia, Carniola, and Friuli* in 1673. *An Account of Several Travels* followed in 1677, with an expanded and collected edition coming out in 1685 as *A Brief Account of some Travels in Divers Parts of Europe*; see C. D. van Strien, *British Travellers in Holland during the Stuart Period: Edward Browne and John Locke as Tourists in the United Provinces* (New York: Brill, 1993), 237–97. At least one reader, Norwich's own Thomas Corie, spotted the collaboration taking place between Sir Thomas and Edward Browne in the 1670s.

[31] There are two manuscript versions in Browne's handwriting, Sloane 1833 and 1871.

[32] In Latin, "*et ne quæ hodie apud nos vigent, interjecto spatio apud alios absolescant, ea institutes et consuedutine clavo quasi trabali figimus*" (Keynes, 3.189; translation 3.197).

experiments" (3.198). Harvey's version of the learned physician, then, has a strong element of modern empiricism that might allow the Royal College to compete with the Royal Society—though Browne does not make this last point. As the speech moves through its praises for benefactors ranging from Henry VIII to Baldwin Hamey and Henry Lord Marquis of Dorchester, Browne celebrates the way in which medical learning has united men of varying social ranks. Indeed, he emphasizes what he identifies as the Stoic measure of a man's value, one which requires that he be viewed without any of the cultural accouterments, birthrights, or "cheats of fortune" that conceal his virtue, genius, and dedication to the advancement of learning against vulgar error. Hamey is especially noteworthy for marshalling his virtues and charms against the dangers that threatened the College in "evil times" (3.200). Dorchester is extensively praised for having recognized that pedigree was hardly enough to count him among the heroes of medicine and philosophy (3.201).[33]

Browne's most sensitive pieces of advice to Edward involve the care with which a physician must assess and work with the personalities of his patients. As he himself ages, Browne becomes especially fascinated by geriatric patients, not least those who bother to seek out medical care even at an exceptionally advanced age. He concerns himself with eye disease, spectacles, and cataracts for his older patients, complaining to Edward that the "ignorance of chirurgeons" in such operations creates opportunities for "so many mountebanck & stage quacksalvers"—often plying their wares in the marketplace outside Browne's home—to trick their unassuming senior patients (Keynes, 4.113).[34] On one occasion, in December 1678, the city of Norwich requested that Browne intervene in the case of "Blind Balliston," whose eyes, particularly one, could in fact be cured with charitable assistance from the citizens.[35] At times, Browne shows interest in rethinking the received opinion about old age: "Some thinck that great Age superannuates persons from the use of physicall meanes: and that at a hundred yeares of age tis ether a folly or a shame to use meanes to live longer, and yet I have knowne many send to mee for their severall troubles at a hundred yeares of age" (4.144). In another letter, he notes the irony with which "intermitting pulses" are considered more perilous for the young than for the old (4.171).

In Browne's notebooks, there are several copies of an observation involving the difficult case of a centenarian, Elizabeth Michell of Yarmouth, "4 foot and an half high, very leane, very poore, and Living in a meane roome without ordinary accomodation" (Keynes, 3.243).[36] Choosing the right approach to her cure entails a moral as well as a medical calculus: "Though I am ready to extend my charity unto her yet I should be loath to spend a peece of Ambregris I have upon her, and to afford her 6 graines for every dosis, till I found some effect thereof, though that bee

[33] Cf. Browne's account of the Roman Marcus Plætorius (Keynes, 4.387).

[34] For spectacles, see Keynes 3.245.

[35] NRO MF RO 72/3, 37r–38v.

[36] Copies exist in MS Rawl. Letters D.58, f. 14; Rawl. Letters D.58, f. 15; and Sloane 1833, f. 24. The hand of the Sloane version is Edward's.

esteemed a specifick in her condition" (3.243). Clearly Browne is unsure whether ambergris will help the poor woman with her condition; what seems unstated is precisely why Browne is unwilling yet to attempt the "esteemed" remedy—is it that ambergris is too precious, that the patient is fragile and old, or simply that the case itself is sufficiently peculiar to warrant caution? Browne found the case interesting enough for Edward to present it to the Royal Society in February 1672.[37]

In another letter, Browne appears to criticize the long-lived for leaving their aging children without inheritance (Keynes, 4.176–7). For the most part without passing judgment himself, however, Browne purveys an interest in these "Macrobii and longlivers" reflective of Bacon's fascination with questions of longevity, and prompts generalizations such as Browne's notation that older people in Norwich tend to rank among the poorest. This latter point leads Browne to think once again about charity, including his personal experience of the virtue in his son Thomas's tendency to donate money to the poor on a regular basis. This association—between Thomas's charity and medical care for the elderly—returns to the letters in November 1680, when Browne relates the story of "a poore woeman of a hundred and five yeares old next Christmasse" who "sent her water unto mee and seems to be under the common distemper" (4.168). While his daughters have been charitable to this woman who "dwells in one of the towers of the wall," Thomas alone is said to have relieved a recently deceased centenarian whose death has coincided with that of the old Elizabethan "who wayted on the Earl of Leicester" and told Browne so much about Elizabeth's visit to Norwich (4.168–9).

The letters to Edward testify to Browne's own aging, in difficult combination with the ceaseless demands of his profession. In September 1680 Browne tells his son that "I have been often at Sprowston" in an effort to get a handle on rampant illness there (Keynes, 4.159), yet other letters make it clear that Browne himself has been ailing. In April 1677 he reports "a payne in my loynes wch makes mee unable to go or stand. I have often had it for 2 or 3 dayes" (4.77). On January 26, 1679, father wrote son that "my feet are very weake & somewhat swelld. I could make a shift to stand with croches, & I am fayne to write in my bed, so that perhaps I had not writt unto you this cold day, butt that I could not well avoyd it" (4.91). Sometimes Browne's afflictions are commonplace, as is the case with the vexing rheum that he developed during a bout of "sharpe" weather in April 1679. In the last years of his father's life and beyond, Edward felt a strong obligation to help Browne's patients when his father could not, in one case noting of the Le Gros family that "my father Sir Thomas Browne having been long Physitian to their family, I thought my self bound to take great care" of a gentleman from their ranks.[38]

In addition to a heightened interest in geriatric medicine, Browne continued to be fascinated by the challenges of gynecology and obstetrics emphasized at Montpellier. "I have made use of this succulus, or quilt, in woemen of hard labour

[37] See Birch, *The History of the Royal Society*, 3.8.

[38] Sloane 1878, letter to an undisclosed recipient, 18r.

or much griped in labour or troubled with wind," he notes in August 1679 (Keynes, 4.87). Regarding his consultation with Edward on a case of "*prolapsus uteri*" in Mrs Baxter, Browne characterizes the patient as "a very good Gentlewoeman . . . wife unto a very good Ingenuous gentleman & prettie botanick," then goes on to describe the patient's appearance, to offer suggestions for analogous afflictions, to inquire about the waxed corks used in such cases, and to discuss the advisability of her travel to Bath (4.123). In one tricky case of excessive blood flow, Browne at first rules out the possibility that the respectable Mrs Suckling has somehow contracted venereal disease, not least because her husband also has a "cleere & good reputation" for virtue; yet by letter's end he is cautioning Edward that "shee is like to bee in a great perplexity if you should positively tell her there is any thing of the Lues in it," adding that "I never knewe her husband complayne of any trouble about him" (4.220).

Browne pays careful attention to the health of mothers and children. On September 16, 1680, for instance, he advises his son to study Bartholinus's treatise on pregnancy, "for you cannot chuse butt meet with many questions from woemen with child" (Keynes, 4.164). According to Norwich city records, Browne also assisted poor parents with their children's ailments. In March 1672, the Court Books record that "David Brand's child [is] to have a chirugeon [*sic*] to view its sores, and to discourse Sir Thos. Browne thereabouts and report his opinion." On September 3, 1673, the Court Books add that "a collection is to be made in St. George Colegate, &c. for charge of Daniel, son of Anne Brande, to travel to London to be touched for the King's Evil and that Dr. Browne's certificate is to be obtained to Dr. Knights."[39]

Some cases and patients required considerable delicacy from the attending physician. In May 1679, Browne and Edward consulted regarding a former gonorrhea patient who had been experiencing "some payne in the genitals and swelling and gleeting, as he calld it, at the penis," and he was also having trouble with weak erections. "Do all with the best secrecy," Browne suggests, "for that will give him best content" (Keynes, 4.107–8). In fact, Browne seems to specialize in the tactful handling of what he calls "meticulous" and "complaining" patients, those whose psychological engagement with their health becomes a major factor in how the physician proceeds. Alderman Wisse, for instance, "is a meticulous doubting man of a good nature, & unwilling to offend God or man, & seldome without thoughts to perplex himself & making his life the more unconfortable"; his is a "busie" and "unquiet" brain. As Wisse plans to consult Edward, Browne advises that his son "encourage him in those disturbed thoughts. I am fayne to compose him sometimes by good counsell & rationall argument; the truth is hee is a very honest inoffensive person & his owne foe most, butt hee is very temperate & sober, & I wish him health & wellfare" (4.108–9). Other difficult patients—those who are excessively fearful or "complayning"—include Lady Churchman, whom Browne finds "weake & disper-

[39] Court Books, 129–31; NRO MF RO 72/3, 252v. Cf. Charles Williams, *The Treatment of the Sick in Norwich During the Seventeenth Century* (Norwich: Fletcher and Son, 1903); and Williams, *The Barber-Surgeons of Norwich* (Norwich: Jarrold and Sons, 1896), 28.

ited & despondent & even despayring ever to go to London agayne." "I conforted her to some good satisfaction," father tells son, yet "I conceave shee did butt half beleeve my predictions of her recovery in time" (4.146). One patient, appropriately named Mr Payne, requires great patience, since he "abounds in questions & doubts, & is soone discouraged & apt to laye hold of any words & to argue agaynst himself or any remedies." Worried that this melancholy man has been "full of perverted imaginations attended with feare of everything which concerned himself or hee could apply unto it," Browne emphasizes the value of the physician's forbearance when the patient has become "sollicitous" (i.e. highly disturbed) "& querimonious & wearying of all his freinds" (4.221). Of another difficult patient, Dr M., Browne apologizes to Edward that he has proved "so suspensory, irresolute and dilatory" yet urges his son to persist in patience with this "good nature[d]" man (4.125–6).

Some patients are far simpler in Browne's estimation, providing a self-evident moral exemplum. This is especially true of the heavy drinkers, including Thomas Peck who reportedly "dranck dayly a quart bottle of clarett before dinner, one at dinner and one at night," and even more with company (Keynes, 4.58). "Happy is the temperate man," Browne concludes in the mode of Leiden's combination of medicine and morality. Then there is Robert Hutchinson, who spent a day in June 1675 drinking "a gallon of Brandie burnt and sweetend" on a binge at "the Wheatsheaf in St. Peters in Norwich." Although Hutchinson recovered a week later, he happily had developed "a great louthing of brandie after." What seems interesting to Browne about the case, however, is that a fellow drinker consumed the same beverage in the same quantity but suffered far less, though Browne draws no conclusions about whether this was despite or because of his consumption of beer after the brandy (3.276). Here the precision of a medical observation vies with moral generality for dominance in Browne's notes.

In such cases of contemporary excess, as well as in the matter of geriatric patients, Browne often concerns himself with the discomposure or spoliation of brains. Of the elderly Marquis of Dorchester, Browne worries that a "mistaken draught of the opiat left some ill impression upon his brayne" (Keynes, 4.171). Regarding Peck he remarks that "if hee had lived a litle longer hee would have utterly spoyled his brayne & been lost unto all conversation" (4.58). In the geriatric cases, Browne is concerned about the onset of senility, with the loss of intellection, wit, conversation, and sensation that can afflict the elderly. Sometimes, however, the discomposure of the brain is not so easily explained, though it is often chalked up to melancholy or hypochondriacal obsession. Of Mr Bishop, Browne asserts that "surely his brayne is not right"; as for Mr Hombarston, "whenever his brayne is distempered," he "resolves upon a journey to London, & there showes himself, acts his part & returnes home better composed, as hee did last time" (4.60). With Mr Peirce, Browne discusses "some stupor in his brayne," a condition accompanied by vertigo and "confusion," and he advises Edward to take "a great care . . . to secure his brayne, least hereafter hee may fall suddenly Apoplecticall, & therefore issues on the shoulders may bee good preventives, and sometimes purging, & drincks also not purging" (4.143). Browne is especially worried that Peirce will lose "his speech & animal"—that is, mental—faculties.

Among the other diseases that Browne's letters focus on, one is the subject of his dissertation, smallpox; Browne is pleased to read Sydenham's new, even "paradoxical" interpretation of the disease and its treatment, but also fearful that the incidence of smallpox has never been higher. In a related matter, since in both cases the question arises about whether the disease can be contracted twice, he is especially concerned about quartan ague, interpreting the evidence of patients who appear to have contracted it twice by drawing a distinction between "legitimate or genuine" and "spurious" versions (Keynes, 4.90). In the case of the quartan ague, Browne models the way in which observations should verify reason (4.89). With agues in general, he concerns himself with the seasons of disease; he seems more interested in time, and its effect on wind and weather, than in place as a factor in pathology.[40]

In prescribing for his patients, Browne is open to medicaments from around the world, for instance, to the ginseng secured by the East India Company (Keynes, 4.100). The long distance to be traveled by exotic medicines such as cortex gives rise to concerns that commercial fluctuations will leave physicians and apothecaries in short supply of crucial materials (4.172). For the most part, though, his methods of curing are highly conventional, a bent in his practice that leads him to challenge a claim set forth by Christopher Love Morley that a particular distemper is new (4.155). Allowing for the way in which changes in human habits and diet can create "more irregular or worse symptoms," Browne still calls on his memory to characterize the disease as often a problem "after a droughty hot summer." Consulting physicians such as John Ellis, who wrote to Browne in December 1677, continue to frame their questions in terms of the humors.[41] Browne offers largely standard herbal prescriptions in keeping with the *Pharmacopoeia* regulating London practice, for instance reminding Edward of the purging to be gained from "Agaric, Rhubarb, Senna, & spina," with guidelines regarding the profile or age of the patient as well as the season that calls for a particular purge (4.97). Concerning cases of the stone, Browne is especially cautious, as we learn from a letter in the Isham family reporting the death of Sir Edward Walpole: "Goddards Dropps had very ille effects gave him convulsions and a numbness that he was a most sad spectacle a Month before he died... Dr. Browne and all his other Phisitions was very much against his taking the Dropps and he himself was not of opinion they could do him good till the Lord Townshend advised him to take them."[42] With stone, as in all matters of health, Browne places heavy emphasis on the adjustment of diet, regimen, and behavior. He is constantly concerned about the "6 non-naturalls" of his patients (4.205), but has less to say about bleeding, perhaps because he considers it the purview of the surgeon; even so, he does mention situations in which he must decide about its appropriateness—in one case, with regard to his young grandson (4.193).

[40] See Keynes 4.97 and 4.146. Cf. his concern about the changing seasons at 4.158.

[41] MS Rawlinson D.391, f. 107.

[42] Quoted in A. Batty Shaw, "The Norwich School of Lithotomy," 227; the letter was sent from Judith Isham to her father Sir Justian Isham.

In keeping with the eclecticism of his favorite authors such as Sennert and Rivière, Browne sometimes factors in chemical components of medical treatments, as he does in arguing that the "nitrosity" of Epsam waters "may bee beneficiall and help to fix or compose the volatility of [a patient's] blood and spirits" (Keynes, 4.187–8). Mercury is included in his remedy for venereal disease (4.220). On at least one occasion, Browne entertains the use of sympathetic medicine: "I have found the pulvis sympatheticus very successfull, shee bleeding upon it and wrapping up some of it in a double or trebble cloath and keeping it about her" (4.168). And he can come across as open to empirical practitioners—he recalls one in London, "who made a powder of Bezoar, musk & Amber & gave it to bee snuffed up into the nostrills in the toothach" (4.173)—as well as to new ideas. His modus operandi—adapting the presuppositions of learned medicine to the ever changing advancement of learning—is epitomized in his gift to Edward in 1682 of "a stick with the figure of a naked man, wherein may bee seen all the veynes of the body which were used to bee opened by the ancients and also by the modernes, with directions in Latin, how & in what cases." Telling Edward that he has had the device for the whole of his medical career, father encourages son to have it updated and improved (4.217).

Over the course of his letters, Browne mentions his responsibility for signing certificates qualifying patients for the treatment by the king's touch of their scrofula, that is, the inflammations caused by tuberculosis.[43] He was obviously supportive of patients being touched by the king, and never expresses "the slightest suspicion of incredulity,"[44] but he focuses his remarks on the role that medical practitioners—Edward first, then the king's surgeons—should play in the rite. The same applies to his remark in September 1680, that "divers go from hence to be touched, butt what chirurgeons are there I yett understand not, nor what physitians attend his Majestie" (4.165). This too is not unusual, for standard accounts of the cure included contributions to health from adjustments in regimen, from pharmaceuticals, and from surgical operations.[45] All the same, Browne's support for the royal touch was turned into royalist propaganda two years after his death in John Browne's *Adenochoiradelogia: Or, an Anatomick-Chirurgical Treatise of Glandules & Strumaes, Or Kings-Evil-Swellings. Together with the Royal gift of Healing, or Cure thereof by Contact or Imposition of Hands, performed for above 640 Years by our Kings of England* (1684).

In defending the royal touch, John Browne includes among the testimonials from "many Persons of Quality" a story of conversion from nonconformity and iconoclasm to a belief in the ritual power of the monarchy:

> A Nonconformists Child in *Norfolk*, being troubled with Scrophulous Swellings, the late deceased Sir *Thomas Brown*, of *Norwich* being consulted about the same, His

[43] See Marc Bloch, *The Royal Touch: Sacred Monarchy and Scrofula in England and France*, trans. J. E. Anderson (London: Routledge & Kegan Paul, 1973, first published in French, 1961); and Raymond Crawfurd, *The King's Evil* (Oxford: Clarendon Press, 1911). See also O'Day, *The Professions in Early Modern England*, 215–16.

[44] Crawfurd's words, *The King's Evil*, 104.

[45] Crawfurd, *The King's Evil*, 123.

> Majesty being then at *Breda* or *Bruges*, he advised the Parents of the Child to have it carryed over to the King (his own Method being used Ineffectually:) the Father seemed very strange at his advice, and utterly denyed it, saying, The Touch of the King was of no greater efficacy than any other Mans. The Mother of the Child adhering to the Doctors advice, studied all imaginable means to have it over, and at last prevailed with her Husband to let it change the Air for three Weeks or a Month; this being granted, the Friends of the child that went with it, unknown to the Father, carried it to *Breda*, where the King touch'd it, and she returned home perfectly healed.[46]

It is impossible to say how much, if any, of this narrative is true. It harks back to the time just before the king's return to England at the Restoration, when the royal touch, kept alive in Charles II's exile, was significant to those Royalists "desirous of reviving the monarchical religion in men's hearts." Its cultural currency was significant once again during the heated disputes over the Exclusion Crisis, the immediate context of John Browne's work. The passage treats the royal touch as a last, miraculous, recourse after the failure of ordinary medical practice. Yet more importantly, it credits the experience of that miracle with the power to convert nonconformists from the error of their ways: the father, having learned the source of his child's newly regained health, "became so amazed, that he threw off his Nonconformity, and exprest his thanks in this method; *Farewel to all Dissenters, and to all Nonconformists: If God can put so much Virtue into the King's Hand as to Heal my Child, I'll serve that God and that King so long as I live with all Thankfulness*" (188–9). Attributing this story to "an eminent Person," John Browne clearly believes that Sir Thomas's support for the royal touch is all the more valuable in the fight against nonconformist enthusiasm because, like Boyle—who also legitimized the rite[47]—Browne was thought to epitomize the perfect reconciliation between piety and skepticism.

Over the 1670s and into the 80s, Browne and Edward were constantly sharing and consulting on their patients, and it is in this capacity that they seem equal partners rather than mentor and student. This tendency to collaborate often reinforces the fact that the Browne medical practice considerably overlaps with the extensive and intricate Browne social circles. For instance, whenever Browne writes about illness in the Burwell family whom Dorothy and he visited together in September 1680 (Keynes, 4.68–9, 4.159), or when he is keen to make sure that Edward mentions his father's referral of their case to the patients, Browne purveys the social and familial dimensions of his medicine.[48] As he lamented the institutionalization of partisanship in contemporary culture, Browne resisted its power by emphasizing friendship, company, dinner parties, and conversation to the very end of his life. In one revealing note, he jotted that he "cannot fancy unto [himself] a more acceptable representation or state of things then if I could see all my best freinds,

[46] John Browne, *Adenochoiradelogia*, 187–8.

[47] Crawfurd, *The King's Evil*, 143.

[48] For a study of Browne's social network, see Toynbee, "Some Friends of Sir Thomas Browne"; for evidence that Browne's sister Mary and her daughters came to Norwich to live near him after 1651, see Morris, "Cradock, Amherst and Howell: A Link between the Selbys of Ightham and Sir Thomas Browne of Norwich," *Archaeologia Cantiana* 102 (1985), 11–18.

and worthy acquaintance of fortie yeares last past, upon the stage of the world at one time" (Keynes, 3.273). In other notes, Browne derives medical queries from classical readings for the purposes of "daylie recreation" and recalls those precious "evening howers" when a physician's "affayres afford [him] the conversation of studious & learned freinds" (3.204). Browne's fondest memories often involve such conversation, some from early days such as his meetings with Robert Hues at Oxford, but also from his years in Norwich. In one letter, he urges Edward to read Latin poetry, recalling that "Sr John Knyvett & Sr Philip Gawdie of Harling were so well versed" in Roman poets "that they never came butt they would have 2 or 3 howers discourse with mee about them" (4.179).

It is commonplace for the letters to record an encounter with an old friend, and the Brownes are forever entertaining a wide circle of friends for dinner, with Browne purveying a strong conviction that hospitality—"a kind & heartie reception" rather than an elaborate table or a gourmet diet—is one of the keys to health and happiness.[49] Hospitality, the warmth of family life, and the good public work of medicine are wrapped up in the simplest ways in the letters, especially in matters of cookery. The letters are apt to report on a good recipe concocted by Lady Browne (for instance, Keynes, 4.136), but Browne reinforces the need for culinary delights to be reconciled with genuine welcome and sobriety (4.134–6). Both his appreciation for good flavor and his opposition to hyper-delicacy prompt Browne to reject a "dayntie" dish known as "Inspinne" and consisting of a deer's rectum "being broiled or fryed" with the "gutt... turned side outward" (4.153). Allowing that he has encountered it "at some gentlemens tables," Browne finds a gag reflex unknown to the author of *Religio*; in short, "my stomack went agaynst it." In a satirical vein, he skewers social ambition by way of the dinner table: "As for L.M. hee may lord it at his owne Trivet, butt if hee hath an ambition to come unto this bourd; hee must bee content to eat out of the sight of the grand salade, to bee spoaken unto by a crier, & at the best to sitt butt a Ledger at the Table" (3.283).

Although friendship often assumes the nomenclature of kinship in the letters, Browne took distinctive pleasure in, and felt acute pain about, the affairs of his immediate family. His son Thomas was still very much a presence in Browne's family life: the social event of dining, like acts of charity, prompted memories of the deceased second son. In a letter on the culinary and medical benefits of pickles, Browne recalled that the only one in the household to like Indian pickles was the adventurous Thomas, "who at severall times eat them at meales" (Keynes, 4.160). In January 1681, Browne remembered his younger son's mastery of Juvenal and Persius while he was serving in the English navy at sea (4.179). Browne does not mention in the extant letters the death of his daughter Mary in 1676.[50] But she was the only one of Browne's children, six of whom were buried in St Peter Mancroft, to have her own memorial stone, one bearing the Browne family arms: "Here lyeth the body of Mary Browne who died on the 26th of September 1676. Daughter of Sir

[49] See for instance Keynes 4.74, 4.132–33, with quotation on 4.135.

[50] Because no funeral was included in the parish register, Wilkin speculated that Mary did not reside with her parents.

Thomas Browne Knight and Doctor of Physick and Dorothy his wife."[51] While the parish register conveys the mundane details of death in the family—Browne paid ten shillings each for the groundbreaking in the burials of a grandchild in 1673 and of Mary in 1676, his letters convey a controlled yet intense sorrow over the death of children in the family. "We are all sad for the losse of litle Tom at Islington," he writes Edward regarding the death of one of Anne's children,[52] then offers a short essay on the grief that parents must face in these situations (4.162). In worrying about his daughter Anne, Browne understands that context can heighten melancholy. Living away from home, in St James Clerkenwell, London, then afterwards in Shiplake before settling in Hurst, Berkshire, Anne continued to cause the family concern, in part because her husband was held by Browne to be too addicted to "drinck and company," and in part because of her children's health throughout the 1670s. A monument in the church at Hurst marked the gravesite of their little five-year-old daughter Frances, who died September 15, 1678.[53] Anne herself would be buried there on April 2, 1698.

From time to time in letters to Edward, Browne's daughter Frances was also spoken of as sending her good wishes. Baptized on September 5, 1662, Frances would marry John Bosville on November 19, 1687.[54] In the letters we are offered a glimpse of her personal strength when amid the report of a flu productive of a whooping cough and vomiting, Browne tells Edward that Frances has not allowed the sickness to prevent her "from going to morning and evening prayers which wee daylie have at our owne parish church" (Keynes, 4.193). Yet nothing delights Browne more in his last years than the two figures, daughter Elizabeth and grandson Tomey, who come to serve as surrogates for Thomas. In September 1680, Tomey forged the link between himself, Elizabeth, and Thomas when he discovered some of Thomas's belongings around the house: "Betty sometimes tells him stories about him, so that hee was importunate with her to write his life in a quarter of a sheet of paper & read it unto him & will have still some more added" (4.163).

Betty's similarity to her late brother Thomas included their mutual penchant for the graphic arts. As her father reports, Betty was ready and able to draw the kidney of a seal (Keynes, 4.56), but she herself weighs in on her depiction of a stork fed snails and frogs by her father (4.151). Browne was especially moved by Betty's strength of character, another point of connection to the deceased Thomas: "My daughter Betty who is very seldome out of health, though shee sitts often in cold wether 5 or 6 howers together in her closett reading & praying, & in old [all]

[51] The monument is now partly hidden by Victorian stalls. Blomefield recorded a memorial stone for Mary "below the rails, in the church of St. Peters, Norwich" (see Wilkin, 1.xcviii; and Blomefield, *Essay Towards a Topographical History*, 2.635). The text of the monument is given in Benjamin Mackerell, *History of the City of Norwich Both Ancient and Modern* (typescript of manuscript history from 1737 in NRO MS 78/1).

[52] The parish register for St James Clerkenwell records the birth of her son Thomas on January 29, 1677.

[53] See Wilkin, 1.cv–cvi.

[54] The marriage took place at St Benet Paul's Wharf; see Robbins on Thomas Browne, *ODNB*.

wethers & seasons never omitts to go to church, sundayes & weekedayes, to sermons & prayers in our parish, fell into a very extreme waye, whereof God bee thancked shee is now newly recovered" (4.102). Elizabeth and her father were also drawn together by their love of books; in December 1679, as he informed Edward that the cold weather made the fireplace a welcome spot in the house, Browne reported that Betty had been reading to him Ricaut on Turkish emperors (4.145); and in her own commonplace book, we find that list of tomes which she read aloud to her father "at nights till she read them all out"—a list so impressive and daunting as to seem almost impossible. The list has clearly favorite genres: travel writing, history, biography, and sermons, many of these books in folio. The histories include English chronicles but also studies of China, Turkey, Naples, and Venice; the travel adventures alone cover the entire world. Among the biographies there are some usual suspects: Plutarch's *Lives* and Foxe's *Book of Martyrs*. But in its final entry, the list gives way to open-ended variety: "Many other Books, Treatises, discourses of severall kinds, which may amount unto halfe the quantety of halfe the books in folio, which are before set down" (3.331–2). If like her mother Betty had an intensely private spiritual life, her reading notes are different from Dorothy's. While Dorothy's notes in the family commonplace book were intensely focused on sermons, Betty's entries were highly eclectic.[55] Some of the entries are politically charged—a powerful royalist speech by Lord Chief Justice Scrogg in praise of King Charles I, for instance, delivered to the Commons during Scrogg's impeachment by the Whigs in 1680–1[56]—while others are more personal: an anagram on a name, or an epitaph on her nephew William Fairfax, attributed to Aphra Behn. While Betty includes a good range of poets—Richard Corbett, Katherine Philips, Henry Wotton, and Juvenal—she also appears to have rewritten contemporary secular verses with Christian themes.[57]

With her marriage to Captain George Lyttleton on December 19, 1680, Betty's subsequent travel abroad deepened her connections to her deceased brother Thomas, a point not lost on Browne when his daughter set off for her new home on the Island of Guernsey. "Thy letters are still our best divertion," Browne writes to his daughter in June 1681, "I am sure their Passes not a day that we are not severall times talking of you" (Keynes, 4.194). Browne sends her news of the family, especially of Tomey, but also praise for that description of the great rocks seen in her voyage across the Channel that puts her father in mind of Thomas (4.197). Browne comforts his daughter that "Almighty God is Omnipotent everywhere in his Mercys," but he also urges her always to remember that her family will never forget her. There are benefits to be found on Guernsey, Browne tells Edward, not least the delicious fish and seafood that Elizabeth has enjoyed already (4.198). But there are also fear and loneliness. The first comes in the shape of a ship cast away, the "uncomfortable sight" of

[55] See Bullard, "'A bright Cœlestiall Mind,'"; and Victoria Burke, "Contexts for Women's Manuscript Miscellanies: The Case of Elizabeth Lyttleton and Sir Thomas Browne," *The Yearbook of English Studies* 33 (2003), 316–28.
[56] See Burke, "Contexts for Women's Manuscript Miscellanies," 326.
[57] See Burke, "Contexts for Women's Manuscript Miscellanies," 321.

which Browne helps his daughter to assimilate, first noting that it is no foreign or "strang" experience for the people of East Anglia, then praising her for her prayers for the beleaguered before finally converting the tragedy into a moral allegory: "Some wear away in Calmes, some are Caried away in storms: we Come into the World one way, there are many gates to goe out of it. God give us grace to fit and prepare our selves for that Necessity, and to be ready to leave all when and how so ever he shall call" (4.200). It is a message that Browne had already given his son Thomas; for Elizabeth, Browne extends his allegory into rules for holy living, arguing that it is crucial to pray during health when we are somewhat in charge of the course of our days rather than waiting for times of sickness which "may Choak our devotions" and thwart us with their unpredictability (4.200). On the other hand, he would tell Edward in January 1682, long periods of good health are apt to make us forget about God, for which reason providence "mercifully interposeth some admonitions & rubbes to make us consider our selves, & to carry a warie hand in our affayres of all kinds" (4.202).

Betty returned home to visit her family prior to her father's death, a visit that began on May 29, 1682. Eventually, she would have an important role to play in the posthumous publication of his later works. With her return home, Browne found that the world still had the capacity to surprise him, given Betty's stories of the peculiar ways in which the people of Guernsey managed to keep their oysters fresh during their sales over several days (Keynes, 4.231). Through the 1670s her presence was especially felt from her role in raising her nephew Tomey, Edward's son, who spent long stretches of his childhood with his grandparents and aunts in Norwich. In April 1677, a letter testifies to the boy's liveliness but also to the way in which Elizabeth and Frances prepare him for sleep with the music of their fiddle (4.76). "When wee send away our letters," Edward is told, Tomey "scribles a paper and will have it sent to his sister, and sayth shee doth not knowe how many fine things there are in Norwich." Like the uncle with whom he becomes fascinated, Tomey is capable of doing good schoolwork, but his dynamism and lust for life entail that some special pains must be taken to keep him still long enough to read or cipher. Browne's letters are filled with Tomey's vibrancy, at times his hyperactivity (4.86). It is Dorothy who most clearly indicates how much grandfather adores his grandson: "I bles god your Tomey is very well: goos to scolle and is a very good Boy and delights his grandfather when hee coms home" (4.88). In other letters over these years, Tomey is found carefully setting conditions on the valentines that Dorothy, Elizabeth, and Frances will give him (4.93); receiving a gift from Captain Le Gros, who is said to have known Anne in France (4.96); piled high with acquisitions from the fair (4.103); "much longing for his briches" (4.122); suffering from fever (4.126); happily dirty from play (4.137); ashamed of recent bad behavior; struggling with his studies and "spending much of this time with grandfather" (4.140); recycling tall tales which he has heard from Will Bunne "in the kichen in London," with some of them "pretty long" (4.143); off to see a play "at the Red lyon hard by" (4.172) or the bears on display (4.202); excited over the coming of Guild Day (4.82); eager for the figure of the tumbler to fill out his set of puppets (4.212); the playmate of a footboy (4.193); having to be persuaded to take "some purging [medicine] and clysters readily" (4.193); preferring the sweet bottoms in their glasses of cider (4.203), learning manners from the awesome Madame Cobbe (4.221), or rushing in to tell his grandfather about a comet's appearance "in the yard" (4.178). Like Betty, Dorothy Browne tells Edward, Tomey "delights to read [to his] Grandfathar and I when he coms from schole" (4.160). In Browne's final years, then, childhood as well as senescence offered distinctive lenses through which to see the never-quite-familiar world. To the end, Browne cherished generation and all living things, so much so that his fascination with senescence involved mainly a reconsideration of how the very old might still care about their health in the face of traditional bias against their doing so.

Browne's physical and mental worlds were also rich and alive with a wide range of animals that appealed to him from books or made their way around his yard. He wished to know about the camel's hump but he also missed his lost hedgehog and her "2 yong ones" (Keynes, 4.68). The deer roaming the park at Woodstock receive more attention in a letter to Edward than the famous sickness and penitence of Lord Rochester in residence there. On the smaller end of the spectrum is the spider described as "large & round & finely marked green, and even allmost as bigge as the figures inclosed drawne by your mother, for your sisters dared not doe it" (4.159). The final letters of his life are dominated by the life and death of an ostrich in Edward's care—a last meditation on the wonderful ways in which nature shows off.

Indeed, Browne's major contribution to the advancement of learning in these years came in the form of his provision of written and graphic material for John Ray's work on birds, a book to which he refers in the discussion of the ostrich (Keynes, 4.205–6).[58] In a variety of works, Ray thanked Browne for the gift of some natural specimen or depiction thereof, such as the egg "having the perfect signature of a Duck swimming upon it" whose picture Browne had sent Ray "some years before" 1673, with a testimonial that the signature "was natural."[59] But it was Ray's continuation of Francis Willughby's master work on birds that drew Browne's richest contribution.[60] For the *Ornithologia*, Ray would cull out Browne's notes and images for specimens otherwise omitted by or unknown to Willughby and Ray, but already in the epistle to *A Collection of English Words*, Ray was detailing Browne's contribution: "among some Pictures of Birds which I have received from the Learned and deservedly Famous Sr. *Thomas Brown* of *Norwich*, I find two or three English Birds by me omitted, as whereof I was not then certain."[61] Ray also included Browne's careful descriptions (of a stork, for instance), which featured a precise attention to color, measurements, behavior, sound, and feeding habits, at

[58] See Charles E. Raven, *John Ray, Naturalist: His Life and Works* (Cambridge: Cambridge University Press, 1950), 116–17.

[59] John Ray, *Observations topographical, moral, & physiological* (1673), 237. Cf. Browne's gift of a double egg to the Royal Society as recorded in Nehemiah Grew's *Musæum Regalis Societatis* (1681), 78; as well as his gift of an elephant's leg bone (32).

[60] For a brief discussion, see F. D. Hoeniger and J. F. M. Hoeniger, *The Growth of Natural History in Stuart England from Gerard to the Royal Society*, 49–54.

[61] John Ray, *A Collection of English words not generally used* (1673), letter to reader.

least in captivity; indeed Ray remarks that while Browne may have "all parts of learning," he is "especially" skillful "in natural History."[62] Yet no doubt Browne's discontent about Ray's tardiness in returning the colorful drawings of birds was heightened by the fact that this work had been a family affair too (Keynes, 4.216), a collaboration between father, daughters, and Dorothy.[63]

For Browne, weather reports, tied as they are both to medical concerns and to a sense of divine providence, could be arresting as well. In one way at least, Browne's concern about the weather resembles his preoccupation with news of England and the world. When, for instance, he details the complicated affairs played out among imperial electors, the French, and the Swedes, Browne shows his desire to master the ultimately unpredictable and volatile energies and motions of the world. In both cases, Browne seeks out patterns yet also has to admit strangeness, confusion, and anxiety. On November 27, 1674, he wrote in his notebook of a "darke thicke miste" that enveloped Norwich, England, and Holland as well (Keynes, 3.240–2). On the one hand, there was nothing unusual about such an event, since "it be not strange to see frequent mistes, Clowdes and raynes in England, as many ancient describers of this country have noted." But at least three factors make this mist a matter for "Candid Considerations." First is the possibility that mist can somehow change, either in size ("it was of larger extent then mists are commonly apprehended") or in causation (for instance, "by unwholesome and sordid manufactures"). For another, even if the mist is the same as always, there is the possibility that modern observers will come to understand its nature better than before, by close attention to "the atomes and particles" which "admit the light." Third, contemporary observers must continue to factor in the role of divine dispensations in weather as in human affairs. Even in the essay on mist, Browne is mindful of the miraculous clouds on display in the Old Testament. In a note fretful about excessive rain and cold, Browne worries not just about his inability to rent out his marsh property "for so much as will defray their charges" but also about God's judgments against the people of Norfolk (3.265).

The Browne family's association with and appreciation for travel helped situate their domestic advancements of learning within a worldwide adventure. From the early 1660s, Browne had received from a Norwich minister, Mr Escaliot, an explosive account of life in Surat, India. Filled with narratives of violence and terror, the letters read at times like prosaic versions of Dryden's heroic dramas, yet they are interspersed with anthropological surveys of the people, their beliefs and customs as well as with information about fruits, weather, and topography.[64] The final fragment of a letter was concluded with a note in Browne's hand, that his "louing friend," Escaliot, had "dyed in the Indies, and so I lost the antiquities and varities which hee had obtained for mee" (Wilkin, 1.442). A similar combination of adventure with the material benefits of travel to curious learning sometimes came through in Edward's letters as well, as for example in a letter from Vienna in which son first reports to father about the toll taken by "hard service" on the health of

62 Ray, *The Ornithology* (1678), 286. 63 Cf. Raven, *John Ray*, 338.
64 Wilkin prints these letters in *Works* 1.424–42; a copy is included in Sloane 1861, ff. 5–21.

good old Captain Macdougal, then details the catalogue of phenomena—from vitriol and antimony to manuscripts and coins—which he has sent from his travels homeward to the Royal Society and to his father (Wilkin, 1.446–9).

In his final years, Browne especially enjoyed compilations such as the *Philosophical Transactions* where in one issue, a reader comes across recent microscopic studies with their speculation that insects might outnumber human beings; extraordinary bouts of weather in Gascony; and accounts of a "flying man," of coal mines and "Astronomicall observations" (4.142). In June 1682, he took pleasure in another "philosophicall collection…sent mee from Dr Briggs," with items on "a monstrous Animal vomited up," on "a newe Theorie of vision communicated to the R.S. by Dr Briggs" and on "a voyage made to the South terra incognita, extracted from the Journall of captaine Abel Jansen Tasman" (4.229). When he lamented the fact that "I have not seen a philosophicall collection a long time," he expressed how much the constant supply of reading material from London—of news, monographs, and collections—was essential to his happiness. But the miscellaneous character of his own late writings also clarify his understanding that the advancement of learning must be slow, fitful, and fragmentary.

2. MISCELLANEOUS TRACTS

Browne's notebooks are chockablock with ancients such as Athenaeus, the biographers Plutarch, Suetonius, and Ammianus Marcellinus, Aristotle on animals, Strabo, Ptolemy, and Pliny on geography. And he is reading them actively, looking for inconsistencies or enigmas that require his—and Edward's—attention (Keynes, 3.303–32). Certain ancient episodes—such as Hannibal's amazing trek from Carthage into the Italian peninsula—are especially equipped to stimulate Browne's imagination (3.311–12). Yet also strong is Browne's desire for a masterly overview, for instance in his proposal "to compose an historicall Calendar affixing unto each day the famous battles, Actions, event[s], & occurrences wch Authentick accounts & best records affoord from Ancient & not to late deliverie, wch may daylie serve to receive & mind the greatest memoriall of Time." Cultivated in his years at Winchester, this aim at a comprehensive history accrues the added benefit of illustrating a certain unevenness with which human life unfolds; for it "may bee observed how thinne some days, how full some others have been in the great concernes of the world & somme dayes sufficient to afford the discourse of a just volume" (3.317). Here then is the historical version of microscopy, one revealing the unexpected plenitude of a single day. Nor does Browne omit scripture—biblical scholarship is still a concern of his—or church history, the benefits of which would be a fresh look at the history of piety.

With books forever at hand no matter what the field of inquiry, Browne also fills his notebooks with experiments that pursue key physical properties as well as various animal and plant specimens. In the vein of a less orderly version of Bacon's *Sylva Sylvarum*, Browne's notebooks compile a wide range of proposed experiments such as these: "To trie the experiment of killing of a frogge by dropping tarre upon his head & back"; "Whether hydropicall persons swell most in the increment of the moone"; "Whether the urines of healthfull persons have a very good odour, if unsound, not so" (Keynes, 3.272). One comes across chemical experiments such as the production of silver caustic (3.276–7); animal queries, for instance about "whether shortwinded horses will not plunge their mouths deep into water when they drinck, butt drinck like oxen sipping" (3.282), or about the direction in which an elephant farts (3.349). Mineral inquiries were always important to Browne, for instance in his question "whether Ice bee to bee found in subterraneous cavities & deepe caves in the earth" (3.295). So too were investigations of astral phenomena such as comets, of physiognomy, human anatomy, cooking, women's health, climate, gardening and botany, shells, insects, tides, bones, egg signatures, and physical properties such as motion (e.g., "what kind of motion sliding is"), impetus, coagulation, metamorphosis, distillation, insemination, digestion, condensation, ebullition, magnetism, congealment, the trajectory of plant growth, and fermentation.[65] Sometimes Browne is recommending an experiment, such that his letters to Edward but also his notebooks are overflowing with incitements to further scholarship and exploration. In one letter from February 1681, he urges his son to explore the voice of a hound, but especially to pursue the question of whether animals aside from human beings possess hymens (4.181). Often, however, Browne is recording his own experiences and experiments, as he does in his two-year observation of "the exquisite sense & the vivacity" of red worms in a glass (3.364). To test for the presence of natural antipathies, he reports introducing "a moll, a toade, & a viper in one glasse," after which "within half an hour the moll eate up half the viper leaving the tayle and harder parts, destroyed the toad, eat part of the entralls, dyed the next day" (3.366).

It is common for Browne to provide a sense of exactly where an observation has taken place, as he does in noting that "in a meadow I use in this citty, besett about with sallowes, I have observed there to growe upon their bare heads builders, corants, gooseberries, cynocrambe, Rasberries, barberries, bittersweet, elder, hawthorne" (Keynes, 3.378). Observation is not enough for him, however. In his experiments with grafting, Browne generalizes a key point that pervades his queries and experiments, namely, his support of Bacon's belief that nature could be understood fully only if forced outside or beyond its normal workings, and only if pursued across the widest possible range of individual specimens. Throughout these notes, Browne predominantly takes it for granted that nature often works in uneven and diverse ways, and that an insistence on the underlying geometry of providence will not advance learning to the extent that the careful observation of exceptions will, a case that he makes in particular with regard to seeds and the generation of plants (3.380–1). This is not at all to say that Browne has abandoned

[65] For examples, see Keynes, 3.294–302, 272–82, 347–400, 432–62. Browne's study of processes such as coagulation interested his correspondents too; see Henry Power's allusion to Browne's "vitale coaguli" in Sloane 1393 (39r); Sloane 1378 (352r–53r), with a letter from G. Hutton to Power; and Sloane 496, Power's *Historia Physica Anatomica* (1666), which notes that Browne's theory of coagulation is related to his interest in digestion.

his belief in nature's sense of purpose; far from it, nature's capacity to make "provision" by means of variation is as remarkable to Browne as the intricacy of the microscopic. Browne's notes also testify to his belief that human intervention can provoke nature into revealing itself, and even alter nature for the better. He makes the latter point with the simple example of the artichoke, which agriculture has made both more accessible and "of a milder & better tast" (3.396).[66]

In strictly human affairs, Browne finds a far greater tendency toward coincidence, randomness, promiscuity, and misprision, a point already noted in his desire for a historical calendar illustrative of thin and thick days. With human events, statistical probability was the new form of prophecy, and it was this type of stochastic insight which an early biographer attributed to Browne, who was uncommonly accurate in making predictions without any regard for "Presages or Superstitions" (Browne, *Posthumous Works*, xxxvii). In the notebooks, one finds jottings about "observable" days involving "a concurrence of accidents" beyond the control of human agency—for instance, "That Charles the Fift was crowned upon the daye of his nativitie caryeth no unmachable consideration, butt that hee tooke King Francis prisoner upon that day was a concurrence of accidents wch must make that day observable" (Keynes, 3.285). Browne was more elaborate about the human capacity for mistakes and chance occurrences. "Transcriptionall errata's, ignorance in some particulars, expedition, inadvertency," he complained, "make not only moales butt wennes in learned workes wch notwithstanding being judged by their better parts admitt not of reasonable disparagement" (3.286). In such cases, he maintains, forgiveness is in order. But Browne is less kind in his assertion that human perception generally misses the mark by fastening on appearances (3.287). Bacon had argued that time was like a river in which the substantial was usually submerged, and Browne seems to agree, shifting the metaphor to optics and to target practice (3.287). All in all, Browne is keenly aware, any advancement of learning is bound to be roughly and rudely borne, the forward march of history no more to be stipulated than the everyday acts of human perception.

The miscellaneous characteristics of Browne's thinking and writing in the last period of his life were heightened by virtue of the fact that he was often responding to an occasional inquiry by a learned friend. But these tendencies also reflect a paradox that Browne developed in the wake of Bacon's reforms of learning. On the one hand, Bacon believed that fragmentary discourse—the essay, the aphorism—was more desirable than a finished, polished work for capturing knowledge which was still broken but actively and attentively in the making. Indeed, while Browne favored the "rationall discoverie of things" (such as "the line of the middle motion of the planets") over their "simple detections" (in the case of the Indies, for instance), he made the striking point that the latter can be the result of efforts "often casuall, & secondary unto intention" (Keynes, 3.287). On the other hand, the endless, inventive human capacity for error was also productive of fragmentation of the kind that

[66] Browne's strong commitment to gardening is vividly illustrated in the extensive list of seeds planted in his garden that he recorded for the year 1667, complete with notes on where in the yard they were placed (Keynes, 3.397–400).

Browne's contemporaries often associated with the multiplication of languages after the debacle of the Tower of Babel, and which Browne himself argued had occurred even before that event. Browne's piecemeal writings work in both directions, as generative seeds of new learning but also as the fractured record of human haplessness. But his constant revision of his manuscripts suggests a conviction that human endeavor can get things right, either once again or anew. In raising "many questions" about guardian angels in his notebook, Browne captured both states of affairs in concluding that "viators may dispute but comprehensors must determine" (Keynes 3.244, Sloane MS 1848, f. 174). (See Figure 11.1.)

The essays or epistles brought together posthumously as *Certain Miscellany Tracts* include two pieces having to do with prophecy. The eleventh tract re-creates ancient views of oracles by means of categories that recall contemporary debates over witchcraft.[67] A key upshot of this study is that the oracles were so misleading as to need excuses, in contrast to the secret wisdom and justice of God "which makes Riddles unto us in the tragicall ends of many noble persons & families" (Keynes, 3.97). The gap between human propositions and divine dispositions was a point also made powerfully in Browne's notebooks, in which he remarked how "in vayne wee seeke to satisfie our soules in narrow theories & close apprehensions of the divine essence from the revealed word"; for although "wee have an happy sufficiency in our owne natures to apprehend the will & pleasure of god delivered in holy scripture," it is beyond our "capacitie to comprehend or reach his nature," with awe "being the act of the creature & not of god, who doth not admire [i.e. wonder at] himself" (3.291). In the final part of the tract, Browne elaborates on the limits to human knowledge, declaring that our minds are contained beneath an "Arch" outside of which angels or "Spirits" have a monopoly on knowledge. In the second tract on prophecy, Browne has been asked to decipher an old and enigmatic prediction, a burden which at first he appears unwilling to shoulder. Yet having dismissed obscure prophecies as of no interest to him, and rejected the "pretended spirit of Divination," he proposes to his unnamed friend a rationalized version of forecasting human events, "not built upon fatal decrees, or inevitable designations, but upon conjectural foundations, whereby things wished may be promoted, and such as are feared, may more probably be prevented" (3.102).

In the other miscellaneous tracts, Browne ranges across a set of natural and artificial phenomena of interest to curious friends such as Sir Nicholas Bacon and William Dugdale. The difficulties of the Bible are confronted once again in the long study of the "several plants mention'd in Scripture," in which Browne offers exegesis based on biblical scholarship as well as a botanical survey. A similar study reviews "the fishes eaten by our saviour with his disciples after his resurrection from the dead" (Keynes, 3.53).[68] To Evelyn, Browne addresses a tract on coronary plants; to an unnamed recipient, he proffers answers to specific questions about the fish called halec and mugil; about a bird sent along with the query (among other birds), and about the cicada, an inquiry that seems to test Browne's patience since the bird in question is the familiar hoop-bird, the cicada has been covered in *Pseudodoxia*,

[67] Sloane 1839; Keynes, 3.95.

[68] This tract was published also by itself in 1684.

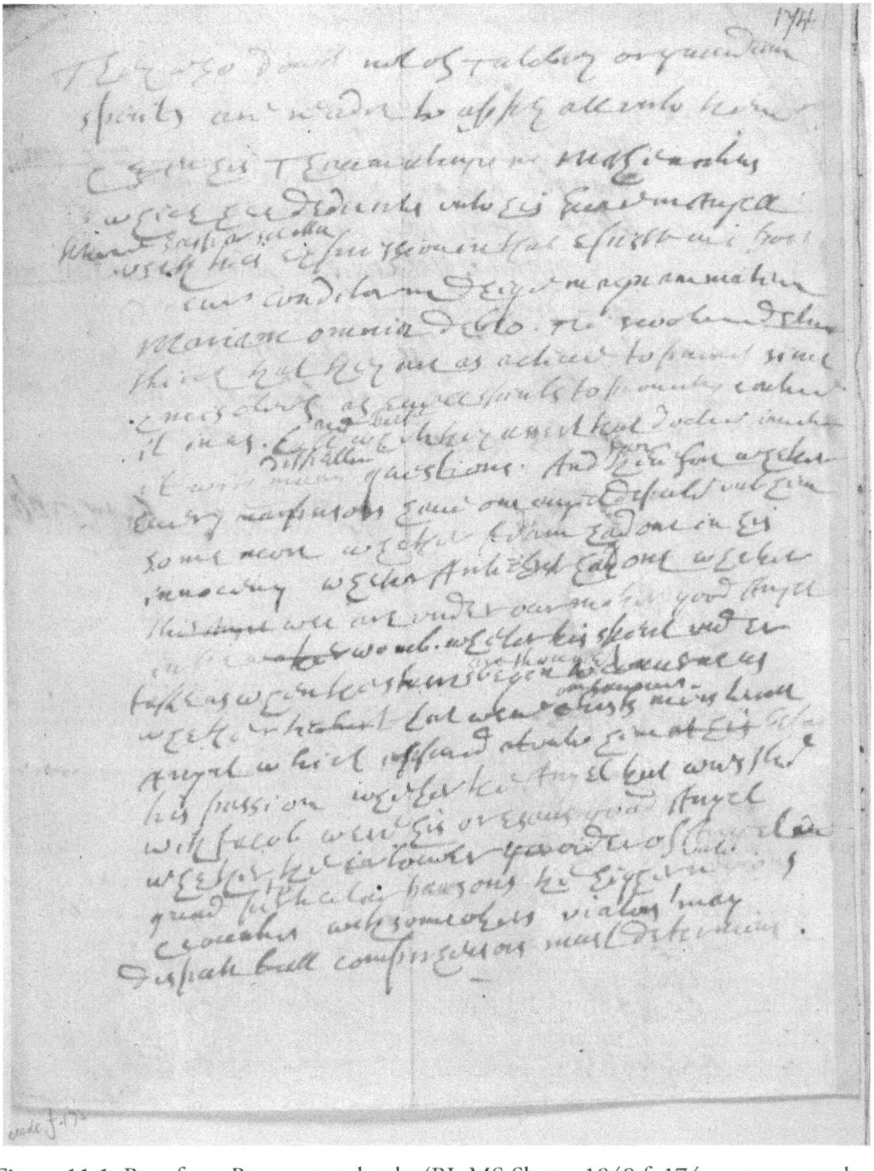

Figure 11.1 Page from Browne notebooks (BL MS Sloane 1848 f. 174, entry on tutelary angels). Reproduced with the permission of the British Library.

and the questions overall are "not of difficult Resolution, or of great moment" (3.59). An essay on the relatively recent history of falconry reveals an interest in veterinary medicine which also appears in Browne's notebooks and stimulates him to recall some dramatic scenes in Norfolk when, for instance, a wild fowl proved so weary that it could be "taken with Dogs, and some knock'd down with Staves and Stones" (3.63).

The essays included in the *Tracts* show Browne's interest in the history of music and poetry, again with varying levels of enthusiasm. A study of cymbals provides Browne with an occasion for thanking the inquirer for a book of hymns, to which he appends his own English rendering of a "Turkish Hymn translated into French out of the Turkish Metre." Browne enjoys imagining the Islamic context of this hymn's performance (Keynes, 3.65–6). Indeed, Browne's reason for keeping this essay so short is that "I can say but little where I understand but little" (3.66). Far otherwise is the short essay on "ropalic or gradual verses," a form of prosodic wit which features five-word lines moving from a single up to five syllables. Although Browne's papers include anagrams, they also bid his farewell to such wit. So too in the tract, Browne informs his inquirer that "though I may justly allow a good intention in this Poem presented unto you, yet I must needs confess, I have no affection for it; as being utterly averse from all affectation in Poetry, which either restrains the phancy, or fetters the invention to any strict disposure of words" (3.67).

Browne's willingness to offer additional witticisms is explained in part by his fascination with comparative linguistics, a subset of which is his interest in translation. Not surprisingly, the tract "of languages and particularly of the Saxon tongue" is one of the longer essays. It begins with Browne's speculation that a variety of languages had developed naturally even before the Tower of Babel, since the differentiation of languages followed from a dispersion of people who spoke according to "their humours, inventions, necessities, and new objects" (3.70). For Browne, the current multiplicity of languages is made all the more impressive by the discovery that in America alone there are so many "of no affinity unto each other; and even in their Northern Nations and incommunicating Angles... their Languages are widely differing" (Keynes, 3.70). Not only does language in general tend to multiply, but a single language such as English is highly changeable, as a study of Old Saxon shows. And Hebrew, that language which "religious obligation" has so carefully preserved, is not so perfect or permanent as some seekers after God's preferred idiom would maintain (3.72).

A number of different seventeenth-century interests interact in Browne's tract. There is Bacon's critique of the "Idol of the Marketplace," according to which linguistic usage distorts human perceptions of the natural world, for instance by advancing multivalent words or even words that name nothing real whatsoever. As part of a desire to correct such distortion and to advance learning, savants were also eager either to locate or to concoct a universal language which could be shared by all humankind and would avoid the slippages and deceptions of ordinary languages. But Browne's focus on Saxon reflects his antiquarian commitment to historical precision, since the birth of Anglo-Saxon studies in his lifetime derived from a growing wariness about the mythologies making up for the woeful lack of evidence in regard to British cultures prior to the arrival of the Germanic peoples. Browne's tract is clearly most obliged to this antiquarian interest, stressing that historical "confusion, admixtion and corruption" of languages that have arisen over time in even those distant places, China for instance, where mythologizers of language might be tempted to posit unity. Indeed, in stressing the sheer variety of languages, Browne argues that linguistic families are far more useful for getting a handle on the phenomena than is the ideal of "one common original" (Keynes, 3.73). And imperial conquest, far from simply imposing a single language on many people, tends to create linguistic mixtures as surely as it deprives native peoples of their own language. No matter how remote a culture, Browne insists, no matter how narrowly confined "in Angles and inaccessible corners," it remains the case that "surely no Languages have been so straitly lock'd up as not to admit of commixture" (3.74). As a guide to sorting out the durable from the promiscuous in a language, he divides between two sets of the parts of speech: on the one hand are the mixable ones, the nouns, adjectives, and certain verbs; on the other, one finds "the distinguishing and lasting part of a Language" in "the great Body of Numerals, auxiliary Verbs, Articles, Pronouns, Adverbs, Conjunctions and Prepositions" (3.76). Just as he strives to pinpoint the distinguishing features of a bird, Browne guides his correspondent through the highly complicated variations and mixings of language with a clue as to what makes each one discrete if not unique. As he admits later in the letter, the "trouble" created by language strikes the learned as both wearisome and delightful, especially since a knowledge of dialects, while challenging, permits an understanding of Rabelais and of rich, witty literature more generally, as well as an enjoyment of human variation that comes most immediately to the traveler (3.81). Indeed, in his tract on a geographical question about Troas, Browne notes that places change and develop in a manner similar to languages (3.91).

In the *Miscellany Tracts* the most extraordinary combination of melancholy and jocundity is found in *Musæum Clausum, or Bibliotheca Abscondita, containing some remarkable books, antiquities, pictures & rarities of several kinds, scarce or never seen by any man now living* (Keynes, 3.109). As a parody of the penchant for collecting the miscellaneous, Preston explains, this tract might bear a certain resemblance to more straightforward works such as *Pseudodoxia*, in which Browne stresses "the critical importance of restorative, regenerative compilation and investigation";[69] yet there is a melancholy, if also comical, inverse side to this Baconianism in Browne's way of thinking, an indictment of the rage for collecting that will form a part of Browne's posthumous reputation. Although the older Browne no longer so readily looks to the hieroglyphs or geometries of nature as a vantage from which to comprehend patterns of divine providence or of a universal moral law, this dissatisfaction with fragmentation or miscellany helps account for his continuing desire to view the world from above, at a distant prospect from which a sage, experienced philosopher can formulate the maxims to be found in *Christian Morals*.

Like the other tracts, *Musæum Clausum* takes the form of a letter, possibly to Walter Charleton. Thanking his addressee for having sent a "noble Catalogue of Books, Rarities and Singularities of Art and Nature" recording a collection of curiosities like the one in Browne's own house or like the many cabinets throughout

[69] Preston, *Browne and the Writing of Early Modern Science*, 155–7. See also Bent Juel-Jensen, "*Musaeum Clausum, or Bibliotheca Abscondita*: Some Thoughts on Curiosity Cabinets and Imaginary Books," *Journal of the History of Collections* 4 (1992), 127–40.

Europe, Browne is confident that his recipient has never glimpsed the items produced by Browne's own fancy, their elusiveness a testimony both to the collector's desire and to his folly. From *Religio* to his notes on Athenaeus, Browne articulates his desire for certain lost works as agonizingly crucial links to a deeper and fuller understanding of the past, and in his fanciful museum, some of the titles are lovingly detailed, including works written by Ovid in exile, "an Ancient British Herbal" but also a herbal covering the plants in the sea, and a precise account of Hannibal's "march out of Spain into Italy" (Keynes, 3.109–10). Many of Browne's major interests are included: travel, geography, medicine, magic, dream lore, ancient history, and biblical history, for example. A lost treatise by Epicurus on piety would help explain a point ventured in *Religio*, why the sect of philosophers held responsible for spreading atheism in fact had their own brand of profound religious belief. Several of the items show Browne's interest in the prospect of one famous author responding to another, including Seneca's supposed correspondence with St Paul, Galen's commentary on the plague in Thucydides, a commentary by King Alfred on Aristotle's writings about plants, and another by Dioscorides the herbalist on Hippocrates. In addition to tragedies written by Diogenes the Cynic and the philosophy of Confucius translated into Spanish—that is, examples of the kinds of books which expand or enrich knowledge of famous persons—some of the titles promise an access to the highest wisdom, including "King Solomon de Umbris Idæarum" and "the Prophecy of Enoch" (3.112). In both these tantalizing cases, Browne explains the indirect, and possibly unreliable, means by which he has heard of these precious volumes.

From books, Browne moves to "Rarities in Pictures," including all manner of antiquarian curiosities: Europe's "purposely awry" towers, ancient musical instruments, and submarine phenomena, for instance. In wishing for images of various battles, Browne captures the conditions—in moonlight, snow, or ice—in which the fight took place. From Browne's vantage, some of the scenes depict exotic places, a nocturnal fair in Arabia or a fire in Constantinople. Some show famous historical scenes in what for him would be familiar places, for instance "Vercingetorix the Gaul submitting his person unto Julius Cæsar," or Hannibal taking his elephants over the Rhone river. Some of the scenes bear witness to horrors: to a mother hanging herself, to "singular inhumanities in Tortures," or to the look on Thyestes's face when he learns that "he had eaten a piece of his own Son." Some are drawn from ancient texts while others are modern scenes: "A Picture of the noble Entertain and Feast of the Duke of Chausne at the Treaty of Collen, 1673, when in a very large Room, with all the Windows open, and at a very large Table he sate himself, with many great persons and Ladies; next about the Table stood a row of Waiters, then a row of Musicians, then a row of Musketiers." Browne is drawn to faces, to "passionate" ones, to white ones painted "in the Æthiopian hue excelling the original White and Red Beauty," to a deformed one "expressed in a notable hard Face," or to caricatures inscribing animal features in famous visages. Some of the scenes are simple, "A Vestal Sinner in the Cave with a Table and a Candle", some are playful, "An Elephant dancing upon the Ropes with a Negro Dwarf upon his Back." There are still lifes including the "exquisite

Piece…with a Dish of Pisces Fossiles, garnished about with the little Eels taken out of the backs of Cods and Perches", but also expansive dramas such as the "large Picture describing the Siege of Vienna by Solyman the Magnificent" (Keynes, 3.112–16).

The fanciful collection turns finally to "Antiquities and Rarities of several sorts." Not surprisingly, Browne features medals, engravings, inscribed stones, decorated eggs, jewels, crosses, and medicines. There are the remains of Father Crispin from the Cordelier vault which Browne toured in Toulouse; an ostrich egg painted with "that famous Battel of Alcazar, in which three Kings lost their lives"; and "the Skin of a Snake bred out of the Spinal Marrow of a Man." Among the medical specimens, Browne includes a wonderful East Indian remedy for melancholy, as well as a list "of the most effectual and wonderfull Roots in Nature." There are sensuous delights, including "a transcendent Perfume made of the richest Odorates of both the Indies," but also humorous bits such as the Homeric mock-battle between the frogs and mice "neatly described upon the Chizel Bone of a large Pike's Jaw." Some items offer the worst treachery known to history, for instance in an ointment that created "the great and horrible Plague of Milan." Some are meant to create wonder, though with varying degrees of dubiousness: Browne clearly cherishes the description of "a Glass of Spirits made of Æthereal Salt, Hermetically sealed up, kept continually in Quick-silver; of so volatile a nature that it will scarce endure the Light, and therefore onely to be shown in Winter, or by the light of a Carbuncle, or Bononian Stone." Here is the kind of strange hieroglyph about which the learned Fortunio Liceti liked to write. Yet when Browne details the "large Agath" with an anamorphic picture of a Centaur, his conclusion that King Pyrrhus used such a device to "find out Apollo and the nine Muses" soon has to contend with the concluding irony: "He who knows where all this Treasure now is, is a great Apollo. I'm sure I am not He." Here the putatively universal hieroglyph proves more elusive than the infinite variety of human desire and the unpredictability of human history (Keynes, 3.116–19).

Browne's simple valediction to the recipient of this extraordinary catalogue serves as a reminder that the Baconian emphasis on collaboration in learning offers some consolation to the melancholy that arises from the imperfections of human knowledge and the ridiculousness of human wishes. In the 1670s, Browne's embodiment of the spirit of the Baconian enterprise is, however, best summed in a first-hand testimonial made to his ethos in a collection of Bacon's writings, *Baconiana*, in which Thomas Tenison revisits the misattribution to Browne of *The Nature's Cabinet Unlock'd* by an author whose ignorance and arrogance directly contradict Browne's profound learning, ingeniousness, and "true Humility," for "as [Browne] is a Philosopher very inward with Nature, so he is one who never boasts of his Acquaintance with her."[70]

Letters written in 1672–73 to John Aubrey contain biographical information especially about Oxonians such as Richard Corbett, Thomas Lushington, and

[70] Thomas Tenison, in *Baconiana, or, Certain Genuine Remains of Sr. Francis Bacon* (1679), 76–7.

Browne himself, as well as some notes on the physical remains of Roman antiquity in Norfolk. As the postscript of one of the letters reveals, Aubrey has visited Browne and his family in Norwich, regarding which Browne expresses regret at having been prevented, surely by professional demands, from properly entertaining his guest. Of his works, Browne includes "some miscellaneous tracts which may bee published," but he seems to overestimate the scope of his influence in the list of languages into which *Religio* has been translated: "Latin, French, Italian, High and low Duch."[71] Listing *Hydriotaphia* and *Garden of Cyrus*, he also notes that *Pseudodoxia* has been "translated into Duch 4 or 5 yeares ago" (4.376).[72] Browne is clearly pleased to be reaching outward from Norwich into the world of learning, as in his Oxford days he had imagined that Camden and his followers would do. And the learned world continues to reach out to him. Given his reputation for universal learning, requests for his assistance flowed in from scholars struggling with the knottiest of learned problems but also from those with a personal motive for seeking a random piece of information, as was the case when in April 1673, Aubrey urged Browne to secure for him the horoscope of an old friend with whom Aubrey had come to loggerheads.[73]

In the 1670s and 80s, testimonials to Browne's prominence in English intellectual culture continued to appear in a variety of forms. Between 1675 and 1678, Cambridge scholar Joshua Barnes versified his praises for the knight and physician in a manuscript poem, one which begins with an epigraph from Homer in praise of physicians, then extols Browne's combination of religion and medicine as well as his conquest of vulgar errors. In 1676, another Cambridge man, James Duport, included a panegyric to Browne in his published *Musae Subsecivae*, his focus resting on both *Religio* and *Pseudodoxia*.[74] More privately, in a notebook associated with George Villiers, second Duke of Buckingham, a compiler cribbed a considerable number of "sentences" from *Religio Medici*.[75]

In the final ten years of his life, Browne's stature as a pious naturalist dedicated to the advancement of learning was enshrined in the 1672 publication of the "sixth and last edition" of *Pseudodoxia*, "corrected and enlarged by the Author, with many Explanations, Additions and Alterations throughout." In this volume, published by Nathaniel Ekins, was included *Religio Medici*, also said to be "corrected and

[71] For the importance of Holland in the history of *Religio*, see Cornelis W. Schoneveld, *Intertraffic of the Mind: Studies in Seventeenth-Century Anglo-Dutch Translation with a Checklist of Books Translated from English into Dutch, 1600–1700* (Leiden: Brill, 1983), 1–28.

[72] The translator was Johann Grindal; see Keynes, *Bibliography*, 61. It would be translated into German in 1680 by Christian Knorr, Baron of Rosenroth; see Keynes, *Bibliography*, 63; and Philip Brady, " 'Nor Let the Hard Words Fright Yee'—on the Fearless Translator Christian Knorr von Rosenroth," *German Life and Letters* 47 (1994), 233–41.

[73] The man was a local historian named Thomas Gore; see Anthony Powell, *John Aubrey and His Friends* (London: Heinemann, 1963), 148–9; a month earlier Aubrey had complained about the illegibility of Browne's letters.

[74] On Barnes, see Frank Stubbings, "A Latin Verse Epistle of Joshua Barnes to Sir Thomas Browne," *Cambridge Bibliographical Society* 10 (1991), 86–91. For Duport, see Keynes, *Bibliography*, item 279 on 194.

[75] See *Plays, Poems, and Miscellaneous Writings Associated with George Villiers, Second Duke of Buckingham*, ed. Robert D. Hume and Harold Love (Oxford: Oxford University Press, 2007), 2.155.

amended," together with Digby's *Observations*, themselves evidence that Browne was sympathetic to critique of his own thinking from the leading lights of his generation. Yet a postscript to the reader of *Pseudodoxia* advertised that the author's revisions to his work were "compleat and perfect," so that there would be no "future Enlargements."[76] Whether the postscript was correct in characterizing the various changes to 1672 edition as "very many," they are certainly noticeable in their updates of scholarship. In the "digression concerning Blacknesse," Browne introduced the most advanced thinking on the nature of color, concluding the first paragraph with the observation that "though colours of bodies may arise according to the receptions, refraction, or modification of Light; yet are there certain materialls which may dispose them unto such qualities" (1.524). As Westfall has pointed out, Newton's work on the spectrum had just been set forth in the *Philosophical Transactions* of February 1672.[77] Regarding the manufacture of porcelain dishes, Browne reports that "the latest account hereof may be found in the voyage of the Dutch Embassadors sent from *Batavia* unto the Emperour of China, printed in *French* 1665" (Robbins, ed., *Pseudodoxia Epidemica*, 1.136). The recent work of Sir George Ent on the toadstone is enlisted together with invitations for the readers to conduct their own experiments (1.211–12), while microscopic observations are brought to bear on the constitution of fiery sparks (1.247) as well as on the "black and atramentous spots or globules" on the horns of snails (1.239).[78] Conclusions on the "double-headed Serpent" or "Amphisbæna" must wait on the author's "advantage to behold or have an iterated ocular testimony concerning such as are sometimes mentioned by *American* relators" (Robbins, 1.218).

In addition to scholarly updates, Browne's revisions to *Pseudodoxia* demonstrate his continuing close attention to matters of content and style. His biblical scholarship informs a paragraph inserted on "the twelve stones in Aarons brestplate" (1.139–40), while his fascination with geography joins forces with research on religious history in discussions of Lot's visit to Sodom (1.585) and of Alexander's journey into Persia (1.603). An interest in poetry gives rise to a quotation from Dante's *Paradiso* on St John the Evangelist (1.563). On the naturalist front, Browne's own experiments with moles are offered in a final paragraph to the eighteenth chapter of Book 3 (1.235–36). Chemical interests make a brief appearance in the chapter on chameleons, with reference to the "nitrous Spirit" of air (1.246), while Browne's advice on future research is added to the discussion of glowworms (1.284). For the 1672 edition, Browne works especially hard at correcting the various treatments of animal excretion: one elaboration of "pissing animals" is simply cut (1.169), as is a later passage on animal waste (1.243); but the treatment of urination in toads is carefully adjusted to reflect the author's own "examination" (1.209).[79] Browne adds one entire, if short, chapter, on pictures of the hanging Haman (1.421–3), an insertion which occasions not just biblical and classical scholarship but also a heady reference, by way of Edward's travels, to "a very old

[76] 1672 edition, **3r. [77] See Westfall, *Sir Thomas Browne's Revisions*, 202–3.

[78] See Westfall, *Sir Thomas Browne's Revisions*, 221, 238–42.

[79] See Westfall, *Sir Thomas Browne's Revisions*, 236–7.

manuscript of *Genesis*, now kept in the Emperors Library at Vienna; and accordingly set down by the learned Petrus Lambecius, in the second Tome of the description of that Library" (1.422). In stylistic revisions, Browne persists in his earlier attempts to simplify, clarify, and make more accessible the extensive learning of *Pseudodoxia*. For instance, he adds an English translation by Sir Robert Stapleton of a passage from Juvenal (1.592).

In his final years, Browne remained steadfast in his commitment to capturing everything that could be known about the little world of Norfolk but also about the great world beyond its borders. And his concern for home and family motivated a further development in his writing, one clearly on display in his letters to his children, but also in the major revisions that he made to *Letter to a Friend*: Browne is eager to distill his accumulated wisdom into maxims—to offer his children and their children a view from above the world's labyrinthine ways as well as a careful record of the localities in which those ways ramified in nature and art alike. In turn, this desire to leave a philosophical and spiritual, as well as a learned legacy prompts Browne to take final stock of the world within himself, one now more than twice the age that it was in *Religio Medici*.

3. CATHEDRAL AND SPIRE

Browne's lovingly antiquarian survey of the monuments of Norwich Cathedral was deemed unworthy of learned attention by his posthumous editor, Thomas Tenison, who opined that it was a private endeavor regarding a subject of insufficient interest to a fine antiquarian. Yet in fact Browne had worked long and hard at his survey, beginning it in the early 1660s then leaving the work in two distinctive manuscript versions dated 1679 and 1680, the latter given the name *Repertorium* (that is, repository, storehouse, or catalogue) and carefully revised.[80] During the civil war period, the cathedral had been especially targeted for abuse which helped to account for the strong feeling conveyed by Thomas Searle in his "Catalogue of All the Deans of the Cathedral Church of Norwich, 1660," in which he exclaimed that "the late most heathenish and tyrannical oppression and persecution begun here AD 1641 and ended May 8, 1660. Gloria Deo in excelsis."[81] (See Figure 11.2.)

While Browne used the *Repertorium* to applaud the cathedral's new pavement, its replacement organ, "fayre well tuned...and afterward paynted and beautifully

[80] The two are bound together in NRO MS 21270. While both are in Browne's hand, the 1679 is much shorter (nineteen pages) and lacks the title. Changes in 1680 range from the very small—"becometh" changed to "becomes," a comma inserted—to substantial insertions, including the concluding prospect from the spire. There is also a third related manuscript, Bodl. Tanner 445, f. 36. The work was first published in the *Posthumous Works* of 1712. For a brilliant reading of the work, see Jonathan F. S. Post, "Miscellaneous Browne Among the Tombs of Norwich Cathedral," in Barbour and Preston, eds., *Sir Thomas Browne: The World Proposed*, 258–75. Browne informed Aubrey in 1672 that he had commenced the work shortly after the Restoration.

[81] The quotation from Searle as well as this account are from Atherton and Morgan, "Revolution and Retrenchment," in *Norwich Cathedral*, ed. Atherton et al., 557, 559.

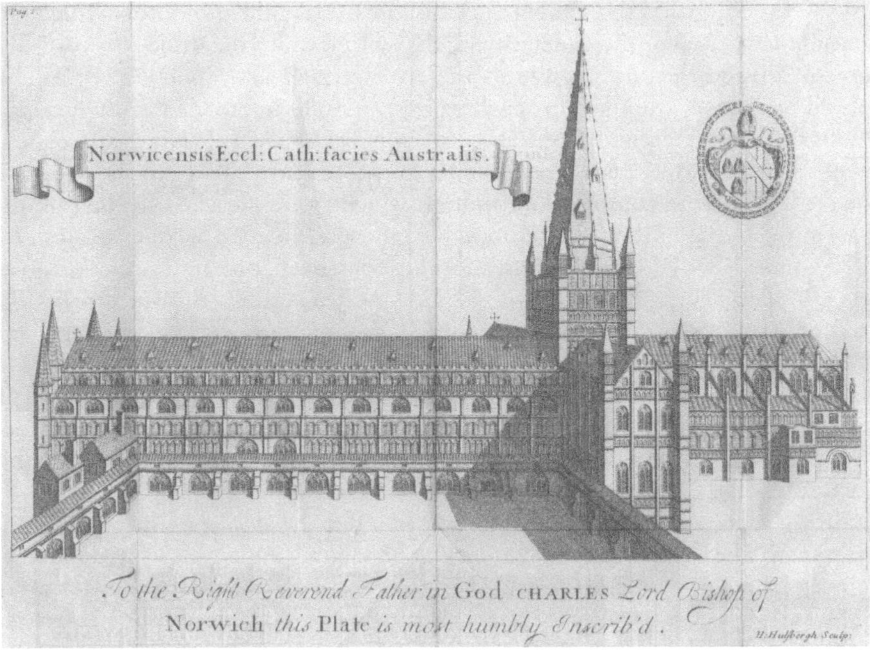

Figure 11.2 Norwich Cathedral: from Sir Thomas Browne's *Posthumous Works*. Reproduced with the permission of the Rubenstein Rare Book & Manuscript Library, Duke University.

adorned," and the friends who had made these beneficences possible, he also praised "our worthy and Honord Diocesan," Anthony Sparrow, whose fragile health Browne knew about only too well, and those contemporary clergymen, from the rector of Heigham, his friend John Whitefoot, to deans and prebends of serious worth and learning from Herbert Astley to John Sharp, Humphrey Prideaux, and several others. The health of the church was recovering to be sure, but these ministers would have to do their level best to defend against any threatening relapse.

For his part, Browne bestowed on his work the powerful sense that, far from ossified markers of status, the monuments and tombs of the cathedral activated in the visitor to the cathedral the living experience of place and time. For one thing, Browne foregrounds the two oral sources of his history, "John Wright a clark above 80 yeares old, and also . . . Mr John Sandlin one of the Quire, who lived in the reigne of Queen Elizabeth" (Keynes, 3.123). For another, as Jonathan Post has argued, Browne leads the reader on a tour of the cathedral in a manner "less bounded by the hierarchical, socially restrictive assumptions often at work in these antiquarian texts, and more akin to the essaying (and assaying) practices of the itinerant traveler."[82] The consequence of this approach is not just that Browne is constantly situating our position in the cathedral, beginning his tour in the south

[82] Post, "Miscellaneous Browne," 263.

aisle. Greater urgency, though not anger, is infused into the project by virtue of its constant awareness of the damage wrought by time and vandalism; indeed, while most of this destruction is owed to the civil war and its iconoclasts, Browne is moved to change "troubles" to "civill warres" in 1680 in order to distinguish the 1640s from more recent opposition between political parties.[83] Not just accouterments but entire experiences have been undone by recent strife—Browne re-creates the setting of those combination sermons which "were preached in the summer time at the crosse in the Green yard, where there was a good accommodation for the Auditors" (3.141). But the most shocking consequence of the destruction arises when a place is simply "left voyd" (3.124). When he can, Browne stresses the accomplishments of the persons memorialized in monuments, the scenic perceptions of the visitor, and even the onetime presence of clergymen who are buried elsewhere or in an uncertain location. Even where the stress is placed on objects in the cathedral, Browne's discovery of those items as he makes his way on the tour "can make the cathedral seem a cabinet of curiosities" as much as a resting place for the dead.[84]

Browne does not flinch from the recognition that the erasure of the past in some measure will be irreversible, no matter what his labors. The advanced age of his oral sources is both a boon and a peril. The site of an entire chapel, Heydon's, cannot be located with any certainty (Keynes, 3.139). And while some of Browne's written sources—John Foxe, for instance—are obvious and accessible, it is also clear that he has spent ample time trolling in the chapter archives. On occasion, the quick repetition of the phrase "is said" serves as a reminder that oral tradition, while precious, can also be tenuous (3.126–7). If the civil war is responsible for senseless violence and rapine, it also strikes Browne as the source of "confusion" (3.128). Even so, he is careful to explain why a monument or its inhabitants mattered in Norwich history. The monument to "Miles Spencer Doctor of Lawe" was the place where "men used to trie their mony" and where "the chapter demanded their Rents" (3.123). Bishop Parkhurst underwent exile during the reign of Queen Mary, we learn from his inscription, and he was "a person of great esteeme & veneration in the Reygne of Queen Elizabeth" (3.124). In the north aisle, the charitable deeds of laymen such as Sir James Hobart are heralded side by side with those of clergymen such as Bishop Walter Hart; in these paeans to charity, Browne's verbs ring forth—built, beautified, and paved—as action seems to spring from the stones. One bishop, Henry le Spencer, lived an adventurous life as a soldier facing "Clement the Anti-pope" as well as "the Rebellious forces of Litster the Dyer in Norfolk" (3.129). But if Spencer's is a storied life, Browne is apt to find greater, if quieter, value in the peaceful. Even Richard Montagu, the combative focus of controversy in the 1620s, is celebrated for his learning, library, and writings especially in church history, as well as for the all too human "quartan ague" which Browne

[83] See Post, "Miscellaneous Browne," 264–5.

[84] Post, "Miscellaneous Browne," 266. For the interweaving of discursive and architectural history, see Anne M. Myers, *Literature and Architecture in Early Modern England* (Baltimore, MD: Johns Hopkins University Press, 2013).

may well have treated in his first years as a Norwich physician. There are Richard Corbett with his wit and eloquence; four Elizabethan bishops who, in the words of John Harington, "lived as Bishops should do, and were not warriars like B. Spencer their predecessor"; and of course Browne's beloved Hall and Reynolds, humble, patient, affable, pious, and assiduous. Nor is the record of human life wholly appealing on the tour, for in the case of Bishop Antonie de Beck, we find a "person of an unquiet spirit, very much hated, and poysond by his servants" (3.131).

Throughout the tour, notable local families are as pertinent to that story as the clergy, and indeed the clergy from such families have their arms and escutcheons as surely as the laity have their share of charitable deeds. In fact, Browne's only deviations from the direction of the walking tour arise when, in discussing a certain family, he offers a quick survey of where else—in the cathedral but also in the county and beyond—they are honored. At moments like these, when charity gives way to genealogy, Browne appears to care about social status and hierarchy a great deal, pausing at one point simply to list the names of families, with special attention paid to those "so many noble and ancient families in these parts" who were abundantly "enterred in the churches and chappells of the monasteries and Religious howses of this citty" (Keynes, 3.135). In a passage left in the manuscript, he even goes so far as quietly to hint at his own entrance into this class of worthy family, since he has "had particular reason to take notice" of the visit from Charles II, who knighted Browne (3.143).

Yet Browne's re-creation and preservation of Norwich society, culture, and history are scarcely if ever nostalgic. In his old age, he finds that family is oriented toward the future as much as the past. In breathing life into the bones and ghostly vestiges of centuries gone by, he is eager to stress the restored and continuing vitality of his world. In a manuscript passage, he follows up news of the death of Dean Herbert Astley with his successor, "my honor'd freind Dr John Sharp" who is "a person of singular worth, and deserved estimation, honour, and love of all men," and whose prebends are "worthy persons, learned men, and very good Preachers" (Keynes, 3.143). Perhaps old Bishop Hall is stirring once again. Another small way in which Browne looks to the future is in his notice that the "strong and handsome fabrick" of the chapel of St John the Evangelist is now the local grammar school—indeed, manuscript records from the history of this institution are mentioned by Browne and would be included in the first edition of *Repertorium* in *Posthumous Works*.[85] That Browne was concerned with the vitality of childhood education is evinced not just in the letters to his own children but also in his donations to Winchester and Cambridge.[86] When the Free School makes its appearance in *Repertorium*, old manuscripts interact with what for Browne is the continuing vitality of Winchester phrases, of Martial and Horace with good notes from

[85] For background, see Saunders, *A History of the Norwich Grammar School*, 290–2.

[86] In the late 1670s, Browne donated £12 to Winchester for a new school building, and he also made a gift to Trinity College, Cambridge, for a new library. Whether he is the Thomas Browne who gave £130 for the reparation of Christ Church, Oxford, has been a matter of debate. See Wilkin, *Works*, 1.c; and also see Bodl Rawinlinson MS D.391, 15r, 17r.

modern scholars, and of classical wisdom transformed by the living, breathing advancement of learning in the gardens and laboratories of Norwich families.

The vitality of contemporary life in Norwich is one of the last things Browne stresses in *Repertorium*. While visitors to cities often ventured first to the highest vantage point from which to take in the whole, Browne concludes his survey of Norwich Cathedral with a journey up its spire. In his notebooks, he had observed in 1663 that during the steeple's reparation, the mason William Brigstow had measured it at "one hundred and five yards & two foote, 14 yards higher then Grantham steeple and about as much higher then St. Pauls London" (Keynes, 3.268). In *Repertorium*, however, Browne celebrates the beauty as well as the height of the spire, acknowledging but also undercutting the higher reach of Salisbury's. In a flourish of civic pride, he notes how "sometimes a long streamer has been hanged" from an upper window "upon the Guild or Maiors daye" (3.142). With the reparations underway after the Restoration, it even became possible for "divers persons" to climb "to the top of the pinnacle," a progress that Browne unfolds before lingering on a description of the weathercock.[87] Finally, there is the glorious view of the city and countryside: "From the top," Browne concludes, "there is a prospect all about the countrey. Mourshold hill seemes lowe & flat ground. The castle and high buildings do very much diminish. The River lookes like a dich. The citty with the streets make a pleasant showe, like a garden, with severall walks in it" (3.142).

From this rarely visited height, the world below is not just diminished in size; it is complexly modified in value as well. The more natural items in Browne's view take his harder hits: the commercial pulse of the city, the river Wensum, has lost its beauty and nobility; a noteworthy hill suddenly appears "lowe & flat." By contrast, artifice takes on a heightened significance.[88] Even if the word "show" might suggest deceptiveness, the diversity of the city appears more carefully crafted, patterned, and sanitized by human agency than it might to those citizens passing along the streets and lanes. At one and the same time, the vision of and from the spire is a reminder of just how much human art can accomplish or repair, yet quietly evokes a sense of how fleeting or unreliable our perception of greatness can be when observed from a transcending vantage. As such, the vista has the feel of the way in which Browne talked about dreams, as well as the need that he felt later in his life for the kind of transcendent, universal moral perspective that he sought to create in *Christian Morals*.

In *Religio Medici*, we have seen, Browne prized the liberation of his intellectual faculties in the experience of dreaming, and he cherished the ways in which dreams could transform his penchant from melancholy to comedy. In that same passage, he lamented the way in which dreams had a way of evaporating from the waking dreamer's memory. On one occasion Browne recorded the thoughts that had occurred to him upon waking from "a good mornings dreame," perhaps enlisting the standard view that the morning was an especially prosperous time for good

87 See Post, "Miscellaneous Browne," 275.

88 I owe this point to Claire Preston.

dreams (Keynes, 3.279). In an extended essay on dreaming, Browne could be harsher, not only lamenting how much time we squander with "the brother of death" but also discrediting dreams as the fragmentary and "phantasticall objects wherin wee are confessedly deceaved" (Keynes, 3.230).[89] "The day supplyeth us with truths," he argued, "the night with fictions and falshoods, which unconfortably divide the natural account of our beings." Clearly sleep was no ally to the erasure of vulgar errors in the advancement of learning, and no relief to the melancholy mind. The challenge, then, was rightly to prepare oneself for sleep, "to compose the phantasticall spirit" so that our rest is not perturbed.

Browne acknowledges that some dreams come to us from divine, angelic, and demonic points of origin, and that "if there bee Guardian spirits, they may not bee unactively about us in sleepe, butt may sometimes order our dreames, and many strange hints, instigations, or discoveries which are so amazing unto us, may arise from such foundations" (Keynes, 3.230). Here is the fanciful altitudinous Browne of *Religio*. But the thrust of his essay on dreams is to naturalize them, to treat them (as Bacon had done with imagination itself in *Sylva Sylvarum*) as natural and artificial specimens for careful analysis. Browne offers guidelines for interpreting the symbolic language of dreams, translating the "naturall fundamental" underneath each thought into "symbolicall adaptation" and "their fundamentall sence & mysterie of similitude." As hieroglyphs, then, dream images transfer the natural into distinctively social or human meanings. Browne is also interested in the ways in which dreams might be used to predict and even to shape the future. "When Alexander going to beseidge Tyre dreampt of a Satyre," he notes with reference to the Greek characters of the key term, "it was no hard exposition for a Grecian to say, Tyre will bee thine" (3.231). If ultimately dreams are too delusional for us to order our lives by, then their best service to our welfare stems from their role in our self-knowledge. Dream so that you may see yourself, Browne argues, for the genuinely virtuous and noble are unlikely to act viciously or "pitifully" once asleep (3.232).

In the final paragraphs of his essay on dreams, Browne quips that the exaggeration typical of our "vaporous state of sleepe" makes it difficult for Democritus to dream of his favorite concept, the miniscule atom. If dreams "enlarge" the objects of our lives, then they operate in reverse of the view from Norwich spire and indeed of the best moral philosophy, which tends to diminish all that earthly triviality about which we tend to care too much. As we navigate through the course of our lives, the moral status of dreams is finally uneven: on the one hand, casuists will be needed to help us discern their spiritual importance, yet "human lawe regards not noctambulos." As far as the law is concerned, in dreams you can do unto your neighbor anything you wish (Keynes, 3.233). Having reminded the reader—perhaps an inquirer along the lines of those addressed in the *Miscellany Tracts*—not to overvalue dreams, Browne concludes the essay with a flourish of received opinions about them: "That some have never dreamed is as improbable as that some have never laughed. That children dreame not the first half yeare, that

[89] See E. S. Merton, "Sir Thomas Browne's Interpretation of Dreams," *Philological Quarterly* 28 (1949), 497–503.

men dreame not in some countries, with many more, are unto mee sick mens dreames, dreames out of the Ivorie gate, and visions before midnight" (3.233). In short, the deluded fantasies of vulgar error have invaded dream lore as much as they have our understanding of minerals and animals.

Among the pieces included in the *Posthumous Works*, one little essay by Browne emphasizes the vanity of wishing that one's life, or history in general, had worked out differently. In the 1712 edition, the essay is entitled "Concerning the too nice Curiosity of censuring the Present, or judging into Future Dispensations." In the *Miscellany Tracts*, Browne had concerned himself with a rationalized prophecy, with probable prediction based on current knowledge. And as a physician and a moralist, he was constantly concerned with the art of living—with the ways in which we can compose our physical and mental health. But this is an essay about regret and longing—about living in the future contingents that are already past and nullified. "We have enough to do rightly to apprehend and consider things as they are, or have been," he begins, "without amusing our selves how they might have been otherwise, or what Variations, Consequences and Differences might have otherwise arose upon a different Face of things, if they had otherwise fallen out in the State or Action of the World."[90] Among several examples from history, Browne reverts to one of his favorite episodes, the march of Hannibal against Rome in the Second Punic War. Apt to find the greatest drama in Hannibal's progress with elephants and armies, Browne betrays his own wonderment about what might have been if Hannibal had accomplished what he came so close to doing. In this case, Browne shifts from the vanity of human wishes to his concern that history must have some order lest all human life amount to the chaos of civil war. From the conviction that history can be mastered and even anticipated by the wise and observant, Browne concludes with an emphasis on providence and Christian teleology (Browne, *Posthumous Works*, 24).

The resistance to longing for an alternative course of events springs from two motivations for Browne, then. On the one hand, the physician and naturalist, the man of practical moral advice and keen for full knowledge of what is true and real, finds that there is more than enough to worry about in the world as we have it. Browne understands that the earth is subject to change, of course; his letters to Dugdale are clear on this matter. Yet he is grateful that actual rather than imaginary change falls under the purview of the advancers of learning. On the other hand, Browne looks at history from the spire as well as from within the aisles. There must be a set pattern to events, for a belief in divine providence and in a universal rational morality makes it necessarily so, even if one's cherished son has been prematurely killed in dubious battle. In *Christian Morals*, a continuation yet drastic rewriting of *Religio Medici*, Browne seeks to help future generations negotiate between the moral and spiritual spire and, far beneath, the transitory, crooked ways of human existence. From the spire one might see the garden-like order of the human city that the streetwalker will miss. The danger is that from that distance,

[90] Browne, *Posthumous Works*, 23. Wilkin published this piece in 4.251–52. Copies appear in Sloane 1885 and 1869. Cf. also Sloane 1879, 37r–v.

the works and monuments, the vitality and variety of life on earth, will begin to seem like a dream from which the wise man has awakened, only to realize that he neither cares about, nor has access to, the vulgar errors left behind. Yet on waking from a "good mornings dreame" recorded in his notebooks, Browne found that a universalizing maxim sprang to mind and eased him back into the world of time, change, and mortality: "*ad quem Animi statum ut perveniamus, oportet ut Nullismo studeamus, ut nihil nos in oculis nostris videamur*" (Keynes, 3.279). This warning reminds Browne that no matter what condition or position we attain in life, it behooves us to focus on the state of worthlessness so that we will appear as nothing in our eyes. Here the experience of dreaming has taught Browne something about humankind as well as himself, but what remains unclear from the jotting is whether the maxim derives from, or serves to castigate, the happiness of dreaming.

4. *CHRISTIAN MORALS*

In *Christian Morals*, Browne expresses dissatisfaction with that contempt for the world which creeps slightly into the conclusion of *Repertorium*. Given "this courtly and splendid world," he explains, the rejection of money or honor is "an obsolete affectation of bravery," and "such contempt of the world out of date." The cynicism which prompted Diogenes to mock Alexander the Great is wholly at odds with "the genius of latter times, unto whom contempt of the world is the most contemptible opinion." Browne will have further advice for those seeking to cope with the uneven or unfair distribution of favors, but moroseness is one step away from the backbiting calumny and malice which he repeatedly associates with the devil.[91] In the third part, Browne once more argues against contempt for the world, but this time more complexly. While it is true that Seneca "spoke too meanly of that state of being which placeth us in the form of men," Browne acknowledges that the value of human life is undercut by our unwillingness to repeat our lives over again. Yet contempt for the world is at cross purposes with itself, since "the great advantage of this mean life is thereby to stand in a capacity of a better" (Roberts, ed., *Christian Morals*, 190–1). Even if on a regular basis Browne praises full happiness and "reality" in heaven at the expense of an existence filled with illusions and vices on earth, his *Christian Morals* is unwilling to embrace contempt and eagerly guides readers in how to live most completely and meaningfully.

Guidance begins with three allegories for the course of our lives. For one, the pursuit of virtue requires inner combat or a spiritual militia and armor, a notion to which Browne recurs throughout the work.[92] This motif is connected to the exhortations to heroic virtue that are especially prominent in the early sections. In the very first paragraphs, the virtue at which we should aim is heralded in uncompromising terms: its essential goodness should be entirely unsullied by wrong

[91] *Sir Thomas Browne's Christian Morals*, ed. S. C. Roberts (Cambridge: Cambridge University Press, 93–4. Hereafter referred to in parentheses as Roberts.

[92] See Roberts, ed., *Sir Thomas Browne's Christian Morals*, 65, 81, 90–1.

intentions or mitigating circumstances, nor should our service to God be confined to "the popular forms and common level of virtues" (65). Reason's victory over the passions must be triumphant (65), and anyone seeking to "be heroically virtuous" will not wait until old age reduces the challenges of overcoming lust (66). So too must our piety be sincerely offered during times of health, not just worked up during periods of illness (67). Sometimes this elevated and purified virtue takes on a Christian identity, for instance when Browne urges a gospel righteousness that requires a higher morality than the law requires (74), a notion to which he returns in directing Christians to outdo even the Stoics in moral excellence (181–2). But the "old ethicks and the classical rules of honesty" still play a strong part in Browne's insistence that the truly virtuous and rightly rational will "eye well those heroes who have held their heads above water, who have touched pitch and not been defiled, and in the common contagion have remained uncorrupted" (75). Moral focus requires that we work for the Stoic's absolute self-governance—without which we are automatons (91–2)—and for those virtues possessed by Jesus that are despised by the madcap world. What is more, it entails that such heroes are always more virtuous than the world will ever know, and even that virtue is essentially solitary, not communal (81–3).

On one occasion, Browne literalizes—and even nationalizes—his image of militant virtue in a manner that recalls his idealization of his son Thomas. Arguing that there are two types of biography, Plutarch's of ancient warriors and Diogenes Laertius's of ancient philosophers, Browne privileges the former for its focus on the "heroical vein of mankind . . . in the soldiery, and courageous part of the world" (*Roberts*, 109–10). In this point, as in others, one glimpses the origins of *Christian Morals* in Browne's family notebooks, here with the recognition not only that Edward helped in the translation of Plutarch's lives but also that Browne may well have wished that such an endeavor might make his elder son more like his late younger. But it is also an incongruous moment—partly because of its nationalism, but also because it serves to remind readers that heroic virtue cannot afford to be a simply solitary affair after all, since the soldier is a bountiful, generous, and loyal friend.

Indeed, the proudly Stoic and militant heroism of virtue is also criticized from the vantage of a more prudent, casuistic virtue whose keynotes are resourcefulness, charity, a good nature, patience, self-improvement, civility, forgiveness, friendship, and humility. For this tendency, Browne provides the two other allegories for the course of our lives. One is closely related to son Thomas's adventures in the navy:

> In this virtuous voyage of thy life hull not about like the ark, without the use of rudder, mast, or sail, and bound for no port. Let not disappointment cause despondency, nor difficulty despair. Think not that you are sailing from Lima to Manillia, when you may fasten up the rudder, and sleep before the wind; but expect rough seas, flaws, and contrary blasts; and 'tis well, if by many cross tacks and veerings you arrive at the port. (*Roberts*, 64)

The course of our lives is not as cataclysmic as the flood during which Noah was required simply to hunker down in his vessel. Our situation is not so drastic, but in many ways it is more demanding, since we must face the inevitable storms of our

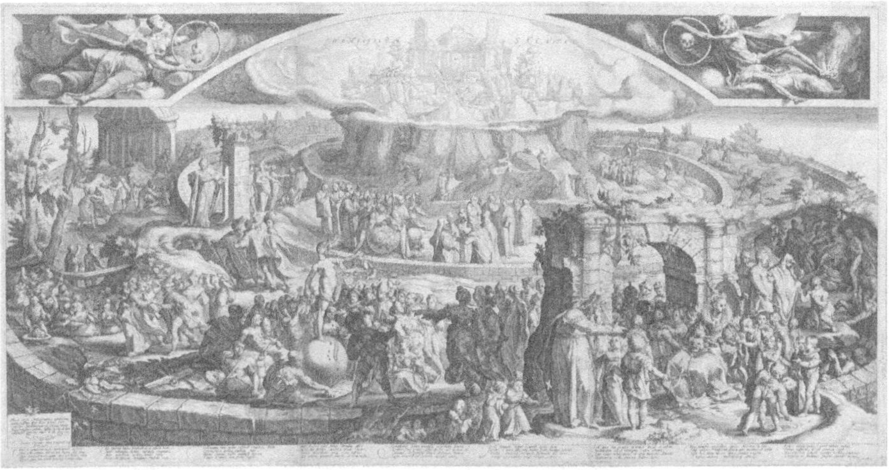

Figure 11.3 Tabula Cebetis, Cabinet des Estampes du Rijksmuseum, print maker Jacob Matham, Objectnummer RP-P-OB-27.329, date 1593. Reproduced by permission of the Rijksmuseum, Amsterdam.

seas with all the intelligence and resources at our disposal. Even though this metaphor gives way immediately to one of readiness for combat, its stress on wise and resourceful navigation is more intimately related to the third allegory for life with which Browne begins, one derived from so-called Cebes's table. (See Figure 11.3.)

"Consider whereabout thou art in Cebes's table," he advises, "or that old philosophical pinax of the life of man: whether thou art yet in the road of uncertainties; whether thou hast entred the narrow gate, got up the hill and asperous way, which leadeth to the house of sanity; or taken that purifying potion from the hand of sincere erudition, which may send thee clear and pure away unto a virtuous and happy life" (Roberts, 63–4). Over the course of Browne's life, the "table" in question had assumed both textual and graphic forms. Most schoolboys knew the Greek dialogue attributed to Cebes, widely assumed in Browne's day to be Plato's interlocutor from Thebes, though the work was in fact Hellenistic. It was the kind of oft-translated moral piece that English schoolchildren might encounter first in the vernacular, then afterwards again in Latin translation and the original Greek. Appearing together with Epictetus's *Enchiridion* and Theophrastus's *Characters*, it had been published in English during the very year in which Browne set out for Winchester, and his library contained a Greek and Latin edition, again bundled with Epictetus, from 1651, about the time that Edward was commencing his education. But whereas the dialogue involves the explanation of a painting said to be in the Temple of Saturn, Browne also encountered a graphic rendition of the "pinax" in Leiden's anatomy theater.[93] The dialogue's exhortation for serious

[93] See chapter 6 in this volume; and Scheurleer "Un amphithéâtre d'anatomie moralisée," 255, 258–9.

pupils to memorize its lessons was reinforced by the ease with which the three concentric enclosures in the table lend themselves to a mnemonic device. In *Christian Morals*, Browne's tripartite structure parodies, without neatly replicating, the triad of the table.

Not only was the *Tabula Cebetis* considered useful for the education of children; it offered, moreover, an allegory of that education. Nor were the lessons to be learned always easy ones; unlike the perfect circle of Padua's botanical garden, or the concentric circles of the Ptolemaic cosmos, the table's circularity did not simply or obviously indicate a good, orderly, and providential cosmos, and it could even serve as the emblem of utmost deception and fragility, like fortune's globe (featured in the allegory) or the bubble (also seen in the Leiden anatomy theater). Yet the outmost circle was clearly meant to suggest comprehensiveness, both in its subject (the course of human life) and lessons. One crucial paradox of the lessons on offer in the allegory was that the method of right living is at once obvious and enigmatic, so that what we might intuit virtually the moment we come naked into the world amounts to much the same truth that we come to understand through long, difficult, and complicated experience. Thus the peril of riddling in the *Pinax* is comparable to the Sphinx, a wrong answer to which spells perdition. Yet elsewhere in the narrative, that which seems difficult (the climb to true understanding and bliss) proves only briefly arduous, with agreeable helpmates on hand to assist us even in that initial difficulty, just as the dialogue itself is meant to be a relatively palatable version of moral philosophy for children. The long experience is certainly necessary insofar as we cannot possibly hold on in life to the spirit of wisdom with which we entered; what is less clear is whether experience manages to give us much that we did not already have.

In the dialogue, the throng of humanity is ready to make its way through the gate of the first enclosure when they encounter an old man called Genius. In the Leiden engraving, those moving toward the entrance are children; the old man (advanced wisdom available to the youngest life) is eager to give the children the right method to pass through their lives, but they are instantly distracted by a lady called Imposture, so much so in fact that they cannot pass through the gate into life without encountering her, and the dialogue even suspends our hearing of what it is that old Genius has to say. Indeed, the drink of error and ignorance that Imposture proffers must be consumed in some measure by all entrants, the difference being only one of degree.

Transformed into adolescents in the engraving, the children appear out the other side of the gate in the company of courtesans who, in the dialogue, embody opinions, desires, and pleasures. Such delightful but treacherous companions, divided between social and internal causes, are extensively treated in Browne's own work. Readers are urged to gain "a triumph over [their] passions" (Roberts, 65); to resist covetousness (71), envy (75), and wrath (77). Part two opens with a warning away from false pleasure, but also with advice on the moderating calculus by which one might find the secret to healthy delight (111–13). In keeping with the allegory, Browne's take on opinion is more complex. While divided theories and opinions can lay no certain claim to truth, he argues, they can be managed so as to contribute to our moral and spiritual well-being. In a debate over whether we have "guardian spirits," for instance, it is morally better to assume that we do. We have a capacity, that is, to pick up debates by a luminous and virtuous handle or by a dark and sinister one. It also serves our purpose to exaggerate the magnitude of evil, since it is precisely the subtlety of some evils that make them so dangerous (147–8). So too Browne advises his charges about the lady standing on a globe or "round stone"[94] in Cebes's table, Fortune, towards whom the youth are ushered in the engraving. There is no getting far into life without passing by the place from which Fortune thrusts out her treasures, blindly and unpredictably, at the eager crowd of suitors there, some churchmen, others noblemen, but none sure of Fortune's rewards. As early as the fifth paragraph of the first part, Browne announces the vicissitude of fortune, then over the course of the work he parses the method by which one should approach both prosperous and adverse fortune. A recurring theme is our need to make the best of adversity, not least by attending closely to those providential proddings and hints, as well as to the historical examples, that can instruct us in the benefits of affliction (Roberts, 99–100).

While the theme of fortune's vicissitude persists into the second enclosure, with voyagers squandering their fortune and ending up a slave to those who once courted them, Browne also shows interest in the specific courtesans whom the travelers encounter near the second portal, including Incontinence, Luxury, Avarice, and Flattery. In one passage he insists that it is far better "to live richly than die rich," especially if one spends wealth on good works (Roberts, 70–1). Acknowledging that "flattery is a juggler, and no kin unto sincerity," he especially eschews self-flattery, however (88–9). After all, the vices of the second portal belong to the category which Browne describes as "the gaping vices of intemperance, incontinency, violence and oppression" (125). The ancient philosophers did well loudly to reject these flaws, since this helped to cover the fact that they were "blindly peccant in iniquities of closer faces, were envious, malicious, contemners, scoffers, censurers, and stuft with vizard vices, no less depraving the ethereal particle and diviner portion of man." Indeed, the real problem with self-praise is that it covers this more insidious set of vices, one deemed by Browne to be singularly inhumane and devilish (124–5). With contemporary England as a den of such mutual scoffing between Guelphs and Ghibellines, Browne moves away from heroic, self-arrogating virtue toward charity, humility, a sociable disposition, forgiveness, and a dedication to self-inspection and improvement. Indeed, a campaign against malice is waged throughout the work. The social emphasis of virtue requires a casuistry that heroic virtue would disdain: we see Browne's efforts to defend this concession in the exhortation that readers "Comply with some humours, bear with others, but serve none. Civil complacency consists with decent honesty. Flattery is a juggler, and no kin unto sincerity" (88).

Friendship figures intermittently among the social virtues in *Christian Morals*, not least because, for Browne, the judgment of the judicious friend is more useful

[94] 1616 translation by John Healey, with the title *Cebes his Table*, 116.

than either self-flattery or whimsical outside opinion (Roberts, 126–7). So too figure family and affection. On two occasions when he exhorts men to avoid female vices, misogyny taints Browne's redrawing of the table (102–3, 166). Yet while the dialogue tends to treat children as an indifferent benefit of fortune, and ignores the prospect of marriage altogether, Browne allows that family can have a moral bearing on us, and that marital love has careful providential support. So long as "generous honesty, valour, and plain dealing" be typical of one's family, ancestors, or countrymen, Browne argues, it is worthwhile to identify with them, so long as we "rest not under the expired merits of others" (103–4).

Time and again, Browne defends the healing power of kindness against a vengeful, carping world. He urges readers not to become obsessed with the evils that have been done to them and to dismay their foes with forgiveness (Roberts, 164–7). In advertising these good-natured virtues, he once again includes a single section in which a specifically English instance is advertised. Having once again praised a sociable "disposition" which comprises "plain and down-right dealing minds, humility, mercy, charity, and virtues acceptable unto God and man," he argues that an orientation against malice will "make natural royalists, obedient subjects, kind and merciful princes, verified in our own, one of the best-natur'd kings of this throne" (137). If this passage seems to attribute the engrained strife of the 1670s to the Whigs, it also leaves open the possibility that obdurate kings, or malicious Tories, are not in fact "natural royalists" (137). One cannot be good natured without an impulse to obey a monarch; but support for monarchy does not ensure that one supports "friendly society." More elaborately, in emphasizing the importance of choosing company carefully, Browne helps his reader steer between social contagion and private melancholy: "Unthinking heads, who have not learn'd to be alone, are in a prison to themselves, if theye be not also with others: whereas, on the contrary, they whose thoughts are in a fair, and hurry within, are sometimes fain to retire into company, must needs have sometimes bad company" (158). Yet it is important to note that while Browne is obviously worried about the malicious erosion of friendly society, he is also fearful that Restoration culture has denigrated the value of solitude, and this same paragraph concludes with a panegyric to the godly advantage found in "the society of thyself." In such an internal world, the imagination can see beyond the bounds of a dark room so that a person "may lie, like Pompey and his sons, in all quarters of the earth; may speculate the universe, and enjoy the whole world in the hermitage of himself. Thus the old Ascetick Christians found a paradise in a desert, and with little converse on earth held a conversation in heaven; thus they astronomiz'd in caves, and though they beheld not the stars, had the glory of heaven before them" (158–9).

It remains unclear whether the claims made by truth and those made by charity can be reconciled in hope for the future of learning. Browne allows that "some have digged deep, yet glanced by the royal vein; and a man may come unto the Pericardium, but not the heart of truth" (Roberts, 117). Yet the thrust of the paragraph suggests that close is not nearly enough. Browne does proceed to recommend that we replace pedantry with good judgment and that we supplement the guidance of nature with our tireless industry. Even if we cannot read the substance of truth, the assiduous pursuit of learning from the vantage of one's own good judgment will render one "the substantial man" (119). In the fifth paragraph of Part 2, Browne encapsulates the ideal approach to study: "Let thy studies be free as thy thoughts and contemplations: but fly not only upon the wings of imagination; join sense unto reason, and experiment unto speculation, and so give life unto embryon truths, and verities yet in their chaos" (119). Nothing like this can be found in Cebes's table. Joining the imaginative flights of *Religio Medici* with the rational-cum-empirical method of *Pseudodoxia*, Browne addresses "the ingenious world" rather than the carping one; applauds the "noble eluctation of truth": and embraces a Baconian hope in the future advancement of learning while paying his profound respect to "the endeavours of Aristotle" so sadly squandered for centuries "in repetitions and transcriptions sealing up the book of knowledge" (119–21). This is the Browne eager to cultivate our seminal learning into a new life, yet also the Browne sorrowful over any seemingly irrecoverable loss of knowledge. Thus he longs for the "just historical accounts of that unparallel'd world" before Noah's flood, the erasure of which by the flood sadly means that "what hath escaped our knowledge, falls not under our consideration; and what is and will be latent, is little better than non-existent" (144–5).

The difficulty in establishing a morally legitimate scholarship finds little assistance from the allegory of Cebes, which maintains that scholarly learning is largely irrelevant to or indifferent within the search for virtue, truth, and beatitude.[95] In one passage, Browne seems to agree that while speculation, imagination, and theory may produce "innocuous" mistakes, it is the "perversity of will" that endangers our souls (Roberts, 80). Familiar from the distinction between error and heresy in *Religio Medici*, this notion seems to go further in *Christian Morals* toward a segregation of intellectual from moral enterprises. From time to time, Browne's efforts to Christianize the allegory of education border on contempt for the struggles of living that lead him to a climactic act of self-quotation. Over the course of *Christian Morals*, he urges readers to keep divine mercy in the forefront of their daily thoughts (85–6); to look everywhere in history, nature, and everyday life, even in unexpected places for signs of that mercy (123, 132–3, 160–1); to direct their winged thoughts at the paradoxes of resurrection according to which gardens spring from graves (135); to prepare for their deaths and to do all they can to avoid eternal punishment (140–1); to realize that there is no substantial glory, not even in the sun, outside of heavenly beatitude (162–3), and to cherish the prospect of that eternal reality that will erase the histrionic misery of human existence (188–9). Dismayed that God's patience has allowed the world to last so long (192–4), Browne posits for a moment that the world is in decline and that, with limited spaces available in heaven, it might make sense to "hasten to make one of that already much filled and abbreviated list to come" (197). Thus Browne prepares us for his version of the goal of Cebes's allegory, a remote domicile of blessedness glimpsed in the cloudy area at the top of the engraving.

[95] Healey, trans., *Cebes his Table*, 125–6; 156–7.

In the allegory, the seeming impossibility of that final goal, gained through a "little gate" and by way of "inaccessible cliffes," is mitigated by the hope that only a little toil is in fact required to reach vistas of great beauty and ease. Both Cebes and Browne do concern themselves with sloth or "sluggishnesse" in the face of difficulty.[96] But both the allegory and Browne offer the possibility of modes of experience which will ease our troubles along the way. In the table, two strong, welcoming women, called Continence and Tolerance in the 1616 translation, reach out their hands to assist the "Trauelers that come that way" (Healey, 129). Browne's happier route to a heavenly vista requires a far rarer, indeed a heavenly, experience whose bliss "we have elsewhere declared," that is, at the conclusion of *Hydriotaphia*: "And if... any have been so happy, as personally to understand christian annihilation, extasy, exolution, transformation, the kiss of the spouse, and ingress into the divine shadow, according to mystical theology, they have already had an handsome anticipation of heaven; the world is in a manner over, and the earth in ashes unto them" (Roberts, 200). If this mystical negation of created things implies that the value of life's education is rendered null and void, the act of self-quotation reinforces just the opposite lesson: that only through the accumulated and evolving experience of a human life can one be sure that one understands what is the spirit of life uttered at the outset. In the passages that the work shares with *Letter to a Friend*, in word choices such as "hieroglyphicks" (25), and with sentences suspended like so many others in *Pseudodoxia*, Browne continues to remind his familiar reader that *Christian Morals* comprises the work of a lifetime. And indeed *Christian Morals* makes a powerful case for the value of longevity. Very rarely concerned with death per se, Browne keeps returning to the phases of our lives and is especially supportive of a life comprising all the ages and phases through which human beings progress.

In these testimonials to the complete life, Browne jettisons bold heroism for "prudence," and the militancy of virtue is traded in for a medical odyssey. In *Cebes his Table*, medical metaphors and analogies figure prominently. Conscience requires a purge, for instance (Healey, 127), while true instruction depends on a cure (134). While Browne shares other metaphors with the dialogue—ships and wild animals, for instance—in addition to converting the dialogue itself into a metaphor, it is this medical one that most informs his appreciation for the stages of life. In the third part, he insists that we "confound not the distinctions of thy life which nature hath divided; that is, youth, adolescence, manhood, and old age: nor in these divided periods, wherein thou art in a manner four, conceive thyself but one" (Roberts, 155). Once we agree to live our own lives, the stages of that life are not as smooth as a stream but as crucially divided as the stages in the cure of a disease. Thus we must "let each distinction have its salutary transition, and critically deliver thee from the imperfections of the former; so ordering the whole, that prudence and virtue may have the largest section" (155). Paradoxically, old age itself is the haven of health.

[96] Healey, trans., *Cebes Table*, 129; Roberts, ed., *Sir Thomas Browne's Christian Morals*, 104.

Browne proceeds to celebrate the sanity of old age in exhorting us not only to give elderly wisdom its proper space in life but also to extend the scope of that wisdom backwards into the earlier stages (Roberts, 156). Ideally of course, the end might touch the beginning so that we might know the meaning of life even before we start it. In keeping with this notion of an essential (if elusive) moral vision, Browne encourages us to seek out epitomes of virtue, all the virtues in a nutshell or the seminal virtues which sprout into secondary ones (149–50). Yet he also makes the case that human dignity and self-composure finally require the fullest experience of our lives, that we have just the one "uniterable" opportunity at making our way through the table, and that the duration of human life, if experienced intensely and attentively, affords us ample opportunity to understand what human life essentially and always is (187, 198–9). So it is that we are neither to scorn the stumblings, imperfections, and "obliquities" of our youth nor to despair at the "prospect" of an even more dreadful old age (122). It is simply the case that we must know how to grow old, a concern far more prominent in *Christian Morals* than the fleeting gesture at a *memento mori.*

On several occasions, Browne offers guidance in growing old. All of history—"the general map of time"—is epitomized in a life of long duration. Although we realize in old age that our life repeats the actions of our ancestors, this does not mean that we have lived in vain. Indeed Browne expatiates on the benefits of old age. In arguing that experience breeds deep understanding and acute judgment, Browne operates between a conventional paean to the wise old man and the Baconian claim that axioms can only ever truly be built from a mass of particularities. As Browne suggests, there is nothing either entirely new or entirely old under the sun. The "varieties" of men may well be the same as the ancients possessed, and the vicissitudes of the present may well recycle those of the past. Yet Browne does not seem to be saying that discovery is merely a symptom of one's perspective. As monstrosities—deviations from the normative—convert into singularities to be situated in patterns, Browne hints at a possibility that he more boldly declared in *Religio*: that long life may well allow us to see what no one has seen before.

Browne's focus is also decidedly inward on "the variation" of oneself, a point to which he returns in the section:

> Such a portion of time will afford a large prospect backward, and authentick reflections how far he hath performed the great intention of his Maker; whether he hath made good the principles of his nature, and what he was made to be; what characteristick and special mark he hath left; to be observable in his generation; whether he hath lived to purpose or in vain; and what he hath added, acted, or performed, that might considerably speak him a man. (Roberts, 185)

Much of the language here is conventional of course: providence has a purpose, a vocation, for each of us, and all of us must fulfill that intention in order to lay claim to our human dignity. But Browne not only stresses the value of long life in our personal pursuit and realization of vocation; he also asserts that an individual can place a stamp on the world that is his or her very own.

Browne is not finished with his praise for longevity, which ends up raising the possibility for a different type of hope. In one of the very last sections, he notes the happiness of those who grow old in virtuous times, precisely because such a state of affairs gives them hope for the future of their children (Roberts, 195). For "good men's wishes extend beyond their lives, for the happiness of times to come, and never to be known unto them" (196). It is a charitable notion that revises *Religio*'s focus on the dead: "And, therefore, while so many question prayers for the dead, they charitably pray for those who are not yet alive; they are not so enviously ambitious to go to heaven by themselves; they canot but humbly wish, that the little flock might be greater, the narrow gate wider, and that, as many are called, so not a few might be chosen" (196). Ignoring Bacon's anxiety over the difference between false and true hope, Browne nonetheless seems to believe at last that hope is the most precious of the theological virtues, though he does not say whether he is living in virtuous times. Close to the end of his table, in the penultimate paragraph, he exhorts his readers—and his children—once again to learn as much as they can about the world so that they may say of their lives that "in some manner" they "lived from the beginning" and endured "to be as old as the world" (198–9). In this final but important way, Browne has learned "how great is humane hope" (136).

Yet with hope comes ceaseless responsibility—the burden of improving one's knowledge right to the end. In a manuscript passage associated with *Christian Morals*, Browne elaborates on the way in which proficiency requires constant improvement and change, for "Time brings not only frequent repentance in actions butt iterated resipiscency in opinions thoughts and notions. euen of what I now apprehend I haue no settled assurance These are my present thoughts this night in England, what they will proue to morrowe, when I arise toward china . . . may bee yet to determine."[97] The strain of conflict between hope and contempt—between resourcefulness and abnegation—in *Christian Morals* is powerfully captured in the drafts of the work that Browne left behind. On one side of a page we find a letter from one Mary Browne eager for further assistance from the physician whose previous efforts against her back and stomach pains are needed again for the aches in her "head and bones" but also for her wind, "fits," and fevers. On the other side of the page are Browne's holograph revisions of the wisdom to be on offer in *Christian Morals*. The attempt to relieve the human condition, both physically and spiritually, is never complete, far from it. On another page, a letter from Mary Well beseeches medicaments for her blister-covered father, and on its verso, Browne is still hard at work on the question of whether angels protect us from harm.[98] Both sets of remedies entail ceaseless effort; neither can be completed in this world; and each exacts from Browne his full attention to detail in the full knowledge that his

[97] See Arno Löffler, "Sir Thomas Browne at Work: An Unpublished Early Section of 'Christian Morals,'" *Notes and Queries* 218 (1973), 391–2. Browne's work at revising *Christian Morals* has been corroborated recently by discoveries of manuscript scraps at Uppsala University, Sweden: Waller MSS gb-00334 and gb-0033.

[98] Sloane MS 1848, 173–4.

efforts might not just falter but backfire: patients might and would die, and readers might find more distress than comfort in the singularity of Browne's religion.

5. BROWNE'S DEATH

In his last years, little facts about Browne testify to the ways in which his concerns and values remained steady, even as he accumulated and recalibrated his learning and experience. In September 1680, in keeping with his longstanding loyalty to the rites of his mother church, he pledged one pound per annum, over and above his normal Easter amd reparation rates, to cover the costs of "the reading of prayers morning and evening according to the use and custome of the Church of England."[99] Browne's dedication to his profession and faith alike was symbolized especially poignantly by one last simple transaction: having followed the wishes of members of the cathedral chapter to seek out a lease for his little meadow in the close, Browne set his seal on the lease in December of 1681.[100] Found between the meadow of Francis Measey to the east, by the ground and orchard of Benjamin Richards to the west, by Francis Corie's pasture to the south, and abutting the causey leading to the river ferry to the north, the meadow offered the naturalist a various amplitude of flora for contemplation: "In a meddow I use in this citty, best about with sallowes, I have observed there to growe upon their bare heads builders, corants, gooseberries, cynocrambe, Rasberries, barberries, bittersweet, elder, hawthorne" (Keynes, 3.378). But as Browne walked from the market through Tombland into the close at its southwest corner, then along the south side of the cathedral close itself, he not just traversed the cityscape of virtually his entire adult life but entered into a bounded microcosm in which the wide range of his life's interests was encapsulated. From the south side of the close, Browne had a panoramic view of the cathedral building, its elongated and variegated structure suggestive of the creativity and fragility of human history. This history was at once ordinary and extraordinary, vulnerable to erasure and destruction but also sturdily resilient and, in some measure, reparable.[101] Inside, he knew, its windows and bosses,[102] as well as its monuments, elaborated and patterned the comic and tragic dimensions of a providential yet also a messy and monstrous world history by which he had been fascinated for so long.

Walking along the south side of the cathedral, Browne would hear bells not unlike those that had moved him in his travels according to *Religio Medici*, and these sounds would lead his eyes up the tower where, midway, the viewer glimpsed a "strange geometric richness,"[103] including circles in two rows of five but surrounded

[99] NRO PD 26/84(s).

[100] See NRO DCN 48/21/152. Wilkin and Keynes thought that the request for a lease had been in vain.

[101] For reparation and gentrification of the close after the Restoration, see Gilchrist, *Norwich Cathedral Close*, 231–5.

[102] See Gilchrist, *Norwich Cathedral Close*, 86–9.

[103] Nikolaus Pevsner and Bill Wilson, *The Buildings of England: Norfolk 1: Norwich and North-East* (London: Penguin, 1997), 188.

by a quincunx of four turrets around the middle spire. Rising above history, yet not fully transcendent were the mediatory hieroglyphs that Neoplatonists had often posited between the divine and the human in an art that Browne had long since believed joined God to nature and man. Where was nature itself in all this? It was all around Browne in the meadows, trees, river, and horses, symbolized by the cock on the spire but also in itself moving around the spire in the shape of those clouds and birds in flight o altitudo. It is no wonder that Browne loved the cathedral close, or that he sought out the lease for a little meadow whose walls and fences, ditches, gates and posts he promised to keep in good repair.

Browne himself was becoming part of history. On the Continent in 1680, Christian Knorr van Rosenroth was placing Browne in a dialogue with philosophers such as Descartes, Leibniz, and the Cambridge Platonist Henry More, this in an effort to rebut Cartesian mechanism and to support a Neoplatonic interaction between the divine one and the earthly many.[104] At home in England, in his manuscript observations on *Religio Medici*, Charles Dodd recorded the fact that Browne had written the work "a few years before ye civil warrs" and situated its legacy within the rise of latitudinarianism.[105] A variety of naturalists, from John Ray to Edward Tyson, took Browne as their Christian hero.[106] While an anonymous elegy on George Thomson in 1677 used "Religio Medici" as a byword for a "right true Christian" death, Christopher Merrett directed his readers to the famous Dr Browne for the character of a complete physician-cum-naturalist.[107] It is likely that when, on November 2, 1682, Henry Atherton lamented the passing of "a more modern Hippocrates both of this Age and Nation, who amongst other sweet Odours to perfume his Memory, hath this, that he was *In toto Vitae statu Christianus*," it was Browne to whom he was referring.[108] Browne's death made the news in *The True Protestant Mercury*, which on October 25 let its readers know that on the 19th, the nation had lost "the Eminently Learned and Loyal Sir Thomas Browne, Doctor of Physick, well known by his Learned Works, particularly his *Religio Medici* so well approved of at home, and Translated into most Languages abroad."[109] Either coy or blithely unaware in ignoring continental upset over Browne's first work, the obituary fudged the number of languages into

[104] See Erich Achermann, "Order in the Vortex: Christian Knorr von Rosenroth as Compiler and Translator of Thomas Browne, Jean d'Espagnet, Henry More, Gottfried Wilhelm Leibniz and Antoine le Grand," trans. Kathryn Murphy and Doris Einsiedel, in Murphy and Todd, eds., "*A man very well studyed*," 247–72.

[105] Birmingham Archdiocesan Archives Dodd MS Z5/2/35/53.

[106] See for instance John Edwards, *A demonstration of the existence and providence of God* (1696), part 1, pp. 54, 212; part 2, pp 3, 146; Edward Tyson, translation of J. Swammerdam, *Ephemeri Vita* (1681), A2r–v; and Tyson, *Phocæna, or the Anatomy of a Porpess, Dissected at Gresham College*, 1680, epigraph.

[107] *An Elegy upon the Death of the Much Lamented, Able and Learned Physician Dr Thomson* (1677). I am grateful to Claire Preston for this reference. For Merrett, see *The Character of a Compleat Physician, or Naturalist* (1680), and Mary Ann Lund's discussion in "The Christian Physician," in Murphy and Todd, eds., "*A man very well studyed*," 238.

[108] Preface to Atherton's *The Christian Physician* (1683); Lund persuasively makes this case in her eponymous essay "The Christian Physician," in Todd and Murphy, eds., "*A man very well studyed*," 239.

[109] Quoted in Lund, "The Christian Physician," 239.

which the *Religio* had been rendered. What mattered was that in death, Browne could finally begin to serve as an English institution rather than a problematic singularity.

On December 2, 1679, with Nicholas Bickerdike, Anthony Mingay, and Augustine Briggs Jr. as his witnesses, Browne drew up his will. Therein he left "all my Lands, Leases, and tenements, all my bonds, bills, moveables, money, plate, Jewells, and all my goods whatsoever" to his executrix Dorothy, who was entrusted with making "liberall maintenance and portions for my deare daughters Elizabeth Browne and Frances Browne, excepting such Lands and tenements as were assigned and made over unto my sonne Edward Browne upon marriage, and to bee entred upon a yeare after my decease" (Keynes, 4.403). The two unmarried daughters—Elizabeth would marry a year later—were made executrixes in the event of Dorothy's predeceasing Browne. Although Browne thus drew up his will for the sake of his family, his daughter Elizabeth treated *Christian Morals* as his last testament to the world. In her dedication to the Earl of Buchan, she states that in gratitude for the Earl's support of her family, "there is no Form of Acknowledgment in our Power, more worthy of your Lordship's Acceptance, than this Dedication of the last Work of our Honoured and Learned Father."[110] According to the preface of John Jeffrey, archdeacon of Norwich, Elizabeth Lyttleton "had lived with her father when it was composed by him; and who, at the time, read it written by his own hand" (61). Jeffrey as well as Lyttleton offered "testimony" that the work was authentically Dr. Browne's own and final. In his copy of the work, Jeffrey noted that Browne "was writing this Book AD 1680."[111]

Clearly Browne's family and friends were keen to protect and to promulgate the legacy inscribed in *Christian Morals*, whose title may well have not been Browne's own. According to Bishop Kennett, Edward had especially "missed the choicest papers" from the box of Browne manuscripts belatedly returned to him by Thomas Tenison, who had culled out the *Miscellany Tracts* from it. Recording the opinion of Elizabeth Lyttleton, Kennett also noted that the children saw *Christian Morals* as "a continuation of [Browne's] *Religio Medici*, drawn up in his elder years, and which his son Dr. Brown had now intended to publish." Elizabeth herself would persist in the search for this manuscript until it was finally uncovered in 1715.[112] Yet, as Robbins points out, John Jeffery and Elizabeth alike realized that there was such a "contrast between the imperative precepts in *Christian Morals* for living and dying and the thirty-year-old Browne's 'soft and flexible sense'" that readers might be suspicious of the attribution—hence their testimonials to Browne's authorship.[113]

In the last years of his life, Browne could look to the successes of Edward as a part of his legacy. Not only were Edward's travel writings well-received, but his medical

[110] Roberts, ed., *Sir Thomas Browne's Christian Morals*, 59.

[111] Thomas Willard, "John Jeffrey's Copy of *Christian Morals*," *Bibliographical Record of America* 92 (1998), 81–4; quotation at 82.

[112] Keynes, *Bibliography*, 119; and Willard, "John Jeffrey's Copy of *Christian Morals*," 82.

[113] Robin Robbins's entry on Sir Thomas Browne in *ODNB*.

career was prosperous. Indeed, some of his patients (Lord Rochester, King Charles) had the very highest profile, and Edward continued to receive prominent offices from the London medical establishment. Having become a lecturer in Surgeons' Hall in 1675, Edward was made a Censor to the Royal College in 1678, and a physician in St Bartholomew's Hospital a month before his father's death. Yet Browne had always known that a reliance on the future of one's family was a fragile hope, not just because of the impermanence of memory but also because of the ways in which misfortune, early death, and moral decline were such pervasive realities in the fallen world. Browne could not have known, though it would not have surprised him to learn, that his male family line would be terminated "within thirty years of his decease," and that his beloved grandson Tomey, also a physician, would perish in 1710 thanks to a drunken fall from his horse.[114] Most of Edward and Henrietta's many children died in infancy, with only Tomey and his sister Anne outliving their father who died in 1708 at Northfleet, according to one acquaintance "in the dignity of President" and "in better Circumstances than I expected."[115] Having been made her mother's executrix in the 1680s, Elizabeth Lyttleton would live until 1736 when her will, made in the parish of St James, Westminster, would clarify her long-standing association with the Tenison family but also her desire to be buried privately. [116] From the vantage point of her kinsman Edward Tenison, Elizabeth carried on the Browne legacy of Christian charity, for in bequeathing her fifty pounds, he requested that she use ten of those pounds for the purchase of twenty Bibles to be distributed by her to the poor as Betty saw fit.[117]

Having occurred a day earlier, Browne's death was announced by Thomas Townshend on October 20, 1682. In a letter to Horatio, Lord Townshend at Raynham Hall, Norfolk, he reported "the worst newes" that "Sr. Tho: Browne is dead, & as hee lived in an eaven temper without deep concerne with how the world went, & was therein very happy so hee dyed like a wise old philosopher." The scene of his death was given as follows:

> Hee fell ill on Saturday, like a feavor. All the phisitions in towne came to him, Hee understood the busines himself, & sayd hee had a payne cross his stomack that nothing could remove, that hee must dye, & would take nothing neither phisick nor cordiall, but with all quietnes & christian meekness dyed yesterday, & is now pronounced a great & happy man in his life & death.

For Townshend, Browne's death marked the end of a great era in learning: "All scholars allow him to have the most curious Learning of all sorts & that his fellow is not left." As all the physicians, no matter what their politics or religion, gathered

[114] See *ODNB* pieces on Edward Browne and his son Tomey Browne by, respectively, Kees van Strien and J. F. Payne, rev. Michael Bevan. Quotation from Wilkin, *Works*, 1.civ.

[115] William Dobyns to Sir William Trumbull, September 4, 1708, vol. 1, part 2 of *Report on the Manuscripts of the Marquess of Downshire* (Royal Commission on Historical Manuscripts; London: H. M. Stationery Office, 1924), 860.

[116] Both Dorothy's and Elizabeth's wills are in the Consistory Court of the Archbishop of Canterbury.

[117] Tenison's will in the Consistory Court of the Archbishop of Canterbury.

to assist this patient, Townshend suggests that together with political partisanship, scholarship was being partitioned—fractured—so that Browne's encyclopedic wisdom would no longer be possible.[118] With Browne's burial taking place in St Peter Mancroft on October 24, a belief that Browne's age at death was 77 reinforced the notion that his life, like his learning, made up a perfect circle, with birth and death occurring on the same day of the year.[119]

Townshend's perception that Dr Browne lived "without deep concerne with how the world went" was not entirely just, as Townshend's own account suggests: Browne had diagnosed his condition, presumably with an interest in its remedy, before resolving on death. Yet in his posthumous reputation, the notion that Browne was not really a creature of this world would soon reappear in an insidious form as fecklessness—not a good quality for a physician to have. This attack would join company with an equally pernicious opposite: that his putative atheism rendered Browne all too worldly. Already in the last years of his life, scholars, especially German ones, had begun to debate whether Browne was an atheist.[120] Yet at home in the first of the Norwich monuments to Browne, the one pointing to the gravesite in his parish church, he was memorialized with a few basic biographical facts—the Cheshire origin of his father's family, his education at Winchester and Oxford—then with a celebration of his excellence in medical practice, in having written *Religio*, *Pseudodoxia*, and "other" works, and in his worldwide fame as a most pious, learned, and honest man. Erected under the direction of his "most sorrowful" ("*mœstissima*") and "affectionate" wife of "41 years," this monument was a modest opening gambit in the long competition over Browne's afterlife.[121]

In the English postscript to the Latin inscription on the monument, Browne was said to have died in the 46th year of his residence in Norwich and in the 77th year of his life. With no birth date given aside from the year 1605, this would seem to support Browne's own claim to Aubrey that he had been born on November 19th—with the implication that he was a month shy of 77 years old at death. Yet the phrasing of his final age was sufficiently ambiguous to enable an alternative to thrive, namely, that Browne had died on his birthday, October 19, and that the arc of his life formed a perfect circle. In some respects, everyday existence at the end of his life must have seemed circular to Browne, since Mancroft featured among its residents a large portion of the city's drapers, mercers, and grocers, the type of tradesmen among whom the young boy had grown up in London.[122] The basic geography and chief sights of Norwich itself had altered little since the late 1630s.

[118] For Townshend's letter, see Keynes's *Bibliography*, vi; it was discovered at Raynham Hall by T. S. Blakeney.

[119] John Jeffrey noted the date in his copy of *Christian Morals*; see Willard, "John Jeffrey's Copy of Christian Morals," 82. It is not clear whether this is right: on one occasion, Browne gave his own birthday as November 19.

[120] See Tobias Wagner, *Examen Elencticum Atheismi Speculativi* (1677), 11, 15, which argues that Browne was atheistic.

[121] See Wilkin, *Works*, 1.xxxix for the monument.

[122] Pound, *Tudor and Stuart Norwich*, 66–7.

Yet over the course of the seventeenth century so very much had changed, not just about the great worlds of learning, politics, and religion, but also inside the little world of Browne himself. As he made plain in *Christian Morals*, Browne believed in the value of an individual's change and growth over all the phases of his life. Nothing illustrates Browne's capacity for change more clearly than his long devotion to Dorothy, a far cry from the youth who in *Religio* had been so suspicious, even disdainful of marital love. Having died on February 24, 1685, at the age of 63, Dorothy Browne received her own testimonial among the monuments in the parish church of St Peter Mancroft: in her grave we find "The prison of a bright celestial mind, | Too spacious to be longer here confined; | Which after all that virtue could inspire, | Or unaffected piety require, | In all the noblest offices of life, | Of tendrest benefactress, mother, wife, | To those serene abodes above is flown, | To be adorned with an immortal CROWN."[123] In praising the spaciousness of her mind together with her unflinching dedication to the duties of everyday existence, the author of these verses clearly believed that in Dorothy Mileham, Sir Thomas Browne had found the most agreeable partner for moving through those final circles in the Cebes table of his life. Dorothy's epitaph was inscribed next to her sermon notes in the family commonplace book,[124] and on the monument still to be seen in the parish church of St Peter Mancroft, the arms of her family were impaled with those of the Brownes. Their monuments facing one another in the sanctuary near the altar, with husband on the south side and wife on the north, Dorothy had done more than anyone or anything else to confirm the qualities of versatility and alchemical transmutability that were recorded on the brass plate affixed to her husband's coffin.[125] But family, Browne had always worried, was a fragile means of finding one's way into futurity: whereas Thomas Townshend would ask in 1705 to be buried "in the same vault on the altar wherein my ever dear wife is interred, next to Sir Thomas Browne, her uncle," the eighteenth-century records pertaining to St Peter Mancroft lament that "None of Browne's family" were "willing to repair his vault in the altar, which by length of time the joists over it were much decayed."[126] And when Dorothy was buried, it was a neighbor, Mrs Wenman, and not one of her own children, that paid for the breaking of the ground.

One of the last mentions of Browne while he was still alive appears in a letter from Lord Yarmouth to his wife in 1682, one reporting a visit paid to Sir Thomas whom the earl had found at home on the marketplace in a house full of women: Mrs Peirce and her daughter, Mrs Needham, and Colonel Harbord's wife "who came downe staires to see me."[127] This image of Browne resonates with the prospect that in a world driven (for Edward) by ambition, for the late Thomas Jr. by military valor, and increasingly for masculine political culture by bitter rivalry and partisanship, it was the women in his life who surrounded the aging physician with the civility, flexibility, and good-heartedness for which he had always longed.

[123] Wilkin, *Works*, 1.civ. [124] See Bullard, "'A bright Cœlestiall Mind.'"

[125] The plate, recovered in the nineteenth century, is on display in St Peter Mancroft.

[126] In NRO MS 78/1 (Benjamin Mackerell, *History of the City of Norwich Both Ancient and Modern*, typescript of manuscript history from 1737), 1.175.

[127] BL Additional MS 36988, 195v.

Conclusion

Chasing the Butterfly

In the years just after his death, Browne was often cited but not always understood. In 1699, for instance, an account of a murder trial invoked his authority on the question of floating bodies, only to remark of the passage in *Pseudodoxia Epidemica* that "I don't understand it my self, but he hath a whole Chapter about it."[1] But Browne's learning was also subject to ridicule. In 1683, just a year after Browne's death, a physician named Gideon Harvey lashed out at his colleagues in the profession of learned medicine with a satire entitled *The Conclave of Physicians, Detecting their Intrigues, Frauds, and Plots, against their Patients.* Twenty years earlier, Harvey's *Archelogia philosophia nova* had included a section called *Religio Philosophi, or Natural Theology*, one in a number of attempts to capitalize on the fame of Browne's *Religio Medici*. Yet in 1683, Harvey told a story about Sir Thomas Browne which converted his curious learning into a case of gross medical negligence:

> Some Physicasters by reputing themselves Virtuoso's, Mathematicians, Philosophers, and witty Cracks, have insinuated this Enthymeme to the Commonalty, that therefore they must necessarily arrive to the top of their profession; for since their porous Brain was capable to imbibe such knotty Mysteries, it's not improbable, they might easier suck up the quintessence of the Art of Medicine. To this Category belonged that famed Doctor of Norw. who being Posted away from his House with a Coach and Four to a Sick Gentleman in the Countrey, an unhappy gawdy Butterfly thwarted the Coach, upon which a halt was made, and the Doctor with the assistance of the Coach-driver, hunted so long, until they had him under the broad brimm'd Beaver.[2]

Having snared his colorful prey with the help of the coachman, Harvey's Browne is keen to lecture his collaborator "upon the admirable Structure, Shape, Organs, and colours of the Butterfly, particularly upn the transparent yellow, of which colour a Cap would better have fitted him than the black Velvet one" (50). As flighty as the butterfly, the virtuoso Browne shows such an ardent and exact attention to what Harvey considers trivial details that natural history doubles as ridiculous, quixotic flights of fancy.[3]

[1] *The Tryal of Spencer Cowper, Esq., John Marston, Ellis Stevens, and William Rogers, gent.* (1699); quoted in Killeen, *Biblical Scholarship*, 150.

[2] Gideon Harvey, *The Conclave of Physicians Detecting their Intrigues, Frauds, and Plots, against their Patients* (2nd edn., 1686), 49–50.

[3] For the Restoration caricature of the virtuoso as "foolish pedantic," see Craig Ashley Hanson, *The English Virtuoso: Art, Medicine, and Antiquarianism in the Age of Empiricism* (Chicago: University of Chicago Press, 2009), 4–5.

The satire continues when Browne arrives at the home of his would-be patient in search of another background against which to display his specimen. There he finds "the new Widow accosting him with the information, *That her dear Husband had passed through many*" of his fits with the "*help of a Cordial, and so probably might this, had she not, wretched Creature as she was! expected his coming to prescribe another.*"[4] The anecdote ends with a jesting speculation about whether Browne, deprived of his fee, was required to walk all the way home.

Harvey's anecdote of the irresponsible Dr Browne was rejected by at least two authors in the 1680s. In *A Dialogue between Philiater and Momus* (1686), an anonymous pamphleteer connected Harvey's penchant for extreme calumny and destructiveness to the effects of a civil-war mentality (3). At times emulating the irenic rhetoric of *Religio Medici*—"I could never wish any Personal ill to another man, because he differs from me in judgment," he explains (7)—Philiater defends Browne against a hypocritical Momus who has dared to co-opt Browne's title in *Religio Philosophi* (101).

In defending Browne against Gideon Harvey, *A Dialogue between Philiater and Momus* has more trouble juggling the sensible with the imaginative Browne. "You do not well," Philiater chides Momus, "to let that same *Religio Medici* run so mightily in your head. There is more Sense, and Religion too in a Paragraph of that Book, than in all your fantastical, raw, and yet borrowed conceits of Natural Theology" (211). At one and the same time, *Religio Medici* concentrates good sense into its paragraphs yet has a way of "mightily" encouraging volatility or pretensions in unstable wits. As Philiater elaborates the latter point, "*Religio Medici* is a serious thing, consisting of very Uncommon Notions, and such as every paltry Pretender is not a competent Judge of" (211). "Uncommon Notions" carries considerable weight in an age in which latitudinarian and rational religion tends to appropriate Lord Herbert's "common notions," that minimal slate of tenets in which all legitimate religions share and through which they might find peace. For Philiater, only the very few should attempt to engage with Browne's singular vision of religious truth, lest his heroic stature be reduced to quixotic ravings and ridiculousness. To ensure that Browne not appear too strange, Philiater generalizes his hero's capacity for the unusual yet, in doing so, purveys the complexity of what Browne was coming to mean for English cultural debates in the late seventeenth century. Browne represents an especially challenging case of what amounts to the general tendency of physicians and natural philosophers to be distrusted with religious matters for two distinctive reasons: they soar too high into the mysteries yet they also speak so bluntly about religion that they strike the contentious as having abandoned religion altogether.

In another response to Harvey, a poem entitled *Gideon's Fleece* from 1684, an author calling himself "a Friend to the Muses" manages to highlight what is at stake for contemporaries in the butterfly episode. The subtitle of the poem, "The Sieur De Frisk, An Heroick Poem," anticipates that the poet—now believed to

[4] Harvey, *Conclave of Physicians*, 50.

have been Thomas Guidott—is subjecting Harvey to the abuse of a mock-heroic. Joining Philiater in attributing Harvey's outburst to spite and malice, Guidott deems the story of Browne and the butterfly no more than an incredible romantic fiction.[5] The effect of this critique is to make Harvey the quixotic author rather than Browne the mock-heroic virtuoso foolishly hunting down a poor butterfly. Yet with the outgrowth of his imitators, appropriators, and critics in the decades after his death, Browne became a pawn in a complex cultural mediation involving the extent to which a culture of good sense can retain the heroic boldness and forceful imagination of pre-civil war English writing without lapsing into the excesses—at best fanciful, at worst demonical—that had unleashed then prospered in the civil war and Interregnum. This attempt to locate a sensible boldness in Browne is on par with the heralding of the heroic virtuoso by mid-seventeenth-century cultural brokers such as Walter Charleton,[6] and with critical efforts made most notably by Dryden to harmonize moderate good sense with heroic boldness or elevation in writers such as Chaucer as well as in political and religious leaders.

The relationship between Browne the man of sense and Browne the man of bold or "uncommon" imagination often becomes vexed in the work of his posthumous readers. While Gideon Harvey might depict the fanciful Browne as ridiculously flighty, it was far more usual for critics to entertain the possibility that his extraordinary wit had pushed Browne into the territory of heresy and atheism. Although the charges of and defenses against Browne's atheism were especially prevalent in German works,[7] one prominent English author, Charles Blount, stressed and celebrated the connection between Browne's rationalism and his innovative thinking about scripture. In *The Oracles of Reason* (1693), Blount enlisted Browne's assistance in a defense of Gilbert Burnet's scriptural criticism. "Justly admired as well by Foreigners as his own Country-men, upon the Account of his Knowledge in all Gentile sorts of Literature," Browne has admitted "his many Doubts and Scruples" regarding certain "Passages in the Mosaic History."[8]

On occasion, Browne's early posthumous reputation was linked to *Pseudodoxia*, which clearly cast him as a man of sense. In J. D.'s *A Memorial for the Learned* (1686), Browne's encyclopedia is included among those works of history and natural history that are sufficiently useful to deserve encapsulation. In Thomas Blount's *A Natural History* (1693), *Vulgar Errors* is the Browne work which matters. Nonetheless, in late seventeenth- and early eighteenth-century constructions of Browne's legacy, *Religio Medici* was emphatically the star. Vague imitation had of course commenced long before his death: setting aside a separate tradition of the *Religio*

[5] Thomas Guidott, *Gideon's Fleece, or, The Sieur de Frisk: An Heroick Poem* (London, 1684), 4, 20.

[6] See Charleton, *The Immortality of the Human Soul*, intro. J. M. Armistead (New York: AMS Press, 1985), 18.

[7] See Jacob Friedrich Reimmann, *Historia Universalis Atheismi* (1725), 446–8; J. Franciscus Buddeus, *Theses Theologicae de Atheisme* (Utrecht, 1737); and especially Elias Fredericus Heister, *Apologia pro Medicis* (Amsterdam, 1736).

[8] Charles Blount, *The Oracles of Reason*, facsimile edition introduced by John Valdimir Price (London: Routledge/Thoemmes, 1995), 2–3.

Laici, which owed as much if not more to Lord Herbert as to Browne, Browne's title alone was converted into *Religio Jurisconsulti* (1649), *Religio Bibliopolæ* (1691), *Religio Libertini* (1712), *Religio Militis* (twice, in 1672 and again in 1690), and *Religio Clerici* (1681). Such imitations continued to thrive after Browne's death, for instance in *Religio Jurisprudentis* (1685), though relatively few of the imitators engaged with Browne's work in any direct or extensive fashion. Rather, imitators often evoked Browne's presence for their own purposes. Vulgarization also brought with it significant changes in the scope of Browne's appeal.[9] Although in *Religio Stoici* George MacKenzie might criticize Browne for his "university style," Browne's posthumous circulation came to include coffee-house venues and a female readership too.[10] Beyond titles, a few of Browne's parodists intervened on the question of his relevance for a culture in which good common sense and bold, uncommon imagination needed a new covenant with one another. If culture were reduced to common sense, then the human capacity for heroic greatness and intellectual nobility would be severely compromised, a moral state of affairs analogous to commercial cheapening. Yet the experience of civil war had underscored the horror that results from a culture too vulnerable to aspiration and mania. And if the man of sense could degenerate into an atheist, the singular imagination could lapse into fanatic heresy.

Among his posthumous interpreters, Browne's attraction came from both his sensible and altitudinous tendencies, and so did his dangers. In *Religio Jurisprudentis* (1685), Mark Hildesley begins with a version of Browne's opening gambit regarding the religion of physicians, admitting that, having read his title, some of his "Perusers" will "presume, that a Person of that Character, commonly is little or nothing acquainted with, or at least ties not himself up to the Rules and Practises of real Virtue and Religion" (A5r). But in shifting the strange generic features of Browne's book into a simpler manual of advice to his son, Hildesley maintains that the religion of jurisprudence adheres to "a Man of Sense or Prudence, a Man of moral Conduct, that distinguishes well between, and judges well of Right and Wrong." It is in fact this capacity for moral good sense which distinguishes the jurisprudent from the vulgar.[11]

A conjunction of "moderate" and "uncommon" Christianity headlines John Dunton's *The New Practice of Piety; Writ in Imitation of Dr. Browne's Religio Medici: or, The Christian Virtuoso: Discovering the Right Way to Heaven, Between all Extreams* (1705). For Dunton, the marriage of boldness and peaceful moderation amounts to the very essence of "Heroick" virtue (A3r), a heroism that he finds reincarnated

[9] Daniela Havenstein, *Democratizing Sir Thomas Browne: Religio Medici and Its Imitations* (Oxford: Clarendon Press, 1999).

[10] See Havenstein, *Democratizing Sir Thomas Browne*, 73, 87 for commercialization; 32 (for MacKenzie) and 86 (for women). For Browne in the coffee houses, see discussions of John Dunton in Havenstein, 45–52; and (with special regard to *Pseudodoxia*) William C. Wright, "Sir Thomas Browne's *Pseudoxia* [*sic*] *Epidemica* and English Coffee House Journalism," *Journal of Popular Culture* 12 (1978), 36–41.

[11] Mark Hildesley, *Religio Jurisprudentis* (1685), A5v.

in John Locke. The imitation of Browne is undertaken to resist the current trend toward official severity, dissenting hyper-scrupulousness, and overall divisiveness in religious culture (A4r). Thus Browne serves as a model of sense, reason, and moderation which should not be mistaken for trimming or lukewarmness but should be cultivated against the dominance of zeal, fanaticism, and contentiousness in contemporary times (B1r–B1v). Yet Browne is not reducible to moderate sense: he is also singled out for his "Uncommon" ideas, albeit in this context with the concession that these tend to be mistakes whose only benefit is their unusualness. Dunton struggles in his attempt to construct Browne as just the right combination of bold speculation and practical boundaries. A key to this struggle lies in Dunton's claim that the benefit of Browne derives chiefly from his mode of self-knowledge. With self-knowledge, bold speculation and practical good sense can safely congregate (Dunton, *New Practice of Piety*, 2).

Browne's boldness received its share of criticism from putatively reasonable divines in the last decades of the seventeenth century. In *Religio Clerici*, an anonymous writer took aim at Browne's "Hyperbolick strains" while John Tillotson expressed dismay at Browne's affection for impossible mysteries.[12] As Havenstein notes, however, Tillotson's attack prompted his own editor, Thomas Birch, to attempt a reconciliation between the two men, arguing that Browne really meant apparent impossibilities and that his words "should be looked upon as a verbum ardens, a rhetorical flourish, and a trial of skill with Tertullian."[13] This impulse, to use Browne as a critical means of retaining the human capacity for heroic intellection and awesome faith within the context of a culture of good sense, was more important to Browne's posthumous reputation than attacks from one side that argued that he was not reasonable enough, or from the other that claimed that Browne had ridden his naturalizing reason straight into irreligion. One of the best examples of this mediation between sense and boldness is *Religio Bibliopolæ in Imitation of Dr. Browns Religio Medici* (1691), a work assigned on its title page to Benjamin Bridgewater but in fact a collaboration with John Dunton.[14] In this work, however, Dunton and his collaborator are fully prepared to indict Browne when his bravado goes too far—on the strength of his faith and on his criteria for "more Bold and Noble" faith in others (36–7). Although *Religio Bibliopolæ* does not explicitly say so, there is the suggestion in passages such as this one that the true marriage between good sense and the "strange and unexpected" (17) in human life and thought eluded Browne as a product of an age that had produced the civil war.[15]

For these early transmitters of Browne's reputation, Browne was a butterfly, lovely, complex, and metamorphic, so elusive as to demand that biographers pin him down

[12] Havenstein, in *Democratizing Sir Thomas Browne*, quotes both *Religio Clerici* and Tillotson, 18.

[13] Havenstein, *Democratizing Sir Thomas Browne*, 18–19.

[14] For authorship, see Almonte C. Howell, "John Dunton and an Imitation of the *Religio Medici*," *Studies in Philology* 29 (1932), 442–62. For a full discussion, see Havenstein, *Democratizing Sir Thomas Browne*, 45–70.

[15] Dunton, *The Art of Living Incognito* (1700), 33, quoted in Havenstein, *Democratizing Sir Thomas Browne*, 49.

against just the right backdrop yet so delicate as to embarrass the awkwardness and rudeness of the capture.[16] No wonder then that although *The Works of the Learned Sir Thomas Browne* (1686) included no prefatory material, the *Posthumous Works* (1712) began with two biographical essays in order to capture and hold Browne's spirit. The first, an anonymous "life," devotes a little space to a narrative, based on Anthony Wood, of Browne's early life, education, and travels, as well as "the Persuasions of Sir *Nicholas Bacon* of *Gillingham*, Sir *Justinian Lewyn*, and Sir *Charles Le Gross* of *Crostwick*" that he settle in Norwich. In replacing Wood's reference to Lushington from this list of associates on a cancel sheet of the book, the biographer or publisher appears to have been following someone's wishes to distance Browne from transgression and heresy.[17] And indeed the greatest part of the biography is concerned with Browne's immediate transmission and reception: the anonymous biographer quotes Browne's own statement of his reasons for publishing *Religio Medici*; scoffs at the criticisms of Alexander Ross, "whose Name alone sufficiently evinces that his Book was not worthy of the least Notice"; and mentions the "general Reception" awarded *Pseudodoxia*. Anonymous quotes at length Merryweather's letter recounting his efforts to publish the Latin translation of *Religio*, in which letter he mentions how "a good Part of Christendom" is now familiar with Browne's work and how he, Merryweather, has persisted against opposition to Browne's supposed "Exorbitant Conceptions in Religion." In a series of concluding gestures, Browne's reception is bolstered by his association with learned men, "who often writ to him for Solutions of very Critical and Abstruse Points of Literature; and his Answers to them always contain'd some very uncommon and curious Remarks"; by his honors from the Royal College and King Charles II; by his humble yet judicious invitation to criticism of *Pseudodoxia*; and by his being "a steadfast Member of that Church, whereof he had so Nobly express'd himself in his Writings."

Whereas the anonymous biographer focuses on reception, John Whitefoot devotes his "MINUTES for the Life of Sir Thomas Browne" to his longtime friend's character. Browne's honor as a physician is his starting point. Just as John Wollaston's 1734 portrait of Browne would be included in a series of great physicians,[18] Whitefoot quotes Ecclesiasticus 38:1 on the divinely bestowed power to heal that renders physicians honorable even among kings (xxiv). Transitioning quickly through the king's show of honor in knighthood, as well as the learned world's admiration for Sir Thomas, Whitefoot pauses for a page or so to express the difficulties that any biographer faces, and he makes the case also pursued by John Dunton that Browne excelled in self-knowledge. Since Browne has not left a much-to-be-desired autobiography in the tradition of wise men from Moses, Josephus, and Marcus Aurelius to Joseph Hall, Whitefoot does the best he can with his long

[16] For early biographies, see Jeremiah S. Finch, "Sir Thomas Browne: Early Biographical Notices, and the Disposition of His Library and Manuscripts," *Studies in Bibliography* 2 (1949–50), 196–201.

[17] See Finch, "Sir Thomas Browne: Early Biographical Notices," 199.

[18] The series includes Thomas Willis, Walter Charleton, William Harvey, Francis Glisson, Thomas Sydenham, and Theodore Turquet de Mayerne; see Wayne Craven, "John Wollaston: His Career in England and New York City," *American Art Journal* 7 (1975), 19–31, at 22.

and intimate knowledge of the subject, not with the facts of Browne's life—we are given only one for the whole of his pre-Norwich years—but with his appearance, ethos, social persona, and intellectual habits (xxv–xxvii). Thus we learn about Browne's hair color and complexion (brown), his height and body weight (moderate), his dress (plain) as well as the astonishing capacity of his understanding, which is said to have comprised the whole celestial and terrestrial world, "as if he had been by Divine Providence ordained Surveyor-General" (xxviii). When Whitefoot turns to praise Browne's extraordinary memory, the character sketch seems to find a sudden restraint, as though the biographer would not want to mythologize or deify his greatness. In this humbler vein, Browne is said to have a "Capacious and Tenacious" memory, but one "not so Eminent as that of *Seneca*, or *Scaliger*." Similarly, his control over the passions was not absolute—"That was a Privilege of Original Perfection, forfeited by the Neglect of the Use of it"—and his relationship to one passion, wonder or "Admiration," was especially complex, having both "more, and less" as his "uncommon Knowledge" familiarized him with more "rarities" than men commonly encounter (xxix–xxx).

As Whitefoot's characterization unfolds, this tendency to proclaim yet also to modify Browne's greatness dovetails with early eighteenth-century attempts to herald Browne as a sensible hero. Having measured Browne's cheer according to a "sensible Rate," Whitefoot proceeds to forge a marriage between his subject's "Modesty" or industry and his singularity of discourse, "never Trite or Vulgar." Yet even Browne's conversation is imperfect, for guests often found themselves "deceived in their Expectation . . . by the Briskness of his Writings": "so free from Loquacity, or much Talkativeness, that he was something difficult to be engaged in any Discourse" (xxxi). Despite Browne's considerable knowledge of languages, it has to be admitted that he had neglected "the Oriental Languages, which never were vernacular in this Part of the World" (xxxiii).

In the final sections of his notes, Whitefoot normalizes Browne by stressing the domestic bliss of his marriage—with husband and wife sharing "a kind of Natural Magnetism" and symmetry (xxxii)—as well as by claiming that his four surviving children are "all of them remarkably Partakers of his Ingenuity and Vertues" (xxxii). Whitefoot posits a consistency in Browne's devotion to that Church of England which Grotius had agreed was the world's best. We learn that Browne "attended the Publick Service very constantly, when he was not withheld by his Practice," that he "read the best English Sermons he could hear of, with liberal Applause," and that, like the young author of *Religio Medici*, he "delighted not in Controversies" (xxxiv). The patience that he showed in the face of a painful death was remarkable yet not theatrical, lacking "any Pretence of Stoical Apathy, Animosity, or Vanity of not being concerned thereat, or suffering no Impeachment of Happiness" (xxxv). That is, his fortitude was all the more meaningful because he was a vulnerable and sensible human being. Whereas Browne is paraphrased as having claimed on his deathbed that as a physician he "had often triumphed over the King of Terrors in others, and given many Repulses in the Defence of Patients," such heroic grandeur gives way in the final hour to the "Meek, Rational, and Religious Courage" with which he took "his own Turn" with "the Will of God" (xxxv). Other qualities are similarly brought down, just a little, to the size of human imperfection: his desire for warm dress at all times of the years belongs somewhere between quirkiness and medical lore, with the best that can be said of it proving to be that Browne did not take the tendency to absurd extremes (xxviii). His liberality to his children—allowing two sons and two daughters to travel on the Continent—is also deemed an "Indulgence"; similarly, his overall generosity in charity and "House Entertainments" meant that "he left a comfortable, but no great Estate." Returning appropriately to Browne's intellect, Whitefoot makes the somewhat surprising case that in other circumstances, Browne's vast knowledge of history "would have made [him] an extraordinary Man for the Privy-Council, not much inferior to the Famous *Padre Paulo*, the late Oracle of the *Venetian* State" (xxxvi–xxxvii). Thus Browne's uncommon features end up firmly planted in the political world of savvy and prudence, much as his oracular mode is not divinely inspired prophecy but the far more worldly skill of "*Stochastick*" prediction (xxxvii).

Like so many of his contemporaries, Whitefoot is eager to protect Browne's extraordinariness from the monstrous extremes against which the sensible arbiters of cultural heroism were doing combat. Yet this did not mean that these arbiters wanted a divorce from heroism or from a heroic Browne. In *Spectator* 177, Joseph Addison praised Browne's expressions of that sociable virtue, charity, as "heroic" in the "noble heat" of its "sentiments."[19] In *Spectator* 487, he reverted to *Religio*'s paean to intellectual liberation within dreams as a testimony to the "wonderful... sprightliness and alacrity" that the soul might experience in sleep. In the quotation which follows, early eighteenth-century readers encountered Browne in his soaring "fancies," utterly transformed from his everyday melancholy into a comedic state far above or beyond himself and indeed "above mortality." Offering no final comment on the passage, Addison goes on a little later to praise Browne again for the way in which his dreaming showed devotion in "a very particular manner heightened and inflamed." Browne's extraordinary dreams, the *Spectator* allows, might not be available to every "constitution," yet its power is sufficient to prompt questions for the reader about whether surreal illusions—a beggar dreaming himself kingly—might amount to a legitimate alternative reality.[20]

The most complex eighteenth-century endeavor to ground Browne's heroic fancy was Samuel Johnson's. As James Lill has argued, Johnson's "Life of Browne," affixed to the second, 1756, edition of *Christian Morals*, ultimately defends its subject's piety and embraces his ethical center. But along the way, Johnson's responses can range from skeptical to envious.[21] Influenced as Johnson was by Browne's prose style,[22] he was prone to baulk at Browne's more extraordinary opinions, not least the one according to which his seemingly

[19] *The Works of the Right Honourable Joseph Addison*, notes by Richard Hurd (London: Bohn, 1854), 3.36.

[20] Hurd, *Right Honourable Joseph Addison*, 4.2–3.

[21] James Lill, "A Lesson in Futurity: Johnson's 'Life of Sir Thomas Browne,'" *The Notre Dame English Journal* 15 (1983), 39–50; see 40.

[22] John Courtenay mocked Johnson's writing as "Form'd on Brown's turgid Latin-English style" (quoted in Havenstein, *Democratizing Sir Thomas Browne*, 184).

standard seventeenth-century life was credited with miraculous or fabulous dimensions. As Lill points out, Johnson's response was to normalize this claim to the extent that he could—"there is, undoubtedly, a sense, in which all life is miraculous"—yet his conclusion that "the wonders probably were transacted in his own mind" relegates Browne's fancy to a source in self-love that reduces its conviction of an exceptional life to commonplace delusion.[23]

In the shape that Johnson bestowed on Browne's life, the sensible older man grew out of his abnormal, paradoxical, and fanciful youth. Indeed, Johnson's Browne is almost normalized in his all too human tendency to illustrate that grand gestures and aspirations prove quixotic:

> To speak inadequately of things really and naturally great, is a task not only difficult but disagreeable; because the writer is degraded in his own eyes by standing in comparison with his subject, to which he can hope to add nothing from his imagination: but it is a perpetual triumph of fancy to expand a scanty theme, to raise glittering ideas from obscure properties, and to produce to the world an object of wonder to which nature had contributed little. To this ambition, perhaps, we owe the Frogs of Homer, the Gnat and Bees of Virgil, the Butterfly of Spenser, the Shadow of Wowerus, and the Quincunx of Browne. (Roberts, ed., *Sir Thomas Browne's Christian Morals*, 23)

Here at least in chasing butterflies, Browne takes his place in the mock-history of great poets, not in the annals of irresponsible physicians. But readers, if not patients, must still beware, since "a reader, not watchful against the power of his infusions, would imagine that decussation was the great business of the world, and that nature and art had no other purpose than to exemplify and imitate a Quincunx" (24).

Johnson also generalizes the reasons for Browne's stylistic tendencies—the seventeenth century was an age in which the English language "was considered by every writer as a subject on which he might try his plastick skill, by moulding it according to his own fancy" (Roberts, 48). But it is the one other contemporary invoked for comparison by Johnson—Milton—that proves to rank among one of the most revealing observations in the biography. Like Latinate Milton, though both more heterogeneously and less disturbingly, Browne imported "a multitude of exotick words" and "a tissue of many languages" into the vernacular (48–9). It is at this point that Johnson chooses to concede Browne's exceptionality: "He must, however, be confessed to have augmented our philosophical diction; and in defence of his uncommon words and expressions, we must consider, that he had uncommon sentiments" (49). In unfolding his "uncommon sentiments," we are told, Browne innovated with an ardent language "by venturing to the utmost verge of propriety," taking "flights which would never have been reached, but by one who had very little fear of the shame of falling" (49). Moving quickly to a defense of Browne's piety, Johnson allows this Icarian image to stand without criticism. At the edge of propriety, Johnson suggests, Browne attempted to accomplish the most difficult of human tasks—to forge a place for human greatness that somehow remained within reach of the general human condition. For Johnson there is surely something genuinely

[23] Lill, "A Lesson in Futurity," 42, quoting *Rambler* 21.

heroic in this fearless, impassioned adventure. "He may, perhaps, in the ardour of his imagination, have hazarded an expression, which a mind intent upon faults may interpret into heresy," Johnson adds a little later, but in the context of the whole, Browne self-evidently deserved his place "among the most zealous Professors of Christianity." And though Johnson does not discuss *Christian Morals*, the work to which his biography serves as an entrée, it afforded Johnson's contemporaries with an extension of the *Religio* that accentuated how Browne's youthful exuberance had matured into a universal and sober vision of the human condition.

By the end of the eighteenth century, Browne was considered good matter for the education of the young: in June 1771, the *Gentleman's Magazine* recommended *Pseudodoxia Epidemica* for its potent capacity "to excite their curiosity, to put them upon thinking and enquiring, & to guard them against taking anything upon trust from opinion or authority."[24] Not long after this recommendation, Browne's reputation began to soar. "In the first half of the nineteenth century," Robin Robbins has noted, "appreciation of Browne's style and imagination reached its highest pitch since the seventeenth among readers and writers such as Lamb, Coleridge ('a brain with a twist'), Leigh Hunt, Hazlitt, De Quincey, Southey, and Carlyle, some praising quaint whimsy and fanciful humours, others finding depth of thought."[25] Yet in the first century after his death, Browne's readers struggled with an inwardly conflicted, and in some ways a more holistic, understanding of his life, mind and writings, that spoke powerfully of the palpable aftershocks of the very civil war through which Browne had lived. In 1748, then again in 1780, the *Biographia Britannica* passed along an appreciation from *A Century of Short Characters of Books and Authors* which encouraged readers to embrace Browne, extravagancies and all:

> The *Religio Medici* may pass for a treatise, on which it is extremely hard to pass any judgment. It is to weak heads, perhaps, a dangerous, to proper judges a most salutary counselor...It is a noble representation of human nature as it is, and who can be untouched at the sight of what so nearly concerns him? It is a brave attempt to bring down those subjects, which have been supposed to be superior to man's intellects, within the view of his reason; and though not near enough to acquaint him with their nature, yet within such a space as to delight him with their prospect. Who then that considers this, but must own an obligation to the author? If singularities, prejudices, extravagancies, wild excursions, and sometimes gloomy reflections, strike us, let us strictly examine whether the fault lies in us or in him; we ought not too readily to exalt our own, at the expence of his judgment. If we meet with strange thoughts, free remarks, disagreeable discoveries, let us bring them to the touchstone of truth, and remember, that though anatomies of human bodies are frequent, yet we are rarely called to the dissection of a human soul.[26]

Browne's heroism is considered a cause for celebration here, even if its Promethean temerity might seem to some timorous readers ill-advised. This "brave" adventure is not sanitized for sensible consumption, for it has to be said that Browne confronts

[24] H., "On Vulgar Errors," *The Gentleman's Magazine* 41 (1771), 251–2, at 251.

[25] Robin Robbins's entry on Sir Thomas Browne in *ODNB*.

[26] Andrew Kippis, *Biographia Britannica*, 2nd edn. (London: 1780), 628–9, in the notes. For information about earlier editions, see Donovan et al., *Sir Thomas Browne and Robert Burton*, 23.

us with a strange, even frightening imaginative world. Yet if we are ready to relegate his wild singularity to a realm outside the human, we are sorely mistaken. For whatever Browne's shocking impact on our "heads," the disturbance derives from the simple fact that we are unaccustomed to looking so intimately at our own inner selves. Browne's anatomy of the human is indeed a monumental effort to return our very own souls into the viewing range of our reason. Like Columbus, the apology continues, Browne brings us bizarre tales of a foreign realm which proves to be our very own earth at long last.

Whether or not Johnson was right to question the fabulous or miraculous character of Browne's life, the author of *A Century of Short Characters of Books and Authors* has decided that Browne was the most courageous and illuminating of humanity's heroes. In the nineteenth century, it seemed obvious to at least one reviewer of Wilkin's wonderful edition that Browne's "record is not in restless actions, but in adventurous and roving thoughts."[27] And in portraying Browne as a "humorist," sympathetic to, if also opinionated about all creation, Walter Pater recognized that to get Browne right, one had to start with the strange, vexed legacy of Origen's father kissing the breast of his sleeping child but find one's way into a love of the open air.[28]

In a copy of the 1658 double volume comprising *Hydriotaphia* and *The Garden of Cyrus*, a nineteenth-century reader transmitted the opinion expressed of Browne in *The Quarterly Review* that "There is perhaps no other writer of our own or of any other country whose intellect had so perfectly assimilated all its stores of learning. His feelings seem always to have ended in meditations; & his meditations on the other hand always brung with them a subdued but vivid feeling."[29] If by the early nineteenth century Browne's sensibility could thus be lauded as singularly admirable, in the eighteenth century lovers of *Religio Medici* could still capture how the lay theologian had decisively altered English religious and intellectual culture. In the manuscript of *Religio* that the Reverend T. Shrigley donated to Browne's own Pembroke College in 1783, an eighteenth-century hand, perhaps Shrigley's own, heralded the work as "The Inestimable Treasure," the phrase that back in the sixteenth century was commonly called upon to praise the Bible.[30] Browne's style in *Religio Medici* has been noted for its Biblical cadences; but the note in the Pembroke manuscript suggests much more—that Browne wrote a book that might heal the human spirit even more than those scriptures over which whole wars had been fought.[31]

[27] Sir Edward Bulwer Lytton, "Sir Thomas Browne's Work (a review of Wilkin's edition)," in the October 1836 *Edinburgh Review*, 1–35; at 4.

[28] Walter Pater, "Sir Thomas Browne," *Macmillan's Magazine* 54 (1886), 5–18.

[29] The copy of 1658 is in the Newberry Library, Ruggles 42; the reviewer is commencing an evaluation of two French works describing the cemeteries and catacombs of Paris; see *The Quarterly Review* 21 (April, 1819), 360.

[30] For this phrase and the Bible, see Femke Molecamp, "'Of the incomparable treasure of the Holy Scriptures': The Geneva Bible in the Early Modern Household," in Matthew Dimmock and Andrew Hadfield, eds., *Literature and Popular Culture in Early Modern England* (Burlington, VT: Ashgate, 2009), 121–36.

[31] For Browne and the Bible, see William Whallon, "Hebraic Synonymy in Sir Thomas Browne," *English Literary History* 28 (1961), 335–52; and Havenstein, *Democritizing Sir Thomas Browne*, 161–8.

Bibliography

MANUSCRIPTS

Archdiocesan Archives, Birmingham

Dodd MS Z5/2/35/53 (Charles Dodd's remarks on *Religio Medici*)

Archivio storico dell'Università, Padua

MS 29/30 (Matriculation records by nationality)
MS 241 (Cronaca del bidello generale artista Bernardo Muneghina, 1620–34)
MS 347/44 (Acts of the School of Medicine, 1631–34)
MS 465 (Matriculation records for divinity and medicine)
MS 680 (Acta universitatis artistarum, 1632–43)
MS 697 (Matricolazioni degli scolari artisti 1633)

Bodleian Library, Oxford

Additional B.82 (Thomas Lushington sermons)
Auct F.5.31 (medieval manuscripts donated by Thomas Clayton)
Bodl. 591 (medieval manuscripts donated by Thomas Clayton)
E.Mus 19 (manuscripts donated by Thomas Clayton)
Eng d 3615 (Thomas Hughes's commonplace book)
Eng th.f.14 (Thomas Lushington sermons)
Lister 3 (Lister family papers)
Malone 19 (Oxford poetic miscellany with Winchester and New College associations)
MS chronology of Oxford events in 1620s
OUA NEP supra/register N (Tomlins lectureship in anatomy, Oxford University)
OUA NEP/supra/register Q (Browne's certificate of incorporation)
OUA register of congregation, 1622–1630 (Browne's supplication for degrees)
OUA SP/2 (Oxford matriculation records and fines)
Rawlinson B.211(*The True Church, Further Vindicated in An Answere to A Book intituled Religio Medici. By An Authour in Distresse*)
Rawlinson D.62 (*Religio Medici*)
Rawlinson D.109 (Browne papers)
Rawlinson D.391 (Browne papers)
Rawlinson D.810 (eulogy for Thomas Clayton)
Rawlinson E.95 (notes on sermons of Thomas Lushington)
Rawlinson Letters D.58 (Browne papers)
Rembert Dodoens's *Herbal* (manuscript annotations; shelfmark 50.d.25)
Selden supra 81 (Degory Wheare letter to Thomas Clayton)
Tanner 73/1 (Henry Briggs letter to Samuel Ward)
Tanner 445 (*Repertorium*)
Tanner 466 (poems written by Winchester pupils on the occasion of the visit of Prince Charles)
Wood D.18 (William Knights scandal)

British Library, London
Additional MS 1756 (Sir Thomas Dutton in Ireland)
Additional MS 5233 (Browne papers)
Additional MS 19253 (The Letter Book of Philip Stanhope, Earl of Chesterfield, 1657–1712)
Additional MS 31021 (records pertaining to Waterhouse's workhouse in Halifax)
Additional MS 36988 (St Peter Mancroft records from the eighteenth century)
Additional MS Section B 27,448 (Paston papers)
Evelyn Collection MS 33 (commentary on Lucretius)
Lansdowne 489 (incomplete manuscript of *Religio Medici*)
Sloane MS 161 (diary of Thomas Gooch)
Sloane MS 175 (recipe book including some of Browne's recipes)
Sloane MS 496 (Henry Power, *Historia Physica Anatomica*, 1666)
Sloane 1378 (Henry Power papers)
Sloane 1393 (Henry Power papers)
Sloane 1827 (Browne papers)
Sloane 1833 (Browne papers)
Sloane 1838 (Browne papers, translation of Proclus's *Elementa Theologica*)
Sloane 1839 (Browne papers)
Sloane 1843 (Browne papers)
Sloane 1848 (Browne papers)
Sloane 1861 (Browne papers)
Sloane 1862 (Browne papers)
Sloane 1869 (Browne papers)
Sloane 1871 (Browne papers)
Sloane 1875 (Browne papers)
Sloane 1878 (Browne papers)
Sloane 1879 (Browne papers)
Sloane 1885 (Browne papers)
Sloane 1906 (Browne papers)
Sloane 1911–13 (Browne papers)
Sloane 4062 (Browne correspondence)
Sloane 4067 (Browne correspondence)
Sloane 4077 (Browne correspondence)

Cambridge University Library, Cambridge
Dd.2.34 (medical notebook)
Dd.2.41 (medical notebook)
Dd.3.10 (medical notebook)
Dd.3.21 (medical notebook)

Cardiff Central Library, Cardiff, Wales
MS 1.160 (Dean Christopher Wren's annotation copy of *Religio Medici*)

Cheshire and Chester Archives
Arderne Collection, ref. DAR/C/91/5 (property transactions pertaining to Browne and his uncle)

City Archives, Montpellier
MS GG 95 (Livre des comptes de l'Hopital St Eloi)

Corpus Christi College, Oxford
CCC MS 263 (Brian Twyne's seventeenth-century notes on anatomy)
CCC MS 288 (Lushington's recantation sermon)
CCC MS 301 (records of Oxford life in the 1620s)

Derbyshire Record Office
D231 M/E 507 (title deeds for Okeover family estates)
D231 M/T 407 (title deeds for Okeover family estates)

Ewelme Hospital Foundation, Oxfordshire
MS D.D. Ewelme d.9 (EA 3) (audits for the hospital)

Folger Shakespeare Library, Washington, DC
MS V.a. 344 (notebook of Sir John Cotton)

Lancashire Record Office
QSB/1/170/60 (Lancashire Courts of Quarter Sessions)
QSB/1/170/64 (Lancashire Courts of Quarter Sessions)
QSB/1/170/69 (Lancashire Courts of Quarter Sessions)

Lehigh University, Pennsylvania
Ref: SC S 828.3 B884r (*Religio Medici*)

Leiden City Archive
231/ONA293 no. 89/8-6-1624 (records pertaining to Richard Monck)

Leiden University, Universiteitsbibliotheek, Leiden, The Netherlands
ASF 9 (Volumina Inscriptionum)
ASF 260 (Acta Senatus Academici Rectore)

London Metropolitan Archives
CLA/002/01/1 (Common Serjeant's book 1586–1614)
P69/MIC4/B/005/MS02895/002 (church warden's records for St Michael le Querne)
P69/MIC4/D/008/MS00805 (deeds and leases from St Michael le Querne parish)
Repertories 31, 36, 40, 138 (Court of Aldermen, deliberations regarding the estate of Browne's father)

Memorial Library, University of Wisconsin, Madison: Daniel and Eleanor Albert Collection
Manuscript collection of writings/lectures from Montpellier medical faculty, including the longest work (90 leaves), a work on gynecology, "De virginum affectibus"; 20 leaves of George Scharpe's lecture "Tractatus de febre purpurata"; Ranchin's *De Morbis ac symptomatis acutissmis*

Mercers' Hall, London
Acts of Court 1595–1629, Mercers' Hall, London
List of Members of the Mercers' Company from 1347 (1915, typescript, Mercers' Hall)

Millennium Library, Norfolk Heritage Centre, Norwich
Copy of Paris edition of Latin *Religio Medici* with "hæreticus" written on front, Colman Collection
Corrected copy of Browne's *Pseudodoxia Epidemica/Religio Medici* (1672), Colman Collection
John Evelyn's copy of *Certain Miscellany Tracts,* Colman Collection

Montpellier Medical School, France
MS 20 (Matricules)
MS S 10 (Liber congregationum)

National Archives, Kew
ADM 7/778 (records of the wounded in the Battle of the Texel, 1673)
ADM 33/97 (records of naval officers and soldiers on the *St George,* Third Dutch War)
Papers of the Privy Council
SP 14 (State Papers Domestic, James I)
SP 63 (State Papers Ireland, Elizabeth I to George III)

Newberry Library, Chicago
MS Case G.35 (anonymous seventeenth-century travel guide to Italy)
Ruggles 42 (annotated copy of Browne, *Hydriotaphia/Garden of Cyrus,* 1658)

New College, Oxford
1091 (William Laud correspondence, visitation of Winchester College)
1094 (scrutiny papers, Winchester College elections)

Norfolk Record Office, Norwich
Archdeacon's transcriptions of parish records
Assembly Book, 1642–68
Cathedral financial records of the Chapter
Extracts from the Court Books of the City of Norwich, 1666–88
Microfilm parish registers for Burlingham St Peter; St George Tombland; St Peter Parmentergate; St Michael at Plea
NCR Case 16b (Norwich policies on medical services to the poor)
Norfolk and Norwich Archaeological Society Collection, C3/7 (Browne letter to Susan Hare)
NRO BL/Y/1/21 (Paston papers)
NRO B/Y/2/27 (Paston papers)
NRO BL/Y/2/48 (Paston papers)
NRO BL/Y/2/57 (Paston papers)
NRO BL/Y/2/60 (Paston papers)
NRO BL/Y/2/68 (Paston Papers)
NRO C3/2/3/5/13 (autograph letter from Browne to Thomas Knyvett)
NRO CON 21, 1663–66 (Browne's certificate for a patient)
NRO DCN 24/3 (the chapter book of Norwich Cathedral)
NRO DCN 48/21/152 (Browne's lease of a meadow)

NRO DCN 107/3 (reports of civil war Norwich)
NRO KNY 750–84 372x5 (Knyvett family papers)
NRO LEST P/10 (L'Estrange family papers)
NRO LEST P/12 (L'Estrange family papers)
NRO LEST P/20 (L'Estrange family papers)
NRO LEST supp 25ii/1/25A–25L (L'Estrange family papers)
NRO MC 107/1 (letter from William Heveningham to his mother)
NRO MC 1628/1 1828X1 (travel journal of Willem Shellinks)
NRO MC 2577/2/6 984x6 (church warden records, St Peter Mancroft)
NRO MC 2577/6/9/1–3 984x7 (Browne as trustee for property transaction)
NRO MF RO 72/3 (Norwich city's use of Browne's medical services)
NRO MF RO 81/4, 1654–1666 (Norwich policies on the poor)
NRO MS 4504 55x7 (passages to be added to 1643 *Religio Medici*, with prefatory matter by A. B. and Browne)
NRO MS 19926 (deed between Justinian Lewin and Edward Mileham)
NRO MS 78/1 (Benjamin Mackerell, *History of the City of Norwich Both Ancient and Modern*, typescript of manuscript history from 1737)
NRO MS 21267 (*Religio Medici*)
NRO MS 21268 T134D (*Religio Medici*)
NRO MS 21270 (*Repertorium*)
NRO MS KIM 9/3 (Wodehouse family papers)
NRO MS Y/L 13/17 (letter by George Harper concerning Browne's medical services)
NRO NCR Case 13a (Norwich hearth tax records)
NRO NCR 13c/2/2 (Solemn League and Covenant in Norwich)
NRO NCR Case 20c (assessments poor rates)
NRO NCR Case 71c (Norwich collections for the forces of Sir Thomas Fairfax)
NRO PD 26/71 (St Peter Mancroft records)
NRO PD 26/84(s) (Browne's payments for reading of prayers)
NRO PD 26/308 (St Peter Mancroft records)
NRO PD 26/725 (St Peter Mancroft, churchwarden accounts)
NRO Rye MS 9/1 (antiquarian study of Norwich market)
NRO Rye 72/284 (letters to and from Thomas Knyvett)
NRO WKC 7/6/1–77 404x1 (Hobart family letters)

Osler Medical Library, Montreal
Niche 1, B884r 1600z (*Religio Medici*)

Oxfordshire Record Office
Dash/IX/i/19 (name index)

Pembroke College, Oxford
Manuscript copy of *Religio Medici*
63/1/1 (letter of September 11, 1661 from Browne to Dugdale, with thanks for the latter's gift of the second volume of *Monasticon Anglicanum*)

Prerogative Court of the Archbishop of Canterbury, London
PROB 11/379 (will of Dorothy Browne, March 17, 1685)
PROB 11/550 (will of Thomas Tenison, archbishop of Canterbury, 23 January 1716)
PROB 11/679 (will of Elizabeth Lyttelton, September 3, 1736)

Princeton University, Princeton, NJ
Taylor Collection RTC01 (autograph letter from Browne to Thomas Knyvett)

Queen's College, Oxford
QC MS 390 (Thomas Crosfield's diary)

Royal College of Physicians, London
MS-COLEG/208/1 (the *Consilia medica* of George Colebrook)

Royal Library, Copenhagen, Denmark
GKS 218 and 219 folio (trans. of *Pseudodoxia Epidemica* into Danish by Gabriel Acheleye Knudsen, 1652)

Uppsala University, Uppsala, Sweden
Waller MSS gb-0033 (Browne's holograph revision of a piece of *Christian Morals*)
Waller MSS gb-00334 (Browne's holograph revision of a piece of *Christian Morals*)

Yale University, Beinecke Library, New Haven, CT
OSB Shelves B1115 (satirical verses possibly by Edward Browne)

Printed

Aberth, John. *The First Horseman: Disease in Human History*. Upper Saddle River, NJ: Prentice Hall, 2007.

Abraham, Lyndy, ed. *Arthur Dee's Fasciculus Chemicus*. Trans. Elias Ashmole. New York: Garland, 1997.

Abrenethy, Adam. *Quæstiones IV Cardinales*. Montpellier, 1609.

Achermann, Erich. "Order in the Vortex: Christian Knorr von Rosenroth as Compiler and Translator of Thomas Browne, Jean d'Espagnet, Henry More, Gottfried Wilhelm Leibniz and Antoine le Grand." Trans. Kathryn Murphy and Doris Einsiedel. In Murphy and Todd, eds. "*A man very well studyed*." 247–72.

Addison, Joseph. *The Works of the Right Honourable Joseph Addison*. Notes by Richard Hurd. 6 vols. London: Bohn, 1854–56.

An Address from the Gentry of Norfolk and Norwich to General Monck in 1660: Facsimile of a Manuscript in the Norwich Public Library. Intro. Hamon Le Strange, notes by Walter Rye. Norwich: Jarrold & Sons, 1913.

Addy, J. "The Uncontrollable and Ungovernable Parish of Halifax in the Seventeenth Century." *Transactions of the Halifax Antiquarian Society* (1993), 36–42.

Ainsworth, Henry. *The Communion of Saincts*. 1607.

Allen, D. E. "Christopher Merrett." *ODNB*.

Allen, Don Cameron. *The Star-Crossed Renaissance: The Quarrel about Astrology and Its Influence in England*. Durham, NC: Duke University Press, 1941.

Allen, Phyllis. "Scientific Studies in the English Universities of the Seventeenth Century." *Journal of the History of Ideas* 10 (1949), 219–53.

Alpers, Svetlana. *The Art of Describing: Dutch Art in the Seventeenth Century*. Chicago: University of Chicago Press, 1983.

Anatole, Christian, ed. *Pèire Godolin 1580–1649: Actes du Colloque international Université de Toulouse-Le Mirail, 8–10 mai 1980*. Toulouse: Service des publications de l'Université, 1983.

Anderson, R. C., ed. *Journals and Narratives of the Third Dutch War*. London: Naval Records Society, 1946.

Andrewes, Lancelot. *Works of Lancelot Andrewes*. 11 vols. Oxford: John Henry Parker, 1854; reprinted in New York: AMS, 1967.

Anon. "The Life of Sir Thomas Browne, Kt." In Browne. *Posthumous Works of Sir Thomas Browne* (1712), i–xxiii.

Anselment, Raymond. "Smallpox in Seventeenth-Century English Literature: Reality and the Metamorphosis of Wit." *Medical History* 33 (1989), 72–95.

Appleby, John H. "Arthur Dee." *ODNB*.

——"Arthur Dee and Johannes Bánfi Hunyades." *Ambix* 24 (1977), 96–109.

——"Dr Arthur Dee: Merchant and Litigant." *Slavonic and East European Review* 57 (1979), 32–55.

——"Some of Arthur Dee's Associations before Visiting Russia Clarified." *Ambix* 26 (1979), 1–15.

Arber, Edward. *The Story of the Pilgrim Fathers, 1606–1623 A. D.: As Told by Themselves, Their Friends, and Their Enemies*. Boston: Houghton, Mifflin, 1897.

Archer, Ian. "Material Londoners?" In Orlin, ed. *Material London*, 179–87.

——*The Pursuit of Stability: Social Relations in Elizabethan London*. Cambridge: Cambridge University Press, 1991.

Aristotle. *The Complete Works of Aristotle*. Ed. Jonathan Barnes. 2 vols. Princeton, NJ: Princeton University Press, 1984.

Astruc, Jean. *Mémoires pour server a l'Histoire de Montpellier*. Paris, 1767.

Atherton, Henry. *The Christian Physician*. 1683.

Atherton, Ian. "Edward Reynolds." *ODNB*.

——et al., eds. *Norwich Cathedral: Church, City and Diocese, 1096–1996*. London: Hambledon, 1996.

——and Victor Morgan. "Revolution and Retrenchment: The Cathedral, 1630–1720." In Atherton et al., eds. *Norwich Cathedral*. 540–75.

Atkinson, Tom. *Elizabethan Winchester*. London: Faber and Faber, 1963.

Aubrey, John. *Brief Lives*. Ed. Andrew Clark. 2 vols. Oxford: Clarendon Press, 1898.

——*Natural History of Wiltshire*. Intro. K. G. Ponting. Newton Abbot: David & Charles Imprints, 1969.

Aylmer, G. E. "Seventeenth-Century Wykehamists." In Roger Custance, ed. *Winchester College: Sixth-Centenary Essays*. Oxford: Oxford University Press, 1982. 281–311.

Baldwin, T. W. *William Shakspere's Small Latine & Lesse Greeke*. 2 vols. Urbana: University of Illinois Press, 1944.

Banga, J. *Geschiedenis van de Geneeskunde... in Nederland*. Leeuwarden: W. Eekhoff, 1868.

Bangs, J. D., ed. and intro. *The Auction Catalogue of the Library of Hugh Goodyear, English Reformed Minister at Leiden*. Utrecht: HES Publishers, 1985.

Barbato, Bartolomeo. *Il Contagio di Padova nell'Anno M.DC.XXXI*. Rovigo, 1640.

Barbour, Reid. "Dean Wren's *Religio Medici*: Reading in Civil War England." *Huntington Library Quarterly* 73 (2010), 263–72.

——"The Hieroglyphics of Skin." In Barbour and Preston, eds. *Thomas Browne: The World Proposed*. 279–95.

——*Literature and Religious Culture in Seventeenth-Century England*. Cambridge: Cambridge University Press, 2001.

——"Thomas Browne's *A Letter to a Friend* and the Semiotics of Disease." *Renaissance Studies* 24 (2010), 407–19.

——"Thomas Browne, the Quakers, and a Letter from a Judicious Friend." In Anne Dunan-Page and Clotilde Prunier, eds. *Debating the Faith: Religion and Letter Writing in Great Britain, 1550–1800*. Dordrect: Springer, 2013. 37–48.

Barbour, Reid. "The Topic of Sir Thomas Browne's Dissertation." *Notes & Queries*, 54 (2007), 38–9.
——and Claire Preston, eds. and intro. *Sir Thomas Browne: The World Proposed.* New York: Oxford University Press, 2008.
Barclay, Alexander. *Shepheards Kalender.* 1656.
Barge, J. A. J. *De Oudste Inventaris der Oudste Academische Anatomie in Nederland.* Leiden: H. E. Stenfert Kroese, 1934.
Bargrave, Robert. *The Travel Diary of Robert Bargrave, Levant Merchant (1647–1656).* Ed. Michael G. Brennan. London: The Hakluyt Society, 1999.
Barnes, W. H. "Browne's *Hydriotaphia* with a Reference to Adipocere." *Isis* 20 (1933), 337–43.
Barrett, Robert W., Jr., *Against All England: Regional Identity and Cheshire Writing, 1195–1656.* Notre Dame, IN: University of Notre Dame Press, 2009.
Barringer, Christopher. "The Changing Face of Norwich." In Rawcliffe and Wilson, eds. *Norwich since 1550.* 1–34.
Bartholin, Caspar. *De studio medico inchoando, continuando et absolvendo consilium breve atque extemporaneum.* Hafniae, 1628.
Bartholin, Thomas. *De peregrinatione medica/On Medical Travel.* Trans. Charles D. O'Malley. Lawrence: University of Kansas Libraries, 1961.
Baskerville, Thomas. "Account of Oxford." Ed. Humphrey Baskerville. *Collectanea*, 4th series. Oxford: Oxford Historical Society, 1905.
Batty Shaw, Anthony. *Norfolk & Norwich Medicine: A Retrospect.* Norwich: Norwich Medico-Chirurgical Society, 1992.
——"The Norwich School of Lithotomy." *Medical History* 14 (1970), 221–59.
——*Sir Thomas Browne of Norwich.* Norwich: Jarrold & Sons, 1982.
——"Sir Thomas Browne's Meadow." *Notes and Queries* 216 (1971), 295–99.
Baumel, Jean. *Montpellier au Cours des XVIe et XVIIe Siècles: Les Guerres de Religion, 1510–1685.* Montpellier: Causse et la Grande Revue, 1976.
Bavinck, H. ed. *Synopsis Purioris Theologiae.* Leiden: Didericum Donner, 1881.
Beecheno, F. R. "The First Residence of Sir Thomas Browne in Norwich." *Eastern Daily Press* (Norwich) February 20, 1912, 210.
Beecheno. F. R., ed. *The Norwich Subscription for the Regaining of Newcastle, 1643.* In *Norfolk and Norwich Archaeological Society* 18 (1913), 149–60.
Beier, Lucinda McCray. *Sufferers & Healers: The Experience of Illness in Seventeenth-Century England.* New York: Routledge & Kegan Paul, 1987.
Beik, William. *Absolutism and Society in Seventeenth-Century France: State Power and Provincial Aristocracy in Languedoc.* Cambridge: Cambridge University Press, 1985.
Bénézet, Jean-Pierre. "La Thériaque de Montpellier." In Rioux, ed. *Le Jardin des Plantes de Montpellier.* 143–7.
Bentley, William, and Samuel Midgley. *The History of the Town and Parish of Halifax.* 1789.
Berensmeyer, Ingo. "Rhetoric, Religion and Politics in Sir Thomas Browne's *Religio Medici.*" *Studies in English Literature* 46 (2006), 113–32.
Bernard, Edward. *Catalogus Librorum MSS. Angliae & Hiberniae.* Oxford, 1697.
Berry, André. *Anthologie de la poésie occitane.* Paris: Stock, 1961.
Bertolli, Franco, and Umberto Colombo. *La Peste del 1630 a Busto Arsizio.* Busto Arsizio, Bramante Editrice, 1999.
Beukers, Harm. "Clinical Teaching in Leiden from Its Beginning until the End of the Eighteenth Century." In H. Beukers and J. Moll, eds. *Clinical Teaching, Past and Present.* Amsterdam: Rodopi, 1989. 139–52.
——"Studying Medicine in Leiden in the 1630s." In Murphy and Todd, eds. "*A man very well studyed.*" 49–64.

Biddle, Martin. "The Bishop of Winchester and the Foundation of the Order of the Garter." In Martin Biddle et al. *King Arthur's Round Table: An Archaeological Investigation.* Woodbridge, Suffolk: Boydell Press, 2000. 513–18.

Biggs, Noah. *Matæotechnia Medicinæ Praxeos.* 1651.

Bingham, C. W., ed. *Private Memoirs of John Potenger.* London: Hamilton Adams, 1841.

Birch, Thomas. *The History of the Royal Society.* 4 vols. London, 1756–57.

Birken, William. "The Social Problem of the English Physician in the Early Seventeenth Century." *Medical History* 31 (1987), 201–16.

Bloch, Marc. *The Royal Touch: Sacred Monarchy and Scrofula in England and France.* Trans. J. E. Anderson. London: Routledge & Kegan Paul, 1973, first published in French, 1961.

Blomefield, Francis. *An Essay Towards a Topographical History of the County of Norfolk.* 11 vols. London, 1805–1810.

Blount, Charles. *The Oracles of Reason.* Facsimile edition intro. John Valdimir Price. London: Routledge/Thoemmes, 1995.

Blount, Thomas. *Glossographia: or a Dictionary Interpreting All Such Hard Words.... now used in our refined English Tongue.* 1661.

Blount, Sir Thomas Pope. *A Natural History.* 1693.

Bonnet, Hubert. "Pierre de Belleval et sa Dynastie." In Rioux, ed. *Le Jardin des Plantes de Montpellier.* 25–33.

Borgherini-Scarabellin, M. "La Vita Privata a Padova nel secolo XVII." *R. Deputazione veneta di storia patria, Miscellanea*, 3rd series, vol. 12, 1917.

Bouwsma, William J. *Venice and the Defense of Republican Liberty: Renaissance Values in the Age of the Counter Reformation.* Berkeley: University of California Press, 1968.

Boyer, Allen. *Sir Edward Coke and the Elizabethan Age.* Stanford, CA: Stanford University Press, 2003.

Boyle, Robert. *Certain Physiological Essays.* 1661.

Brady, Philip. "'Nor Let the Hard Words Fright Yee'—on the Fearless Translator Christian Knorr von Rosenroth." *German Life and Letters* 47 (1994), 233–41.

Bray, Alan. *The Friend.* Chicago: University of Chicago Press, 2003.

Brennan, Michael, ed. *The Origins of the Grand Tour: The Travels of Robert Montague, Lord Mandeville, 1649–1654; William Hammond, 1655–1658; Banaster Maynard, 1660–1663.* London: The Hakluyt Society, 2004.

Brenner, Kurt. *Montpellier.* Trans. Phillp Mattson. Heidelberg: HVA, 1990.

Brenner, Robert. *Merchants and Revolution: Commercial Change, Political Conflict, and London's Overseas Traders, 1550–1653.* Princeton, NJ: Princeton University Press, 1993.

Brereton, William. "Travels in Holland, the United Provicnes, England, Scotland and Ireland M.DC.XXXIV–M.DC.XXXV." Ed. Edward Hawkins. In *Remains Historical & Literary... of Lancaster and Chester.* Chetham Society, 1844.

Bridgewater, Benjamin, and John Dunton. *Religio Bibliopolæ in Imitation of Dr. Browns Religio Medici.* 1691.

Briggs, Robin. *Early Modern France 1560–1715.* Oxford: Oxford University Press, 1977.

Broadway, Jan. *"No historie so meete": Gentry Culture and the Development of Local History in Elizabethan and Early Stuart England.* Manchester: Manchester University Press, 2006.

Brockliss, L. "Seeing and Believing: Contrasting Attitudes towards Observational Autonomy among French Galenists in the First Half of the Seventeenth Century." In W. F. Bynum and Roy Porter, eds. *Medicine and the Five Senses.* New York: Cambridge University Press, 1993. 63–84.

Brosse, Guy de la. *Description du Jardin Royal des Plantes medecinales.* Paris, 1636.

Brown, Horatio. *Inglesi e Scozzesi all'Università di Padova dall'anno 1618 sino al 1765.* Venice: C. Ferrari, 1921.

Browne, Edward. *An Account of Several Travels.* 1677.

——*A Brief Account of some Travels in Divers Parts of Europe.* 1685.

——*A brief account of some travels in Hungaria, Servia, Bulgaria, Macedonia, Thessaly, Austria, Styria, Carinthia, Carniola, and Friuli.* 1673.

——"Journal of a Visit to Paris in the Year 1664." Ed. Geoffrey Keynes. *Saint Bartholomew's Hospital Reports* 56 (1923), 1–34.

Browne, John. *Adenochoiradelogia: Or, an Anatomick-Chirurgical Treatise of Glandules & Strumaes, Or Kings-Evil-Swellings. Together with the Royal gift of Healing, or Cure thereof by Contact or Imposition of Hands, performed for above 640 Years by our Kings of England.* 1684.

Browne, Thomas, Sir. *Certain Miscellany Tracts.* 1683.

——*Christian Morals.* Ed. John Jeffery. 1716.

——*Christian Morals.* With a life and notes by Samuel Johnson. 1756.

——*Hydriotaphia Urne-Buriall and The Garden of Cyrus.* 1658.

——*A Letter to a Friend.* 1690.

——*Posthumous Works.* 1712.

——*Pseudodoxia Epidemica.* 1646.

——*Pseudodoxia Epidemica.* 1650.

——*Pseudodoxia Epidemica.* 1658.

——*Pseudodoxia Epidemica.* With *Hydriotaphia* and *Garden of Cyrus.* 1669.

——*Pseudodoxia Epidemica... Together with Religio Medici.* 1672.

——*Religio Medici.* 1642a.

——*Religio Medici.* 1642b.

——*Religio Medici.* 1643.

——*Religio Medici.* Latin edition. Trans. John Merryweather. Leiden, 1644.

——*Religio Medici.* Latin edition. Trans. John Merryweather. With new preface by a Catholic. Paris, 1644.

——*Religio Medici.* Latin edition. With notes by Levin Nicolas von Moltke of Mecklenburg-Schwerin. 1652.

——*Religio Medici.* With annotations by Thomas Keck. 1656.

——*Religio Medici.* 1659.

——*Religio Medici, Dat is: Noodwendige beschryvinge van Mr. Thomas Browne.* Dutch edition. Trans. Abraham van Berckel. 1665.

——*La Religion du Medecin: C'est à dire: Description necessaire par Thomas Brown, Medecin renommé à Norwich; touchant son Opinion accordante avec le pur service Divin d'Angleterre.* French edition. 1668.

——*Religio Medici.* 1669.

——*Religio Medici.* With *Pseudodoxia Epidemica.* 1672.

——*Religio Medici.* 1678.

——*Religio Medici.* 1682.

——*Religio Medici: Or, The Christian Religion, As Professed by a Physician.* 1736.

——*The Works of the Learned Sir Thomas Browne.* 1686.

Buddeus, Johannes Franciscus. *Theses Theologicae de Atheismo et Svperstitione.* Utrecht, 1737.

Bullard, Rebecca. "'A bright Coelestiall Mind': A New Set of Writings by Lady Dorothy Browne." *Huntington Library Quarterly* 71 (2010), 99–122.

Burke, Peter. *The Historical Anthropology of Early Modern Italy: Essays on Perception and Communication.* New York: Cambridge University Press, 1987.

—— *Venice and Amsterdam: A Study of Seventeenth-Century Élites.* London: Temple Smith, 1974.

Burke, Victoria. "Contexts for Women's Manuscript Miscellanies: The Case of Elizabeth Lyttleton and Sir Thomas Browne." *The Yearbook of English Studies* 33 (2003), 316–28.

Burnette, Arianne. "Joan Carlile." *ODNB.*

Burton, Robert. *The Anatomy of Melancholy.* Ed. Floyd Dell and Paul Jordan-Smith. New York: Tudor, 1927.

Butler, Samuel. *Hudibras.* Ed. John Wilders. Oxford: Clarendon Press, 1967.

Butlin, R. A. "Land and People, c. 1600." In T. M. Moody et al., eds. *A New History of Ireland, III: Early Modern Ireland, 1534–1691.* Oxford: Clarendon Press, 1976. 142–7.

Bylebyl, Jerome J. "Commentary on Loris Premuda's Influence of the Nineteenth-Century Vienna School on Italian Medicine: The Roles of Padua and Trieste." In Lloyd G. Stevenson, ed. *A Celebration of Medical History.* Baltimore, MD: Johns Hopkins University Press, 1981. 200–11.

—— "The School of Padua: Humanistic Medicine in the Sixteenth Century." In Charles Webster, ed. *Health, Medicine and Mortality in the Sixteenth Century.* Cambridge: Cambridge University Press, 1979. 335–70.

Calendar of State Papers Domestic, of the Reign of Charles I. Ed. John Bruce et al. 23 vols. London, 1858–97.

Calendar of State Papers Domestic, of the Reign of James I. Ed. Mary Anne Everett Green. 4 vols. London, 1857–59.

Calendar of the State Papers Relating to Ireland . . . 1625–1632. Ed. Robert Pentland Mahaffy. London: Stationery Office, 1900.

Calimani, Riccardo. *The Ghetto of Venice.* Trans. Katherine Silberblatt Wolfthal. New York: M. Evans, 1987.

Calvi, Giulia. *Histories of a Plague Year: The Social and the Imaginary in Baroque Florence.* Trans. Dario Biocca and Bryant T. Ragan, Jr. Berkeley: University of California Press, 1989.

Calvin, John. *Institutes of the Christian Religion.* Ed. John T. McNeill, trans. Ford Lewis Battles. 2 vols. Philadelphia: Westminster Press, 1960.

Camdeni Insignia. 1624.

Campbell, Gordon, and Thomas N. Corns. *John Milton: Life, Work, and Thought.* Oxford: Oxford University Press, 2008.

Carlton, Charles. *The Court of Orphans.* Leicester: Leicester University Press, 1974.

Carmichael, Ann G., and Arthur M. Silverstein, "Smallpox in Europe before the Seventeenth Century: Virulent Killer or Benign Disease?" *Journal of the History of Medicine and Allied Sciences,* 42 (1987) 147–68.

Carpenter, Nathanael. *Achitophel, or, the picture of a wicked politician.* 1629.

—— *Philosophia libera, triplici exercitationum decade proposita.* 1621.

Carter, E. H. *The Norwich Subscription Books: A Study of the Subscription Books of the Diocese of Norwich 1637–1800.* New York: Thomas Nelson & Sons, 1937.

Carter, John. "Sir Thomas Browne's Autograph Corrections." *The Library,* 4th series, 19 (1938/9), 492–3.

Carter, John, ed. *Urne-Buriall and The Garden of Cyrus.* London: Cassell & Co, 1932.

Castiglioni, Arturo. "The Medical School at Padua and the Renaissance of Medicine." *Annals of Medical History,* n.s., 7 (1935), 214–27.

Catel, Guillaume. *Mémoires de l'histoire du Languedoc curieusement et fidèlement recueillis de divers auteurs.* Toulouse, 1633.

Cawley, Robert Ralston, and George Yost. *Studies in Sir Thomas Browne.* Eugene: University of Oregon Press, 1965.

Cebes his Table. Trans. John Healey. 1616.

Chadwick, Henry. *Boethius: The Consolations of Music, Logic, Theology, and Philosophy.* Oxford: Clarendon Press, 1981.

Chalmers, Gordon Keith. "Effluvia, The History of a Metaphor." *PMLA* 52 (1937), 1031–50.

——"The Lodestone and the Understanding of Matter in Seventeenth-Century England." *Philosophy of Science* 4 (1937), 75–95.

——"Thomas Browne, True Scientist." *Osiris* 2 (1936), 28–79.

——"Three Terms of the Corpuscularian Philosophy." *Modern Philology* 33 (1935–36), 243–60.

Chambers, David, and Brian Pullan, eds. *Venice: A Documentary History, 1450–1630.* Toronto: University of Toronto Press, 2001.

Chaplin, Arnold. "A History of Medical Education in the Universities of Oxford and Cambridge, 1500–1850." *Proceedings of the Royal Society of Medicine* 12 supplement (1920), 83–107.

Charleton, Walter. *The Immortality of the Human Soul.* Intro. J. M. Armistead. New York: AMS Press, 1985.

——*A Ternary of Paradoxes.* 1650.

Chevalier, A. G. "Medical Teaching at Montpellier." *Ciba Symposia* 2 (1940), 408–11.

Cheynell, Francis. *The Man of Honour, Described in a Sermon, Preached before the Lords of Parliament, In the Abbey Church at Westminster, March 26,1645.* 1645.

Cholvy, Gérard, ed. *Historie de Montpellier.* Toulouse: Privat, 1984.

Cipolla, Carlo M. *Faith, Reason, and the Plague in Seventeenth-Century Tuscany.* Trans. Muriel Kittel. Ithaca, NY: Cornell University Press, 1979.

——*Fighting the Plague in Seventeenth-Century Italy.* Madison: University of Wisconsin Press, 1981.

Ciscato, Antonio. *Gli Ebrei in Padova (1300–1800).* Bologna: Forni, 1967.

Clark, Donald Lemen. *John Milton at St Paul's School: A Study of Ancient Rhetoric in English Renaissance Education.* New York: Columbia University Press, 1948.

Clark, Sir George. *A History of the Royal College of Physicians of London.* 3 vols. Oxford: Clarendon Press, 1964.

Clark, Stuart. *Thinking with Demons: The Idea of Witchcraft in Early Modern Europe.* Oxford: Oxford University Press, 1997.

Clarke, A. W. Hughes, and Arthur Campling, eds. *The Visitation of Norfolk Anno Domini 1664 Made by Sir Edward Bysshe.* Norwich: Norfolk Record Society, 1934.

Clay, J. W. "Dr Henry Power, of New Hall, F.R.S." *Transactions of the Halifax Antiquarian Society* 1917, 1–28.

Cliffe, J. T. *The Yorkshire Gentry: From the Reformation to the Civil War.* London: Athlone Press, 1969.

Cochrane, Eric. "The Renaissance Academies in their Italian and European Setting." In *The Fairest Flower: The Emergence of Linguistic National Consciousness in Renaissance Europe.* Florence: Firenze Presso l'Accademia, 1985. 21–40.

Cogswell, Thomas. *The Blessed Revolution: English Politics and the Coming of War, 1621–24.* New York: Cambridge University Press, 1989.

Colie, Rosalie L. "Dean Wren's Marginalia and Early Science at Oxford." *The Bodleian Library Record* 6 (1960), 541–51.

——"Sir Thomas Browne's 'Entertainement' in XVIIth Century Holland." *Neophilologus* 36 (1952), 162–71.

A Collection of Modern Relations of Matter of Fact Concerning Witches & Witchcraft upon the Persons of People. 1693.

Collinges, John. *Provocator Provocatus.* 1654.

Collop, John. *The Poems of John Collop.* Ed. Conrad Hilberry. Madison: University of Wisconsin Press, 1962.

Colón, A. R. *Nurturing Children: A History of Pediatrics.* Westport, CT: Greenwood Press, 1999.

Colvin, Howard. "Inigo Jones and the Church of St Michael le Querne." *The London Journal* 12 (1986), 36–9.

Conti, Brooke. "*Religio Medici*'s Profession of Faith." In Barbour and Preston, eds. *Sir Thomas Browne: The World Proposed.* 149–67.

Cook, A. K. *About Winchester College, To Which is Prefixed "De Collegio Wintoniensi" by Robert Mathew.* London: Macmillan, 1917.

Cook, Harold J. *The Decline of the Old Medical Regime in Stuart London.* Ithaca, NY: Cornell University Press, 1986.

——*Matters of Exchange: Commerce, Medicine, and Science in the Dutch Golden Age.* New Haven, CT: Yale University Press, 2007.

—— *Trials of an Ordinary Doctor: Joannes Groenevelt in Seventeenth-Century London.* Baltimore, MD: Johns Hopkins University Press, 1994.

Corbett, Richard. *Poems of Richard Corbett.* Ed. J. A. W. Bennett and H. R. Trevor-Roper. Oxford: Clarendon Press, 1955.

Corfield, Penelope. "A Provincial Capital in the Late Seventeenth-Century: The Case of Norwich." In Peter Clark and Paul Slack, eds. *Crisis and Order in English Towns, 1500–1700: Essays in Urban History.* London: Routledge & Kegan Paul, 1972. 263–310.

Corie, Thomas. *Correspondence of Thomas Corie, Town Clerk of Norwich, 1664–1687.* Ed. Robert H. Hill. Norwich: Norwich Record Society, 1956.

Cornford, Margaret E. *Paul's Cross: A History.* London: SPCK, 1910.

Cornish, Vaughan. *The Churchyard Yew and Immortality.* London: Frederick Muller, 1946.

Cozens-Hardy, Basil, and Ernest A. Kent, *The Mayors of Norwich 1403 to 1835 being Biographical Notes on the Mayors of the Old Corporation.* Norwich: Jarrold, 1938.

Crakanthorpe, Richard. *Introductio in metaphysicam.* 1619.

Crane, Mary Thomas. *Framing Authority: Sayings, Self, and Society in Sixteenth-Century England.* Princeton, NJ: Princeton University Press, 1993.

Craven, Wayne. "John Wollaston: His Career in England and New York City." *American Art Journal* 7 (1975), 19–31.

Crawfurd, Raymond. *The King's Evil.* Oxford: Clarendon Press, 1911.

Creighton, Charles. *A History of Epidemics in Britain.* 2 vols. London: Frank Cass, 1965.

Cremonini, Cesare. *De calido innato.* Leiden, 1634.

Crossley, A. "Early Modern Oxford." In Alan Crossley, ed. *The Victoria History of the County of Oxford. Volume IV: The City of Oxford.* Oxford: Oxford University Press, 1979.

Crossley, E. W. *The Monumental and Other Inscriptions in Halifax Parish Church.* Leeds: John Whitehead, 1909.

Cullen, L. M. *The Emergence of Modern Ireland: 1600–1900.* New York: Holmes & Meier, 1981.

Cunningham, Andrew. "Sir Thomas Browne and *Religio Medici*: Reason, Nature and Religion." In Ole Peter Grell and Andrew Cunningham, eds. *Religio Medici: Medicine and Religion in Seventeenth-Century England.* Aldershot: Ashgate, 1996. 12–61.

Curry, Patrick. "John Heydon." *ODNB.*

Curtis, Mark H. *Oxford and Cambridge in Transition, 1558–1642: An Essay on Changing Relations between the English Universities and English Society.* Oxford: Clarendon Press, 1959.

Custance, Roger, ed. *Winchester College: Sixth-Centenary Essays.* Oxford: Oxford University Press, 1982.

D. C. "Sir Thomas Brown." *European Magazine* 40 (1801), 89–90.

D'Aigrefeuille, Charles. *Histoire de la Ville de Montpellier depuis son origine jusqu'à notre temps.* 4 vols. Marseille: Laffitte Reprints, 1976.

Dale, Bryan. "Shibden Dale and Sir Thomas Browne's *Religio Medici*." *Bradford Antiquary* 1 (1896), 45–57.

Dandy, J. E., ed. *The Sloane Herbarium.* London: British Museum, 1958.

Daniel, George. *The Selected Poems of George Daniel of Beswick, 1616–1657.* Ed. Thomas B. Stroup. Lexington: University of Kentucky Press, 1959.

Darley, Gillian. *John Evelyn: Living for Ingenuity.* New Haven, CT: Yale University Press, 2006.

Daston, Lorraine, and Katharine Park. *Wonders and the Order of Nature, 1150–1750.* New York: Zone Books, 1998.

Datta, Kitty Scoular. "Sir Thomas Browne and *Vox Norwici*." *Notes and Queries* 231 (1986), 461.

Davidson, Peter. "The Jesuit Garden." In O'Malley, ed. *The Jesuits II.* 86–107.

Davis, Dorothy. *Fairs, Shops, and Supermarkets: A History of English Shopping.* Toronto: University of Toronto Press, 1966.

Dawson, John Charles. *Toulouse in the Renaissance.* New York: Columbia University Press, 1923.

Day, John. *Concio ad Clerum, Preached at St Mary's Oxford, 1612.* Oxford, 1612.

De Beer, E. S. "The Correspondence between Sir Thomas Browne and John Evelyn." *The Library*, 4th series, 22 (1941–42), 103–6.

——"An Uncollected Poem by Waller." *Review of English Studies* 8 (1932), 203–5.

Dear, Linda Allen. *Academic Theories of Generation in the Renaissance: The Contemporaries and Successors of Jean Fernel (1497–1558).* PhD thesis Warburg Institute, London, 1990.

Dear, Peter. *Discipline and Experience: The Mathematical Way in the Scientific Revolution.* Chicago: University of Chicago Press, 1995.

Debus, Allen G. "Sir Thomas Browne and the Study of Colour Indicators." *Ambix* 10 (1962), 29–36.

——ed. *Medicine in Seventeenth Century England.* Berkeley: University of California Press, 1974.

Delalain, Jules. *Les pénitents blancs et les pénitents bleus de la ville de Montpellier: leur origines, leur histoire, leur reglès.* Montpellier: Jean Martel Ainé, 1874.

Delmas, Paul. *Sept Siècles D'Obstétrique à la Faculté de Médecine de Montpellier.* Montpellier: Librairie Coulet, 1927.

Delort, André. *Mémoires inédits d'André Delort sur la ville de Montpellier au XVIIe siècle.* Marseille: J. Martel, 1876–78.

Demaitre, Luke. *Leprosy in Premodern Medicine: A Malady of the Whole Body.* Baltimore, MD: Johns Hopkins University Press, 2007.

Dempster, Thomas. *Historia ecclesiastica gentis Scotorum, sive, de scriptoribus Scotis.* 2 vols. Edinburgh: Andreas Balfour, 1829.

Denonain, Jean-Jacques. "Les Problèmes de L'Honnête Homme vers 1635: *Religio Medici* et les *Conférences* du Bureau d'Adresse." *Études Anglaises* 18 (1965), 235–47.

——"Le reître et le jouvenceau." *Caliban* n.s. 1 (1965), 7–20.
——ed. *Une Version Primitive de Religio Medici par Sir Thomas Browne.* Publications de la Faculté d'Alger 36, 1958.
Derham, W., ed. *Philosophical Experiments and Observations of the late Eminent Dr. Robert Hooke... And Other Eminent Virtuoso's in his Time.* London, 1726.
Des Chene, Dennis. *Life's Form: Late Aristotelian Conceptions of the Soul.* Ithaca, New York: Cornell University Press, 2000.
De Vic, Dom. Claude, and Dom J. Vaissete. *Histoire Generale de Languedoc.* Reprinted Osnabrück: Otto Zeller, 1973. Vol. 11.
Dexter, Henry Martyn, and Morton Dexter. *The England and Holland of the Pilgrims.* New York: Houghton, Mifflin and Company, 1905.
A Dialogue between Philiater and Momus. 1686.
Digby, Anne. *Making a Medical Living: Doctors and Patients in the English Market for Medicine, 1720–1911.* Cambridge: Cambridge University Press, 1994.
Digby, Sir Kenelm. *Observations vpon Religio Medici.* 1643.
Dixon, C. W. *Smallpox.* London: J. & A. Churchill, 1962.
Dobell, P. J. *Books of the Time of the Restoration.* London: P. J. and A. E. Dobell, 1920.
Donovan, Dennis G. et al. *Sir Thomas Browne and Robert Burton: A Reference Guide.* Boston: G. K. Hall, 1981.
Doody, Margaret. *Tropic of Venice.* Philadelphia: University of Pennsylvania Press, 2007.
Downame, George. *Abrahams Tryall: A Sermon Preached at the Spittle, in Easter weeke, Anno Domini, 1602.* 1607.
——*Lectures on the XV. Psalme: Read in the Cathedrall Church of S. Paule in London.* 1604.
——*Two Sermons, The One Commending the Ministerie in Generall: The Other Defending the Office of Bishops in Particular.* 1608.
Dulieu, Louis. *La Médecine a Montpellier.* 4 vols. Avignon: Les Presses Universelles, 1983.
——*La Pharmacie à Montpellier: de ses origines à nos jours.* Avignon: Les Presses Universelles, 1973.
Dunton, John. *The New Practice of Piety; Writ in Imitation of Dr. Browne's Religio Medici: or, The Christian Virtuoso: Discovering the Right Way to Heaven, Between all Extreams.* 1705.
Dutt, William A. *Some Literary Associations of East Anglia.* London: Methuen, 1907.
Dymond, David. *The Norfolk Landscape.* London: Hodder and Stoughton, 1985.
Earle, John. *Microcosmography.* Ed. Harold Osborne. London: University Tutorial Press, 1933.
Eccles, Audrey. *Obstetrics and Gynaecology in Tudor and Stuart England.* Kent, OH: Kent State University Press, 1982.
Eddington, Arthur J. *The First Fifty Years of Quakerism in Norwich.* London: Friends' Historical Society, 1932.
Edelstein, Emma J., and Ludwig Edelstein. *Asclepius: A Collection and Interpretation of the Testimonies.* 2 vols. Baltimore, MD: Johns Hopkins University Press, 1945.
Eden, Kathy. *Friends Hold All Things in Common: Tradition, Intellectual Property, and the Adages of Erasmus.* New Haven, CT: Yale University Press, 2001.
Edwardes, Edward J. *A Concise History of Small-Pox and Vaccination in Europe.* London: H. K. Lewis, 1902.
Edwards, John. *A Demonstration of the Existence and Providence of God.* 1696.
Edwards, Karen L. "Engaging with Pygmies: Thomas Browne and John Milton." In Barbour and Preston, eds. *Sir Thomas Browne: The World Proposed.* 100–17.

Ekkart, R. E. O. *Athenae Batavae: De Leidse Universiteit, 1575–1975*. Leiden: University of Leiden Press, 1975.

An Elegy upon the Death of the Much Lamented, Able and Learned Physician Dr Thomson. 1677.

Ellis François, Martha J. "The Social and Economic Development of Halifax, 1558–1640." *Leeds Philosophical and Literary Society* 11 (1966), 217–80.

——"A Study in the Manorial History of Halifax Parish in the Sixteenth and Early Seventeenth Centuries." *The Yorkshire Archælogical Journal* 40 (1961), 250–64; 420–42.

Endicott, Norman J. "Browne's *Letter to a Friend*." *TLS*, September 15, 1966, 868.

——"Sir Thomas Browne as 'Orphan,' with Some Account of His Stepfather, Sir Thomas Dutton." *University of Toronto Quarterly* 30 (1960–61), 180–210.

——"Sir Thomas Browne, Montpellier, and the Tract 'Of Languages.'" *TLS* August 24, 1962, 645.

——"Sir Thomas Browne's *Letter to a Friend*," *University of Toronto Quarterly* 36 (1966–7), 68–86.

——ed. *The Prose of Sir Thomas Browne*. Garden City, NY: Anchor, 1967.

England and Scotland Vnited. 1647.

Erasmus, Desiderius. *The Praise of Folly*. Trans. and ed. Clarence Miller. New Haven, CT: Yale University Press, 1979.

Evans, John T. *Seventeenth-Century Norwich: Politics, Religion, and Government, 1620–1690*. Oxford: Clarendon Press, 1979.

Evelyn, John. *The Diary*. Ed. E. S. De Beer. 6 vols. Oxford: Oxford University Press, 1955.

——*Sylva*. 1664.

Ewing, Majl. "A Note on the Sir Thomas Browne–Sir William Dugdale Letters." *Philological Quarterly* 21 (1942), 425–7.

Favour, John. *Antiquitie Triumphing ouer Noueltie*. 1619.

Favre, Albert. "Sir Thomas Browne, *Pseudodoxia Epidemica*: Révélation d'une Personnalité? Le Livre V." *Études Anglaises* 42 (1989), 140–50.

Feingold, Mordechai. "The Humanities." In Tyacke, ed. *The History of the University of Oxford: Volume IV*. 211–358.

——"The Mathematical Sciences and New Philosophies." In Tyacke, ed. *The History of the University of Oxford: Volume IV*. 359–448.

——*The Mathematicians' Apprenticeship: Science, Universities and Society in England, 1560–1640*. Cambridge: Cambridge University Press, 1984.

Fernel, Jean. *The Physiologia of Jean Fernel (1567)*. Trans. John M. Forrester, intro. and notes John Henry and Forrester. Philadelphia: American Philosophical Society, 2003.

——*Jean Fernel's On the Hidden Causes of Things*. Trans. and ed. John M. Forrester, intro. and notes John Henry and Forrester. Boston: Brill, 2005.

Ferrari, Ciro. *L'Ufficio della Sanità di Padova nella Prima Metà del Sec. XVII*. Venice: A Spese della Società,1910.

Ferrari, Giovanni Battista. *De florum cultura*. Rome, 1633.

Fichtner, Gerhard. "Padova e Tübingen: La Formazione Medica nei Secoli XVI e XVII." *Acta Medicae Historiae Patavina* 19 (1972–73), 43–62.

Ficino, Marsilio. *Three Books on Life*. Ed. and trans. Carol V. Kaske and John R. Clark. Binghamton, NY: Center for Medieval and Early Renaissance Studies, 1989.

Figurovski, N. A. "The Alchemist and Physician Arthur Dee." *Ambix* 13 (1965), 35–51.

Finch, Jeremiah S. "Early Drafts of the *Garden of Cyrus*." *PMLA* 55 (1940), 742–9.

——"A Newly Discovered *Urn Burial*." *The Library*, 4th series, 19 (1938/9), 347–53.

——"The Norfolk Persuaders of Sir Thomas Browne: A Variant Copy of the 1712 Posthumous Works." *Princeton University Library Chronicle* 11 (1949–50), 199–201.

——*Sir Thomas Browne: A Doctor's Life of Science and Faith.* New York: Henry Schuman, 1950.

——"Sir Thomas Browne: Early Biographical Notices, and the Disposition of His Library and Manuscripts." *Studies in Bibliography* 2 (1949–50), 196–201.

——ed. *A Catalogue of the Libraries of Sir Thomas Browne and Dr Edward Browne, His Son.* Leiden: E. J. Brill, 1986.

Finch, Jonathan. "The Monuments." In Atherton et al., eds. *Norwich Cathedral.* 467–93.

Fincham, Kenneth. "Material Evidence: The Religious Legacy of the Interregnum at St George Tombland, Norwich." In Kenneth Fincham and Peter Lake, eds. *Religious Politics in Post-Reformation England: Essays in Honour of Nicholas Tyacke.* Rochester, NY: Boydell, 2006. 224–40.

——ed. *Visitation Articles and Injunctions of the Early Stuart Church.* Vol 2. Rochester, NY: Boydell, 1998.

Findlay, Alison. "Sexual and Spiritual Politics in the Events of 1633–34 and *The Late Lancashire Witches.*" In Robert Poole, ed. *Lancashire Witches: Histories and Stories.* Manchester: Manchester University Press, 2003. 146–65.

Findlen, Paula. "Sites of Anatomy, Botany, and Natural History." In Katharine Park and Lorraine Daston, eds. *Cambridge History of Science: Volume 3: Early Modern Science.* New York: Cambridge University Press, 2006.

Firth, J. D.'E. *Winchester College.* London: Winchester Publications, 1949.

Fletcher, J. M. "The Faculty of Arts." In McConica, ed. *The History of the University of Oxford: Volume III.* 157–99.

Foster, Joseph. *Alumni Oxonienses.* 4 vols. Oxford: Parker and Co., 1891.

Fox, George. *The Journal of George Fox.* Ed. Nigel Smith. New York: Penguin, 1998.

Fracastoro, Hieronymus. *Contagion, Contagious Diseases and Their Treatment.* Ed. and trans. Wilmer Cave Wright. New York: G. P. Putnam's Sons, 1930.

Frank, Robert G., Jr. *Harvey and the Oxford Physiologists: A Study of Scientific Ideas.* Berkeley: University of California Press, 1980.

——"Medicine." In Tyacke, ed. *The History of the University of Oxford: Volume IV.* 505–58.

French, Roger. "Harvey in Holland: Circulation and the Calvinists." In Roger French and Andrew Wear, eds. *The Medical Revolution of the Seventeenth Century.* New York: Cambridge University Press, 1989. 46–86.

Fuller, Thomas. *The History of the Worthies of England.* 1662.

Funkenstein, Amos. *Theology and the Scientific Imagination from the Middle Ages to the Seventeenth Century.* Princeton, NJ: Princeton University Press, 1986.

Galen. *Selected Works.* Trans. and intro. P. N. Singer. New York: Oxford University Press, 1997.

Garside, M. W. "The Social History of Halifax in the Seventeenth Century." *Transactions of the Halifax Antiquarian Society* (1923), 65–99.

Gayton, Edmund. *The Religion of a Physician.* 1663.

Geis, Gilbert, and Ivan Bunn. *A Trial of Witches: A Seventeenth-Century Witchcraft Prosecution.* New York: Routledge, 1997.

Gentilcore, David. *Healers and Healing in Early Modern Italy.* New York: Manchester University Press, 1998.

Gerard, John. *The Herbal or General History of Plants.* Facsimile of 1633 enlarged edition. New York: Dover, 1975.

Germain, A. *La Faculté de Théologie de Montpellier.* Montpellier: Boehm et Fils, 1883.
Gibson, Kenneth. "George Downame." *ODNB.*
Gilbert, Neal W. *Renaissance Concepts of Method.* New York: Columbia University Press, 1960.
Gilchrist, Roberta. *Norwich Cathedral Close: The Evolution of the English Cathedral Landscape.* Rochester, NY: The Boydell Press, 2005.
Glynn, Ian, and Jenifer Glynn. *The Life and Death of Smallpox.* London: Profile, 2004.
Gogelein, A. J. F., and R. E. O. Ekkart. *Leidse universiteit 400.* Amsterdam: Rijksmuseum, 1975.
Goldgar, Anne. *Tulipmania: Money, Honor, and Knowledge in the Dutch Golden Age.* Chicago: University of Chicago Press, 2007.
Goldie, Mark. "Andrew Crooke." *ODNB.*
Goodall, John A. A. *God's House at Ewelme: Life, Devotion, and Architecture in a Fifteenth-Century Almshouse.* Burlington, VT: Ashgate, 2001.
Gouk, P. M. "Music." In Tyacke, ed. *History of the University of Oxford: Volume IV.* 621–40.
Gowland, Angus. *The Worlds of Renaissance Melancholy: Robert Burton in Context.* Cambridge: Cambridge University Press, 2006.
Grafton, Anthony. *Athenae Batavae: The Research Imperative at Leiden, 1575–1650.* Leiden: Primavera Pers, 2003.
Grassby, Richard. *The Business Community of Seventeenth-Century England.* Cambridge: Cambridge University Press, 1995.
Graves, Rolande. *Born to Procreate: Women and Childbirth in France from the Middle Ages to the Eighteenth Century.* New York: Peter Lang, 2001.
Green, Lawrence D., ed. and trans. *John Rainolds's Oxford Lectures on Aristotle's "Rhetoric."* Newark: University of Delaware Press, 1986.
Gregory, John. *Gregorii Posthuma: or, Certain learned tracts.* 1650.
Grell, Ole Peter. "The Attraction of Leiden University for English Students of Medicine and Theology, 1590–1642." In C. C. Barfoot and Richard Todd, eds. *The Great Emporium: The Low Countries as a Cultural Crossroads in the Renaissance and the Eighteenth Century.* Amsterdam: Rodopi, 1992. 83–104.
Grell, Ole Peter, and Andrew Cunningham, eds. *Health Care and Poor Relief in Protestant Europe, 1500–1700.* New York: Routledge, 1997.
Grendler, Paul F. *The Universities of the Italian Renaissance.* Baltimore, MD: Johns Hopkins University Press, 2002.
Grew, Nehemiah. *Musæum Regalis Societatis.* 1681.
Grey, Elizabeth, Countess of Kent. *A choice manual of rare and select secrets in physick and chirurgery.* 1653.
Griffiths, Elizabeth, ed. *William Windham's Green Book, 1673–1688.* Norfolk Record Society 66 (2002).
Guenée, Simonne. *Les Universités Françaises des origines à la révolution.* Paris: Picard, 1982.
Guibbory, Achsah. "Sir Thomas Browne's *Pseudodoxia Epidemica* and the Circle of Knowledge." *Texas Studies in Language and Literature* 18 (1976), 486–99.
Guidott, Thomas. *Gideon's Fleece, or, The Sieur de Frisk: An Heroick Poem.* London, 1684.
Guiraud, Louise. *Études sur la réforme à Montpellier.* Montpellier: Louis Valat, 1918.
Gunther, R. T. *Early British Botanists and Their Gardens.* Oxford: Oxford University Press, 1922.
H. "On Vulgar Errors." *The Gentleman's Magazine* 41 (1771), 251–2.
Hactenus Inaudita. London, 1663.

Hafenreffer, Samuel. *Pandocheion aiolodermon.* 1630.

Hakluyt, Richard. *Voyages and Discoveries.* Ed. and intro. Jack Beeching. Baltimore, MD: Penguin, 1972.

Halifax Daily Courier & Guardian.

Hall, Joseph. *The Works of Joseph Hall, D.D.* 12 vols. Oxford: D. A. Talboys, 1837.

Hall, Marie Boas. "Thomas Browne Naturalist." In Patrides, ed. *Approaches to Sir Thomas Browne.* 178–87.

Hall, R. F. *Studies in Sir Thomas Browne's Letter to a Friend.* MLitt diss, Oxford University, 1972.

Hall, Thomas. *The Beauty of Holiness.* London, 1655.

Hall, Thomas S. *Ideas of Life and Matter: Studies in the History of General Physiology, 600 B.C.–1900 A.D.* 2 vols. Chicago: University of Chicago Press, 1969.

Hamper, William, ed. *The Life, Diary, and Correspondence of Sir William Dugdale, Knight.* London: Harding, Lepard, and Co., 1827.

Hanson, Craig Ashley. *The English Virtuoso: Art, Medicine, and Antiquarianism in the Age of Empiricism.* Chicago: University of Chicago Press, 2009.

Hanson, T. W. "John Brearcliffe, the Antiquary." *Transactions of the Halifax Antiquarian Society* (1908), 321–48.

——"Minutes of Halifax Workhouse." *Halifax Antiquarian Society* (1921), 77–96.

——"The Multure Hall." *Transactions of the Halifax Antiquarian Society* (1935), 1–19.

——"Nathaniel Waterhouse, Great Halifax Benefactor." *Halifax Antiquarian Society* (1919), 73–104.

Harington, Sir John. *Nugæ antiquæ.* London, 1792.

Harney, Martin P., SJ. *The Jesuits in History: The Society of Jesus through Four Centuries.* New York: The America Press, 1941.

Harris, W., ed. *Nicholas Pynnar's 1618–19 Survey of Ulster.* In *Hibernica: Or, some Antient Pieces relating to Ireland.* Dublin, 1770.

Hartlib, Samuel. *Hartlib Papers: A Complete Text and Image Database of the Papers of Samuel Hartlib (c. 1600–1662) Held in Sheffield University Library.* Sheffield: Humanities Research Institute, 2002.

Harvey, Elizabeth D. "The Touching Organ: Allegory, Anatomy, and the Renaissance Skin Envelope." In Elizabeth Harvey, ed. *Sensible Flesh: On Touch in Early Modern Culture.* Philadelphia: University of Pennsylvania Press, 2003. 81–102.

Harvey, Gideon. *The Conclave of Physicians Detecting their Intrigues, Frauds, and Plots, against their Patients.* 2nd ed. 1686.

Harwood, Winfred A. "The Household of Winchester College in the Later Middle Ages, 1400–1560." *Proceedings of the Hampshire Field Club Archaeological Society* 59 (2004), 163–79.

Havenstein, Daniela. *Democratizing Sir Thomas Browne: "Religio Medici" and Its Imitations.* Oxford: Clarendon Press, 1999.

Hayes-McCoy, G. A., ed. *Ulster and Other Irish Maps c. 1600.* Dublin: Stationery Office, 1964.

Healy, Simon. "Sir Arthur Ingram." *ODNB.*

Heaton, Herbert. *The Yorkshire Woollen and Worsted Industries from the Earliest Times up to the Industrial Revolution.* 2nd ed. Oxford: Clarendon Press, 1965.

Heideman, Margaret Ash. "*Hydriotaphia* and *The Garden of Cyrus*: A Paradox and a Cosmic Vision." *University of Toronto Quarterly* 19 (1949–50), 235–46.

Heister, Elias Fredericus. *Apologia pro medicis.* Amsterdam, 1736.

Henderson, John. *The Renaissance Hospital: Healing the Body and Healing the Soul.* New Haven, CT: Yale University Press, 2006.

Heninger, S. K., Jr. *Touches of Sweet Harmony: Pythagorean Cosmology and Renaissance Poetics.* San Marino, CA: Huntington Library, 1974.

Herbert, William. *The History of the Twelve Great Livery Companies of London.* London: Published by the Author, 1836–37.

Herendeen, Wyman H. "William Camden." *ODNB.*

—— *William Camden: A Life in Context.* Rochester, NY: The Boydell Press, 2007.

Heylyn, Peter. *Theologia veterum, or, The summe of Christian theologie, positive, polemical and Philological, contained in the Apostles Creed.* 1654.

Hickson, Mary Agnes. *Ireland in the Seventeenth Century.* 2 vols. London: Longmans, Green & Co., 1884.

Hildesley, Mark. *Religio Jurisprudentis.* 1685.

Hill, George. *An Historical Account of the Plantation in Ulster at the Commencement of the Seventeenth Century, 1608–1620.* Intro. John G. Barry. Shannon: Irish University Press, 1970.

Hobbs, Mary. *Early Seventeenth-Century Verse Miscellany Manuscripts.* Brookfield, VT: Scholar Press, 1992.

Hobbes, Thomas. *Critique du "De Mundo" de Thomas White.* Ed. Jean Jacquot and Harold W. Jones. Paris: Vrin, 1973.

Hoeniger, F. D., and J. F. M. Hoeniger. *The Growth of Natural History in Stuart England from Gerard to the Royal Society.* Charlottesville: University Press of Virginia, 1969.

Holmes, Martin. *Elizabethan London.* London: Cassell, 1969.

Höltgen, Karl Josef. "Browne's *Letter to a Friend.*" *TLS* October 20, 1966, 966.

Homer. *The Iliads of Homer Prince of Poets.* Trans. George Chapman. 1611.

Hopkins, Donald R. *The Greatest Killer: Smallpox in History.* Chicago: University of Chicago Press, 2002.

——*Princes and Peasants: Smallpox in History.* Chicago: University of Chicago Press, 1983.

Hopper, Andrew. "The Civil Wars." In Rawcliffe and Wilson, eds. *Norwich since 1550.* 89–116.

Hopper, Florence. "Clusius' World: The Meeting of Science and Art." In Tjon Sie Fat and de Jong, eds. *The Authentic Garden.* 13–36.

Horowitz, Elliott. "Processions, Piety, and Jewish Confraternities." In Robert C. Davis and Benjamin Ravid, eds. *The Jews of Early Modern Venice.* Baltimore, MD: Johns Hopkins University Press, 2001. 231–47.

Horrox, Rosemary, and Sarah Rees Jones, eds. *Pragmatic Utopias: Ideals and Communities, 1200–1630.* Cambridge: Cambridge University Press, 2001.

Houghton, Walter E., Jr. "The English Virtuoso in the Seventeenth Century." *Journal of the History of Ideas* 3 (1942), 51–73, 190–219.

Houseman, J. W. "Notes and Comments on Halifax Churchwardens' Accounts, 1620–1714." *Transactions of the Halifax Antiquarian Society* (1925), 137–67.

Hovenden, Robert, ed. *A True Register of all the Christeninges . . . in the Parishe of St. James Clarkenwell.* Harleian Society Publications vols. 9–10, 13, 17, 19–20. London, 1884–93.

Howell, Almonte C. "John Dunton and an Imitation of the *Religio Medici.*" *Studies in Philology* 29 (1932), 442–62.

Howell, James. *Epistolæ Ho-Elianæ.* 1645.

——*A German diet.* 1653.

Hubberthorn, Richard. *The Testimony of the Everlasting Gospel Witnessed through Suffering.* 1654.

Hughes, J. Trevor. "The Browne Family at Upton by Chester." *Cheshire History* 39 (1999–2000), 2–6.

——"The Childhood of Sir Thomas Browne: His Relationship to His Mother and Stepfather." *London Journal* 23 (1998), 21–9.

——"Dr Henry Power (1626–1668): The Medical Practice of a Halifax Physician." *Transactions of the Halifax Antiquarian Society* 11 (2003), 56–67.

——"George Scharpe, c.1581–1637: A Scots Doctor at Montpellier." *Scottish Medical Journal* 47 (2002), 40–3.

——"Henry Power (1626–1668) of New Hall, Elland and Experiments on Barometric Pressure." *Transactions of the Halifax Antiquarian Society* 10 (2002), 14–26.

——"The Medical Education of Sir Thomas Browne." *Journal of Medical Biography* 9 (2001), 70–6.

——"Sir Thomas Browne, Shibden Dale and the Writing of *Religio Medici*." First published *Yorkshire History Quarterly* 5 (2000), 89–94; included in Hughes. *Essays in Medical Biography*. Oxford: Rimes House, 2008. 40–50.

——"Sir Thomas Browne's Knighthood." *Norfolk Archaeology* 43 (1998–99), 326–31.

Hughes, Shaun F. D. "Sir Thomas Browne and Iceland." *English Renaissance Prose* 1 (1987), 25–47.

Huisman, Frank. "Medicine and Health Care in the Netherlands, 1500–1800." In Klaas van Berkel et al., eds. *A History of Science in the Netherlands: Surveys, Themes, and Reference*. Leiden: Brill, 1999. 239–78.

Huisman, Tim. *The Finger of God: Anatomical Practice in Seventeenth-Century Leiden*. Leiden: Primavera Pers, 2009.

——*A Theatre for Anatomy: The Leiden Theatrum Anatomicum, 1594–1821*. Leiden: Museum Boerhaave, 2002.

Hull, William. *Repentance not to be repented of*. 1612.

Huntley, Frank Livingstone. "Browne's Masterpiece, *Vulgar Errors*." In *Essays in Persuasion: On Seventeenth Century English Literature*. Chicago: University of Chicago Press, 1981. 86–96.

——"Dr. Thomas Lushington (1590–1661), Sir Thomas Browne's Oxford Tutor." *Modern Philology* 81 (1983), 14–23.

——"The Occasion and Date of Sir Thomas Browne's *A Letter to a Friend*." *Modern Philology* 48 (1950–1), 157–71; reworked in *Essays in Persuasion: On Seventeenth Century English Literature*. 114–25.

——"The Publication and Immediate Reception of *Religio Medici*." *The Library Quarterly* 25 (1955), 203–18.

——*Sir Thomas Browne: A Biographical and Critical Study*. Ann Arbor: University of Michigan Press, 1962.

——"Sir Thomas Browne and His Oxford Tutor: or, Academic Guilt by Association." *The History of Ideas News Letter* 2, no. 3 (1956), 50–3.

——"Sir Thomas Browne: The Relationship of *Urn Burial* and *The Garden of Cyrus*." *Studies in Philology* 53 (1956), 204–19.

Huston, K. Garth. "Sir Thomas Browne, Thomas le Gros, and the First Edition of *Pseudodoxia Epidemica*, 1646." *Journal of the History of Medicine* 25 (1970), 347–8.

Hutton, Leonard. "Antiquities of Oxford." In Charles Plummer, ed. *Elizabethan Oxford: Reprints of Rare Tracts*. Oxford: Clarendon Press, 1887.

Hutton, Matthew. *The Correspondence of Dr. Matthew Hutton, Archbishop of York*. Ed. Timothy Hutton and Matthew Hutton. Publications of the Surtees Society, 1843.

Huygens, Constantijn. *De Briefwisseling van Constantijn Huygens, 1608–1697.* Ed. J. A. Worp. 5 vols. The Hague: M Nijhoff, 1911–17.

Imperiale, Giovanni. *Musæum Historicum et Physicum.* Venice, 1640.

——*Le Notti Beriche.* Venice, 1663.

——*Pestis Anni MDCXXX Historico-Medica.* Vicenza, 1631.

Imperiale, Giovanni Vincenzo. *Viaggi.* Ed. Anton Guilio Barrili. Genoa: Società ligure di storia patria, 1898.

Ingle, H. Larry. *First Among Friends: George Fox and the Creation of Quakerism.* New York: Oxford University Press, 1994.

Irvine, William Fergusson. "Sir Thomas Browne, Author of *Religio Medici.*" *Chester Sheaf,* 3rd series, 3 (September, October, November, 1899), 100, 107–8, 118–19.

——ed. *A Collection of Lancashire and Cheshire Wills... 1301–1762.* The Record Society 30 (1896).

Israel, Jonathan. *The Dutch Republic: Its Rise, Greatness, and Fall, 1477–1806.* Oxford: Oxford University Press, 1995.

J. D. *A Memorial for the Learned.* 1686.

Jackson, Thomas. *The Works of Thomas Jackson, D.D.* 12 vols. Oxford: Oxford University Press, 1844.

James I, King of England. *A Proclamation for the confirmation of all Authorized Order.* 1615.

Jardine, Nicholas. "Keeping Order in the School of Padua: Jacopo Zabarella and Francesco Piccolomini on the Offices of Philosophy." In Daniel A. Di Liscia et al., eds. *Method and Order in Renaissance Philosophy of Nature: The Aristotle Commentary Tradition.* Burlington, VT: Ashgate, 1997. 183–210.

Jay, George Branwhite, ed. *The First Parish Register of St. George of Tombland, Norwich (A.D. 1538–1707).* Revised William Hudson. Norwich: Agas H. Goose, 1891.

Johns, Adrian. "Henry Power." *ODNB.*

Johnston, Arthur. *Musa Latina Aberdonensis.* Ed. Sir William Duguid Geddes. 3 vols. Aberdeen: New Spalding Club, 1895.

Jones, J. R. *The Anglo-Dutch Wars of the Seventeenth Century.* New York: Longman, 1996.

Jong, E. de. "Nature and Art: The Leiden Hortus as 'Musaeum.'" In Tjon Sie Fat and de Jong, eds. *The Authentic Garden.* 37–70.

Jonge, H. J. de. *Daniel Heinsius and the Textus Receptus of the New Testament.* Leiden: Brill, 1971.

——"The Study of the New Testament." In Scheurlee and Meyjes, eds. *Leiden University in the Seventeenth Century.* 65–109.

Jordan, W. K. *The Charities of Rural England, 1480–1660.* New York: Russell Sage Foundation, 1962.

Josten, C. H., ed. *Elias Ashmole (1617–1692): His Autobiographical and Historical Notes, His Correspondence, and Other Contemporary Sources Relating to His Life and Work.* 5 vols. Oxford: Clarendon Press, 1966.

Joubert, Laurent. *Popular Errors.* Ed. and trans. Gregory David de Rocher. Tuscaloosa: University of Alabama Press, 1989.

——*The Second Part of the Popular Errors.* Ed. and trans. Gregory David de Rocher. Tuscaloosa: University of Alabama Press, 1995.

——*Treatise on Laughter.* Trans. and ed. Gregory David de Rocher. Tuscaloosa: University of Alabama Press, 1980.

Juel-Jensen, Bent. "*Musæum Clausum, or Bibliotheca Abscondita*: Some Thoughts on Curiosity Cabinets and Imaginary Books." *Journal of the History of Collections* 4 (1992), 127–40.

Kaplan, Benjamin J. *Divided by Faith: Religious Conflict and the Practice of Toleration in Early Modern Europe.* Cambridge, MA: Harvard University Press, 2007.

Keck, Thomas. *Annotations upon Religio Medici.* In *Religio Medici.* 1656.

Keene, Derek. *Winchester Studies 2: Survey of Medieval Winchester.* Vol. 2, i, part I. Oxford: Clarendon Press, 1985.

Keene, Derek, and Vanessa Harding. *Historical Gazetteer of London before the Great Fire, Part I, Cheapside.* London: Institute for Historical Research, University of London, 1987.

Keevil, J. J. *Medicine and the Navy, 1200–1900.* 3 vols. London: E. & S. Livingstone, 1957–1961.

Kellett, C. E. "Sir Thomas Browne and the Disease Called the Morgellons." *Annals of Medical History,* n.s., 7 (1935), 467–79.

Kendall, Hugh P. "The Plague in Halifax Parish." *Halifax Antiquarian Society* (1931), 3–26.

Kendrick, Christopher. *Utopia, Carnival, and Commonwealth in Renaissance England.* Toronto: University of Toronto Press, 2004.

Kennedy, Ross. "Robert Loveday." *ODNB.*

Kessler, Eckhard. "The Transformation of Aristotelianism during the Renaissance." In John Henry and Sarah Hutton, eds. *New Perspectives on Renaissance Thought: Essays in the History of Science, Education and Philosophy: In Memory of Charles B. Schmitt.* London: Duckworth, 1990. 137–47.

Ketton-Cremer, R. W. *Felbrigg: The Story of a House.* London: Rupert Hart-Davis, 1962.

——*Forty Norfolk Essays.* Norwich: Jerrod, 1961.

——*Norfolk in the Civil War: A Portrait of a Society in Conflict.* Hamden, CT: Archon Books, 1969.

——*Norfolk Portraits.* London: Faber and Faber, 1944.

Keynes, Geoffrey, ed. *The Commonplace Book of Elizabeth Lyttelton, Daughter of Sir Thomas Browne.* Cambridge: Cambridge University Press, 1919.

——ed. *The Works of Sir Thomas Browne.* 4 vols. London: Faber & Faber, 1964.

Killeen, Kevin. *Biblical Scholarship, Science and Politics in Early Modern England: Thomas Browne and the Thorny Place of Knowledge.* Burlington, VT: Ashgate, 2009.

——"The Politics of Painting: *Pseudodoxia Epidemica* and Iconoclasm." In Barbour and Preston, eds. *Sir Thomas Browne: The World Proposed.* 188–205.

King, David. *The Medieval Stained Glass of St Peter Mancroft, Norwich.* Oxford: Oxford University Press, 2006.

King, Lester. *The Road to Medical Enlightenment, 1650–1695.* New York: American Elsevier, 1970.

Kippis, Andrew. *Biographia Britannica.* 2nd ed. London, 1780.

Kirby, Thomas Frederick. *Winchester Scholars.* London: Henry Frowde, 1888.

Klestinec, Cynthia. "Civility, Comportment, and the Anatomy Theater: Girolamo Fabrici and His Medical Students in Renaissance Padua." *Renaissance Quarterly* 60 (2007), 434–63.

——"A History of Anatomy Theaters in Sixteenth-Century Padua." *Journal of the History of Medicine and Allied Sciences* 59 (2004), 375–412.

——*Theaters of Anatomy: Students, Teachers, and Traditions of Dissection in Renaissance Venice.* Baltimore, MD: The Johns Hopkins University Press, 2011.

Knighton, C. S. "John Bowle." *ODNB.*

Kohn, George Childs, ed. *Encyclopedia of Plague and Pestilence from Ancient Times to the Present.* Rev. ed. New York: Facts on File, 2001.

Kooi, Christine. *Liberty and Religion: Church and State in Leiden's Reformation, 1572–1620.* Boston: Brill, 2000.

Kroon, J. E. *Bijdragen tot de Geschiedenis van het Geneeskundig Onderwijs aan de Leidsche Universiteit 1575–1625.* Leiden: S. C. Van Doesburgh, 1911.

Krueger, Robert, ed. *The Poems of Sir John Davies.* Oxford: Clarendon Press, 1975.

Kuhn, Heinrich C. *Venetischer Aristotelismus im Ende der aristotelischen Welt: Aspekte der Welt und des Denkens des Cesare Cremonini (1550–1631).* New York: Peter Lang, 1996.

Laget, Mireille. *Naissance et Conscience de la Vie: Procréation, Enfantement, Obstétrique en Languedoc aux XVIIe et XVIIIe Siècles.* Thesis, Sorbonne, 1980.

Lamping, A. J. *Johannes Polyander: Een dienaar van Kerk en Universiteit.* Leiden: Brill, 1980.

Lane, Frederic C. *Venice: A Maritime Republic.* Baltimore, MD: Johns Hopkins University Press, 1973.

Lawrence, Thomas. *Mercurius centralis.* 1664.

Lawson, John, and Harold Silver. *A Social History of Education in England.* London: Methuen, 1973.

Lazzaro, Claudia. *The Italian Renaissance Garden: From the Conventions of Planting, Design, and Ornament to the Grand Gardens of Sixteenth-Century Central Italy.* New Haven, CT: Yale University Press, 1990.

Le Clerc, Joannes. *Disputatio Medica Inauguralis, De Melancholia.* Leiden, 1633.

Le Loyer, Pierre. *A Treatise of Specters.* 1605.

Leach, Arthur F. *Educational Charters and Documents 598 to 1909.* Cambridge: Cambridge University Press, 1911; republ. New York: AMS, 1971.

——*A History of Winchester College.* London: Duckworth & Co., 1899.

——*Milton as Schoolboy and Schoolmaster.* Folcroft, PA: Folcroft Library Editions, 1976.

Leonard, E. M. *The Early History of English Poor Relief.* Cambridge: Cambridge University Press, 1900.

Le Roy Ladurie, Emmanuel. *The Ancien Régime: A History of France, 1610–1774.* Trans. Mark Greengrass. Oxford: Blackwell, 1996.

—— *The Peasants of Languedoc.* Trans. John Day. Urbana: University of Illinois Press, 1974.

Letts, Malcolm. "Sir Thomas Browne and Witchcraft." *Notes and Queries,* 11th series, 5 (1912), 221–3.

Lewis, Elizabeth. "A Sixteenth-Century Painted Ceiling from Winchester College." *Proceedings of the Hampshire Field Club Archaeological Society* 51 (1995), 137–65.

Lewis, Gillian. "The Faculty of Medicine." In McConica, ed. *The History of the University of Oxford: Volume III.* 213–56.

Liceti, Fortunio. *Allegoria Peripatetica.* 1630.

——*De anima physice non propensa dialogus.* 1637.

——*De animarum rationalium immortalitate: Aristotelis opinionem diligenter explicantes.* 1629.

——*De anima subiecto corpori.* 1631.

——*De feriis altricis animae.* 1631.

——*De monstrorum natura, caussis, et differentiis.* 2nd ed. 1634.

——*De natura & efficientia luminis.* 1640.

——*De quesitis per epistolas.* 1640.

——*Hieroglyphica.* 1653.

Lill, James. "A Lesson in Futurity: Johnson's 'Life of Sir Thomas Browne.'" *The Notre Dame English Journal* 15 (1983), 39–50.

Lindeboom, G. A. *Dutch Medical Biography.* Amsterdam: Rodopi, 1984.

Lister, John. "History of Shibden Hall." *Halifax Antiquarian Society* (1910), 109–32.

——"History of Shibden Hall." *Halifax Antiquarian Society* (1923), 101–22.

——"History of Shibden Hall." *Halifax Antiquarian Society* (1926), 1–11.

Löffler, Arno. "Sir Thomas Browne at Work: An Unpublished Early Section of *Christian Morals.*" *Notes and Queries* 218 (1973), 391–2.

Lohr, Charles H. *Latin Aristotle Commentaries, vol 2, Renaissance Authors.* Florence: Leo S. Olschki, 1988.

The London Gazette. 1671.

Lough, John. *France Observed in the Seventeenth Century by British Travellers.* Boston: Oriel Press, 1985.

Loveday, Robert. *Letters Domestick and Forrein, to Several Persons, Occasionally distributed in Subjects Philosophicall, Historicall & Morall.* 1659.

Lowe, John. *The Yew-Trees of Great Britain and Ireland.* London: Macmillan, 1897.

Lund, Mary Ann. "The Christian Physician." In Murphy and Todd, eds. "*A man very well studyed.*" 229–46.

Lushington, Thomas. *Logica analytica.* 1650.

—— *The Resurrection Rescued from the Souldiers Calumnies.* 1658.

Luzzatto, Simone. *Discorso circa il Stato de Gl'Hebrei et in Particolar... Venetia.* Intro. Riccardo Bachi. Facsimile of the 1638 edition, first published 1946, reprinted, Bologna: A. Forni, 1976.

Lyncker, Peter. *Samuel Hafenreffer (1587–1660): Leben, Werk, seine Bedeutung für die Dermatologie.* Dissertation, Eberhard-Karls University, Tübingen, 1966.

Lytton, Sir Edward Bulwer. "Sir Thomas Browne's Work (a review of Wilkin's edition)." In the October 1836 *Edinburgh Review*, 1–35.

MacKinnon, Murdoch. "An Unpublished Consultation Letter of Sir Thomas Browne." *Bulletin of the History of Medicine* 27 (1953), 503–11.

Maclean, Ian. "Heterodoxy in Natural Philosophy and Medicine: Pietro Pomponazzi, Guglielmo Grataroło, Girolamo Cardano." In John Brooke and Ian Maclean, eds. *Heterodoxy in Early Modern Science and Religion.* Oxford: Oxford University Press, 2005. 1–30.

——*Logic, Signs, and Nature in the Renaissance: The Case of Learned Medicine.* Cambridge: Cambridge University Press, 2002.

Macleane, Douglas. *A History of Pembroke College Oxford.* Oxford: Oxford Historical Society, 1897.

——*Pembroke College.* Reprinted London: Routledge/Thoemmes Press, 1998.

MacLysaght, Edward. *Irish Life in the Seventeenth Century.* Dublin: Irish Academic Press, 1979.

Mączak, Antoni. *Travel in Early Modern Europe.* Cambridge: Cambridge University Press, 1995.

Malavialle, L. *Le Bas-Languedoc en 1626 d'après la description du géographe allemande Abraham Golnitz.* Montpellier: Sociéte Anonyme de L'Imprimerie Générale du Midi, 1909.

Malkiel, David Joshua. *A Separate Republic: The Mechanics and Dynamics of Venetian Jewish Self-Government, 1607–1624.* Jerusalem: Magnes, 1991.

Manley, Lawrence, ed. *London in the Age of Shakespeare: An Anthology.* University Park: Pennsylvania State University Press, 1986.

Marchant, Ronald A. *The Puritans and the Church Courts in the Diocese of York, 1560–1642.* London: Longmans, 1960.

Marcus, Leah Sinanoglou. *Childhood and Cultural Despair: A Theme and Variations in Seventeenth-Century Literature.* Pittsburgh: University of Pittsburgh Press, 1978.
Mariani, Paola. "Johann Rhode." In Alessandro Minelli, ed. *The Botanical Garden of Padua, 1545–1995.* Venice: Marsilio, 1995.
Martin, L. C., ed. *Sir Thomas Browne: "Religio Medici" and Other Works.* Oxford: Clarendon Press, 1964.
Masterson, George. *The Triumph stain'd.* 1647.
[Mathew, Tobie?] *Charity Mistaken, with the Want Whereof, Catholickes are Vniustly Charged.* Saint-Omer, 1630.
Mayer, John. *A Commentarie vpon the New Testament.* 1631.
Mayerne, Théodore Turquet de. *Sommaire Description de La France, Allemagne, Italie, et Espagne.* Rouen,1604.
Maxwell, Susan M. "Robert Hues." *ODNB.*
McCabe, Richard, "Joseph Hall." *ODNB.*
McConica James. "Elizabethan Oxford: The Collegiate Society." In McConica, ed. *History of the University of Oxford. Volume III.* 645–732.
——ed. *The History of the University of Oxford: Volume III: The Collegiate University.* Oxford: Clarendon Press, 1986.
McCullough, Peter, ed. *Lancelot Andrewes: Selected Sermons & Lectures.* Oxford: Oxford University Press, 2005.
McDonnell, Sir Michael. *The Registers of St Paul's School, 1509–1748.* London: privately printed, 1977.
McGrath, Patrick. "Winchester College and the Old Religion in the Sixteenth Century." In Custance, ed. *Winchester College: Sixth-centenary Essays.* 229–80.
McLachlan, H. John. *Socinianism in Seventeenth-Century England.* Oxford: Oxford University Press, 1951.
McTavish, Lianne. *Childbirth and the Display of Authority in Early Modern France.* Burlington, VT: Ashgate, 2005.
Meeres, Frank. *A History of Norwich.* Chichester: Phillimore, 1998.
Mège, Alexandre du. *Histoire des institutions religieuses, politiques, judiciares et littéraires de la ville de Toulouse.* 4 vols. Toulouse: Larent Chapelle, 1844–1846.
Mendelsohn, Everett. *Heat and Life: The Development of the Theory of Animal Heat.* Cambridge, MA: Harvard University Press, 1964.
Mercer, Christia. "The Vitality and Importance of Early Modern Aristotelianism." In Tom Sorell, ed. *The Rise of Modern Philosophy: The Tension between the New and Traditional Philosophies from Machiavelli to Leibniz.* Oxford: Clarendon Press, 1993. 33–67.
Mercuriale, Girolamo. *De morbis puerorum.* Venice, 1588.
——*Sixteenth Century Physician and His Methods: Mercurialis on Diseases of the Skin.* Trans. and ed. Richard L. Sutton. Kansas City, MO: Lowell Press, 1986.
Merrett, Christopher. *The Character of a Compleat Physician, or Naturalist.* 1680.
Merryweather, John. *Directions for the Latine Tongue.* London, 1681.
Merton, E. S. "The Botany of Sir Thomas Browne." *Isis* 47 (1956), 161–71.
——"Microcosm, Epitome, and Seed: Some Seventeenth-Century Analogies." *History of Ideas News Letter* July (1957), 54–7.
——"Old and New Physiology in Sir Thomas Browne: Digestion and Some Other Functions." *Isis* 57 (1966), 249–59.
——*Science and Imagination in Sir Thomas Browne.* New York: Octagon, 1949.
——"Sir Thomas Browne as Zoologist." *Osiris* 9 (1950), 413–34.
——"Sir Thomas Browne on Astronomy." *History of Ideas News Letter* 4 (1958), 83–6.

——"Sir Thomas Browne's Embryological Theory." *Journal of the History of Medicine* 4 (1950), 416–21.

——"Sir Thomas Browne's Interpretation of Dreams." *Philological Quarterly* 28 (1949), 497–503.

——"Sir Thomas Browne's Theories of Respiration and Combustion." *Osiris* 10 (1952), 206–23.

Metters, G. A., ed. *The Parliamentary Survey of Dean and Chapter Properties in and around Norwich in 1649.* Norfolk Record Society 51 (1985).

Meursius, Joannes. *Athenae Batavae.* Leiden, 1625.

Michael, Emily. "The Nature and Influence of Late Renaissance Paduan Psychology." *History of Universities* 12 (1993), 65–94.

Midgley, Samuel. *Halifax and its Gibbet-Law Placed in a True Light.* London, 1708.

Mileham, John. "Dame Dorothy Browne and the Family of Mileham of Burlingham." *The Norfolk Ancestor* 2 (1982), 104–9.

Miller, Clarence H. "Seventeenth-Century Latin Translations of Two English Masterpieces: Hooker's *Polity* and Browne's *Religio Medici.*" In Roger Green et al., eds. *Acta Conventus Neo-Latini Abulensis: Proceedings of the Tenth International Congress of Neo-Latin Studies.* Tempe: Arizona Center for Medieval and Renaissance Studies, 2000. 55–72.

Miller, Genevieve. *The Adoption of Inoculation for Smallpox in England and France.* Philadelphia: University of Pennsylvania Press, 1957.

Miller, John. *Cities Divided: Politics and Religion in English Provincial Towns, 1660–1722.* Oxford: Oxford University Press, 2007.

—— *The Restoration and the England of Charles II.* 2nd ed. New York: Longman, 1997.

Miller, Peter N. "Description Terminable and Interminable: Looking at the Past, Nature, and Peoples in Peiresc's Archive." In Pomata and Siraisi, eds. *Historia: Empiricism and Erudition in Early Modern Europe.* 355–97.

Millican, Percy. "The Gawdys of Norfolk and Suffolk." *Norfolk and Norwich Archaeological Society* 26, part 2 (1938), 335–90.

——*Register of the Freemen of Norwich, 1548–1713.* Norwich: Norfolk Record Society, 1934.

Milner, Rev. John. *The History Civil and Ecclesiastical & Survey of the Antiquities of Winchester.* 2nd ed., corrected and enlarged. 2 vols. Winchester, 1809.

Milton, Anthony. *Catholic and Reformed: The Roman and Protestant Churches in English Protestant Thought, 1600–1640.* Cambridge: Cambridge University Press, 1995.

——*Laudian and Royalist Polemic in Seventeenth-Century England: The Career and Writings of Peter Heylyn.* Manchester: Manchester University Press, 2007.

Minadoi, Giovanni Tommaso. *De variolis et morbillis liber unicus.* Padua, 1603.

Modena, Leon, *The Autobiography of a Seventeenth-Century Venetian Rabbi: Leon Modena's 'Life of Judah.'* Trans. and ed. Mark R. Cohen. Princeton, NJ: Princeton University Press, 1988.

Molecamp, Femke. "'Of the incomparable treasure of the Holy Scriptures': The Geneva Bible in the Early Modern Household." In Matthew Dimmock and Andrew Hadfield, eds. *Literature and Popular Culture in Early Modern England.* Burlington, VT: Ashgate, 2009. 121–36.

Molhuysen, P. C., ed. *Bronnen tot de geschiedenis der Leidsche Universiteit.* 2nd part. s'Gravenhage: Martinus Nijhoff, 1916.

Mommsen, Theodor E. *Medieval and Renaissance Studies.* Ed. Eugene F. Rice, Jr. Ithaca, NY: Cornell University Press, 1959.

Moon, Antonia. "'A Fresh Reading of Books': Some Note-Taking Practices of Thomas Browne." In Murphy and Todd, eds. "*A man very well studyed.*" 67–86.

Moore, James. *The History of the Small Pox.* London: Longmans, 1815.
More, Henry. *Observations upon Anthroposophia theomagica, and Anima magica abscondita.* 1650.
More, Sir Thomas. *Utopia.* Ed. and trans. Robert M. Adams. 2nd ed. New York: Norton, 1992.
Morris, G. C. R. "Cradock, Amherst and Howell: A Link between the Selbys of Ightham and Sir Thomas Browne of Norwich." *Archaeologia Cantiana* 102 (1985), 11–18.
——"Sir Thomas Browne's Daughters, 'Cosen Barker,' and the Cottrells." *Notes and Queries* 231 (1986), 472–9.
Mortimer, Sarah. *Reason and Religion in the English Revolution: The Challenge of Socinianism.* Cambridge: Cambridge University Press, 2010.
Mortoft, Francis. *Francis Mortoft: His Book.* Ed. Malcolm Letts. London: Hakluyt Society, 1925.
Moryson, Fynes. *The Itinerary.* 4 vols. Glasgow: James MacLehose and Sons, 1907.
Muir, Edward. *Civic Ritual in Renaissance Venice.* Princeton, NJ: Princeton University Press, 1981.
——*The Culture Wars of the Late Renaissance: Skeptics, Libertines, and Opera.* Cambridge, MA: Harvard University Press, 2007.
Muller, Jeffrey. "Jesuit Uses of Art in the Province of Flanders." In O'Malley et al., eds. *The Jesuits II.* 113–56.
Munday, Anthony. *Camp-bell, or the Ironmongers faire field.* 1609.
——*Himatia Poleos.* 1614.
Munk, William. *The Roll of the Royal College of Physicians of London.* Vol. 1. London: Royal College of Physicians, 1878.
Murison, William, ed. *Religio Medici.* Cambridge: Cambridge University Press, 1922.
Murphy, Kathryn. "'The best pillar of St Francis': Thomas Browne and Samuel Hartlib." In Murphy and Todd, eds. "*A Man very well studyed.*" 273–92.
——"'Between the Paws of a Sphinx': The Contexts of Thomas Browne." In Murphy and Todd, eds. "*A man very well studyed.*" 3–12.
——"'A Likely Story': Plato's *Timaeus* in the *Garden of Cyrus.*" In Barbour and Preston, eds. *Sir Thomas Browne: The World Proposed.* 242–57.
——"'A man of excellent parts': The Manuscript Readers of Thomas Browne's *Religio Medici.*" *TLS* July 4, 2008, 14–15.
Murphy, Kathryn, and Richard Todd, eds. "*A man very well studyed": New Contexts for Thomas Browne.* Leiden: Brill, 2008.
Muskett, J. J. "From a Herald's Letter Book, No. IV." *The East Anglian* 13 (1909), 88–9.
Myers, Anne M. *Literature and Architecture in Early Modern England.* Baltimore, MD: Johns Hopkins University Press, 2013.
Nance, Brian. *Turquet de Mayerne as Baroque Physician: The Art of Medical Portraiture.* New York: Rodopi, 2001.
Napier, Henry Alfred. *Historical Notices of the Parishes of Swyncombe and Ewelme in the County of Oxford.* Oxford: James Wright, 1858.
Naudé, Gabriel. *Gabrielis Navdæi... Epistolæ.* Geneva, 1667.
Nedham, Marchamont. *Medela Medicinæ.* London, 1665.
Needham, Joseph. *A History of Embryology.* Cambridge: Cambridge University Press, 1934.
Nelson, Brent. "The Browne Family's Culture of Curiosity." In Barbour and Preston, eds. *The World Proposed.* 80–99.
Newman, Sir George. *A Century of Medicine at Padua.* London: British Periodicals, 1922.

Niero, Antonio. "I temple del Redentore e della Salute: motivazioni teologiche." In *Venezia e la Peste 1348/1797*. Preface Paolo Peruzza. Venice: Marsilio Editori, 1979. 294–328.

Norton, David. *A History of the English Bible as Literature*. New York: Cambridge University Press, 2000.

Nougaret, Jean. "Les Constructions du Jardin de Pierre Richer de Belleval." In Rioux, ed. *Le Jardin des Plantes de Montpellier*. 97–102.

O'Brien, George, ed. *Advertisements for Ireland*. Dublin: The Royal Society of Antiquaries of Ireland, 1923.

O'Day, Rosemary. "Hugh Robinson." *ODNB*.

—— *The Professions in Early Modern England, 1450–1800: Servants of the Commonweal*. New York: Longman, 2000.

Oerle, H. A. van. *Leiden binnen en buiten de stadvesten*. Leiden: Brill, 1975.

Ogilvie, Brian W. "Natural History, Ethics, and Physico-Theology." In Pomata and Siraisi, eds. *Historia*. 75–103.

—— *The Science of Describing: Natural History in Renaissance Europe*. Chicago: University of Chicago Press, 2006.

Oldenburg, Henry. *The Correspondence of Henry Oldenburg*. Ed. A. Rupert Hall and Marie Boas Hall. 13 vols. (vols. 1–9 Madison: University of Wisconsin Press; vols. 10–11 London: Mansell; vols. 12–13 London: Taylor and Francis), 1965–86.

O'Malley, John W. et al., eds. *The Jesuits II: Cultures, Sciences, and the Arts, 1540–1773*. Toronto: University of Toronto Press, 2006.

Oppenheimer, Jane M. "John Hunter, Sir Thomas Browne and the Experimental Method." *Bulletin of the History of Medicine* 21 (1947), 17–32.

Orlers, J. J. *Beschrijvinge der Stadt Leyden*. 1641.

Orlin, Lena, ed. *Material London, ca. 1600*. Philadelphia: University of Pennsylvania Press, 2000.

Otterspeer, Willem. *Groepsportret met Dame, I: Het bolwerk van de vrijheid: de Leidse universiteit 1575–1672*. Amsterdam: Bert Bakker, 2000.

Overbury, Sir Thomas. "Sir Thomas Overbury's Observations in his Travels, upon the State of the Seventeen Provinces, As they stood Anno Domini, 1609 (published 1626)." In *The Harleian Miscellany*. Vol. 3. London: Robert Dutton, 1809. 97–100.

Oxford Dictionary of National Biography Online (ODNB). Oxford: Oxford University Press, 2004. (http://www.oup.com/oxforddnb/)

Palamedes. "Mr. Sainthill and His Basque Studies." *Notes and Queries*, 9th series, 3 (March, 1899), 201–2.

Palmer, Richard. " 'Ad Una Sancta Perfettione': Health Care and Poor Relief in the Republic of Venice in the Era of the Counter-Reformation." In Ole Peter Grell and Andrew Cunningham, with Jon Arrizabalaga, eds. *Health Care and Poor Relief in Counter-Reformation Europe*. New York: Routledge, 1999. 87–101.

—— "Pharmacy in the Republic of Venice in the Sixteenth Century." In Andrew Wear et al., eds. *The Medical Renaissance of the Sixteenth Century*. New York: Cambridge University Press, 1985. 100–17.

Parr, Johnstone. "Sir Thomas Browne's Birthday." *English Language Notes* 11 (1973), 44–6.

Parry, Graham. *The Arts of the Anglican Counter-Reformation: Glory, Laud and Honour*. Woodbridge, Suffolk: Boydell Press, 2006.

—— *The Trophies of Time: English Antiquarians of the Seventeenth Century*. Oxford: Oxford University Press, 1995.

Pater, Walter. "Sir Thomas Browne." *Macmillan's Magazine* 54 (1886), 5–18.

Patin, Guy. *Naudæana et Patineana*. Paris, 1701.

Patrides, C. A., ed. *Approaches to Sir Thomas Browne*. Columbia: University of Missouri Press, 1982.
——ed. *Sir Thomas Browne: The Major Works*. New York: Penguin, 1977.
Payne, J. F. "Thomas Browne [Browne's grandson]." Revised Michael Bevan. *ODNB*.
Pebworth, Ted-Larry. "Wandering in the America of Truth: *Pseudodoxia Epidemica* and the Essay Tradition." In Patrides, ed. *Approaches to Sir Thomas Browne*. 166–77.
Peck, Linda Levy. *Consuming Splendor: Society and Culture in Seventeenth-Century England*. Cambridge: Cambridge University Press, 2005.
Pellegrini, Francesco. *La Clinica Medica Padovana Attraverso I Secoli*. Verona: La Tipographia Veronese, 1939.
Pelling, Margaret. *The Common Lot: Sickness, Medical Occupations, and the Urban Poor in Early Modern England*. New York: Longmans, 1998.
——"Illness among the Poor in an Early Modern English Town." *Continuity and Change* 3 (1988), 273–90.
——"Medical Practice in Early Modern England: Trade or Profession?" In Wilfrid Prest, ed. *The Professions in Early Modern England*. New York: Croom Helm, 1987. 90–128.
——"Who Most Needs to Marry? Ageing and Inequality among Women and Men in Early Modern Norwich." In Lynn Botelho and Pat Thane, eds. *Women and Ageing in British Society Since 1500*. New York: Longman: 2001. 31–42.
Pelling, Margaret, and Charles Webster. "Medical practitioners." In Charles Webster, ed. *Health, Medicine, and Mortality in the Sixteenth Century*. New York: Cambridge University Press, 1979. 165–235.
Peltonen, Markku. *The Duel in Early Modern England: Civility, Politeness and Honour*. New York: Cambridge University Press, 2003.
Pepys, Samuel. *The Diary of Samuel Pepys*. Ed. Robert Latham and William Mathews. 9 vols. Berkeley: University of California Press, 2000.
Péronnet, Michel. "La théologie à Montpellier durant l'époque moderne." In *L'Université de Montpellier: ses maîtres et ses étudiants depuis sept siècles, 1289–1989*. Montpellier: La Fédération, 1995. 59–70.
Perrott, John. *Battering Rams against Rome*. 1661.
Pevsner, Nikolaus, and Bill Wilson. *The Buildings of England: Norfolk 1: Norwich and North-East*. London: Penguin, 1997.
Philosophical Transactions. May 1669.
Picard, Liza. *Elizabeth's London: Everyday Life in Elizabethan London*. New York: St Martin's Griffin, 2003.
Pine, Martin L. *Pietro Pomponazzi: Radical Philosopher of the Renaissance*. Padua: Antenore, 1986.
Pinon, Laurent. "Conrad Gessner and the Historical Depth of Renaissance Natural History." In Pomata and Siraisi, eds. *Historia*. 241–67.
Platter, Thomas. *Journal of a Younger Brother: The Life of Thomas Platter as a Medical Student in Montpellier at the Close of the Sixteenth Century*. Trans. and intro. Seán Jennett. London: Frederick Muller, 1968.
Plomer, H. R. et al. *A Dictionary of the Booksellers and Printers Who Were at Work in England, Scotland, and Ireland from 1641 to 1667*. London: Bibliographical Society, 1907.
Plooij, D. *The Pilgrim Fathers from a Dutch Point of View*. New York: New York University Press, 1932.
Pol, Elfriede Hulshoff. "The Library." In Scheurleer and Meyjes, eds. *Leiden University in the Seventeenth Century*. 395–459.
Pomata, Gianna, and Nancy G. Siraisi, eds. *Historia: Empiricism and Erudition in Early Modern Europe*. Cambridge, MA: MIT Press, 2005.

Porritt, Arthur. *Halifax as it Was*. Nelson, Lancashire: Hendon, 1973.
Porro, Girolamo. *L'Horti de I Semplici di Padoua*. Venice, 1591.
Porter, Bertha. "Richard Mocket." Revised Glenn Burgess. *ODNB*.
Porter, Edmund. *Θεος Ἀνθρωποφρος: or God Incarnate*. 1655.
Porter, Stephen. "University and Society." In Tyacke, ed. *The History of the University of Oxford: Volume IV*. 25–103.
Post, Jonathan F. S. "Browne's Life: A 'Cabinet of Rarities.'" *English Language Notes* 19 (1982), 313–35.
—— "Miscellaneous Browne among the Tombs of Norwich Cathedral." In Barbour and Preston, eds. *Sir Thomas Browne: The World Proposed*. 258–75.
—— *Sir Thomas Browne*. Boston: Twayne, 1987.
Potter, Christopher. *Want of Charitie Justly Charged*. 1633, rev. ed. 1634.
Pound, John. "Government to 1660." In Rawcliffe and Wilson, eds. *Norwich since 1550*. 35–61.
—— *Tudor and Stuart Norwich*. Chichester: Phillimore, 1988.
Powell, Anthony. *John Aubrey and His Friends*. London: Heinemann, 1963.
Power, Henry. *Experimental Philosophy*. Reprint of 1664 edition, intro. Marie Boas Hall. New York: Johnson Reprint Corporation, 1966.
Premuda, L. and B. Bertolaso. "La Prima Sede dell'Insegnamento Clinico nel Mondo: L'Ospedale di S. Francesco Grande in Padova." *Acta Medicae Historiae Patavina* 7 (1960–61), 61–92.
Prest, John. *The Garden of Eden: The Botanic Garden and the Re-Creation of Paradise*. New Haven, CT: Yale University Press, 1981.
Preston, Claire. "'An Incomium of Consumptions': *A Letter to a Friend* as Medical Narrative." In Barbour and Preston, eds. *Sir Thomas Browne: The World Proposed*. 206–21.
—— *Thomas Browne and the Writing of Early Modern Science*. Cambridge: Cambridge University Press, 2005.
Prestwich, Edmund. *The Hectors, or, The False Challenge: A Comedy*. 1656.
Preto, Paolo. "Le grandi pesti dell'età moderna: 1575–77 e 1630–31." In *Venezia e la Peste 1348/1797*. Preface by Paolo Peruzza. Venice: Marsilio Editori, 1979. 123–56.
Priestley, Ursula. *The Great Market: A Survey of Nine Hundred Years of Norwich Provision Market*. Norwich: University of East Anglia, 1987.
Primerose, James. *Academia Monspeliensis*. 1631.
—— *Partes duæ de morbis puerorum*. Rotterdam, 1659.
Proclus. *The Elements of Theology: A Revised Text*. Trans., intro., and commentary E. R. Dodds. Oxford: Clarendon Press, 1933.
Pullan, Brian. *The Jews of Europe and the Inquisition of Venice, 1550–1670*. Oxford: Blackwell, 1983.
Puppi, Lionello, and Mario Universo. *Le citta nella storia d'Italia: Padova*. Rome: Laterza, 1982.
Raach, John A. *A Directory of English Country Physicians, 1603–1643*. London: Dawsons, 1962.
Rabelais, François. *The Complete Works of François Rabelais*. Trans. Donald Frame. Berkeley: University of California Press, 1991.
Radbill, Samuel X. "Pediatrics." In Allen G. Debus, ed. *Medicine in Seventeenth-Century England*. Berkeley: University of California Press, 1974. 237–82.
Ramsden, Henry. *A Gleaning in Gods Harvest*. 1639.
Ranchin, François. *Commentarius in Hippocratis*. 1618.
—— *Opuscula medica*. 1627.
—— *Opuscules; ou, Traictés divers et curieux en médicine*. 1640.
—— *Traité de la Peste*. 1637.

Ranchin, François. *Tractatus duo posthumi*. 1645.
Randall, John Herman. *The School of Padua and the Emergence of Modern Science*. Padua: Antenore, 1961.
Rappaport, Steve. *Worlds within Worlds: Structures of Life in Sixteenth-Century London*. Cambridge: Cambridge University Press, 1989.
Rashdall, Hastings, and Robert S. Rait. *New College*. London: F. E. Robinson, 1901.
Raven, Charles E. *English Naturalists from Neckam to Ray: A Study of the Making of the Modern World*. Cambridge: Cambridge University Press, 1947.
——*John Ray, Naturalist: His Life and Works*. Cambridge: Cambridge University Press, 1950.
Ravid, Benjamin. "Curfew Time in the Ghetto of Venice." Reprinted in *Studies on the Jews of Venice, 1382–1797*. Burlington, VT: Ashgate, 2003. Separately paginated 237–75.
Rawcliffe, Carole. *Medicine for the Soul: The Life, Death and Resurrection of an English Medieval Hospital, St Giles's, Norwich, c. 1249–1550*. Stroud, Gloucestershire: Sutton, 1999.
Rawcliffe, Carole, and Richard Wilson, eds. *Medieval Norwich*. London: Hambledon and London, 2004.
Rawcliffe, Carole, and Richard Wilson, eds. *Norwich since 1550*. New York: Hambledon and London, 2004.
Ray, John. *Catalogus Plantarum Angliæ*. 1670.
——*A Collection of English words not generally used*. 1673.
——*Observations topographical, moral, & physiological*. 1673.
——*The Ornithology of Francis Willughby*. 1678.
Raymond, Thomas. *Autobiography of Thomas Raymond*. Ed. G. Davies. London: Camden Society, 1917.
Reay, Barry. *The Quakers and the English Revolution*. London: Temple Smith, 1985.
Redondi, Pietro. *Galileo Heretic*. Princeton, NJ: Princeton University Press, 1987.
Redworth, Glyn. *The Prince and the Infanta: The Cultural Politics of the Spanish Match*. New Haven, CT: Yale University Press, 2003.
Reeds, Karen Meier. *Botany in Medieval and Renaissance Universities*. Thesis, Harvard University, 1975.
Reimmann, Jacob Friedrich. *Historia Universalis Atheismi*. 1725.
Report on the Manuscripts of the Family of Gawdy, Formerly of Norfolk. Hist. MSS. Comm. Rep. 1885.
Report on the Manuscripts of the Marquess of Downshire. 6 vols. Royal Commission on Historical Manuscripts, London: H M Stationery Office, 1924–1995.
Reynolds, Edward. *Twenty-Five Sermons Preached upon Several Occasions*. 1663.
Reynolds, Matthew. *Godly Reformers and Their Opponents in Early Modern England: Religion in Norwich, c.1560–1643*. Rochester, NY: Boydell, 2005.
Rhegius, Urbanus. *An Homely or Sermon of Good and Euill Angels*. 1590.
Rhodes, Dennis E. "The Botanical Garden of Padua: The First Hundred Years." *Journal of Garden History* 4 (1984), 327–31.
Rich, Barnabe. *A New Description of Ireland*. London: 1610.
Ridder-Symoens, Hilde de, ed. *A History of the University in Europe*. Vol. 2. Cambridge: Cambridge University Press, 1996.
Riddle, John M. *Contraception and Abortion from the Ancient World to the Renaissance*. Cambridge, MA: Harvard University Press, 1992.
——*Eve's Herbs: A History of Contraception and Abortion in the West*. Cambridge, MA: Harvard University Press, 1997.
Rioux, Jean-Antoine. *Le Jardin des Plantes de Montpellier: 'Les leçons de l'histoire.'* Montpellier: Sauramps, 2003.

——ed. *Le Jardin des Plantes de Montpellier: Quatre siècles d'histoire.* Grauhlet: Odyssée, 1994.

Rivière, Lazare. *Lazari Riverii... Opera Medica Universa.* 1738.

Robbins, Robin. "Browne's Cosmos Imagined: Nature, Man, and God in *Pseudodoxia Epidemica.*" In Patrides, ed. *Approaches to Sir Thomas Browne.* 155–65.

——"Sir Thomas Browne." *ODNB.*

——ed. *Sir Thomas Browne: Pseudodoxia Epidemica.* 2 vols. Oxford: Clarendon Press, 1981.

Robb-Smith, A. H. T. "Cambridge Medicine." In Debus, ed. *Medicine in Seventeenth Century England.* 327–69.

Roberts, S. C., ed. *Sir Thomas Browne's Christian Morals.* Cambridge: Cambridge University Press, 1927; reprinted New York: Kraus Reprint Co., 1969.

Robinson, Hugh. *Annalium mundi universalium.* 1677.

——*I. Preces. II. Grammaticalia Quaedam. III. Rhetorica Brevis.* Oxford, 1616.

Robinson, John, Jr. *Endoxa.* Latin 1656, English 1658.

Robinson, John, Sr. *The Works of John Robinson, Pastor of the Pilgrim Fathers.* Ed. Robert Ashton. London: John Snow, 1851.

Rode, Johan. *De acia dissertatio.* 1639.

——*Observationum medicinalium.* 1657.

——*Scribonii Largi, Compositiones medicae.* 1655.

Rooden, Peter T. van. *Theology, Biblical Scholarship and Rabbinical Studies in the Seventeenth Century: Constantijn L'Empereur (1591–1648), Professor of Hebrew and Theology at Leiden.* New York: Brill, 1989.

Rosen, Adrienne. "Winchester in Transition, 1580–1700." In Peter Clark, ed. *Country Towns in Pre-Industrial England.* New York: St Martin's Press, 1981. 143–95.

Rosenheim, James M., *The Townshends of Raynham: Nobility in Transition in Restoration and Early Hanoverian England.* Middletown, CT: Wesleyan University Press, 1989.

——ed. *The Notebook of Robert Doughty 1662–1665.* Norfolk Record Society 54, 1989.

Ross, Alexander. *Arcana microcosmi, or, The hid secrets of man's body discovered in an anatomical duel between Aristotle and Galen concerning the parts thereof.* 1652.

——*Medicus medicatus.* 1645.

Rossetti, Lucia. *The University of Padua: An Outline of Its History.* Trieste: LINT, 1983.

——ed. *Acta Nationis Germanicae Artistarum (1616–1636).* Padua: Editrice Antenore, 1967.

Ruestow, Edward G. *Physics at Seventeenth and Eighteenth-Century Leiden: Philosophy and the New Science in the University.* The Hague: Martinus Nijhoff, 1973.

Ruhräh, John, ed. *Pediatrics of the Past: An Anthology.* New York: Paul B. Hoeber, 1925.

Rural Houses of West Yorkshire, 1400–1830. London: HMSO, 1986.

Rutledge, Paul. "Doctor Thomas Browne." *Norfolk Archaeology* 44 (2005), 712–13.

Rye, Walter. *Some Historical Essays Chiefly Relating to Norfolk.* Part 6. Norwich: H.W. Hunt, 1928.

——"What Brought Sir Thomas Browne to Norwich?" *Norfolk Antiquarian Miscellany,* 2nd series, 1 (1906), 83–5.

——ed. *Extracts from the Court Books of the City of Norwich, 1666–1688.* Norwich: Norfolk and Norwich Archæological Society, 1905.

Sala, Giovanni Domenico. *Ars Medica.* Venice, 1620.

——*De Alimentis et eorum recta administratione.* Padua, 1628.

Salkeld, John. *A Treatise of Angels.* 1613.

Salmon, J. H. M. "Degory Wheare." *ODNB.*

Salmon, J. H. M. "Precept, Example, and Truth: Degory Wheare and the Ars Historica." In Donald R. Kelley and David Harris Sacks, eds. *The Historical Imagination in Early Modern Britain: History, Rhetoric, and Fiction, 1500–1800.* Cambridge: Cambridge University Press, 1997. 11–36.

Sanna, Vittoria, ed. *Religio Medici: Edizione Critica con Introduzione e Note.* 2 vols. Cagliari: Annali delle Facoltà di Lettere-Filosofia e Magistero dell'Università di Cagliari, 1958.

Saunders, H. W. *A History of the Norwich Grammar School.* Norwich: Jarrold and Sons, 1932.

Savage, Henry. *Balliofergus, or a Commentary upon the Foundation, Founders and Affaires, of Balliol Colledge.* Oxford, 1668.

Sberti, Anton-Bonaventura. *Degli Spettacoli e delle Feste che si facevano in Padova.* Padua, 1818.

Schama, Simon. *The Embarrassment of Riches: An Interpretation of Dutch Culture in the Golden Age.* London: Harper, 1987.

Scharpe, George. *Institutiones Medicae.* 1638.

Scheurleer, Th. H. Lunsingh. "Un amphithéâtre d'anatomie moralisée." In Scheurleer and G. H. M. Posthumus Meyjes, eds. *Leiden University in the Seventeenth Century.* 217–78.

Scheurleer, Th. H. Lunsingh, and G. H. M. Posthumus Meyjes, eds. *Leiden University in the Seventeenth Century: An Exchange of Learning.* Leiden: Brill, 1975.

Schmitt, Charles B. *The Aristotelian Tradition and Renaissance Universities.* London: Variorum, 1984.

——*Aristotle and the Renaissance.* Cambridge, MA: Harvard University Press, 1983.

Schoeck, R. J., ed. *Sir Thomas Browne and the Republic of Letters. English Language Notes* 19 (1982).

Schofield, Bertram, ed. *The Knyvett Letters, 1620–1644.* Norwich: Norfolk Record Society, 1949.

Schofield, John, ed. *The London Surveys of Ralph Treswell.* London Topographical Society, Publication 135, 1987.

Scholder, Klaus. *The Birth of Modern Critical Theology: Origins and Problems of Biblical Criticism in the Seventeenth Century.* Trans. John Bowden. Philadelphia: Trinity Press International, 1990.

Schoneveld, Cornelis W. *Intertraffic of the Mind: Studies in Seventeenth-Century Anglo-Dutch Translation with a Checklist of Books Translated from English into Dutch, 1600–1700.* Leiden: Brill, 1983.

——"Sir Thomas Browne and Leiden University in 1633." Originally in *English Language Notes* 19 (1982), 335–59; reworked in *Sea-Changes: Studies in Three Centuries of Anglo-Dutch Cultural Transmission.* Amsterdam: Rodopi, 1996. 1–30.

——"'The True Anatomy of My Selfe.'" In *Sir Thomas Browne, M.D. and the Anatomy of Man.* Leiden: Brill, 1982. 5–9.

Schouten, Jacob. *Johannes Walaeus.* Assen: Van Gorcum, 1972.

Schwartz, Gary, and Marten Jan Bok. *Pieter Saenredam: The Painter and His Time.* New York: Abbeville, 1989.

Schwarz, Marc L. "Lay Anglicanism and the Crisis of the English Church in the Early Seventeenth Century." *Albion* 14 (1982), 1–19.

Schwyzer, Philip. *Archaeologies of English Renaissance Literature.* Oxford: Oxford University Press, 2007.

Scot, Patrick. *The Tillage of Light.* 1624.

Screech, M. A., ed. and intro. *Richard Mocket, Doctrina et Politia Ecclesiae Anglicanae: An Anglican Summa: Facsimile, with Variants, of the Texts of 1617.* Leiden: Brill, 1995.

Seaton, Ethel. *Literary Relations of England and Scandanavia in the Seventeenth Century.* Oxford: Clarendon Press, 1935; reissued, New York: Blom, 1972.

Sebastian, Anton. *A Dictionary of the History of Medicine.* New York: Parthenon, 1999.

Sellin, Paul R. *Daniel Heinsius and Stuart England.* Leiden: Leiden University Press, 1968.

Sells, A. Lytton. *The Paradise of Travellers: The Italian Influence on Englishmen in the Seventeenth Century.* Bloomington: Indiana University Press, 1964.

Seneca. *Tragedies of Seneca.* Ed. and trans. Frank Justus Miller. 2 vols. Cambridge, MA: Harvard University Press, 1961.

Sennert, Daniel. *Sixth book of Practical Physick.* 1662.

Sessions, W. A. *Henry Howard, The Poet Earl of Surrey: A Life.* New York: Oxford University Press, 1999.

Shannon, Laurie. *Sovereign Amity: Figures of Friendship in Shakespearean Contexts.* Chicago: University of Chicago Press, 2002.

Sharp, David M. *The Church of St Peter Mancroft, Norwich.* Norwich: Jarrold, 1994.

Sharpe, James. *Instruments of Darkness: Witchcraft in England, 1550–1750.* New York: Penguin, 1996.

Sharrock, Robert. *History of Vegetables.* 1660.

Sheils, William, and Sarah Sheils. "Textiles and Reform: Halifax and its Hinterland." In Patrick Collinson and John Craig, eds. *The Reformation in English Towns, 1500–1640.* New York: St Martins, 1998. 130–43.

Shuger, Debora. "The Laudian Idiot." In Barbour and Preston, eds. *Sir Thomas Browne: The World Proposed.* 36–62.

Shurkin, Joel N. *The Invisible Fire: The Story of Mankind's Victory over the Ancient Scourge of Smallpox.* New York: G. P. Putnam's Sons, 1979.

Shurlock, Barry. *The Winchester Story.* Horndean, Hampshire: Milestone, 1986.

Silvaticus, Benedictus. *Consiliorvm et Responsorvm Medicinalivm Centuriæ Qvatvor.* Geneva, 1662.

Silver, Victoria. "'Wonders of the Invisible World': The Trial of the Lowestoft Witches." In Barbour and Preston, eds. *Sir Thomas Browne: The World Proposed.* 118–45.

Siraisi, Nancy G. *Medieval & Early Renaissance Medicine: An Introduction to Knowledge and Practice.* Chicago: University of Chicago Press, 1990.

Sixth Report of the Royal Commission on Historical Manuscripts. London: Eyre & Spottiswoode, 1877.

Slack, Paul. *From Reformation to Improvement: Public Welfare in Early Modern England.* Oxford: Clarendon Press, 1999.

Sloan, A. W. *English Medicine in the Seventeenth Century.* Durham, England: Durham Academic Press, 1996.

Smith, A. Hassell, and D. MacCulloch. "The Authorship of the Chorographies of Norfolk and Suffolk." *Norfolk Archaeology* 36 (1977), 327–41.

Smith, Cyril Eugene. *The University of Toulouse in the Middle Ages: Its Origins and Growth to 1500 A.D.* Milwaukee, WI: Marquette University Press, 1958.

Smith, David L. "Catholic, Anglican or Puritan? Edward Sackville, Fourth Earl of Dorset, and the Ambiguities of Religion in Early Stuart England." *Transactions of the Royal Historical Society*, 6th series, 2 (1992), 105–24.

Smith, J. R. *The Speckled Monster: Smallpox in England, 1670–1970, with particular reference to Essex.* Chelmsford: Essex Record Office, 1987.

Smith, Nigel. *Literature and Revolution in England, 1640–1660.* New Haven, CT: Yale University Press, 1994.

——"Sir Thomas Browne and the Levellers." *Notes and Queries*, n.s., 33 (1986), 421–2.

Smith, R. W. Innes. *English-Speaking Students of Medicine at the University of Leyden.* Edinburgh: Oliver and Boyd, 1932.

Southwell, Thomas, ed. *Notes and Letters on the Natural History of Norfolk... from the Mss. Of Sir Thomas Browne, M.D.... in the Sloane Collection in the Library of the British Museum and in the Bodleian Library, Oxford.* London: Jarrold & Sons, 1902.

Spanio, Michela L. Nichetti. "Accademie Padovane nel Sei e nel Settecento." In *Accademie e Cultura: Aspetti Storici tra Sei e Settecento.* Florence: Leo S. Olschki, 1979. 211–21.

Spitzel, Theophilus. *Theophili Spizelii Scrutinium Atheismi Historico-Ætologicum.* 1663.

Sprague, R. K., ed. *The Older Sophists.* Columbia, SC: University of South Carolina Press, 1972.

Sprott, Samuel Ernest. *Tom Browne's Schooldays: A Study of the Education of Sir Thomas Browne at Winchester College.* PhD diss., Columbia University, 1954.

Sprunger, Keith L. *Dutch Puritanism: A History of English and Scottish Churches of the Netherlands in the Sixteenth and Seventeenth Centuries.* Leiden: Brill, 1982.

Stevens, Charles. *Winchester Notions: The English Dialect of Winchester College.* New Brunswick, NJ: The Athlone Press, 1998.

Stevenson, Matthew. *Norfolk Drollery.* 1673.

Still, George Frederic. *The History of Paediatrics: The Progress of the Study of Diseases of Children up to the End of the XVIIIth Century.* Oxford: Oxford University Press, 1931.

Stoker, David. "'To all Booksellers, Country Chapmen, Hawkers and Others': How the Population of East Anglia Obtained Its Printed Materials." In Robin Myers et al., eds. *Fairs, Markets and the Itinerant Book Trade.* London: The British Library, 2007. 107–36.

Stow, John. *A Survey of London by John Stow.* Ed. Charles Lethbridge Kingsford. 2 vols. Oxford: Clarendon Press, 1908.

Stoye, John. *English Travellers Abroad, 1604–1667: Their Influence in English Society and Politics.* Revised ed., New Haven, CT: Yale University Press, 1989.

Strafford, Thomas Wentworth, Earl of. *The Earl of Strafforde's Letters and Dispatches.* Vol. 1. London, 1739.

Strien, C. D. van. *British Travellers in Holland during the Stuart Period: Edward Browne and John Locke as Tourists in the United Provinces.* New York: Brill, 1993.

Strien, Kees van. "Edward Browne." *ODNB.*

Strode, William. *The Poetical Works.* Ed. Bertram Dobell. London: B. Dobell, 1907.

Stroumsa, Guy G. *A New Science: The Discovery of Religion in the Age of Reason.* Cambridge, MA: Harvard University Press, 2010.

Stubbings, Frank. "A Latin Verse Epistle of Joshua Barnes to Sir Thomas Browne." *Cambridge Bibliographical Society* 10 (1991), 86–91.

Swann, Marjorie. *Curiosities and Texts: The Culture of Collecting in Early Modern England.* Philadelphia: University of Pennsylvania Press, 2001.

——"'Procreate like Trees': Generation and Society in Thomas Browne's *Religio Medici.*" In Barbara Hanawalt and Lisa Kiser, eds. *Nature in the Middle Ages and Renaissance.* Notre Dame, IN: University of Notre Dame Press, 2008. 137–54.

Swart, K. W. *The Miracle of the Dutch Republic as Seen in the Seventeenth Century.* London: H. K. Lewis, 1969.

Tanner, J. R. *A Descriptive Catalogue of the Naval Manuscripts in the Pepysian Library at Magdalene College, Cambridge.* London: Naval Records Society, 1903.

Tapié, Victor-L. *France in the Age of Louis XIII and Richelieu*. Trans. and ed. D. Mc.N. Lockie. New York: Praeger, 1975.

Taylor, D. "Annals of the Parish of Halifax." *Halifax Antiquarian Society* (1972), 107–30.

Taylor, E. G. R. *Late Tudor and Early Stuart Geography, 1583–1650*. London: Methuen, 1934.

Taylor, John, the Water Poet. *Part of this Summers Travels, or News from Hell, Hull, and Hallifax*. 1639.

Temkin, Owsei. *Galenism: Rise and Decline of a Medical Philosophy*. Ithaca, NY: Cornell University Press, 1973.

Tenison, Thomas. *Baconiana, or, Certain Genuine Remains of Sr. Francis Bacon*. 1679.

—— *The Creed of Mr. Hobbes Examined*. 1670.

Tildesley, Miriam L. *Sir Thomas Browne: His Skull, Portraits, and Ancestry*. Reprinted from *Biometrika* 15 for subscribers only, 1923.

Tjon Sie Fat, Leslie. "Clusius' garden: a reconstruction." In Tjon Sie Fat and Jong, eds. *The Authentic Garden*. 3–12.

Tjon Sie Fat, Leslie, and E. de Jong, eds. *The Authentic Garden: A Symposium on Gardens*. Leiden: Clusius Foundation, 1991.

Todd, Margo. *Christian Humanism and the Puritan Social Order*. Cambridge: Cambridge University Press, 1987.

Tomasino, J. P. *Gymnasium Patavinum*. 1654.

——*Illustrium virorum elogia*. 1630.

Toynbee, M. "Some Friends of Sir Thomas Browne." *Norfolk Archaeology* 31 (1957), 377–94.

Toynbee, M., and Gyles Isham. "Joan Carlile (1606?–1679): An Identification." *Burlington Magazine* 96 (1954), 275–7.

A Tryal of Witches at the Assizes Held at Bury St. Edmonds. London, 1682.

Turner, J. Horsfall. *Biographia Halifaxiensis*. Bingley, 1883.

Tyacke, Nicholas. *Anti-Calvinists: The Rise of English Arminianism, c.1590–1640*. Oxford: Clarendon Press, 1987.

——"Science and Religion at Oxford before the Civil War." In Donald Pennington and Keith Thomas, eds. *Puritans and Revolutionaries: Essays in Seventeenth-Century History presented to Christopher Hill*. Oxford: Clarendon Press, 1978. 73–93.

——ed. *The History of the University of Oxford: Volume IV, Seventeenth-Century Oxford*. Oxford: Clarendon Press, 1997.

Tyler, Dorothy. "A Review of the Interpretation of Sir Thomas Browne's Part in the Witch Trial of 1664." *Anglia* 54 (1930), 179–95.

Tyson, Edward. *Phocæna, or the Anatomy of a Porpess, Dissected at Gresham College*. 1680.

——trans. *J. Swammerdam's Ephemeri Vita*. 1681.

Ulvioni, Paolo. *Il Gran Castigo di Dio: Carestia ed epidemie a Venezia e nella Terraferma 1628–1632*. Milan: Franco Angeli, 1989.

Vance, Shona MacLean. "Alexander Read." *ODNB*.

Vaughan, Thomas. *A Brief Natural History... with Refutations of such Vulgar Errours as our Modern Authors have omitted*. 1669.

Vedova, Giuseppe. *Biografia degli Scrittori Padovani*. 2 vols. Padua, 1832–36.

Veendorp, H., and L. G. M. Baas Becking. *Hortvs Academicvs Lvgdvno-Batavvs 1587–1937*. Harlaam: Enschedaiana, 1938.

Venezia e la Peste 1348/1797. Preface by Paolo Peruzza. Venice: Marsilio Editori, 1979.

Venn, John, and J. A. Venn, eds. *Alumni Cantabrigiensis.* Cambridge: Cambridge University Press, 1924.
Vesling, Johann. *De Plantis Aegyptiis observationes et notae ad Prosperum Alpinum.* 1638.
——*Syntagma Anatomicum.* 1647.
The Victoria History of the Counties of England: Hampshire and the Isle of Wight. Westminster: A. Constable, 1900–12.
Villani, Stefano. "The Italian Protestant Church of London in the 17th Century." In Barbara Schaff, ed. *Exiles, Emigrés and Intermediaries: Anglo-Italian Cultural Transactions.* New York: Rodopi, 2010. 217–36.
Villiers, George, second Duke of Buckingham. *Plays, Poems, and Miscellaneous Writings Associated with George Villiers, Second Duke of Buckingham.* Ed. Robert D. Hume and Harold Love. 2 vols. Oxford: Oxford University Press, 2007.
Visentini, Margherita Azzi. "Il giardino dei semplici di Padova: Un prodotto della cultura del Rinascimento." *Comunità* 34 (1980), 259–338.
Vivo, Filippo de. "Pharmacies as Centres of Communication in Early Modern Venice." *Renaissance Studies* 21 (2007), 505–21.
Vltima linea Savilii. 1622.
Vorstius, Adolph. *Aphorismoi Hippocrates.* 1628.
Vox Norwici. London, 1646.
W. T. *Strange and wonderful news from Norwich.* 1681.
Wagley, Mary Frances, and Philip F. Wagley. "Comments on Samuel Johnson's Biography of Sir Thomas Browne." *Bulletin of the History of Medicine* 31 (1957), 318–26.
Wagner, Tobias. *Examen Elencticum Atheismi Speculativi.* 1677.
Walaeus, Johannes. *Iohannis Walæi Oratio Inavgvralis.* Leiden, 1633.
——*Medica Omnia.* 1660.
Walcott, Mackenzie E. C. *William of Wykeham and His Colleges.* London: David Nutt, 1852.
Walker, Obadiah. *Periamma epidemion, or, Vulgar Errours in practice censured.* 1659.
Walker, Walter James. *Chapters on the Early Registers of Halifax Parish Church.* Halifax: Whitley & Booth, 1885.
Wall, Cynthia Sundberg. *The Prose of Things: Transformations of Description in the Eighteenth Century.* Chicago: University of Chicago Press, 2006.
Walsham, Alexandra. *Providence in Early Modern England.* Oxford: Oxford University Press, 1999.
Ward, John. *The Lives of the Professors of Gresham College.* Facsimile of the 1740 edition. New York: Johnson Reprint Corporation, 1967.
Ward, W. E. F. *A History of Mercers' School.* London: Old Mercers' Club, 1971.
Warneke, Sara. *Images of the Educational Traveller in Early Modern England.* Leiden: Brill, 1995.
Waters, D. W. *The Art of Navigation in England in Elizabethan and Early Stuart Times.* New Haven, CT: Yale University Press, 1958.
Watson, Gilbert. *Theriac and Mithridatium: A Study in Therapeutics.* London: The Wellcome Historical Medical Library, 1966.
Watson, John. *The History and Antiquities of the Parish of Halifax, in Yorkshire.* London, 1775.
Watts, Henry. *Dictionary of Chemistry.* London: Green and Co., 1918.
Wear, Andrew. "Religious Beliefs and Medicine in Early Modern England." In Hilary Marland and Margaret Pelling, eds. *The Task of Healing: Medicine, Religion and Gender in*

England and the Netherlands, 1450–1800. Rotterdam: Erasmus Publishing, 1996. 145–69.

Webster, Charles. "The Recognition of Plant Sensitivity by English Botanists in the Seventeenth Century." *Isis* 57 (1966), 5–23.

Webster, John. *The Displaying of Supposed Witchcraft.* 1677.

Webster, Tom. *Godly Clergy in Early Stuart England: The Caroline Puritan Movement, c. 1620–1643.* New York: Cambridge University Press, 1997.

Welsby, Paul A. *Lancelot Andrewes, 1555–1626.* London: SPCK, 1958.

Welsch, Georg. *Exercitatio de vena medinensi, ad mentem Ebnsinae... Cui accedit altera, De vermiculis capillaribus infantium.* 1674.

Wenley, Robert. "Robert Paston and the Yarmouth Collection." *Norfolk Archaeology* 41 (1991), 113–44.

West, William N. "Brownean Motion: Conversation with *Pseudodoxia Epidemica*'s 'Sober Circumference of Knowledge.'" In Browne and Preston, eds. *Sir Thomas Browne: The World Proposed.* 168–87.

Westfall, Tipton Marshall. *Sir Thomas Browne's Revisions in Pseudodoxia Epidemica: A Study in the Development of his Mind.* PhD diss., Princeton University, 1938.

Westwood, Anthony. *De Variolis & Morbillis.* London, 1656.

Whallon, William. "Hebraic Synonymy in Sir Thomas Browne." *English Literary History* 28 (1961), 335–52.

Whitaker, Tobias. *An Elenchus of opinions concerning the cure of the small pox.* London, 1661.

White, P. O. G. "Justinian Lewin." *ODNB.*

Whitefoot, John. *Israel Agchithanes.* 1656.

—— "Some Minutes for the Life of Sir *Thomas Browne.*" In *Posthumous Works of Sir Thomas Browne.* 1712. xxiv–xxxvii.

Whiteman, Anne, ed., assisted by Mary Clapinson. *The Compton Census of 1676: A Critical Edition.* British Academy Records of Social and Economic History, 10. London: Oxford University Press, 1986.

Wild, Robert. *Iter Boreale.* 1668.

Wilkin, Simon, ed. *Sir Thomas Browne's Works.* 4 vols. London: William Pickering, 1836.

Wilkins-Jones, Clive, ed. *Norwich City Library, 1608–1737.* Norfolk Record Society 72, 2008.

Willard, Thomas. "John Jeffrey's Copy of *Christian Morals,*" *Papers of the Bibliographical Society of America* 92 (1998), 81–4.

Williams, C. F. Abdy. *A Short Historical Account of the Degrees in Music at Oxford and Cambridge.* New York: Novello, Ewer and Co., 1893.

Williams, Charles. *The Barber-Surgeons of Norwich.* Norwich: Jarrold and Sons, 1896.

—— "The Pedigree of Sir Thomas Browne." *Norfolk Archaeology* 15 (1904), 109–13.

—— "Residence of Sir Thomas Browne, M.D. at Norwich." *East Anglican,* n.s., 1 (1886), 194–5.

—— *Souvenir of Sir Thomas Browne.* London: Jarrod & Sons, 1905.

—— *The Treatment of the Sick in Norwich During the Seventeenth Century.* Norwich: Fletcher and Son, 1903.

—— "The Will of Thomas Browne, Mercer." *Proceedings of the Norfolk and Norwich Archeological Society* 16 (1906), 132–36.

Williams, Elizabeth A. *A Cultural History of Medical Vitalism in Enlightenment Montpellier.* Burlington, VT: Ashgate, 2003.

Williams, Penry. "From the Reformation to the Era of Reform 1530–1850." In John Buxton and Penry Williams, eds. *New College, Oxford, 1379–1979*. Oxford: New College, 1979. 44–71.

Williams, Phyllis Mary. *Norwich Subscriptions to the Voluntary Gift of 1662*. Norfolk Record Society 1 (1931).

Willis, Thomas. *Dr. Willis' Practice of Physick*. 1684.

Wilson, Arthur. *History of Great Britain, Being the Life and Reign of King James the First*. 1653.

Wilson, Matthew. *Mercy & Truth. Or Charity Maintayned by Catholics*. 1634.

W[inchester] C[ollege] A[rchaeological] S[ociety]. *Winchester, Its History, Buildings and People*. 1913.

Wise, James N. *Sir Thomas Browne's Religio Medici and Two Seventeenth-Century Critics*. Columbia: University of Missouri Press, 1973.

Wolff, Philippe, ed. *Documents de l'Histoire du Languedoc*. Toulouse: Édouard Privat, 1969.

Wolffe, Mary. "George Hughes." *ODNB*.

Wood, Anthony. *Athenae Oxonienses, Fasti*. Ed. Philip Bliss. 4 vols. 1813–1820; reprinted. Hildesheim: Georg Olms, 1969.

Woodward, Michael, and R. L. Rickard, eds. *The Progress Notes of Warden Woodward 1659–1675 and Other 17th Century Documents Relating to the Norfolk Property of New College Oxford*. Norfolk Record Society 22 (1951).

Woolfson, Jonathan. *Padua and the Tudors: English Students in Italy, 1485–1603*. Toronto: University of Toronto Press, 1998.

Wootton, David. *Paolo Sarpi: Between Renaissance and Enlightenment*. Cambridge: Cambridge University Press, 1983.

Worden, Blair. *Literature and Politics in Cromwellian England: John Milton, Andrew Marvell, Marchamont Nedham*. New York: Oxford University Press, 2007.

Worm, Ole. *Breve fra og til Ole Worm*. Ed. H. D. Schepelern. 3 vols. Munksgaard: DSL, 1965–68.

Wotton, Henry. *An Essay on the Education of Children in the First Rudiments of Learning*. 1753.

Wright, Thomas. *The Antiquities of the Town of Halifax in Yorkshire*. Leeds, 1738.

—— *The Autobiography*. Ed. Thomas Wright, grandson. London: John Russell Smith, 1864.

Wright, William Aldis. "The Great Antonio." *Notes and Queries*, 7th series, 4 (1887), 386.

Wright, William C. "Sir Thomas Browne's *Pseudoxia* [sic] *Epidemica* and English Coffee House Journalism." *Journal of Popular Culture* 12 (1978), 36–41.

Yarchin, William. *History of Biblical Interpretation: A Reader*. Peabody, MA: Hendrickson, 2004.

Zelante, Gerardo. *S. Francesco Grande di Padova*. Padua: Messaggero, 1921.

Index